Treating Chronic and
Severe Mental Disorders

Treating Chronic and Severe Mental Disorders
A Handbook of Empirically Supported Interventions

Edited by

STEFAN G. HOFMANN
MARTHA C. TOMPSON

Foreword by David H. Barlow

THE GUILFORD PRESS
New York   London

To Benjamin and Rosemary
—S.G.H.

To Jared and Mark
—M.C.T.

© 2002 The Guilford Press
A Division of Guilford Publications, Inc.
72 Spring Street, New York, NY 10012
www.guilford.com

Paperback edition 2004

All rights reserved

No part of this book may be reproduced, translated, stored in a retrieval system, or transmitted, in any form or by any means, electronic, mechanical, photocopying, microfilming, recording, or otherwise, without written permission from the Publisher.

Printed in the United States of America

Last digit is print number: 9 8 7 6 5 4 3 2

Library of Congress Cataloging-in-Publication Data

Treating chronic and severe mental disorders : a handbook of empirically supported interventions / edited by Stefan G. Hofmann and Martha C. Tompson.
    p. cm.
Includes bibliographical references and index.
    ISBN 1-57230-765-X (hc.)   ISBN 1-59385-098-0 (pbk.)
   1. Psychoses—Treatment—Handbooks, manuals, etc. 2. Psychotherapy—Handbooks, manuals, etc. I. Hofmann, Stefan G. II. Tompson, Martha C.
RC512 .T74 2002
616.89′1—dc21   2002005332

About the Editors

Stefan G. Hofmann, PhD, received his doctorate from the University of Marburg, Germany. He is presently an Assistant Professor of Psychology at Boston University. His research, which has been funded by the National Institute of Mental Health and the National Alliance for Research on Schizophrenia and Depression, focuses on the treatment of anxiety disorders and schizophrenia. Dr. Hofmann is also the coauthor of *From Social Anxiety to Social Phobia: Multiple Perspectives* (2001, Allyn & Bacon).

Martha C. Tompson, PhD, received her doctorate from the University of California, Los Angeles. She is currently an Assistant Professor of Psychology at Boston University. Her research interests include family processes among individuals with severe psychopathology, family-based treatment for mood disorders, and developmental psychopathology. Dr. Tompson was recently awarded an Exploratory/Treatment Development Grant from the National Institutes of Health to develop a family-based treatment for preadolescents suffering from depression.

Contributors

Alan J. Budney, PhD, Department of Psychiatry, University of Vermont, Burlington, Vermont

Phillippe B. Cunningham, PhD, Family Services Research Center, Department of Psychiatry and Behavior Sciences, Medical University of South Carolina, Charleston, South Carolina

Keith S. Dobson, PhD, Department of Psychology, University of Calgary, Calgary, Alberta, Canada

Amy S. Elkavich, BA, Department of Psychiatry, University of California at Los Angeles, Los Angeles, California

Ian R. H. Falloon, MD, DSc, Department of Psychiatry, University of Auckland, Auckland, New Zealand

Ellen Frank, PhD, Department of Psychiatry, University of Pittsburgh School of Medicine, Pittsburgh, Pennsylvania

Arthur Freeman, EdD, Philadelphia College of Osteopathic Medicine, Philadelphia, Pennsylvania

Alison M. Goldstein, MA, Department of Psychiatry, University of California at Los Angeles, Los Angeles, California

John Gunderson, MD, Department of Psychiatry, McLean Hospital, Harvard Medical School, Belmont, Massachusetts

Gillian Haddock, PhD, Department of Clinical Psychology, University of Manchester, and Withington Hospital, Manchester, United Kingdom

Kate E. Hamilton, PhD, Department of Psychology, University of Calgary, Calgary, Alberta, Canada

Nancy S. Handmaker, PhD, Department of Psychology, University of New Mexico, Albuquerque, New Mexico

Scott W. Henggeler, PhD, Family Services Research Center, Department of Psychiatry and Behavior Sciences, Medical University of South Carolina, Charleston, South Carolina

Stephen T. Higgins, PhD, Department of Psychiatry, University of Vermont, Burlington, Vermont

Stefan G. Hofmann, PhD, Department of Psychology, Boston University, Boston, Massachusetts

Gerard E. Hogarty, MSW, Department of Psychiatry, Western Psychiatric Institute and Clinic, University of Pittsburgh School of Medicine, Pittsburgh, Pennsylvania

Kelly Koerner, PhD, Behavioral Technology Transfer Group, Seattle, Washington

Nathaniel S. Kuhn, MD, PhD, Department of Psychiatry, Cambridge Health Alliance, Harvard Medical School, Belmont, Massachusetts

Elizabeth J. Letourneau, PhD, Family Services Research Center, Department of Psychiatry and Behavior Sciences, Medical University of South Carolina, Charleston, South Carolina

Marsha M. Linehan, PhD, Department of Psychology, University of Washington, Seattle, Washington

John C. Markowitz, MD, Department of Psychiatry, Weill Medical College, Cornell University; Department of Psychiatry, Columbia University College of Physicians and Surgeons; and New York State Psychiatric Institute, New York, New York

Leigh McCullough, PhD, Department of Psychiatry, Beth Israel Deaconess Medical Center, Harvard Medical School, Dedham, Massachusetts

David J. Miklowitz, PhD, Department of Psychology, University of Colorado at Boulder, Boulder, Colorado

Peter M. Monti, PhD, Center for Alcohol and Addiction Studies, Brown University, Providence, Rhode Island

Kim T. Mueser, PhD, New Hampshire–Dartmouth Psychiatric Research Center, Concord, New Hampshire

Joseph Nowinski, PhD, Department of Psychology, University of Connecticut, Storrs, Connecticut

K. Daniel O'Leary, PhD, Department of Psychology, State University of New York at Stony Brook, Stony Brook, New York

Tracy A. O'Leary, PhD, Center for Alcohol and Addiction Studies, Brown University, Providence, Rhode Island

Michael W. Otto, PhD, Cognitive-Behavior Therapy Program, Massachusetts General Hospital, and Department of Psychiatry, Harvard Medical School, Boston, Massachusetts

Sarah Pratt, PhD, New Hampshire–Dartmouth Psychiatric Research Center, Concord, New Hampshire

Noreen Reilly-Harrington, PhD, Department of Psychiatry, Harvard Medical School, Boston, Massachusetts

Maria Elena Ridolfi, MD, private practice, Fano, Italy

Michael J. Rohrbaugh, PhD, Department of Psychology, University of Arizona, Tucson, Arizona

Mary Jane Rotheram-Borus, PhD, Department of Psychiatry, University of California at Los Angeles, Los Angeles, California

Varda Shoham, PhD, Department of Psychology, University of Arizona, Tucson, Arizona

Stacey C. Sigmon, MA, Department of Psychiatry, University of Vermont, Burlington, Vermont

Holly A. Swartz, MD, Department of Psychiatry, Western Psychiatric Institute and Clinic, University of Pittsburgh School of Medicine, Pittsburgh, Pennsylvania

Nicholas Tarrier, PhD, Department of Clinical Psychology, University of Manchester, and Withington Hospital, Manchester, United Kingdom

Martha C. Tompson, PhD, Department of Psychology, Boston University, Boston, Massachusetts

Scott T. Walters, MA, Department of Psychology, University of New Mexico, Albuquerque, New Mexico

Teresa Whitehurst, PhD, Graduate School of Education, Harvard University, Cambridge, Massachusetts

Foreword

The last decade has witnessed nothing less than a revolution in the development of psychological interventions. While we have much to learn, and our treatments are no panacea, we now can say with some confidence that, based on currently accepted rules of evidence in our public health effort, we have psychological treatments with proven effectiveness for the majority of mental disorders that so trouble and impair a large proportion of the population. Thus, while we have known for decades about the importance of "common" factors, such as forming an effective therapeutic alliance, and instilling positive expectancies for change and a sense of hope, we can now add to these important ingredients a technology of behavior change that is as good as or better than any other single approach currently available. Recent sophisticated multisite clinical trials across a number of child and adult disorders have demonstrated that psychological treatments alone, or sometimes in combination with new and effective drugs, are at least the equal of other approaches to treatment, such as drugs alone in the short term, and usually far superior in the long term, since psychological treatments are subject to less relapse than other approaches. Add to this the fact that most people would far prefer a psychological treatment in which they may learn new coping skills to an effective drug treatment if given the choice, and we would seem to be entering a golden age for psychological interventions.

Yet there is one overriding barrier that prevents thousands of mental health clinicians from effectively utilizing these powerful new treatments. The infrastructure for dissemination and training of these techniques and strategies is simply not available in all but a few highly specialized centers. Contrast this to the infrastructure available for marketing and disseminating effective new drug treatments when they become available. Overcoming this problem has begun to occupy the best minds in our field working at the level of governmental health care policy on both state and federal levels, as well as in research centers where these procedures are developed, often with the support of federal funds.

As this effort continues, there is one tried-and-true method for informing mental health professionals seeking knowledge about new and effective interventions to better assist their clients: an informed and carefully crafted book pulling together details on a number of diverse treatment protocols. This is such a book. Here, Stefan Hofmann and Martha Tompson have focused on clusters of emerging treatment protocols addressing four of the most severe areas of psychopathology—schizophrenia, addictive behaviors, severe mood disorders, and severe personality disorders. While the public and professionals alike have looked to new developments in psychopharmacology to address these most difficult problems, equally important advances in psychological strategies for these groups have received less attention. Yet whether combined with medication, as in the case of schizophrenia and bipolar disorder, or administered independently, psychological interventions are some of the most powerful tools in our armamentarium to address these difficult disorders. By assembling from around the world some of the leading figures in the development of psychological interventions for these disorders, the editors have provided an invaluable resource to clinicians and students everywhere who hope to increase the effectiveness of their clinical work with these very needy groups of patients.

DAVID H. BARLOW, PhD
Professor of Psychology
Research Professor of Psychiatry
Director, Center for Anxiety and Related Disorders and Clinical Programs
Boston University

Preface

Mental disorders impose a great burden not only on those afflicted with them but also on patients' families, employers, and other friends and affiliates. Such disorders exact their toll by causing serious emotional distress and by reducing the patients' ability to function in the tasks of daily life. By definition, all mental disorders involve significant distress or impairment. Some disorders—such as psychotic disorders, severe personality disorders, overwhelming mood disorders, and substance use disorders—have such an impact on people's lives that they in fact cripple the affected individuals and greatly interfere with the lives of their loved ones. In addition, the costs of these disorders to society, due to the frequent need for costly inpatient treatment, lost wages, lowered productivity, and disability, are enormous. In the treatment of these patients, clinicians are presented with the challenge of addressing devastating symptoms, reducing the need for costly inpatient services, and helping to rebuild shattered lives.

Thankfully, in recent years, the science of mental disorders and their treatment has begun to make important advances in both understanding and treating these severe afflictions. New psychotropic medications as well as efficacious psychological interventions provide new hope for alleviating many debilitating symptoms and enabling patients to regain some order in their lives. On the one hand, drug treatments are easily accessible and widely distributed, because the organizations that developed them have invested deeply in marketing them. Drug companies spend considerable resources disseminating information about their products, including findings on the efficacy of medications, their indications, and strategies for prescribing them in clinical settings. On the other hand, although clinical psychology and psychiatry have also made significant advances in the psychosocial treatment of severe mental disorders, few practitioners are aware of these new treatments, and fewer still are trained to provide them. Psychosocial treatments are frequently developed through academic research rather than commercial "research and development" efforts, and fewer resources are available for aggressive efforts at dissemination of these treatments. Thus, a gap exists between what science has to offer mental health providers, and what mental health providers have at their disposal. With this book, we hope to bridge that gap.

The initial idea for this book grew out of desperation. Our field has developed approaches to treating many of the more severe mental disorders. These approaches are delineated in manual-based treatments of which practitioners could take advantage, if

Contents

I. PSYCHOLOGICAL TREATMENTS FOR SCHIZOPHRENIA — 1

1. Cognitive-Behavioral Family and Educational Interventions for Schizophrenic Disorders — 3
   Ian R. H. Falloon

2. Social Skills Training for Schizophrenia — 18
   Sarah Pratt and Kim T. Mueser

3. Personal Therapy: A Practical Psychotherapy for the Stabilization of Schizophrenia — 53
   Gerard E. Hogarty

4. Cognitive-Behavioral Therapy for Schizophrenia: A Case Formulation Approach — 69
   Nicholas Tarrier and Gillian Haddock

II. PSYCHOLOGICAL TREATMENTS FOR MOOD DISORDERS — 97

5. Cognitive-Behavioral Therapy for Depression — 99
   Kate E. Hamilton and Keith S. Dobson

6. Cognitive-Behavioral Therapy for the Management of Bipolar Disorder — 116
   Michael W. Otto and Noreen Reilly-Harrington

7. Interpersonal Psychotherapy for Unipolar and Bipolar Disorders — 131
   Holly A. Swartz, John C. Markowitz, and Ellen Frank

8. Family-Focused Treatment for Bipolar Disorder — 159
   David J. Miklowitz

9. Treatment of Marital Discord and Coexisting Depression — 175
    K. Daniel O'Leary

10. Treatment of Suicidality: A Family Intervention for Adolescent Suicide Attempters — 191
    Mary Jane Rotheram-Borus, Alison M. Goldstein, and Amy S. Elkavich

III. PSYCHOLOGICAL TREATMENTS FOR SUBSTANCE USE AND ABUSE DISORDERS — 213

11. Motivational Interviewing for Initiating Change in Problem Drinking and Drug Use — 215
    Nancy S. Handmaker and Scott T. Walters

12. Cognitive-Behavioral Therapy for Alcohol Addiction — 234
    Tracy A. O'Leary and Peter M. Monti

13. Twelve-Step Facilitation Therapy for Alcohol Problems — 258
    Joseph Nowinski

14. Couple Treatment for Alcohol Abuse: A Systemic Family-Consultation Model — 277
    Michael J. Rohrbaugh and Varda Shoham

15. Psychosocial Treatment for Cocaine Dependence: The Community Reinforcement plus Vouchers Approach — 296
    Stephen T. Higgins, Stacey C. Sigmon, and Alan J. Budney

IV. PSYCHOLOGICAL TREATMENTS FOR SEVERE PERSONALITY DISORDERS — 315

16. Dialectical Behavior Therapy for Borderline Personality Disorder — 317
    Kelly Koerner and Marsha M. Linehan

17. Multiple Family Group Treatment for Borderline Personality Disorder — 343
    Teresa Whitehurst, Maria Elena Ridolfi, and John Gunderson

18. Multisystemic Treatment of Antisocial Behavior in Adolescents — 364
    Elizabeth J. Letourneau, Phillippe B. Cunningham, and Scott W. Henggeler

19. Cognitive-Behavioral Therapy for Severe Personality Disorders — 382
    Arthur Freeman

20. **Short-Term Dynamic Psychotherapy: Resolving Character Pathology by Treating Affect Phobias** 403
    Nathaniel S. Kuhn and Leigh McCullough

Concluding Remarks 419
Stefan G. Hofmann and Martha C. Tompson

Index 421

I

Psychological Treatments for Schizophrenia

Characterized by psychosis, regression, and both social and occupational dysfunction (American Psychiatric Association, 1994, p. 285), schizophrenia is regarded by many as the prototype of a "severe mental disorder." The impact of schizophrenia on an individual's affect, perception, cognition, behavior, and interpersonal relations is often devastating. In recent years, research on the phenomenology, course, genetics, neurobiology, and psychosocial factors associated with schizophrenia has led to an increasing understanding of its psychopathological processes and has allowed for the development and improvement of treatment strategies. The pathogenesis of schizophrenia has been described using a vulnerability–stress framework (Nuechterlein & Dawson, 1984; Zubin & Spring, 1977). In this model, a latent biological vulnerability in an at-risk person is presumed to be present, and environmental stress acts upon this underlying vulnerabilility. The results of this interaction are expressed as episodes of schizophrenic disorder.

Using the vulnerability–stress model as a framework, optimal treatment for schizophrenia involves a two-pronged approach, addressing both the underlying biological vulnerability to schizophrenia through appropriate pharmacological intervention and the role of life circumstances/stresses through psychological intervention. In the last two decades, tremendous strides have been made in the pharmacological treatment of schizophrenia. The advent of atypical antipsychotics has led to improved symptoms and functioning, and lower levels of debilitating medication side effects for many patients. Frequently, improved pharmacological treatment allows for greater engagement in and benefits from psychological interventions. Reductions in both the positive and negative symptoms of schizophrenia free patients to contribute more to the process of their own rehabilitation through psychotherapeutic approaches. Many challenges remain for clinicians, including helping patients reduce residual symptoms, avoid symptom relapses, lessen life stress, build coping strategies, and establish greater quality of life. Addressing nonadherence to prescribed medications remains a central concern for all clinicians working with patients with schizophrenia and is addressed in each of the interventions described in these chapters.

These four chapters present some of the most strongly supported strategies in the arsenal of empirically supported interventions. Given that many individuals with schizophrenia now reside in their communities, families are frequently called upon to provide assistance and support in their rehabilitation. In such a context, family-based approaches, as described in Chapter 1 by Ian Falloon, play an increasingly important therapeutic role. These interventions involve psychoeducation about schizophrenia and communication and problem-solving skills building in a family context. Over two decades of research and numerous clinical trials underscore the value of family-based treatments for reducing relapse among patients. Patients with schizophrenia often display deficits in life skills. In Chapter 2, Sarah Pratt and Kim Mueser describe social skills–building strategies that help patients develop coping and life skills—an important piece in a comprehensive, rehabilitation strategy. In the long-term recovery from schizophrenia, individual treatment models play an important role. In Chapter 3, Gerard Hogarty describes a long-term, stage-oriented model for the individual treatment of individuals with schizophrenia. In this sophisticated approach, the therapy goals and strategies evolve as the patient slowly recovers, develops new capacities, and can make use of treatment in new ways. Finally, in Chapter 4, Nicholas Tarrier and Gillian Haddock describe how cognitive therapy strategies have been modified for the treatment of individuals with psychotic disorders. Cognitive strategies show great promise for reducing the impact of residual psychotic symptoms and increasing patients' coping. These four chapters represent the "state of the art" in current psychosocial treatment approaches for schizophrenia.

REFERENCES

American Psychiatric Association. (1994). *Diagnostic and statistical manual of mental disorders* (4th ed.). Washington, DC: Author.

Nuechterlein, K. H., & Dawson, M. E. (1984). A heuristic vulnerability/stress model of schizophrenic episodes. *Schizophrenia Bulletin, 10,* 300–312.

Zubin, J., & Spring B. (1977). Vulnerability: A new view of schizophrenia. *Journal of Abnormal Psychology, 86,* 103–126.

1

Cognitive-Behavioral Family and Educational Interventions for Schizophrenic Disorders

IAN R. H. FALLOON

A BRIEF OVERVIEW OF HISTORICAL DEVELOPMENT

Cognitive-behavioral approaches to family therapy emerged more than 30 years ago, with a series of case reports of specific strategies demonstrated as having benefits for specific problems in childhood disorders, such as nocturnal enuresis, aggressive behavior, tantrums, autism, and learning deficits. These case reports focused on training parents to apply specific strategies to reduce the disturbed behavior of young children. The family members were co-opted as members of the clinical team. Prior to training, their best efforts to resolve the disturbed behavior patterns were carefully assessed from a social learning theory perspective, and patterns of family behavior that were thought to promote and sustain the specific disturbances in the child were observed. These early formulations were derived mainly from operant conditioning paradigms and in retrospect appear overly simplistic. Nevertheless, they gave rise to straightforward interventions involving relatively minor changes in the responses of key family members that were often dramatically effective. Most interventions involved training family members to eliminate those responses that were observed to increase the frequency of the disturbed behavior, and to increase those responses that appeared to promote desirable behavior patterns that were incompatible with disturbed behavior. The training involved active learning through guided practice, therapist demonstration, and direct coaching of skills in the home setting. Benefits were measured in simple counts of the frequency of the disturbed responses, both during and between the training sessions.

Development of cognitive-behavioral family strategies for major mental disorders was initiated by Robert Paul Liberman (1970), who used social learning principles to work with adults with mental disorders. In addition to employing an operant conditioning framework in family interaction, he introduced the imitative learning principles of

Bandura and Walters (1963). This included *modeling and role rehearsal* to help family members acquire more effective interpersonal communication patterns. Liberman emphasized the need for developing a collaborative therapeutic alliance with all family members and encouraged therapists to use their own expression of positive reinforcement, usually praise, to support the efforts of all participants. A final contribution involved the provision of straightforward education about mental disorders and their clinical management to all patients and their informal caregivers. This education, often provided in multifamily seminars, became the forerunner of the psychoeducational approaches to family intervention (Falloon & Liberman, 1982).

This early approach was further developed by Gerald Patterson and John Reid and their colleagues in Eugene, Oregon (Patterson, Reid, Jones, & Conger, 1975). They recognized the limitations of the basic operant approaches, particularly when dealing with multiproblem families and with children who showed disturbances in multiple settings, such as home and school. They demonstrated that the behavior of disturbed children was often the culmination of coercive patterns of parent–child interaction, thereby validating the reciprocity concepts that were emerging from the theoretical constructs of the early systems theorists.

In 1975, while on sabbatical, Liberman teamed up with Falloon, Leff, Tarrier, and Vaughn at the Institute of Psychiatry in London. The seminal work on the effects of stressful family interactions and coping with stressful life changes that had been recently completed there by Vaughn and Leff (1976), Brown and Birley (1968), and Tarrier, Vaughn, Lader, and Leff (1979) led to an approach that combined health education with strategies to enhance the management of stresses associated with recovery from schizophrenic disorders. It was hypothesized that stress associated with features of the illness and its treatment, as well as a lack of effective interpersonal skills in managing the stress of reintegration into community life, interacted with a person's biological vulnerability to delay recovery and promote recurrences of schizophrenia. The strength of the family unit in the management of these stresses was considered one of the greatest natural resources to assist patients in the full and lasting recovery from this disorder. Furthermore, high stress in family members living with and caring for recovering patients was considered a major risk to their health and welfare, so that a systemic approach to stress in each household was adopted (Falloon, Boyd, & McGill, 1984).

This work was subjected to intensive research and development on an international level, with outstanding input from Carol Anderson and Gerard Hogarty, Michael Goldstein and David Miklowitz, Christine McGill, Gina Randolph, Shirley Glynn, David Kavagnagh, Kurt Hahlweg, Max Birchwood, Christine Barrowclough, Elizabeth Kuipers, Lyman Wynne, William MacFarlane, Nina Schooler, Kim Mueser, Tilo Held, Marina Economou, Per Borrell, Nisse Berglund, Rolf Grawe, Charles Brooker, Victor Graham-Hole, Rita Roncone, Isabel Montero, Grainne Fadden, and many other superb scientist-practitioners. Major innovations have included the refinement of methods for assessing the strengths and weaknesses of family interaction, the introduction of structured training in problem-solving strategies, and the inclusion of the entire range of research-validated, cognitive-behavioral strategies wherever they are specifically indicated. These innovations are outlined later in this chapter.

CORE THEORETICAL ASSUMPTIONS

The cognitive-behavioral family therapist considers that the family in its many guises constitutes the greatest natural resource for the management of the wide range of stresses associated with personal development and maintaining a productive, satisfying life in our communities. It is all too easy to criticize the family when breakdowns in this vital role appear to contribute to major health or psychosocial problems, whether due to poor physical and emotional nurturance or to a lack of skills in dealing with major life crises, such as bereavement, childbirth, or relationship breakup. In contrast to these dramatic events, the everyday efforts that families contribute to the quality of life of their members may be readily overlooked. However, recent developments in research on the way people cope with stress suggest that the role of the family is crucial in helping people to resolve major stresses in their lives. Furthermore, a series of studies has shown that the way in which a family helps its members cope with stress may be a major factor in the recovery from major physical and mental illnesses (Falloon & McGill, 1985).

Family care extends well beyond the confines of the family home, with continued, extensive support being provided for family members when they are residing in households other than the family home. Vast improvements in telecommunications and modern transportation have enabled people to remain in close contact while at different ends of the earth. The concept of the intimate social network that provides both emotional and physical support for an individual on an everyday basis probably encompasses the notion of a "family" much better than that attributed solely to people sharing a living space, or to those related by birth. Even the homeless person sleeping on the streets may have a close support network of fellow itinerants who are deeply concerned for his or her day-to-day welfare. It is a sad reflection that sometimes people in such situations may receive greater supportive human contact than those living in mansions with relatives, or in the splendid social isolation of modern housing developments.

CLINICAL STRATEGIES

Assessment of the Vulnerability, Stress, and Problem-Solving Capacity in a Family Unit

Many strategies have been used to assess the strengths and weaknesses of family management of stress. Most have been developed from the Camberwell Family Interview and the Expressed Emotion Index that is derived from its scales (Leff & Vaughn, 1985). Because this research approach is rather cumbersome and has limited application in clinical practice, we have adapted a more straightforward approach to family assessment.

Intervention strategies are constructed on a framework of baseline assessment of the index patient and each key family member's goals and problems, with continual review every session. When one member is vulnerable to a major disorder, a range of stressful problems are often evident. Each of these key problems is explored using a problem analysis, which is similar to the functional analysis of classic cognitive-behavioral therapy. At its most straightforward level, this consists of defining the specific contingencies that surround a specific problem. For example, what triggers a family argument, or increases or decreases the intensity of agitated behavior? What happens when a person experiences rejection while attempting to develop a friendship? All the strategies used currently by family members to resolve or cope with these problems are explored. This problem analysis forms the basis for collaborative problem solving to achieve each person's desired personal goals in a more effective and efficient way, preferably generating less stress for all involved.

Each family member is also interviewed individually in order to obtain a broader picture of the setting of the presenting problems than the consensus view provided by a family group. The assessment process also includes attempts to obtain the following:

1. *A therapeutic alliance with all family members.* Factors that may interfere with the therapeutic alliance include paranoid ideas, denial of illness, stigma, demoralization, and fear of the awareness that one has psychotic symptoms. Techniques that may benefit the alliance include "sharing mistrust" with paranoid patients, providing patients who deny their illness with alternative points of view, making admiring and approving comments to demoralized patients, and normalizing experiences for stigmatized patients.

2. *Specific information about each family member's observations, thoughts, and feelings about the key presenting problems.* This includes the level of understanding of the nature and treatment of the index patient's disorder, with particular reference to factors that seem to make the disorder better or worse. A lack in understanding of the nature of the disorder frequently contributes substantially to family stress.

3. *Information about each family member's interaction within the family system.* This includes his or her attitudes, feelings, and behavior toward the other family members; and his or her support for efforts to resolve presenting problems and major stressors, and to assist others in achieving their personal goals.

4. *Information about each family member's function in settings outside the family unit.* This takes into account his or her personal assets and deficits that might be relevant to problem resolution processes.

5. *An assessment of the strengths and weaknesses of the family as a problem-solving unit.* In addition to interviews with each household member, the therapist assesses the collaborative efforts of the family unit in solving everyday problems, resolving stressors, and providing mutual assistance in achieving personal goals. Wherever feasible, these assessments are conducted in the circumstances where the issues arise, usually at home. Such naturalistic observations are invaluable, but they may be too costly for routine practice. Alternatives include having the family tape-record interactions at targeted times and time sampling recordings with automated time switches, and having family members reenact problem situations or family discussions about "hot issues." Nevertheless, at least one home visit is an essential part of the family assessment and usually provides the therapist with an abundance of valuable information that is seldom accessible in clinic-based assessments.

The cognitive-behavioral family therapist is interested in pinpointing not only the setting in which problem behavior is most likely to arise but also the family's past and current efforts to cope with the behavior. Usually, any problem is present only a small proportion of the time and only arises on some occasions when it might be expected. Even when severely depressed or psychotic, a person has extensive periods when his or her main symptoms are not observed. From another view point, most behavior observed in families is positive or neutral (i.e., nonproblematic), and families for the most part have already learned some strategies to cope with the major problems. Thus, the therapist is interested in uncovering the contingencies that exist not only when the targeted problem is quiescent but also when the problem is present but results in minimal distress. It is assumed that although the family may have developed responses to cope with the problem, these coping behaviors are only partially effective, often because family members apply them in an inconsistent manner or do not persist to derive the full benefits from these coping efforts. Where such effective strategies can be pinpointed, the therapist is left with the relatively straightforward task of assisting family members to enhance the efficacy of their preexisting interaction patterns. Such a targeted intervention may take a mere session or two, but the analysis that precedes it may be a much longer process.

6. *An assessment of the quality of everyday life of the family, including an assessment of situations that are desired and avoided.* Major health and psychosocial problems

play havoc with the everyday routine of family living and quality of life. A survey of current activities is contrasted with desired activity patterns. Each family member is invited to describe his or her most frequent activities, as well as the people, places, and objects with which he or she spends the most time. Discrepancies between current and expected activity levels help the therapist pinpoint key areas of dissatisfaction that may assist in defining specific goals related to each family member's quality of life.

Unpleasant situations that family members tend to avoid are also listed. These may vary from simple phobias to various family interactions such as arguments, or discussions about finances or sexual concerns. Feelings of rejection, isolation, frustration, coercion, lack of support, mistrust, and intrusion may be discussed in this content. Family members are asked to provide clear examples of interactions in which they experience these negative feelings. This process may be facilitated by inviting family members to complete daily activity schedules. Otherwise, information obtained by interview may be notoriously unreliable, particularly when the interviewees are highly stressed.

This survey of reinforcing and aversive situations often provides a fascinating picture of the manner in which the everyday activities of family members intertwine in patterns of mutual reinforcement, positively in happy families, and negatively in distressed families, where marked avoidance of intimacy, confrontation, or coercion may predominate. One final use of the reinforcement survey involves the selection of positive reinforcers that may be employed to promote specific behavior change during the intervention phase. Activities, places, people, and objects deemed highly desirable can mediate change when used as specific rewards for performance of targeted behaviors.

7. *Setting personal goals for each family member.* The assessment process is completed by specifying the short-term personal goals of each patient and key family member, and the conflicts and problems that may need to be resolved in order to achieve these goals. Whenever possible, the therapist assists the patients and family members to specify goals that, with their current resources of time, skills, money, and impairment levels, can be readily achieved and maximize the quality of their everyday lives within the next 3 to 6 months. For many people who have felt burdened by a major mental disorder, this process may need to extend over parts of several sessions. Family members may require time to focus on their own personal needs and not have as their sole concern merely seeing improvement in the patient's state.

Education about Specific Disorders

The initial sessions are usually devoted to providing the patient and family with a straightforward explanation of the nature of the disorder and its treatment. Handouts are provided, and the index patient is invited to describe his or her experiences of the disorder and its treatment. The vulnerability–stress theory is outlined as a framework for integrating the benefits of combined biomedical and psychosocial interventions to reduce morbidity. Revision of this education is conducted whenever indicated throughout the treatment process, for example, when participants are reluctant to continue taking the recommended medications, or on occasions when major stresses threaten to overwhelm the family's coping resources and stress responses may be emerging.

The ability to recognize and respond effectively to the earliest warning signs that precede serious episodes of major mental disorders is a core aspect of this education. While these signs are sometimes similar among disorders (e.g., decreased sleep may herald impending episodes of depression, anxiety, or psychosis), each patient must delineate these early warning signs most pertinent to him or her. While research studies have

Variability of Approaches

The manner in which the components of cognitive-behavioral family interventions are combined varies considerably from center to center and case to case. A collaborative education of patients, families, and other caregivers, with attempts to enhance problem-solving effectiveness, is the most prominent feature of all the approaches. Full integration with drug strategies, crisis management, and case management services appears rare, with services often provided somewhat independently of mainstream psychiatry. It is probable that cognitive-behavioral family therapy is most readily applied in settings where it is an integral part of a comprehensive multidisciplinary mental health service rather than a specialized agency (Falloon & Fadden, 1993).

CASE EXAMPLE

Paul, a single, university lecturer in ancient history, age 31, lives in an apartment on the same street as his parents. He enjoys reading background books about his work, listening to jazz, and playing soccer with a group of friends. He currently does not have an ongoing relationship with a woman.

His mother Jenny is 60 and works as a florist. She is very involved in charity work, particularly with a local Buddhist group. His father Patrick, age 65, a recently retired electrical engineer, enjoys home improvement work and continues to do small projects for many of his friends. The mother and father spend little time together and their relationship is devoid of affection. Jenny is highly critical of Patrick for his indifference toward her interests. A younger son, Jack, 23, is completing medical school. He lives with his parents but spends much of his time at the hospital library or with his friends.

Paul first noted difficulties 2 years ago, when he found it difficult to concentrate and organize material for his lessons. He noticed that students and colleagues were looking at him in a strange way and making comments about his sexual orientation. He continued to work for 6 months but found it increasingly difficult. He ceased going out with his friends and spent most of his time in his apartment. His mother took over meal preparation most evenings. She noted that he seemed to be talking with somebody when she arrived at his apartment, but there was never anyone else there. Paul also developed the idea that all his friends had been killed, and that he was in some way responsible.

Assessment

Paul, initially diagnosed as having symptoms of work stress, had 15 sessions with a psychotherapist that were of some limited benefit. Two years after the onset, he was admitted for 15 days to a psychiatric inpatient hospital, where his symptoms of persecutory delusions, hallucinations, and thought interference were considered to meet the criteria for a schizophrenic disorder. He was treated with low doses of antipsychotic medication and most of his cognitive and perceptual difficulties remitted. However, he remained fearful of going out and meeting friends, and still suspected that his colleagues had been involved in a plot to defame him. Neither Paul nor his parents accepted the diagnosis. His father read many books about schizophrenia and its treatment, and although he had doubts about the precise diagnosis, he observed the benefits of the medication and assisted his son in taking his daily dose in the manner prescribed. Paul noted that when he became stressed, he developed a tremor that he considered to be a side effect of his medication—risperidone, 3 mg daily. His principal personal goal was to return to work as soon as possible; a second goal was to find a suitable woman with whom to develop an intimate relationship.

His parents found it very difficult to set personal goals; their overwhelming concern was to help in Paul's recovery. After some time, Jenny set a goal to take a class in art history. Patrick set a goal to play tennis with a friend twice a week. Younger brother Jack did not want to be involved in the program on account of his busy study and social schedule.

The strengths of the family unit were both parents' eagerness to help with Paul's recovery, Paul's good work record and intelligence, his adherence to drug treatment, and adequate financial and material resources. The weaknesses included misunderstanding the nature of the disorder; the mother's belief that Paul would be best treated spiritually, without any medication; poor communication and problem-solving skills as a family unit; a tendency for both parents to be intrusive and overinvolved; marital dissatisfaction between the parents; and the younger brother's refusal to be engaged in any aspects of the program.

Orientation Session

One session was used to outline the principles of the integrated mental health care program. The caseworker summarized the findings of his assessments, described in detail what would happen in each phase of the program, and gave the family members an opportunity to clarify any of their concerns. Jenny wanted to discuss her views about religion and mental illness, but the caseworker reassured her that this would be the focus of the next sessions and that he would be better prepared to discuss this with her then.

Education about the Disorder and Its Treatment

Five sessions were provided initially to clarify misunderstandings about Paul's disorder. After considerable discussion, a consensus was reached that Paul probably had had a schizophrenic episode, possibly precipitated by work stress. Paul and his father agreed that the medication was useful and that it would be a good idea to continue a low dosage as a preventative strategy for at least 12 months. All were convinced that learning more effective skills to solve problems collaboratively would be extremely helpful for Paul's recovery and for family life in general. Jenny remained convinced that if Paul had taken her advice and learned to meditate and relax his mind properly, his disorder would not have emerged.

Early Warning Signs

Two signs were agreed upon as warning signals of an impending psychotic recurrence:

1. Paul's difficulty recalling the key facts that he read in a history book 5 minutes later.
2. Not leaving his apartment for 3 consecutive days.

If either of these signals occurred, it was agreed that Paul or his parents would call the caseworker immediately. They would convene a family meeting and assess any changes (including biological or pharmacological) or stresses that might have triggered these signs, and make a plan to resolve any specific problems that had been detected. Copies of the early warning signs guidesheet were placed in prominent places in Paul's and his parents' apartments, and in the front of his clinical records at the mental health center and his medical record at his family practitioner's office.

Enhancing Problem-Solving Skills

Six sessions were devoted to teaching family members to express their feelings about problems and goals to each other in an open and clear way. Paul and his father had little difficulty with this, but his mother found it extremely difficult to express her own feelings to either her son or her husband. With considerable support and encouragement, she slowly began to tell her husband how sad she felt that they had drifted apart, and how she felt that he had always seemed more devoted to Paul than to her or their younger son. Patrick was able to tell Jenny how difficult it had been for him to see her getting more and more involved with her Buddhist activities, which were of little interest to him and sometimes very irritating. Both agreed to try to work together more on household management and to organize one social or cultural event each week together as a family. Jenny was able to invite Paul to participate in some charitable activities with her group to help him occupy some of his time in a constructive way and perhaps meet some potential new friends.

The family found it relatively easy to learn to use the structured problem-solving approach and apply it in weekly family meetings. These meetings were also attended by the younger brother, who found them useful. He was able to get his family to help him move to his own apartment and was pleased to be invited to share in family activities when he had the time to spare.

Specific Cognitive-Behavioral Skills

Two sessions devoted to the anxiety management module to assist Paul in overcoming his interpersonal anxieties focused on his recontacting his friends in a graduated fashion, using some of the meditation techniques he learned from his mother's Buddhist group.

Three further sessions, using the module on *Learning to Cope Better with Unpleasant Thoughts and Voices*, helped Paul to reevaluate his conclusion that people at his workplace were plotting against him. During the second of these sessions, Paul disclosed that, prior to his admission to the hospital, he had heard voices when nobody had been about, but that rather than bothering him, the voices were often quite helpful, so he had not told anyone about them.

Booster Sessions

When the family had completed 6 months of sessions every 1–2 weeks (18 sessions of 45 minutes each) and developed a regular pattern of convening their own family meetings every Wednesday evening, a comprehensive review of progress was completed. The family, the caseworker, and the treatment team agreed to continue with monthly booster sessions of 30 minutes each to monitor progress and revise any education or skills as needed.

At the end of 12 months, Paul was free of any psychotic or residual symptoms and was spending more and more time assisting his father and mother on their work projects, as well as preparing lessons for the next university term, when he planned to return to lecturing part-time. He had begun dating a girl he met in his mother's group. She had begun making probing inquiries about Paul's situation, and a session was devoted to practice the best ways to respond to these potentially embarrassing questions. Prior to Paul's return to work, another session was devoted to practice interviewing skills for a meeting with the Dean of the Faculty. In both situations, Paul insisted on speaking frankly and openly about his experiences and emphasizing the benefits of his treatment. The role-play practice helped Paul express this in a clear and positive way that improved collaboration with the key people in his life.

His parents' relationship improved considerably. Although both pursued their separate interests, they began to spend pleasurable time together and at the end of 12 months had taken a 3-week cruise that they enjoyed very much. Jenny had begun her art history course, and Patrick was playing tennis regularly at a local club.

Crisis Management

Throughout the 18-month treatment, Paul had minimal psychotic or deficit symptoms. However, a few days prior to his interview with the Dean of the Faculty, he noticed that he was having difficulty concentrating. His mother noted that he was somewhat withdrawn and not participating in his usual pattern of work and social activities. After a brief discussion with his parents, Paul decided to call his caseworker, even though he was due for a booster session in a few days. A crisis session was convened the same day. The probable presence of warning signals was confirmed; biomedical status, medication intake, and symptoms were checked. The consensus was that the probable trigger for the warning signals was Paul's constant worrying about the interview, its outcome, and the consequences. The family problem-solved these issues, planned further practice of the interview, and made a stepwise plan to deal with the most likely possibilities. According to this plan, Paul would continue to engage in his usual weekly activities, increase his use of meditation strategies before the interview, and brainstorm alternative work and career opportunities if the university did not accept his return at this point. His mental state was monitored daily through phone calls to his caseworker.

The plan worked well. Paul experienced a decrease in the intensity of cognitive impairments and resumed his usual activities. His interview went smoothly and he was accepted back to work on a highly optimistic note.

Transfer Back to Primary Care

At the time of the 18-month comprehensive assessment, Paul was working 30 hours per week; he had a blossoming relationship with his girlfriend Jessica and was enjoying evenings at a local jazz club. His parents' relationship was harmonious and all members of the family, including Jessica and brother Jack, had a family meeting each week, followed by a movie, concert, sporting event, or picnic. Over the next 3 months, Paul decreased and finally stopped taking his low-dose medication. The caseworker arranged for continued care, provided by the family practitioner, with continued monitoring of early warning signs and fast-track access to advice from the mental health service as needed. Now, 2 years later, no further crises have emerged, and Paul and his family are functioning extremely well.

Comment

This case study presents the common course of integrated biomedical and psychosocial treatments over 12–24 months for recent-onset psychotic disorders, illustrating the well-documented observation that in the early stages of most schizophrenic disorders, complications such as comorbid conditions (deficit syndromes, anxiety, depression, alcohol and drug abuse, personality disorders), social difficulties of stigma, support group burden, work, and financial and housing problems tend to be minimal. Moreover, those that exist are quite easily resolved by the integrated treatment approach that relies heavily on continued existing social supports, usually the person's family and close friends. The same approach applied a few years later, after one or two further major episodes, can achieve similar outcomes, but the professional resource required to achieve such benefits is many times greater and beyond the capacity of most public health services. For this reason, we believe it is imperative that services provide such approaches in an optimal manner as early as possible in the course of major mental disorders.

ASSESSMENTS OF EFFICACY OF COGNITIVE-BEHAVIORAL FAMILY THERAPY IN MAJOR MENTAL DISORDERS

The effectiveness of cognitive-behavioral family therapy is based on more than persuasive case studies. A substantial body of carefully conducted, controlled trials suggests that these benefits can be achieved in a highly consistent manner and are associated with the application of the previously described treatment strategies.

There are two phases to the assessment of educational approaches. In the first phase, the question that must be answered is "What is the evidence that the specific goals of the education program were achieved in a specific manner?" In the second phase, the question is "Does the achievement of those specific objectives modify the outcome of the disorder in the manner postulated in the formulation of the case?"

Achievement of Specific Goals

The main goal of cognitive-behavioral family therapy approaches in treating major mental disorders is to enhance the problem-solving efficiency of the family unit. Achievement of this goal has been defined in a variety of ways, including direct measures of problem solving (Doane, Goldstein, Falloon, & Mintz, 1985; Doane, Goldstein, Miklowitz, & Falloon, 1986; Hahlweg, Revensdorf, & Schindler, 1984) as well as indirect measures, such as the reduction in household stress and tension (Falloon, 1985; Hogarty et al., 1986; Leff, Kuipers, Berkowitz, Eberlein-Fries, & Sturgeon, 1982; Tarrier et al., 1988).

Cognitive-behavioral family therapy appears able to help most families achieve specific improvements in their problem-solving efficiency. It has compared favorably with individual case management of similar intensity in a controlled study of the long-term management of schizophrenia (Doane et al., 1986). Measures of family problem solving indicated that after the initial, intensive 3-month phase, the number of problem-solving statements in the cognitive-behavioral family therapy condition had trebled, whereas no significant change in the number of family problem-solving statements was noted with the individual approach. Perhaps more significantly, the quality of family problem solving observed by independent assessors who interviewed the families about everyday stressful events showed significant linear improvement over the first 9 months of treatment in families receiving cognitive-behavioral family therapy (Falloon, 1985). However, no benefits were noted for families of patients treated individually. Since similar levels of stress were encountered by families in each condition, it is reasonable to conclude that the cognitive-behavioral family therapy may be associated with specific improvements in family problem-solving functions and consequent stress management.

Furthermore, several studies have used the Expressed Emotion Index to assess changes in household stress contingent upon enhanced problem-solving efficiency (Hogarty et al., 1986; Leff et al., 1982; Tarrier et al., 1988). All have shown a consistent reduction specific to the family intervention in the proportion of families expressing high levels of criticism toward the index patient.

Functional Outcomes

It has been hypothesized that specific changes in problem-solving ability would assist families to cope with a wide range of stressful life situations and be associated with clinical benefits for family members suffering from major mental disorders. There is substantial evidence that cognitive-behavioral family therapy can modify the morbidity associated with schizophrenic disorders (Falloon, Held, Coverdale, Roncone, & Laidlaw, 1999). Fourteen controlled studies completed since 1980 meet minimal standards of research design, with follow-up for at least 1 year. Overall, these studies show that the addition of educational family strategies to optimal case management and long-term drug prophylaxis halves the rate of major clinical exacerbations in people suffering from schizophrenia. This benefit is most notable during the first year after a major schizophrenic episode. Less impressive results are evident when only parts of the approach are provided (Cuijpers, 1999).

In addition to the clinical benefits, studies have shown reductions in social disability, improved work functioning, lowered stress, and improved functioning of caregivers. The reduction in crisis care substantially lowers the overall direct and indirect costs of care (Falloon et al., 1999). Unfortunately, without direct incentives and funding to provide mental health care in this way, such research-based evidence falls on deaf ears. As a result, very few people receive the benefits described in this chapter. Sadly, for most, recovery from schizophrenia remains merely a dream.

CONCLUSIONS

Although the measurement of outcome in this body of research is flawed and the most striking clinical benefits reported are almost exclusively based upon clinical judgments, we can conclude that the quality of this psychosocial research is similar to that employed in drug studies in similar populations. There is good evidence that educational interventions with families caring for people with schizophrenic disorders reduce clinical, social, and family morbidity. Challenges for the future include refining these approaches by delineating the most effective and efficient strategies, integrating them into routine clinical practice, and examining the long-term application of these methods on the course of schizophrenia. A further exciting prospect is the potential for cognitive-behavioral family interventions to provide a basis for early intervention programs that promise to change dramatically the outlook for schizophrenic disorders from one of long-term vigilance and care to that of prevention and cure (Falloon, 1992).

NOTE

1. Now termed "Resource Group" meetings to emphasize that the "family" may be friends, roommates, or any other supportive people who are not relatives.

REFERENCES

Bandura, A., & Walters, R. (1963). *Social learning and personality development.* New York: Holt, Rinehart & Winston.

Brown, G. W., & Birley, J. L. T. (1968). Crises and life changes and the onset of schizophrenia. *Journal of Health and Social Behavior, 8,* 203–214.

Cuijpers, P. (1999). The effects of family interventions on relatives' burden: A meta-analysis. *Journal of Mental Health, 8,* 275–285.

Doane, J. A., Goldstein, M. J., Falloon, I. R. H., & Mintz, J. (1985). Parental affective style and the treatment of schizophrenia: Predicting course of illness and social functioning. *Archives of General Psychiatry, 42,* 34–42.

Doane, J. A., Goldstein, M. J., Miklowitz, D. J., & Falloon, I. R. H. (1986). The impact of individual and family treatment on the affective climate of families of schizophrenics. *British Journal of Psychiatry, 148,* 279–287.

D'Zurilla, T. J., & Goldfried, M. R. (1971). Problem solving and behaviour modification. *Journal of Abnormal Psychology, 78,* 107–126.

Falloon, I. R. H. (1985). *Family management of schizophrenia.* Baltimore: Johns Hopkins University Press.

Falloon, I. R. H. (1992). Early intervention for first episodes of schizophrenia: A preliminary exploration. *Psychiatry, 55,* 1–12.

Falloon, I. R. H., Boyd, J. L., & McGill, C. W. (1984). *Family care of schizophrenia.* New York: Guilford Press.

Falloon, I. R. H., & Fadden, G. (1993). *Integrated mental health care.* Cambridge, UK: Cambridge University Press.

Falloon, I. R. H., Held, T., Coverdale, J. H., Roncone, R., & Laidlaw, T. M. (1999). Psychosocial interventions for schizophrenia: A review of long-term benefits of international studies. *Psychiatric Rehabilitation Skills, 3,* 268–290.

Falloon, I. R. H., & Liberman, R. P. (1982). Behavioral family interventions in the management of chronic schizophrenia. In W. R. McFarlane & C. C. Beels (Eds.), *Family therapy in schizophrenia.* New York: Guilford Press.

Falloon, I. R. H., & McGill, C. W. (1985). Family stress and the course of schizophrenia: A review. In I. R. H. Falloon (Ed.), *Family management of schizophrenia.* Baltimore: John Hopkins University Press.

Hahlweg, K., Revensdorf, D., & Schindler, L. (1984). Effects of behavioural marital therapy on couples' communication and problem solving skills. *Journal of Consulting and Clinical Psychology, 52,* 553–566.

Hogarty, G. E., Anderson, C. M., Reiss, D. J., Kornblith, S. J., Greenwald, D. P., Javna, C. D., & Madonia, M. J. (1986). Family psycho-education, social skills training and maintenance chemotherapy in the aftercare treatment of schizophrenia. *Archives of General Psychiatry, 43,* 633–642.

Leff, J., Kuipers, L., Berkowitz, R., Eberlein-Fries, R., & Sturgeon, D. (1982). A controlled trial of social intervention in the families of schizophrenic patients. *British Journal of Psychiatry, 141,* 121–134.

Leff, J. P., & Vaughn, C. E. (1985). *Expressed emotion in families.* New York: Guilford Press.

Liberman, R. P. (1970). Behavioral approaches to family and couple therapy. *American Journal of Orthopsychiatry, 40,* 106–118.

Patterson, G. R., Reid, J. B., Jones, R. R., & Conger, R. E. (1975). *A social learning approach to family interaction: Vol. 1. Families with aggressive children.* Eugene, OR: Castalia Press.

Stein, L. I., & Test, M. A. (1980). An alternative to mental hospital treatment. *Archives of General Psychiatry, 37,* 392–399.

Tarrier, N., Barrowclough, C., Vaughn, C., Bamrah, J. S., Porceddu, K., Watts, S., & Freeman, H. (1988). The community management of schizophrenia: A controlled trial of behavioral intervention with families to reduce relapse. *British Journal of Psychiatry, 153,* 532–542.

Tarrier, N., Vaughn, C. E., Lader, M. H., & Leff, J. P. (1979). Bodily reactions to people and events in schizophrenia. *Archives of General Psychiatry, 36,* 311–315.

Vaughn, C. E., & Leff, J. P. (1976). The influence of family and social factors on the course of psychiatric illness: A comparison of schizophrenic and depressed neurotic patients. *British Journal of Psychiatry, 129,* 125–137.

2

Social Skills Training for Schizophrenia

SARAH PRATT
KIM T. MUESER

Sustained impairment in one or more major areas of life functioning is not only required for a diagnosis of schizophrenia (over 6 months for DSM-IV) but it also represents one of the most problematic symptoms and is predictive of the course and outcome of the illness (Johnstone, MacMillan, Frith, Benn, & Crow, 1990; Perlick, Stastny, Mattis, & Teresi, 1992; Sullivan, Marder, Liberman, Donahoe, & Mintz, 1990). Common difficulties in psychosocial functioning include problems fulfilling the roles of a worker, student, or homemaker; poor social relationships; inadequately developed leisure and recreational activities; and inability to properly care for oneself (e.g., impaired grooming, hygiene, ability to cook, clean, do laundry, and attend to mental and physical health care needs). Impaired psychosocial functioning often leads to anxiety, low self-esteem, frustration, depression, and social isolation, which may cause exacerbation of the primary symptoms of the illness, low subjective quality of life, and increased risk of relapse (Bellack, Sayers, Mueser, & Bennett, 1994; Penn, Mueser, Spaulding, Hope, & Reed, 1995).

Several factors may be responsible for the functional impairments commonly observed in individuals with schizophrenia. The other symptoms of the illness, namely, positive and negative symptoms and thought disorder, may interfere with the ability to perform the behaviors required for success in a variety of life domains. Characteristic cognitive deficits such as distractibility, impaired information processing, inattention, and poor memory may worsen social competence (Green, 1996; Green, Kern, Braff, & Mintz, 2000; Herz, 1996). The relapsing nature of the illness may make sustained progress in important life spheres particularly difficult. Finally, specific social skills deficits may be responsible for failures in psychosocial functioning. Social skills training (SST) was developed to remediate deficient social skills that are identified as lacking but are required for success in overall psychosocial functioning.

OVERVIEW AND THEORETICAL UNDERPINNINGS

Two models provide the broad theoretical framework for addressing social skills deficits in persons with schizophrenia: the stress–vulnerability model and the social skills model. The *stress–vulnerability model* (Zubin & Spring, 1977) posits that symptom severity and other characteristic impairments of schizophrenia, including psychosocial dysfunction, have genetic and related biological bases (psychobiological vulnerability). The vulnerability, and hence symptom severity and functional impairment, can be decreased by medications, and increased by stress and substance abuse. Stress can impinge on vulnerability, precipitating relapses and contributing to impairments in other domains (e.g., psychosocial functioning). Coping resources, such as the skills taught in SST, can minimize the effects of stress on relapse and the need for acute care (Liberman, Mueser, Wallace, Jacobs, Eckman, & Massel, 1986).

According to the *social skills model*, impaired psychosocial functioning results when individuals either cannot perform social skills adequately or appropriately and display inappropriate behaviors, or do not perform skills they possess when they should (Mueser, 1998). SST involves teaching more effective and appropriate social and interpersonal behaviors, with the goal of improving functioning in major life domains.

Social skills, defined as specific behaviors or cognitive-perceptual abilities that are needed for successful role performance, interpersonal functioning, and gratification of needs (Mueser & Bellack, 1998; Mueser & Sayers, 1992), require successful integration of (1) expressive behaviors (e.g., verbal and nonverbal behaviors such as voice volume, speech rate, content and pitch, eye contact, facial expression, and posture); (2) receptive behaviors (e.g., verbal and nonverbal behaviors related to listening, obtaining clarification, noticing relevant cues); (3) interactive behaviors (e.g., response timing, taking turns in conversation); and (4) social perception (e.g., emotion recognition and perspective taking) (Bellack, Mueser, Gingerich, & Agresta, 1997). Some social skills are universal for all humans (e.g., facial expression of affect), but many are determined by cultural norms and codes of conduct (e.g., business associates in the United States shake hands as a greeting, whereas French business associates kiss one another on each cheek). At the most basic level, social skills include nonverbal behaviors, such as making eye contact while having a conversation, and verbal behaviors, such as expressing a greeting at the beginning of an interpersonal interaction, that are largely taken for granted by members of a social group. More complex social skills, such as negotiating a contract or settling a dispute, require not only simple interpersonal behaviors but also the ability to perceive and interpret social and emotional cues, synthesize inputs with previous experience, and anticipate probable responses to verbal and nonverbal behaviors. Deficiencies in these basic and complex social skills, which are common in individuals with schizophrenia, often lead to dysfunctional social and interpersonal functioning (Smith, Bellack, & Liberman, 1996).

Many basic social skills (e.g., maintaining interpersonal distance) are learned in childhood, with development of behaviors required for adult role functioning gradually acquired in adolescence and early adulthood. Individuals who experience an early onset of schizophrenia are at particular risk for developing social skills deficits if symptoms of the illness or required treatment, especially lengthy hospitalizations, result in their removal from healthy peer groups, social isolation, and reduced opportunity to perform normal, age-appropriate social behaviors. Although level of premorbid functioning is related to subsequent social skills deficits (Mueser, Bellack, Morrison, & Wixted, 1990), even individuals who develop the illness in later adulthood often demonstrate characteristic impairments in performance of skills that were previously included as part of their behavioral repertoires.

Several factors may explain the nonuse of existing or previously existing skills, including (1) psychotic symptoms, which can interfere with the ability to perceive accurately and process social situations; (2) primary negative symptoms, such as alogia, apathy, flat affect, and anhedonia; (3) avoidance or lack of social interactions due to anxiety, negative symptoms, the stigma of mental illness, or living on the margins of society; (4) interference of characteristic neurocognitive deficits, such as inattention, distractibility, poor memory, and impaired executive functioning; or (5) functioning in an environment, such as an inpatient ward of a psychiatric hospital, that may not adequately reinforce performance of socially appropriate behaviors (Bellack et al., 1997; Mueser & Sayers, 1992). It is also conceivable that social skills may be lost simply as a result of chronic lack of use (Mueser & Sayers, 1992; Penn & Mueser, 1996).

ASSESSMENT OF SOCIAL FUNCTIONING AND SOCIAL SKILLS

Social behavior and functioning in individuals with schizophrenia have been operationalized and measured in a number of ways, including the ability to perceive social cues accurately, solve problems, evaluate behavioral alternatives in social situations, comprehend common social interactions, decode facial and vocal expressions of affect, engage in conversations, maintain interpersonal relationships, and attend to personal needs such as grooming, hygiene, and self-care of medical conditions (Bellack et al., 1994; McEvoy et al., 1996; Mueser et al., 1996). Although the nature of social skills deficits and the areas of life functioning that are disturbed are similar among individuals with schizophrenia, the breadth and severity of the deficits may vary considerably. Systematic assessment of social skills and overall social functioning is therefore important to identify individual deficits, evaluate treatment needs, and establish reasonable treatment goals. Some indication of baseline pretreatment skills level and functioning also permits assessment of the effects of treatment, which should be performed periodically, at least once a year. An initial evaluation should include a general assessment of overall social and role functioning, followed by more detailed scrutiny of specific skills deficits that are suggested by identified impairments in functioning (Bellack et al., 1997).

The evaluation should start with identification of any dysfunctional interpersonal behaviors, followed by information gathering relative to the situations in which the dysfunction occurs (Bellack et al., 1997; Heinssen, Liberman, & Kopelowicz, 2000). Social or interpersonal functioning may differ depending on whether the individual is at home or at work, in familiar or unfamiliar places, and in a clinic or in the home. Important situations to assess include social venues that require basic as well as more complex conversational skills, close interpersonal interactions that occur in residential settings, and the workplace. Life skills, such as use of leisure time, grooming and hygiene, care of personal possessions, and money management, should also be evaluated.

Next, the situations need to be analyzed in an attempt to determine the source of the dysfunction and whether environmental factors or underlying social anxiety, as opposed to social skills deficits, may be responsible for failure to perform appropriate behaviors (Bellack et al., 1997). The behavioral skills needed for success in the situations should also be evaluated (Heinssen et al., 2000). Specific social skills deficits should be measured. Finally, insight regarding deficits, motivation for change, and client goals should be evaluated (Heinssen et al., 2000).

Evaluation of Overall Psychosocial Functioning

Information regarding general functioning is best acquired through interviews with both clients and significant others who have firsthand knowledge about performance of social skills and behaviors (Bellack et al., 1997; Mueser & Bellack, 1998). Several standardized instruments may be helpful in structuring such interviews. The Social Behavior Schedule (Wykes & Sturt, 1986), which is administered to a person familiar with the client, assesses domains of interpersonal functioning, such as ability to hold conversations, comfort and appropriateness of behavior in social situations, degree of social contact, and interpersonal strife. The Katz Adjustment Scale (Katz & Lyerly, 1963) includes self-reports, as well as ratings by close informants, and assesses social behavior, use of leisure time, and participation in socially expected activities. The client and family versions of the Social Adjustment Scale–II (Schooler, Hogarty, & Weissman, 1979) elicit information about instrumental role functioning, performance of household chores, finances, relationships with immediate and extended family members, social leisure, friendships and dating, and overall personal well-being. The Life Skills Profile (Rosen, Hadzi-Pavlovic, & Parker, 1989) is completed by a close informant and contains items evaluating self-care, social contact, appropriateness of communications, social responsibility, and social turbulence. The Social Functioning Scale (Birchwood, Smith, Cochrane, Wetton, & Copestake, 1990) is completed on the basis of information provided by a close informant and the client, and assesses seven areas of functioning: social withdrawal, interpersonal functioning, prosocial activities, recreation, level of independence, level of dependence, and employment. The Social-Adaptive Functioning Evaluation (Harvey et al., 1997) was designed as a rating scale for geriatric psychiatric patients but may be used with lower functioning individuals with schizophrenia to assess instrumental and self-care, impulse control, and basic social behaviors, such as conversational skills, social engagement, and participation in treatment. Assessment of basic daily living skills may also be accomplished using the self-report and informant versions of the Independent Living Skills Survey (Wallace, Liberman, Tauber, & Wallace, 2000), which includes questions regarding domains of functioning such as self-care, care of personal possessions, money management, and use of public transportation.

Choice of instrument should be based on a number of factors, including which particular aspects of functioning are of interest, the extent to which the resulting data will be used in treatment planning, and practical issues, such as cost, time, and available staff (Scott & Lehman, 1998). Awareness of neurocognitive impairments and lack of awareness of illness may also influence the decision about whether to rely on self-administered questionnaires or to conduct interviews with knowledgeable informants (Scott & Lehman, 1998).

In addition to the information that may be gathered using these instruments, it is important to obtain an account of the client's interpersonal history, including a subjective impression of the factors that have led to interpersonal difficulties. Interviewers are most likely to obtain honest self-reports and assessments by starting with general, nonjudgmental questions such as "Can you remember the last time you had an argument with someone?", followed by more targeted questions that elicit information about the nature of the problematic psychosocial functioning, typical responses of others, and frequency of difficulties.

Observation of behavior in natural settings, such as the clinic, work site, or home, can provide excellent data regarding functioning and behavior in a variety of real-life situations. The main advantage of this approach is the ecological validity of the assessment and the opportunity to observe a wide range of behaviors for extended periods of time. Naturalistic observation also provides information about the environmental response of others to the client's behavior, which may help to identify individuals who do not suffer skills deficits but instead have little opportunity to display socially appropriate skills or are not reinforced for them. The disadvantages include the time-consuming nature of such an evaluation, the inability to control extraneous factors that may affect skills performance, the reality that some situations are impossible to observe, and the fact that individuals often behave differently when they know they are being observed.

Measurement of Social Skills

After problematic areas of psychosocial functioning have been identified, specific social skills that may be required for success in those areas should be measured. The best way to isolate and evaluate specific social skills is through behavioral observation of role plays (Benton & Schroeder, 1990; Eckman et al., 1992; Mueser & Bellack, 1998; Mueser & Sayers, 1992). Techniques for designing and implementing role plays as part of SST, which also apply to their use in the initial evaluation, are discussed later in this chapter. Role plays used at the initial evaluation should be relatively brief (3 minutes or less) and designed to assess a variety of situations. It is important to develop some type of behavioral rating scheme to quantify performance of skills. For example, target behaviors such as making eye contact, verbal fluency, or body posture may be enumerated and rated using a Likert-style rating with four to six categories. More complex skills such as social perception and cognitive processing ability may be assessed by asking questions after a role play, for example, "If you had done _____, how would the other person have reacted?" or "How did the other person feel when you said _____?"

Role plays are very useful in differentiating skills deficits from other factors that may be responsible for lack of success in important domains of psychosocial functioning. For example, individuals who display appropriate behaviors and skills in the context of the role play but not in natural settings do not have a skills deficit. On the other hand, individuals who cannot perform skills in a brief role play are unlikely to have the ability to perform them in natural settings. Role plays at initial assessment are particularly useful baseline measurements with which future performance of skills may be compared if they are repeated periodically throughout the course of treatment. The standardized nature of a scripted role play also has the advantage of controlling extraneous situational factors that may affect the performance of social skills in real-life settings. Research supports the validity of role-play tests in clients with schizophrenia; therefore, they are strongly recommended as a means of identifying specific deficits in social skills (Bellack et al., 1997; Mueser & Sayers, 1992).

The Role Play Task, which is part of the Social Problem Solving Battery designed by Sayers, Bellack, Wade, Bennett, and Fong (1995), is an assessment tool that consists of six 3-minute standardized role plays enacted with a confederate that evaluate ability to generate solutions to social problems. Information about the ability to initiate and maintain conversations, stand up for personal rights, and use persuasion, negotiation and compromise in an interpersonal context may be obtained from these role plays. For example, one role play requires clients to act out a situation in which the confederate plays the role of a family member with whom they are having a conversation to try to decide on a movie to select in a video store. These role plays should be videotaped for subsequent evaluation of skills performance by a trained clinician. The confederate in the role play should be an individual with whom the client has had minimal or no prior contact (Bellack et al., 1997). Brief role plays, such as those included in the Role Play Task may need to be extended for less impaired clients who demonstrate skills deficits only with longer interactions.

The Response Generation Task is also part of the Social Problem Solving Battery and represents an effective method for evaluating problem-solving ability. Clients begin by viewing several short video segments in which two individuals are having a disagreement. The clinician stops the tape after each segment to ask the client a series of questions about the goals of the individual who was visible on the screen, how the goal could be achieved, and what could go wrong if the strategy identified were implemented.

LOGISTICS AND TREATMENT PROCEDURES

SST programs differ in terms of the specific training techniques used, the content of the curriculum, and practical considerations such as setting, timing, and length of treatment. Nevertheless, most SST programs include a number of common ingredients in one form or another. For example, most utilize a sequential and hierarchical approach to learning, in which complex target behaviors are dissected into constituent elements and introduced in a graded manner. Active teaching techniques based on learning principles such as didactic instruction, behavioral rehearsal, modeling, reinforcement, shaping, corrective feedback, and homework are used to effect change. Increasingly, SST programs include techniques designed to accommodate cognitive deficits commonly observed in schizophrenia. For example, course material is presented slowly, comprehension of instructions is regularly checked, review of previous learning is frequent, and the same information is presented in a variety of formats.

Logistics

Before commencing SST, a number of practical questions must be answered: Who will receive the treatment? How long will the treatment last? Where will the treatment be administered? Who will administer the treatment? How often will the treatment sessions be administered? What will determine the pacing of the treatment? Answers to these questions are in part determined by availability of resources, but they should also be based on the lessons learned from controlled studies of SST.

Treatment Format

SST has most often been administered in a group format, not only because group therapy is generally more efficient and cost-effective, but also because of the inherent benefits afforded by teaching social behavior in a social setting. For example, group members may serve as models of behavior. In line with Bandura's (1977) assertion that similarity to a model increases the strength of beliefs that one can be successful enacting similar behaviors, peer modeling may be more powerful than modeling by the group leader. Group members may also provide one another with feedback about performance of skills. Receiving positive feedback, in particular, from a peer versus the group leader, may have a greater impact because the peer has no obligation to give praise, whereas the group leader strives to provide as many accolades as possible. The group setting provides a venue for socialization and possible friendships, which may help to decrease social isolation among individuals with schizophrenia. Often, members of a social skills group will develop a sense of community in the sessions even if they do not socialize together outside the treatment setting.

Although SST has most often been administered using a group format, individualized treatment programs may be designed for clients who are unable or unwilling to attend group therapy. The advantages of this approach include the ability to pace the presentation of course material according to achievement of individual mastery, the ability to tailor content and teaching techniques to accommodate individual needs, and greater freedom to plan opportunities to practice skills in natural settings. Combining group with individual sessions that may be needed to address specific needs represents the ideal format and maximizes potential for learning.

Group Composition

Decisions about which clients should be invited to receive SST depend on a number of factors, including the goals and content of the program, and information gained from a comprehensive assessment of mental status, functional impairment, and individual needs. Obviously, individuals who are not judged to be deficient in the targeted skills need not be included. Among those who do demonstrate skills impairments, there are almost always differences in the degree of impairment. Ideally, if resources permit, groups should be formed according to degree of impairment, and SST should be administered separately to relatively high- and low-functioning clients. In the absence of such resources, clients with different levels of functioning but social skills deficits in similar areas can be engaged in SST in the same group, with the leader tailoring feedback to each client's individual needs.

Although research on SST has demonstrated that the presence of positive and negative symptoms does not represent a substantial obstacle to learning (Eckman et al., 1992; Marder et al., 1996; Smith et al., 1996), it is best to invite individuals to participate when symptoms are as stable as possible. Individuals who are pervasively preoccupied with positive symptoms of schizophrenia, such as auditory hallucinations or paranoid delusions, may have difficulty attending to material presented in SST groups without extensive prompting. Clients with prominent negative symptoms, such as apathy, alogia, or social withdrawal, may require substantial amounts of encouragement and reinforcement simply to ensure attendance. However, because social skills deficits are strongly correlated with the severity of negative symptoms (Mueser & Bellack, 1998), strenuous attempts should be undertaken to involve such clients in SST groups. Furthermore, research indicates that clients with more severe negative symptoms respond well to SST (Matousek, Edwards, Jackson, Rudd, & McMurry, 1992; Mueser, Bellack, Douglas, & Wade, 1991).

It is important to evaluate potentially disruptive behaviors such as pacing, inappropriate touching, uncontrollable verbalizations (as with a tic disorder), or even snoring. Overall cognitive functioning should be evaluated to alert group leaders to clients who may need special help or checking on comprehension. At a minimum, given implications for the ability to acquire new information, attention span should be assessed. Individuals who cannot maintain a reasonable focus on group material and activities for at least 20 minutes either may not benefit from SST (Liberman, Wallace, Blackwell, MacKain, &

Eckman, 1992) or may require briefer individual training sessions to develop their attention span.

Finally, insight regarding skills deficits and motivation for change are important to evaluate prior to inclusion in an SST group. Poor insight is a relatively common feature observed in individuals with schizophrenia (Amador, Strauss, Yale, & Gorman, 1991). At a minimum, poor insight may negatively impact attendance, group participation, or efforts to practice skills. At worst, however, lack of awareness of skills deficits that produces feelings of resentment, indignation, or anger about being included in an SST group can lead to disruptive behaviors. Meeting with clients individually before an SST group commences can enable leaders to help clients identify personal goals related to participation in the group, thereby instilling motivation for change.

Group Size

Maximization of learning potential should govern decisions about the minimum and maximum number of clients in SST groups. Generally speaking, groups may range in size from 2 to 12 members. Groups of 4–8 people can most readily be offered the ideal balance of individualized attention from group leaders and the opportunity for socialization and feedback from peers.

Evaluation Procedures

In addition to performing a thorough evaluation prior to initiation of treatment, periodic reassessments should occur to ensure that target behaviors and skills are being acquired. Decisions about how skills will be evaluated, and when this will happen, should be made before treatment begins. Outcome criteria based on the goals of the group should also be established prior to the first meeting.

Group Duration

SST groups may be open-ended or time-limited. Many are limited at least in terms of the time required to teach all components of the target skill, if not in terms of an exact number of sessions. Given that SST usually involves presentation of material in a gradual, graded fashion, with more difficult skills building upon previously learned, more basic skills, an open-ended format may be problematic when new members join after training has commenced. In practice, open-ended groups are most feasible when teaching a limited core curriculum that does not build on previously taught skills, such as a brief inpatient SST group that focuses on conflict management, with the targeted skills repeated every several weeks (Douglas & Mueser, 1990). Even in the case of time-limited groups, it is best to decide in advance at what point new group members will need to wait for subsequent administrations of the treatment. Before that point, members who join late should be provided with individualized, catch-up sessions to ensure that they learn all material they may have missed. The time-limited nature of SST groups does not imply that they are brief. In fact, many SST groups last for 2–6 months, and some data in the literature suggest a dose–response relationship such that greater acquisition of skills is related to longer duration of training. Consistent with the idea that schizophrenia is a lifelong illness, Penn and Mueser (1996) recommend that SST be provided for at least 1 year.

Pacing

In general, the pace of the training should correspond to the rate of learning. Learning is demonstrated by successful completion of role plays, *in vivo* exercises, and homework. Ideally, training should not proceed until all clients have achieved mastery of all skills. However, in the case of a large group, this may be unrealistic, and it may be necessary to advance to the next skill when the majority of clients has mastered the skill. It is important for trainers to be attuned to the interest level of the clients. If clients are becoming bored and restless with the group activities, this may be another sign that it is time to move on.

Training Location

Ideally, training should occur in the setting in which the target behaviors are to be used to facilitate generalization of skills. This is generally only feasible when a large enough group of clients either work or reside in the same location. For example, SST with the elderly could be conducted in a community room of a nursing home. Most SST is conducted in a hospital or clinic setting. Accessibility of the facility is a primary consideration in planning an SST group. For example, a facility that is not served by the public transportation system may be undesirable given that many individuals with schizophrenia either do not drive or do not have access to a vehicle.

There are several practical considerations when choosing the physical space in which SST will be administered. The room should contain a blackboard, dry eraser board, or easel, so that course material may be visually displayed. It should be equipped with tables or desks and chairs, and should be large enough to afford space for role plays. Arrangement of furniture in the room should be classroom-style, with chairs in rows facing the front of the room as opposed to the traditional group therapy style of arranging chairs in a circle. The room should be located in a relatively quiet area of the facility that is nonetheless easy to find. It should be simply decorated, with minimal extraneous objects that may represent distractions, such as bulletin boards with written notices or colorful paintings.

Session Duration

Each session should last from 45 to 90 minutes. Anything less than about 40 minutes does not allow for adequate review of previous learning and sufficient time for new learning. It is unrealistic to expect even nondisabled individuals to attend to a learning task for longer than 2 hours without a break. Two or three SST groups may be scheduled on the same day, assuming that adequate breaks are provided between sessions. If possible, SST groups should meet at least twice a week. Frequent meetings help maintain learning, encourage practice of skills, and prevent forgetting of information.

Timing

Setting the time for group meetings is an important consideration in designing an SST program. It is crucial to avoid scheduling groups when appealing, popular recreational activities occur. For example, SST groups on inpatient wards should not conflict with scheduled smoking breaks or recreational activities (e.g., bowling). Early mornings are often problematic for clients who struggle with the sedating effects of medications that may make rising difficult. If groups meet more than once each week, the scheduled time should remain consistent across all days.

Group Leadership

In addition to professionals from a variety of mental health disciplines, including psychologists, psychiatrists, social workers, and nurses, paraprofessionals such as case managers, residential counselors, and occupational or recreational therapists may lead SST groups if they have been adequately trained. The style for delivering course information and performing teaching activities is more important than the professional degree held by the potential group leader. Enthusiasm, good humor, and patience, as well as the ability to stick to structure, ignore (rather than criticize) inappropriate responses, and immediately notice and praise evidence of learning, are particularly important for group leaders.

Leaders should have some familiarity with the principles of social learning theory and behavior modification, and should be able to apply these in the context of teaching skills. A description of many principles of social learning theory used in SST may be found in *Behavior Modification: What It Is and How to Do It* (Martin & Pear, 1996). Experience watching either videotaped sessions or live groups is crucial for individuals who have no experience with the SST approach. Potential group leaders should also review written materials explicating teaching techniques. Supervision of new leaders by experienced experts, if possible, is recommended.

Ideally, groups should be co-led by two individuals. An additional leader may be assigned to assist with activities if the group size is large, but leadership should remain fairly consistent. At any given time, one of the group leaders should be identified as the primary teacher, with the other leader spending session time monitoring group members, providing individualized instruction when needed, and assisting with role plays. Leaders can either rotate responsibilities when new skills or skills components are introduced or maintain the same roles throughout the training.

Attendance

Given the hierarchical nature of learning, attendance is more important at SST groups than at traditional supportive psychotherapy groups. Above all, it is crucial that clients view participation in SST groups as an important component of their personal treatment plans, and that other members of the treatment team share and reinforce this perspective. Planned strategies designed to improve attendance may be necessary. For example, group members may be rewarded for attendance with money, increased privileges (in the case of an inpatient ward), recreational opportunities, food, time with staff, or tokens that may be used to purchase goods in a hospital or clinic "store." Being on time (within 5–10 minutes of the start of group) may also be reinforced or required for clients to collect the attendance reward. Strategies for dealing with poor attendance are discussed later in this chapter.

Training Procedures

SST is a treatment approach based on several principles of social learning theory (Bandura, 1969) and operant conditioning (Skinner, 1953), including the notion that social skills and behaviors are learned by (1) observing and modeling others; (2) attending to the consequences of behaviors, which either promote and reinforce or extinguish them; (3) repeating new material (i.e., overlearning); and (4) generalizing recently learned behaviors to new situations. With regard to modeling, group leaders generally serve as exemplars of appropriate behavior and social skills in all of their interactions with clients. The leaders also model specific skills in role plays, and clients may observe actors modeling targeted skills on videotaped segments.

Positive reinforcement should be given as frequently as possible. This is most often provided in the form of verbal praise for appropriate demonstration of skills, correct responses to questions, attendance, completion of homework, or any other evidence of success with group tasks. Other forms of positive reinforcement include giving tangible rewards (e.g., money, food, privileges, time with staff, recreational opportunities, etc.) for attendance, being on time, or paying attention. Shaping involves reinforcement of successive approximations of target behaviors. Even individuals who demonstrate no success should be praised if they are making an effort. Consistent with the principle of behavior modification that immediate reinforcement will strengthen a response more quickly than delayed reinforcement, reinforcement should be given as soon as positive behavior is noticed. For example, if a client volunteers to be the first person to perform a role play, acknowledge this by saying, "Thank you, it's great that you volunteered to go first." When individuals demonstrate incorrect or inappropriate skills or responses, this behavior should be ignored, based on the theory that unreinforced behavior will be extinguished.

It is important for clients to receive positive reinforcement from their peers as well as from the group leaders. This can be accomplished by initiating a round of applause for a client who has demonstrated success, and eliciting positive feedback about role play performance from the group participants. Although it may seem childish at first to clap when someone has successfully completed a role play, many individuals with schizophrenia have never experienced this type of acknowledgment and truly appreciate it.

Overlearning of course material is accomplished by repeating new information frequently, practicing skills repeatedly in role plays, assigning homework, and asking frequent questions that serve to check on acquisition of knowledge. An inherent goal of SST is that newly acquired skills will be used in real-life situations. Homework and *in vivo* exercises serve as vehicles for encouraging generalization of skills. Other generalization strategies are discussed as the final step in training new skills.

Starting the Group at the First Meeting

The first session sets the tone for the SST group and should begin with introductions, if necessary, followed by an explanation of how the group will differ from traditional insight- or process-oriented psychotherapy groups that the clients may have attended in the past. Leaders should explain, for example, that the group is similar to a course in that it is time-limited and the goal is to learn skills that are to be used to achieve important life goals. A brief description of the teaching techniques that will be used to do this, including didactic instruction, role plays, and homework, should be provided. Leaders may also inform clients, in a general way, of the evidence supporting this method of helping individuals like them to achieve important life goals.

It is particularly crucial that the first group begin on time and that the leaders convey the importance of consistent attendance and avoidance of tardiness. Leaders may accomplish this by asking questions such as "Why is it important for us to start on time?" A clear explanation of the rewards for attendance, if any, should be provided, followed by questions designed to check on understanding of the rules (e.g., "So, do you get the tokens if you are more than 10 minutes late?"). Leaders should stress the importance of attending even if rewards cannot be earned (e.g., if someone is 15 minutes late). This can be achieved by asking questions such as "Why is it important to attend even if you are too late to receive the tokens?" If clients do not mention the important learning that they will miss if they are absent, the leader should add this as a reason for attending. Clients may also be informed that their absence may produce concern on the part of their peers and the group leaders (e.g., "If you don't show up for group, we will worry about you."). Clients should be provided with a list of phone numbers of group leaders and clinic staff, including instructions about which number to call if they cannot make it to group.

Directing the Sessions

Sessions should always begin with a warm greeting from the trainers to welcome and thank clients for attending (e.g., "It's wonderful to see you all today. Thank you for making the effort to be here."). The session should proceed with some questions that serve to remind clients about the overall goal of the group, the specific task that is being worked on, and key information that has been learned. For example, a relapse prevention group may start with questions such as the following: "What is the overall goal of this group?" "What are we working on in this skill area?" "What do we mean by the term 'relapse'?" "Why is it important to monitor warning signs?" The next 5 minutes should be spent reviewing any homework that was assigned. If necessary, 5–15 minutes can then be spent engaging in role plays based on homework assignments. Then, the leader should provide an overview of the goals of the session and proceed for the next 20–30 minutes with the planned activities for the group. The last 5–10 minutes of the session should be devoted to assigning (and individually tailoring, if necessary) new homework.

Steps for Teaching Skills

Several different teaching techniques are used to convey information and practice new skills. One reason for using a variety of techniques to teach the same material is to accommodate different styles of learning. Some individuals learn best by observing, while others learn best by hearing, and still others by doing. In the case of complex social skills, the same teaching techniques should be used in succession for each component of the skill. See Table 2.1 for a summary.

Step 1: Establish a Rationale for Learning the Skill

It is crucial to begin SST by explaining why it is important to learn the skills that will be taught. Whenever possible, it is helpful to elicit the rationale from the group members by asking questions about how learning the skill will be useful. This enables them to take greater ownership of the rationale and may create more motivation to engage in the learning process. In establishing the rationale, trainers should illustrate the practical relevance of the skill to the clients' life and functioning. An example of providing a rationale for the skill "leaving stressful situations" is provided on pages 30–31.

TABLE 2.1. Steps of Social Skills Training

Step 1: Establish a rationale for the skill.
- Elicit reasons for learning the skill from group participants.
- Provide additional reasons not provided by group participants.
- Emphasize relevance of learning skill to achieving important life goals.

Step 2: Discuss the steps of the skill.
- Display the steps of the skill on a board or poster.
- Explain each step.
- Elicit reasons for and importance of each step from group participants.
- Provide additional reasons not provided by group participants.

Step 3: Perform role-play exercises.
- Plan the role play, including script, in advance.
- Explain the value of performing role plays in terms of practicing skills.
- Describe the scenario that will be enacted in the role play.
- Use two leaders to model the role play.
- Encourage group participants to identify when each step was used in the role play.
- Ask group participants to evaluate effectiveness of the role model.
- Check understanding of assigned roles and expectations for performance in role play.
- Elicit a volunteer to perform the role play with the group leader.
- Instruct group participants to observe the volunteer.
- Elicit positive feedback from observers about performance of skills.
- Immediately redirect if negative feedback is offered.
- Provide additional positive feedback.
- Offer one suggestion for how performance of skills could be enhanced.
- Encourage repetition of the same role play, incorporating suggestion.
- Elicit and provide additional positive and corrective feedback.
- Use supplementary modeling, discrimination modeling, and coaching, if necessary.

Step 4: Assign homework.
- Assign a task to be completed in a natural environment.
- Remind group participants of the value of practicing skills in real-life situations.
- Tailor assignments to match level of mastery of the skill.
- Assist group participants with identification of when, where, how, and with whom the assignment may be completed.

Step 5: Use generalization strategies.
- Provide training to staff at treatment facility on techniques used in social skills training.
- Inform staff about what skills to look for and reinforce, and when.
- Invite indigenous community supports to participate as agents of change to encourage and reinforce performance of skills in real-life settings.
- Hold regular meetings with community supports to obtain information about use of skills.

LEADER: Today we're going to work on the skill "leaving stressful situations." Can anyone give me an example of a stressful situation?

BILL: How about if you have to shop in a crowded supermarket?

LEADER: Absolutely. Shopping in crowds can be very stressful. (*Writes "shop in a crowded supermarket" on the blackboard, adding to the list as other examples are provided.*) Can anyone think of other stressful situations?

JILL: When you're busy at work?

LEADER: Excellent example. Any others? . . . Can you think of an example, Susan?

SUSAN: If you are having an argument with someone?

LEADER: Good. How do you feel when you are having an argument with someone?

SUSAN: Usually I get mad.

LEADER: Right. Arguments can often get very heated and cause people to get angry at each other. What happens if an argument continues to the point where people get mad?

BRAD: They could start yelling at each other?

LEADER: Exactly. Sometimes, the longer an argument continues, the more angry people become, and the more stressful the situation becomes. The chance of resolving an argument also decreases the longer the argument continues. What about if you stopped the argument and left the situation instead of yelling?

BILL: You might not be so angry.

LEADER: Very good, Bill. You might not begin to get so upset, and if you leave you might feel calmer. Do you think you would have a better chance of settling the argument if you left or if you stayed?

BILL: If you keep arguing.

LEADER: (*Ignores the incorrect response.*) What do people think?

SUSAN: Better if you leave.

LEADER: Yes. Sometimes the best thing to do when you are in a stressful situation is to leave because remaining can make things worse. If you leave, you can take time to calm down and when you feel less stressed, you can think better and then come back and do a better job of solving the problem. This may help you get along better with people in a variety of situations, which could mean greater success at home, at work, and in interpersonal relationships.

Step 2: Discuss the Steps of the Skill

When initially presenting the skill or skills to be learned, the leader should enumerate and explain all component parts of the skill(s). It is advisable to list these on large poster board or a flipchart, so that they may be displayed when the particular skill(s) components are being addressed in the session. Providing this visual cue assists individuals with memory impairments. The leader should also explain the importance of each step. The following example of discussing the steps of the skill(s) uses the same group working on "leaving stressful situations":

LEADER: There are a number of steps involved in "leaving stressful situations." First, you should figure out whether the situation you are in is stressful. How do you know whether a situation is stressful?

BRAD: If you feel stressed?

LEADER: That's right. What information do you use to decide if you feel stressed?

BRAD: You might feel mad or anxious.

LEADER: Excellent. You would pay attention to your feelings, and you might also be aware of your thoughts and the way your body feels. For example, when you get angry, sometimes you feel tense or hot. Why is it important to take the time to decide whether you are in a stressful situation?

SUSAN: Because you don't want to be in a stressful situation.

LEADER: Good. As we said, staying in a stressful situation can often make things worse, right? So it is a good idea to pay attention to some of the signs that you might be stressed. The next step is to tell the other person in the situation that you are stressed and need to leave. Why do you think it's important to tell the person this?

JILL: So they won't be mad at you?

LEADER: That's right. What might happen if you didn't say anything about how you were feeling?

JILL: The person might be confused.

LEADER: Exactly. If you just walked away without saying anything, the other person wouldn't know what to think. But this way, the other person knows you are feeling stressed. The next step, if you are in a conflict with someone, is to tell the person that you will talk about it more later. Why should you do this?

BILL: So you can settle the problem sometime.

LEADER: Very good. Saying that you would like to continue the discussion later lets the person know you want to reach some kind of solution, that you are not trying to avoid the problem. The last step is actually physically leaving the situation, which can be difficult. Why do you think that is?

BRAD: Because you might want to stay.

LEADER: Good thinking. What could make you want to stay?

BRAD: Maybe if the other person keeps arguing.

LEADER: Yes, that could happen. Even if you tell someone how you feel and that you need to leave the situation, the person may want to continue the argument. So it is important to keep your word and leave. If you follow these steps to "leaving a stressful situation," it is more likely that you will reach a better resolution of the problem and feel calmer than if you stay in the situation.

Step 3: Perform Role-Play Exercises

Role plays are brief, scripted interactions with one of the group leaders that enable clients to demonstrate how well they have acquired and can perform the skills that have been taught. A practice role play that does not necessarily address a targeted skill may be performed before the skills training begins to familiarize clients with the procedure. Chairs and other props should be arranged at the front of the room, so that the role-play area represents a distinct physical space and is the focus of attention. Before starting the task, the leader provides a clear description of what will happen in the role play, including who will play what part, who will start the action, where the scene is occurring, which target behaviors should be performed, the client's goal in the role play, and the length of time for the interaction. The leader asks clients questions about this information to ensure adequate understanding before the role play begins.

Clients are informed that when they are not performing the role play, they need to be paying careful attention to the person who is performing, so that they may give feedback afterward about how well the skills were performed. Clients are invited to provide feedback about not only skills performance but also important verbal and nonverbal communication skills such as eye contact, body posture, energy level, verbal fluency, voice volume, and so on. A list of these behaviors may be provided to prompt clients when they are asked to provide feedback.

The scenario for the role play should be realistic and relevant to the clients' circumstances. Initially, they should be fairly brief, about 30–45 seconds, and should involve only four or five verbal exchanges. The duration and complexity of role plays may be increased if skills permit. The leader uses the same script for each client, so that expectations about each successive role play do not change. However, clients who wish to add some creativity to their role play should not be discouraged from doing so. Allowing individuals some creative license can make the role plays more engaging for the clients who are observing. The leader may need to stray from the script in order to enable some clients to demonstrate skills successfully. For example, if a client playing the role of a therapist is supposed to tell the confederate about warning signs of illness to demonstrate knowledge of the concept but fails to use the phrase "warning signs," the confederate may alter the script, adding, "My friend said something about 'warning signs.' What are those?"

The trainers should demonstrate the role play before clients are asked to perform. Next, volunteers should be elicited to try the role play. Leaders should expect a variety of responses from clients—from enthusiasm to outright refusal. If no one volunteers, the leader should ask an individual who is likely to perform relatively well to begin. Successful performance by a peer may help other clients feel more comfortable about attempting the role play. Suggestions for engaging clients who are reluctant to participate in role plays are provided later in the chapter.

Some clients, particularly individuals with persistent delusions, need to be reminded frequently that the role play is "pretend." The leader should try to facilitate positive behaviors during the role play to maximize subsequent positive feedback for the client. For example, if a client is rambling, the confederate should try to interrupt gently, so that the progress of the role play will be maintained.

Immediately after the role play, the leader should clap and invite the observers to provide a round of applause to the performer. Next, the leader should elicit positive feedback by asking, "What did you like about _____'s role play?" It is important that the client receive feedback from peers before receiving it from the leader. If necessary, comments by the observers may be supplemented with positive feedback from the group leader. If the clients do not spontaneously provide feedback when the general invitation to do so is made, the leader should call on individuals by name. Or specific questions about items on the list of verbal and nonverbal behaviors may be asked. For example, if the leader noticed that the client made good eye contact throughout the role play, one of the observers may be asked, "What did you think of _____'s eye contact during the role play?" It is important to obtain feedback that is behaviorally specific. If an observer states, "I thought _____ did a really good job in the role play," the leader should attempt to acquire more specific feedback by saying, "I agree. _____ did do a good job. Can you tell her what it was, in particular, that you liked about the way she performed the role play?"

If observers offer negative feedback, they should immediately be interrupted and redirected to describe what they liked about the performance. Sometimes a performance is so marginal that it is difficult to elicit much positive feedback. In these cases, the leader must either find some aspect of behavior to reinforce or praise evidence of effort or persistence. For example, "I like the way you stayed with the task and kept trying right to the end."

Corrective feedback should be provided by the leader after sufficient positive feedback has been obtained. This should come in the form of brief, behaviorally specific suggestions that are offered in a noncritical manner. The leader should identify important aspects of behavior that could be altered to improve performance. For example, the leader may say, "One thing that would make your performance in the role play even better is if you _____." The leader should then ask the client to repeat the role play, incorporating the suggestion for improved performance. It is best to provide clients with only one suggestion for improvement at a time, given that it may be difficult or discouraging for them to have to remember to make too many changes in the subsequent role play. The same procedure for eliciting and providing positive feedback should follow the second role play. Leaders should focus their feedback on the skill or behavior targeted for improvement in the second role play.

Leaders may need to use coaching or prompting to help clients succeed in role plays. *Coaching* involves providing verbal prompts during the role play. A leader may, for example, whisper reminders in the client's ear. It is important to check with clients before using this procedure given that this may be uncomfortable for individuals with paranoid delusions. *Prompting* involves using nonverbal signs to cue clients about specific behaviors. For example, the leader might cup her hand around her ear as a cue to increase voice volume. These signs should be explained before the role play begins.

Supplementary modeling by the leader may be used if the client does not seem to be able to incorporate corrective verbal feedback. The leader instructs the client to pay special attention to the demonstration of a particular element of a skill, then models the behaviors that the client had been instructed to perform in the previous role play. After the behavior is modeled by the leader, the client is asked to describe the performance of the skill ("Did you notice when I demonstrated _____?"), and then to repeat the role play. *Discrimination modeling* may be used to highlight a particular behavior or component of a skill. The leader successively models a target behavior, first the way it should be performed and then the way it should not be performed. The incorrect performance of the behavior may be exaggerated to accentuate the difference between the two. The leader should follow up with questions such as "How were the two role plays different?" or "Was I more effective in one role play as compared with the other?" As many as three or four role plays should be conducted, if required, for adequate performance of the target skills. Role plays may need to be simplified for clients who, after the second attempt, continue to struggle with skill performance. Time constraints will likely necessitate going onto the next client after four role plays with the same person have been conducted.

Target behaviors that are to be performed during the role play may be assessed in a number of ways, including frequency counts, Likert-style ratings, or simple ratings of the presence or absence of skills (Bellack et al., 1997; Mueser & Sayers, 1992). The evaluation may be performed by the trainer during the role play or more in-depth analyses of skills may be conducted later, if patients consent to audio or videotaping (Bellack et al., 1997; Mueser & Bellack, 1998). An example of using a role play to demonstrate the skill "leaving a stressful situation" is provided:

LEADER: Now that we have talked about the steps involved in "leaving a stressful situation," we are going to practice following the steps by doing a role play. Tania [Leader B] and I will demonstrate the role play first to show you how to follow the steps. When you do the role play, you are going to pretend that you and Tania are roommates who have a disagreement about whose turn it is to do the dishes. You will pretend to be sitting in the kitchen finishing a glass of soda when Tania comes in to look for a clean glass. When she can't find one, she will tell you it's your turn to do the dishes and then you will disagree about whose turn it is. You will notice that you are feeling tense and angry and tell Tania that you are feeling stressed and need to leave. Then, you should tell her that you want to settle the argument later and you'll come back in an hour or so. Then, you will pretend to leave the room. When you are not performing your role play, I want you to watch and see that all of the steps of the skill are performed (*points to steps on blackboard*). You should also watch for the communication behaviors on the list I just handed out that we used for the practice role play. Are there any questions?

BRAD: Do we all have to do the role play?

LEADER: It would be great if everyone could try. Remember, practicing these skills really makes it easier to use them when you need to in real-life situations. Okay, Tania and I will demonstrate the role play now. (*Moves with Leader B to the front of the room where two chairs are arranged for use in role plays. The role play is then modeled, followed by questions to assess whether clients can identify performance of all steps of the skill.*) Okay, so that was an example of how to leave a stressful situation. Now I'd like to give each of you a chance to practice this skill in a role play. Who would like to go first with Tania?

SUSAN: I will.

LEADER: Great. Thanks or volunteering to go first. Now, what is Susan's role in the role play?

BILL: She is going to sit in the kitchen.

LEADER: Right. She will be sitting, pretending to drink a soda. What is Tania's role?

JILL: She is the roommate who is mad because the dishes are dirty.

LEADER: Good. She is the roommate and is going to walk in and the two will disagree about whose turn it is to do the dishes. Who is going to start the role play?

SUSAN: Tania is going to start talking first.

LEADER: That's right. Okay, let's begin. Remember, the rest of us are watching to see that the steps of the skill are followed. (*Leader B and Susan move to the front of the room to perform the role play*).

LEADER B: Hello. How are you?

SUSAN: I'm okay. And you?

LEADER B: (*Motions to pretend to open a cabinet and look for a glass.*) Okay. Is that the last clean glass you are using?

SUSAN: I guess so.

LEADER B: Look at all of these dirty dishes. How come you haven't washed them yet? It's your turn.

SUSAN: I don't think so. I washed them the last time.

LEADER B: No. You're wrong. I remember washing them the last time. You always forget your turn.

SUSAN: I am starting to get tense and feel stressed. I really need to leave for a while.

LEADER B: So you're just going to leave these dirty dishes?

SUSAN: Well, I am getting very upset and if I don't leave, it will just get worse, so I really have to go. (*Walks to the opposite side of the room, pretending to leave.*)

LEADER: Okay, the role play is over. (*Begins clapping.*) Great job with your role play, Susan. Let's give Susan a round of applause and tell her what we liked about her role play.

BILL: She didn't really make eye contact.

LEADER: Let's give Susan some positive feedback about her role play. Jill, what did you like about the way Susan performed her role play?

JILL: I thought she did a very good job.

LEADER: I agree. Can you tell her, specifically, what you liked about her role play?

JILL: Well (*looking at list of communication behaviors*), she had good voice volume and good body posture.

LEADER: That's great feedback. You're right. She didn't speak too loudly or too softly, and she maintained good posture. What about the first step of the skill?

BRAD: She said she was tense.

LEADER: Yes. That means she was paying attention to her body and her feelings. How about the second step?

BILL: She said she was stressed and needed to leave, and then she did leave.

LEADER: That's right. So that took care of the last step, too. How about the third step, telling the person that you want to talk more later?

SUSAN: I think I forgot that one.

LEADER: Susan, you did a great job of demonstrating how to leave a situation before making things worse. You didn't seem to get too angry, and you did a good job of telling Tania how you were feeling. Your role play could have been even better if you had told Tania that you intended to come back later to talk more about whose turn it was to wash the dishes. I would like you to do the role play again and, this time, remember to tell Tania that you want to talk more later. (*The same role play is enacted again, following the same procedure afterward of eliciting positive feedback and providing constructive criticism and additional role playing if needed.*)

Step 4: Assign Homework

Homework assignments should be clear and include specific instructions for activities that can feasibly be completed in the clients' natural environments. When homework is first assigned, clients should be reminded of the importance and value of practicing new skills in order to become more successful at performing them. All attempts at completing homework assignments should be praised. If clients report that they were minimally successful, or if homework was not completed, leaders should elicit advice from those who had at least some success regarding how to perform the tasks. For example, if an individual in a relapse prevention course did not remember to monitor warning signs, the leader may ask someone who did remember to describe what he or she did to help remember to do the daily ratings. Suggestions for handling repeated noncompliance with homework are provided later in this chapter.

Feedback about homework can provide ideas for new role plays that may be enacted in the session. For example, suggestions from peers about how an individual may have been more successful with a homework assignment can be incorporated into a role play that serves as a means of practicing a close approximation of the situation that will be encountered for homework. Reports about homework also provide important information about the extent to which skills generalize to real-life situations. Homework assignments may be individually tailored to match the mastery level of a skill. If some clients have mastered a skill in homework but others need more practice, the complexity of the assignment should be increased to maintain challenge for the successful individuals and may be simplified for less successful clients. An example of providing a homework assignment is provided:

LEADER: You are all doing a good job in the sessions of practicing the skill "leaving a stressful situation." Now I would like you to try the skill in a real-life situation. So before we meet the next time, I want you to complete a homework assignment. The assignment is to practice leaving a stressful situation. Does anyone have any questions about the assignment?

JILL: What if I don't run into any stressful situations?

LEADER: I don't want you to try to create a stressful situation, but we all encounter situations that are stressful, and it is useful to practice leaving stressful situations when it is necessary. What about when your niece and nephew are fooling around when you are trying to concentrate on a book you are reading? You have said that is stressful.

JILL: Oh, yeah. I get so irritated when they do that. I usually start shouting at them, but maybe I should just go to another room.

LEADER: What about other people? Can you think of stressful situations you might encounter that you might want to practice leaving before making things worse?

BRAD: How about when I get real busy at work?

LEADER: Well, do you think you would be able to leave your cash register if the store has a long line?

BRAD: No. My boss would probably get upset if I just left, but maybe I could practice telling her when I am getting stressed and need to take a 15-minute break.

LEADER: Good idea. It will also give you a chance to practice paying attention to your thoughts and feelings when the store is busy. What about you, Bill?

BILL: Well, my roommate always gets upset with me when I don't feel like going to his grandmother's house with him and we get into a big argument about it. He has been mentioning that he wants to go to her house on Saturday, so I think he'll probably ask me tonight or tomorrow to go with him.

LEADER: Okay. Well, maybe you can practice paying attention to whether you are feeling stressed, and if you notice that you are, you can practice following the other steps of leaving the situation. Susan, what about you. . . . (*Checks with each member of the group to ensure that a situation that could be used for homework is identified.*)

Step 5: Use Generalization Strategies

Most SST is administered in hospital or clinic settings. The skills that are to be learned, however, are intended to be used in other settings, such as in the home, at work, or in public places that serve as venues for social interactions. Generalization of skills, therefore, is an inherent goal of SST, and strategies designed to promote generalization should be included routinely as part of the program. As mentioned, homework assignments may be used to encourage use of skills in the natural environment. Other staff at the hospital or clinic who are familiar with the skills that are being trained and the techniques used in the treatment should be encouraged to reinforce skills that are used outside the classroom setting. Workshops regarding the key principles borrowed from social learning theory and operant conditioning may be offered to provide staff training. Individuals who interact with clients in their living environments, such as family members and residential staff, or case managers who spend time with clients in public places other than the hospital or clinic, should also routinely be included as agents of change.

Individuals in the natural environment are in an ideal position to prompt and reinforce the performance of target behaviors and skills outside the treatment setting, which will facilitate their inclusion in the client's behavioral repertoire. They can report on the demonstration of target behaviors, obstacles to skills performance, and general response of the environment to clients' attempts to practice skills. They may also help set reasonable client goals, monitor longitudinal progress, assist with homework assignments, and provide suggestions for personally relevant role plays. If trainers learn that skills are not being performed in the natural environment, role plays that are similar to clients' real-life circumstances should be practiced in sessions, or homework designed to specifically address the component behaviors should be assigned. Indigenous community supports should be invited to observe an SST session, so that they will feel included in the program. Trainers should also hold regular meetings with community supports to discuss progress toward goals, new skills that are being taught, and suggestions for other behaviors that require attention. The following example uses information obtained from a community support to facilitate use of skills in real-life situations:

LEADER: Brad, in our last meeting with your case manager, we talked about how stressful it was for you when your brother criticized the way you prepared a meal. That sounds like a situation where you could have used the skill "leaving a stressful situation."

BRAD: Well, I tried, but it didn't really work very well.

LEADER: Can you describe what happened?

BRAD: I had worked hard to make supper and then my brother said I overcooked the meat, that it was dry. So, I got upset and told him I was feeling stressed and needed to leave. He told me he could have done a better job, so I told him to cook his own food, and we got into an argument about the right way to cook the food.

LEADER: Why don't we do a role play of the situation and see what happened? Would someone volunteer to play Brad's brother?

BILL: Okay, I will.

LEADER: Thanks, Bill. (*Sets up role play.*) You two pretend to be sitting at the dining room table and Bill, you start the role play by saying that you think the meat is too dry.

BILL: (*Role play begins.*) You overcooked the meat again. It's too dry.

BRAD: I worked really hard on this meal. I am so upset that you criticized my cooking, I need to leave.

BILL: I could have done a much better job than you.

BRAD: Why don't you cook your own food, if you don't like my cooking?

BILL: Because I am busy and it is your job to do the cooking.

BRAD: Well, I don't see you doing much of anything around here.

LEADER: (*Stops the role play.*) Okay, let's stop the role play. Let's give Brad some feedback. What did people like about the way Brad handled the situation?

SUSAN: Well, he asserted himself and didn't let his brother get away with criticizing him.

LEADER: That's true. And you did a good job of telling your brother how his comment made you feel. I noticed that you continued the discussion with your brother after you said you were upset and needed to leave.

BRAD: Well, when we did the role play in class, the other person didn't keep arguing after I said I needed to leave, but my brother kept talking to me.

LEADER: What if you had tried Step 3 of the skill, which would have meant telling him that you were willing to continue the discussion when you returned?

BRAD: I guess I forgot to try that.

LEADER: I would like you to repeat the role play and, this time, try to remember to tell your brother that you would like to finish the conversation when you come back. Bill, do you mind doing the role play again? (*Role plays are repeated until all steps of the skill are incorporated.*)

Other Training Techniques

In addition to the techniques already discussed, problem-solving and *in vivo* exercises may also be used in the context of SST. Problem solving is a tool that clients may use in a variety of situations and life circumstances that extend beyond the target behaviors of SST. Most problem-solving techniques consist of several steps, including definition of the problem that needs to be solved, generation of solutions to the problem, determination of whether the solutions are feasible, evaluation of the advantages and disadvantages of each solution, choice of the solution that is anticipated to be most successful, and development of a plan for implementing it. Trainers should explain that these exercises will provide clients with an opportunity to brainstorm about situations they are likely to encounter in attempting to perform target skills in their environments. Problem-solving exercises can be particularly useful when there seem to be barriers to performance of skills that need to be assessed.

In vivo exercises may be used as a precursor to homework exercises to practice skills with the help of one of the trainers, who accompanies the client to serve as a coach. These can be simple interactions that are performed using staff at the hospital or clinic where the training occurs, or opportunities for clients to begin practicing a skill, with assistance, in a real-life setting. Clearly, the latter requires considerably more flexibility and time on the part of the trainer but can be a valuable step in generalization of skills.

CURRICULUM PLANNING

The skills that are taught in an SST program should correspond to identified deficits in the behavioral repertoires of clients who will receive treatment. Some programs are designed to address very specific behaviors, such as smoking cessation, while other teach more general skills, such as basic conversational techniques. There are several preplanned, commercially available SST packages designed to address common social skills deficits in individuals with schizophrenia. Some provide a basic framework for teaching the skill, while others also include teaching materials, such as client workbooks, manuals with scripts for each session, suggestions for role plays, problem-solving exercises, and homework assignments. Most may be adapted to meet the unique needs of treatment settings. Reference to these packages will provide a sense of how much material can be covered in each session, how many sessions are required for each skill, and how to break skills into their component parts. Initial training in basic skills, such as expressing positive and negative feelings, making requests, listening to others, or perceiving social cues, that serve as a foundation for more complex skills, such as finding a job or structuring leisure time, may be necessary for some clients.

Several manualized skills training modules have been developed by the Clinical Research Center for Schizophrenia and Psychiatric Rehabilitation at UCLA. These modules have been empirically validated and used in several countries around the world (Chambon & Marie-Cardine, 1998; Liberman, 1998; Liberman et al., 1986, 1992, 1998; Liberman, DeRisi, & Mueser, 1989; Schaub, Behrendt, & Brenner, 1998). Among the available modules are symptom self-management, recreation for leisure, medication self-management, community reentry, job seeking, workplace fundamentals, basic conversation skills, and friendship and dating skills, all of which use the same teaching techniques, including didactic instruction, role play, problem solving, homework, and *in vivo* behavioral rehearsal. These modules have demonstrated effectiveness in promoting significant learning of social and independent living skills in individuals with schizophrenia (e.g., Liberman et al., 1998; Marder et al., 1996), and given their user-friendly nature, may be administered by a broad array of mental health professionals.

Preplanned curricula for conversation skills, conflict management skills, assertiveness skills, community living skills, friendship and dating skills, medication management skills, and vocational skills are available in Bellack and colleagues' (1997) *Social Skills Training for Schizophrenia: A Step-by-Step Guide*. The guide includes rationales for the skills, steps of the skills, suggested role play scenarios, and special considerations for teaching each skill. The guide also contains a sample problem-solving worksheet; a sample homework sheet for documenting completion of assignments; a sample rating scale for assessing cooperation, performance, and attention during groups; and a copy of the Social-Adaptive Functioning Evaluation (Harvey et al., 1997), which may be used to evaluate several aspects of social functioning.

Regardless of the materials used, trainers should substantially prepare and preplan group activities. It is advisable to develop a curriculum menu, which is an enumeration of all of the specific component behaviors required for successful completion of the overall skills. Trainers should also devise a lesson plan with tentative timetables for accomplishing group tasks. Flexibility in the lesson plans and timetables is important given the difficulty in anticipating clients' rates of response to the training. Sensitivity to sociocultural factors that may impact skills performance, such as differences in societal norms regarding personal space and proxemics, is particularly important when designing curriculum plans and group activities (Bellack et al., 1997).

Introducing an SST program into the context of an existing system of care requires considerable support from administrators and supervisors. Although SST programs can serve as an adjunct to other services and interventions, they work best when all mental health professionals and staff learn to "speak the same language" and interact with clients similarly. It is also helpful for all staff to be familiar with the skills being taught and when, so that they can recognize and reinforce appropriate performance of skills. Workshops regarding the principles of social learning and behavioral modification may be offered for staff who lack familiarity with this approach. They may find the techniques useful in handling a variety of behaviors, even those that are not the focus of training.

COMMON PROBLEMS ENCOUNTERED IN THE DELIVERY OF SOCIAL SKILLS TRAINING

Before implementing any psychotherapeutic technique or program, clinicians should familiarize themselves with common problems that frequently have been observed in the course of its use with clients. Some problems, such as poor attendance, may be attributable to symptoms of schizophrenia. Other problems, such as noncompliance with homework, may be encountered as a result of the nature of the treatment techniques. Social skills trainers should prepare for the following frequently occurring problems in addition to the two just mentioned: low participation in the group; distractibility and problems with comprehension; disruptive behavior; reluctance to perform role plays; and lack of investment in SST.

Poor Attendance

Poor attendance, with at least one client, is almost certain to occur in any group and represents the greatest barrier to the success of SST at the individual level. Given the substantial rates of treatment noncompliance among individuals with schizophrenia, this problem is not unique to SST. However, because learning is designed to occur in incremental steps, with basic skills providing the foundation for more complex skills, attendance is particularly important in SST.

Negative symptoms of schizophrenia, such as apathy and social withdrawal, play a substantial role in poor attendance. Positive symptoms, such as intrusive auditory hallucinations and delusions, particularly paranoia, may also make it difficult for clients to maintain consistent attendance. The importance of good attendance should be explicitly conveyed to clients at the first meeting of the group. As mentioned, a variety of incentives may be offered to reinforce clients for attendance, including money, increased privileges (in the case of an inpatient ward), recreational opportunities, food, time with staff, or tokens that may be used to purchase goods in a hospital or clinic "store." The leaders should immediately contact clients who miss a group to provide the message that their presence is important enough to warrant concern about an absence, and to ask some nonconfrontational questions about reasons for the absence, as well as to offer assistance in facilitating attendance. Clients should then be invited to attend the next session and reminded of the time and day the group is held.

Individuals who miss several sessions in a row will need individual catch-up sessions to keep pace with the rest of the group. Sometimes describing what was missed in positive terms can create motivation for attending (e.g., "We watched a video that gave us the chance to observe someone learning about what to do when you notice warning signs to prevent having to go back into the hospital"). It may also be necessary to elicit assistance from supports in the community, such as residential counselors, case managers, or family members, to remind frequently absent clients to attend.

The leaders should avoid canceling groups and instead stress the importance of attending all sessions. Backup group leaders should therefore be trained and available to fill in when regular leaders are on vacation or ill. Most importantly, leaders should not give up on absent clients. Clients often appreciate persistent efforts to engage them and may eventually decide to attend with greater frequency.

Low Level of Participation in Group

The same positive and negative symptoms of schizophrenia that interfere with ability to attend groups may also affect clients' ability to participate actively during sessions. Clients who attend but do not seem engaged may also be socially anxious or lack confidence in their ability and may therefore be reluctant to answer questions or complete group tasks. These individuals should be praised generously for any spontaneous attempts at participation. The leader should call on reticent group members to answer specific questions, starting with those requiring only a "yes" or "no" response. Participation may also be reinforced with a tangible reward. The leader is advised not to draw attention to lack of participation, particularly in the context of the group.

Negative Effects of Cognitive Impairments

The characteristic neurocognitive impairments found in many individuals with schizophrenia, including distractibility, poor attention, impaired executive functioning, and memory deficits, affect not only social functioning but also the ability to benefit from SST (see, e.g., Mueser et al., 1991). Some of the packaged SST programs, including the UCLA modules mentioned earlier, were designed to compensate for commonly observed cognitive deficits through reliance on techniques such as repetition, overlearning, and behavioral rehearsal (Liberman et al., 1992). Several other strategies may be used to address cognitive impairments.

As mentioned earlier, the treatment room should be minimally distracting and located in a quiet area of the treatment facility. In addition, it should be arranged to facilitate eye contact with the leader; visual cues such as posters, labels, schedules, and signs may be used to assist individuals with memory impairments. The leader who is not serving as the primary group leader should constantly be scanning the clients and may unobtrusively, gently approach individuals who appear distracted to remind them to focus on the leader. Questions may be directed to individuals who appear distracted to prevent them from drifting away from the work of the group. Shaping procedures that may facilitate learning may be used to improve attention, such as rewarding good eye contact, appropriate responses to questions, or comments reflecting accurate tracking of the group topic, with tokens or positive verbal praise (Heinssen et al., 2000). If clients have trouble paying attention to role plays, the leader should assign them the task of watching for specific target behaviors (e.g., "I want you to report on_____'s eye contact at the end of the role play").

Verbal instructions and information should be conveyed in the form of brief, pointed statements. The leaders should periodically remind clients of the goals of the session in terms of task completion. They should frequently ask clients to repeat instructions, and should ask them questions designed to confirm attention to and comprehension of group material (e.g., "What is my role in the role play?" "What are the goals of this skill area?"). If comprehension appears poor, skills or skill components should be further simplified.

Between-session reviews may be helpful in promoting learning and memory of skills learned in groups (Eckman et al., 1992). Finally, SST may be accompanied by adjunctive therapy targeting skills such as social perception, verbal communication, and cognitive processing that are judged to be important in learning other, more complex skills.

Brenner and colleagues (1994) have developed a rehabilitation program, integrated psychological therapy, that includes enhancement of cognitive functioning as a precursor to skills training. Integrated psychological therapy is a highly structured, manualized treatment divided into five subsections: cognitive differentiation, social perception, verbal communication, social skills, and interpersonal problem solving. Client groups are formed on the basis of results of an overall assessment of cognitive functioning prior to initiation of the treatment. The first three subsections address cognitive impairments and consist of activities, directed by a therapist, designed to combine cognitive operations with social interaction. For example, clients learn to attend better to verbal communications, take in details of a social situation, incorporate information from the environment into an understanding of situations, and solve problems. The fourth and fifth subsections of the program target social interactions and are similar to skills training programs that do not include an explicit focus on enhancing cognitive functioning. Some research indicates that integrated psychological therapy enhances the effects of SST in improving social skills and functioning (Spaulding, Reed, Sullivan, Richardson, & Weiler, 1999).

Reluctance to Role Play

Reluctance to participate in role plays may be due to social anxiety, fear of failure, or primary effects of negative symptoms (e.g., apathy). Sometimes it may be helpful simply to validate clients' feelings about performing a role play (i.e., that many people are initially uncomfortable playing a role before an audience). The leaders should remind reluctant clients that the training setting is a safe place for them to practice their skills without fear of criticism, and that practicing skills, in terms of performing them even better in real-life situations, will lead to achievement of important life goals. They should inform clients that most people become increasingly comfortable the more role plays they perform. Particularly shy clients may prefer to perform their role play near the end of a session, after having had the opportunity to observe others complete the task. Some clients may appreciate the chance to perform their role play first, to prevent accumulation of anticipatory anxiety. Reluctant individuals can be invited to perform at least the first step of a role play. This may increase willingness to perform the remaining steps. As a last resort, the role play may be enacted in the area where the reluctant client is seated if moving into the "spotlight" is too anxiety provoking.

Noncompliance with Homework

There are a variety of reasons that homework may not be completed. Most individuals are simply not used to completing assignments outside the treatment setting and need time to establish a routine for incorporating homework into their lives. When homework has not been completed, the leaders should obtain feedback to try to identify obstacles to its completion. If necessary, homework assignments should be simplified. It is important that early assignments be simple enough to ensure a high likelihood of successful completion. Community supports, which may be very helpful in assisting clients with assignments, should be encouraged to provide immediate reinforcement when homework is completed.

The leaders may need to help clients plan when, where, and with whom homework assignments will be completed. Clients with memory deficits, who may not complete their homework because they have forgotten the instructions, should be instructed to write down assignments. If possible, homework assignments may be done during the group session to demonstrate that they can be completed. For example, if a client in a relapse prevention group has not completed the assignment of rating warning signs on a daily basis, the leaders should help the client perform the rating in the session. It is particularly important when individuals have struggled with homework that the leaders praise even minor efforts at completing assignments.

Disruptive Behavior

Leaders should be prepared to handle disruptive behavior produced by a variety of problems, such as medication side effects, positive symptoms, and thought disorder. A relatively common side effect of antipsychotic medications, akathisia, is manifested by an inner restlessness that causes many individuals to rock, fidget, or even pace. Clients who experience this side effect may benefit from instruction in simple relaxation techniques, such as deep breathing exercises, that may be quietly used in the context of a group session. Drowsiness is another common side effect of antipsychotic and other psychotropic medications. Many of the strategies designed to address distractibility and inattentiveness, such as asking frequent questions and rewarding behaviors (e.g., good eye contact, appropriate responses to questions, or comments reflecting accurate tracking of the group topic), may also help maintain wakefulness.

Clients who are experiencing auditory hallucinations may respond audibly to their inner voices, which can be disruptive to other group members. The leader who is not responsible for the primary teaching may approach such individuals and encourage them to try to remain focused on the group task. Problems with responding to internal stimuli tend to decrease as clients become familiar with the structure of the SST group. Perseveration on a thought or idea is commonly observed among individuals with thought disorders, who may have difficulty shifting to a new topic or ignoring personal concerns that preoccupy their thoughts. Leaders should expect to encounter unrelated comments or perseverations that threaten to derail the work of the group. When this happens, the leaders should immediately redirect clients to the group task (e.g., "Let's try to stay focused on what we were doing, which was _____"). If clients do not respond to redirection but continue to elaborate on their unrelated thoughts or concerns, the leaders should politely suggest that the issue be discussed after the group has concluded (e.g., "That's a very interesting point you are making, but let's wait to talk about that until the end of class. Right now we need to keep working on _____"). If these attempts at redirection for responding to voices or making unrelated statements are still unsuccessful, one of the leaders may ask the disruptive clients to take a short break or to excuse themselves from the remainder of the group for the day, making sure to invite them to return to the next meeting. In rare instances, for example, if symptoms substantially worsen, a client's participation in the group may need to be terminated completely, until a subsequent iteration of the treatment is offered. Decisions involving removals from the group should only be made when the disruptive behavior makes it impossible for other clients to learn or for the leaders to teach.

Lack of Investment in Social Skills Training

Leaders should be aware that clients sometimes reject the notion that SST is warranted, particularly when they are included in groups with much lower functioning clients. They may feel they are faring quite well in comparison with other clients and may lack insight about their own deficits. Or they may not see the connection between their problems and social skills deficits. Sometimes individuals who reject SST because they do not wish to be reminded of their mental illness make critical or sarcastic comments to register their displeasure, attempt to engage the trainer in prolonged conversation about unrelated topics, or otherwise disrupt the group. Some clients object to the teaching techniques, complaining that the frequent repetition of information and simple questions designed to check comprehension feel patronizing.

There are several ways to handle sarcastic comments or complaints that result from a lack of investment in SST. Most importantly, confrontation should be avoided. Some clients find it more palatable to refer to the SST intervention as a "course" or "class" rather than a "group," because the learning rather than the therapy component is emphasized. Group leaders may liken practice in SST to playing a musical instrument; particularly, the fact that easy pieces must be learned before more complex pieces, and the same pieces must be played repeatedly to achieve mastery (Bellack et al., 1997). Reminders to clients regarding the value of what is being taught in terms of achieving important life goals may help focus their attention on desired outcomes.

Higher functioning clients who complain about being grouped with lower functioning clients may be encouraged to assist them with group tasks or be asked to serve as confederates in role plays as a way of increasing their sense of responsibility. Or they may be invited to serve as "consultants" who provide periodic and regular feedback about the process and progress of the group. This feedback should be received outside the context of the group. Increasing the difficulty and complexity of homework and role plays may also make higher functioning clients feel more challenged. Given adequate numbers of clients and trainers, subgroups of higher and lower functioning clients should be created, so that pacing of learning may be appropriately adjusted.

EMPIRICAL SUPPORT FOR SOCIAL SKILLS TRAINING

Controlled research on SST has provided ample evidence that it is effective in improving the skills targeted by the training and, to a large extent, social adjustment and functioning in general (Chambon & Marie-Cardine, 1998; Dilk & Bond, 1996; Eckman et al., 1992; Heinssen et al., 2000; Liberman et al., 1992, 1998; Mueser & Bond, 2000; Wallace, Liberman, MacKain, Blackwell, & Eckman, 1992). A recent review of the SST literature reported that individuals with schizophrenia are capable of learning both simple and complex social behaviors (Heinssen et al., 2000). Evidence for the durability of the knowledge and skills learned as part of SST has been provided by numerous studies demonstrating retention of learning as long as 1 year after conclusion of active treatment (Chambon & Marie-Cardine, 1998; Eckman et al., 1992; Liberman et al., 1992; Marder et al., 1996; Penn & Mueser, 1996; Wallace et al., 1992).

SST has produced particularly robust effects when delivered in combination with prompt response (in the form of medication supplementation) to early warning signs of relapse (Marder et al., 1996). Not surprisingly, the most substantial gains have been obtained when specific behavioral measures that resemble training activities have been used to measure outcome (Benton & Schroeder, 1990). In spite of demonstrated improvements in performance of specific behaviors and overall social adjustment, SST has exerted little direct impact on level of psychopathology or relapse rates (Liberman et al., 1998; Mueser & Bond, 2000; Penn & Mueser, 1996). Successful SST may, however, play a protective role when relapse is stress-related given that it can help individuals feel more assertive and less socially anxious (Heinssen et al., 2000).

SST has been administered to thousands of individuals with schizophrenia in the United States and in several foreign countries, including Great Britain, Germany, France, Italy, and Poland. Positive effects of SST have been observed among relatively stable outpatients, persistently psychotic outpatients, and even acutely ill inpatients (Heinssen et al., 2000). High levels of positive and/or negative symptoms have not represented barriers to skills acquisition (Eckman et al., 1992; Marder et al., 1996; Smith et al., 1996). Kopelowicz, Liberman, Mintz, and Zarate (1997) found that presence of the deficit syndrome (a subtype of negative symptoms that is primary, enduring, and prominent) seemed to interfere with skills acquisition. However, cognitive deficits, which are often associated with the deficit syndrome and may have been responsible for this result, may be responsive to alterations in teaching techniques (Heinssen et al., 2000).

Differential response to SST based on demographic characteristics such as gender, age, and ethnicity has not been systematically evaluated with the exception of two studies, which found that males acquired more social skills than females (Mueser, Levine, Bellack, Douglas, & Brady, 1990; Schaub, Behrendt, Brenner, Mueser, & Liberman, 1998). This is interesting considering evidence that females with schizophrenia generally tend to demonstrate better baseline levels of social skills than males (Mueser, Blanchard, & Bellack, 1995). Descriptive analyses of differential response based on severity of symptoms have been conducted, with general consensus that symptom level is not a significant predictor of skills acquisition. Another case of differential response that has emerged from several studies is the difference in learning of skills depending on degree of cognitive impairment (Kern, Green, & Satz, 1992; Mueser et al., 1991; Silverstein, Schenkel, Valone, & Nuernberger, 1998; Smith, Hull, Romanelli, Fertuck, & Weiss, 1999). Specifically, thought disorder, distractibility, pretreatment attention, and memory deficits have been predictive of skills acquisition or maintenance (Heinssen et al., 2000; Mueser, Kosmidis, & Sayers, 1992; Smith et al., 1996). Based on these findings, the role of cognition in learning, and the prevalence of cognitive deficits in individuals with schizophrenia, SST programs have increasingly focused on addressing both the cognitive impairments and behavioral deficits characteristic of many individuals with schizophrenia (Cook, Pickett, Fitzgibbon, Jonikas, & Cohler, 1996).

Early reviews of controlled studies of SST consistently identified limited generalization of skills as a shortcoming of the approach (Benton & Schroeder, 1990). More recent reviews of the SST literature suggest that some generalization does occur across settings and situations in which trained skills may be applied (Chambon & Marie-Cardine, 1998; Dilk & Bond, 1996; Glynn et al., 2001; Liberman et al., 1998; Smith et al., 1996), particularly when direct strategies designed to improve generalization (e.g., inclusion of community supports) have been included as part of the intervention, and when training has targeted narrowly defined behaviors (Tauber, Wallace, & Lecompte, 2000). It is likely that when generalization has not occurred, it has been due to a lack of positive reinforcement for performance of skills in other settings, or lack of opportunity to demonstrate and thus practice skills learned in SST (Liberman et al., 1998). For example, an individual with schizophrenia who lives alone and has few social contacts due to negative symptoms of apathy, alogia, and anhedonia will likely have little opportunity to practice or receive positive reinforcement for newly learned basic conversation skills.

A review of the literature by Heinssen and colleagues (2000) revealed the following recent developments in the SST approach: (1) greater individualization of training for treatment refractory patients; (2) greater use of contingent reinforcement and shaping procedures to improve acquisition of skills; (3) greater use of strategies designed to account for cognitive impairments that may interfere with learning; (4) inclusion of specific strategies to facilitate generalization of skills across settings and situations; (5) use of techniques to enhance compliance; (6) efforts to target motivation and investment in change; and (7) use of trained paraprofessionals to lead groups. Based on their review, the authors proposed a model of "prescriptive" skills training in which individuals would be matched to treatment based on characteristics such as phase of illness, cognitive processing capability, and receptivity to change. They urged designers of new SST programs to include mechanisms for augmenting the standard teaching techniques to address individual deficits and needs, including, especially, cognitive deficits. They also suggested that the clinical effectiveness of SST might be enhanced if training were administered in the setting in which the skills were to be used, and recommended that future programs include more *in vivo* training and greater involvement of indigenous community supports to act as reinforcing agents.

CASE EXAMPLE

A case example is provided to illustrate the implementation of SST.

Mr. B, a 48-year-old male, was first diagnosed with schizophrenia at age 23, after obtaining a bachelor's degree in physics at the state university. Mr. B had no notable psychiatric problems or functional impairments until the onset of the illness, which was acute and insidious. Although Haldol produced substantial symptomatic relief, the uncomfortable side effects of the medication caused Mr. B to discontinue treatment repeatedly, resulting in almost yearly hospitalizations until Risperdal was started 5 years ago. Since that time, Mr. B has resided in a group home and has required only one brief inpatient stay at the state psychiatric hospital. Mr. B recently moved so that he could live closer to his parents, who are elderly. He scheduled an intake to initiate treatment at the local mental health center in his new community.

The extensive intake interview included many questions about Mr. B's history of psychosocial functioning. The clinician who conducted the interview asked about achievement of developmental milestones, academic performance, adjustment at school, transition to young adulthood and college, friendships and dating, interpersonal functioning, and work history. The Social Adjustment Scale–II (Schooler et al., 1979) was used to evaluate current instrumental role functioning, performance of household chores, ability to manage money, relationships with immediate and extended family members, use of leisure time, friendships and dating, and overall personal well-being. Friendships and dating, relationships with family members, paid work, and use of leisure time were identified as areas in which functioning was marginal. Mr. B's parents were invited to the mental health center for an interview to furnish more detailed information about the history of their son's functional impairments.

After administration of the family version of the Social Adjustment Scale–II, the treatment team learned that Mr. B had lost all of the friendships he had before his first hospitalization. Although he had made some friends during the course of his many hospitalizations, the negative symptoms of schizophrenia, including social withdrawal, anhedonia, and apathy, had steadily increased over the past several years, leading to a solitary lifestyle that included contact only with his parents and the treatment team at the local community mental health center. Mr. B occasionally worked part-time, with his longest tenure (2 months) at his most recent job cleaning bathrooms at local fast-food restaurants.

Observation of Mr. B's behavior during initial interviews with his new case manager, psychiatrist, and therapist pointed to a major deficit in basic communication skills as a potential underlying cause for his deficient psychosocial functioning. Mr. B's performance on the Role Play Task (Sayers et al., 1995) confirmed not only a deficit in communication skills but also difficulty with negotiation and compromise. Additional role plays designed to evaluate even more elementary social skills revealed Mr. B's difficulty expressing negative emotions, listening to others, and making requests.

In addition to pharmacotherapy, case management, and work with a vocational specialist, Mr. B was invited to take advantage of the SST program offered at the mental health center, taught by trained clinicians from a variety of disciplines, including psychology, social work, and occupational therapy. Most used materials from commercially available SST packages adapted to accommodate the population of clients served by the mental health center. All were offered as twice weekly courses lasting from 2–6 months. Mr. B initially received training in basic social skills, such as expressing positive and negative feelings, listening to others, and perceiving social cues. Based on his performance in final role plays, he was referred to the first level of a basic conversations course and a recreation for leisure course.

Mr. B was frequently absent from his groups and infrequently completed homework assignments. A residential counselor from his group home was invited to serve as a support in the community who could encourage attendance and facilitate use of skills learned in the SST courses. She agreed to observe one of the group sessions and meet with the group leader to learn about the principles from social learning theory and behavior modification on which the groups were based. Her participation produced a notable improvement in Mr. B's attendance and completion of homework assignments. After 1 year of SST, Mr. B's psychosocial functioning was reassessed using the Role Play Task; interviews with Mr. B, his parents, his residential counselor, and his case manager; and administration of the patient and family versions of the Social Adjustment Scale–II. Improvements were noted in the quality of his interpersonal relationships and his abilities to listen, start conversations, express positive and negative feelings, and make requests. Given that Mr. B continued to demonstrate impairments in more complex social skills, such as negotiation and compromise, job seeking, and friendship and dating, the treatment team recommended continued SST, with yearly reassessment of skills.

CONCLUSION

Although SST has clearly been demonstrated to be a useful mode of improving social functioning, it should not be viewed as a stand-alone treatment. The ability of antipsychotic medications to control the positive symptoms of schizophrenia continues to make psychopharmacology a crucial aspect of the overall approach to treating the illness. However, SST should be regarded as an essential component in a comprehensive behavioral approach to treating the symptoms and associated impairments of schizophrenia (Heinssen et al., 2000). Widespread inclusion of such an approach in customary care will require a greater partnership between psychiatry and psychosocial rehabilitation (Cook et al., 1996). The future success of SST also depends on commitment to an overarching model of treatment that emphasizes active, directive, positive rehabilitation of disabilities; a dedication of resources required to train group leaders; and involvement of partners in the community (e.g., case managers, family members, or residential counselors) to encourage and reinforce use of skills. When combined with ongoing monitoring of symptoms, assertive community treatment, and responsive psychopharmacology, SST promotes positive social functioning by providing individuals with the tools to negotiate and advocate for themselves, to confront situations that require information processing and decision making, and to maintain interpersonal relationships that can serve as important sources of psychosocial support.

REFERENCES

Amador, X., Strauss, D., Yale, S., & Gorman, J. M. (1991). Awareness of illness in schizophrenia. *Schizophrenia Bulletin, 17*, 113–132.

Bandura, A. (1969). *Principles of behavior modification.* New York: Holt, Rinehart & Winston.

Bandura, A. (1977). Self-efficacy: Toward a unifying theory of behavioral change. *Psychological Review, 84*, 191–215.

Bellack, A. S., Mueser, K. T., Gingerich, S., & Agresta, J. (1997). *Social skills training for schizophrenia: A step-by-step guide.* New York: Guilford Press.

Bellack, A. S., Sayers, M., Mueser, K. T., & Bennett, M. (1994). Evaluation of social problem solving in schizophrenia. *Journal of Abnormal Psychology, 103*, 371–378.

Benton, M. K., & Schroeder, H. E. (1990). Social skills training with schizophrenics: A meta-analytic evaluation. *Journal of Consulting and Clinical Psychology, 58*, 741–747.

Birchwood, M., Smith, J., Cochrane, R., Wetton, S., & Copestake, S. (1990). The Social Functioning Scale: The development and validation of a new scale of social adjustment for use in family intervention programmes with schizophrenic patients. *British Journal of Psychiatry, 157*, 853–859.

Brenner, H. D., Roder, V., Hodel, B., Kienzle, N., Reed, D., & Liberman, R. P. (1994). *Integrated psychological therapy for schizophrenic patients (IPT).* Seattle, WA: Hogrefe & Huber.

Chambon, O., & Marie-Cardine, M. (1998). An evaluation of social skills training modules with schizophrenia inpatients in France. *International Review of Psychiatry, 10*, 26–29.

Cook, J. A., Pickett, S. A., Fitzgibbon, G., Jonikas, J. A., & Cohler, J. J. (1996). Rehabilitation services for persons with schizophrenia. *Psychiatric Annals, 26*, 97–104.

Dilk, M. N., & Bond, G. R. (1996). Meta-analytic evaluation of skills training research for individuals with severe mental illness. *Journal of Consulting and Clinical Psychology, 64*, 337–346.

Douglas, M. S., & Mueser, K. T. (1990). Teaching conflict resolution skills to the chronically mentally ill: Social skills training groups for briefly hospitalized patients. *Behavior Modification, 14*, 518–547.

Eckman, T. A., Wirshing, W. C., Marder, S. R., Liberman, R. P., Johnston-Cronk, K., Zimmerman, K., & Mintz, J. (1992). Technique for training schizophrenic patients in illness self-management: A controlled trial. *American Journal of Psychiatry, 149*, 1549–1555.

Glynn, S. M., Marder, S. R., Liberman, R. P., Blair, K., Wirshing, W. C., Wirsching, D. A., & Ross, D. (2001). Supplementing clinic based skills training for schizophrenia with manualized community: Nine month follow-up effects on social adjustment. *Schizophrenia Research, 49* (Suppl.), 261.

Green, M. F. (1996). What are the functional consequences of neurocognitive deficits in schizophrenia? *American Journal of Psychiatry, 153*, 321–330.

Green, M. F., Kern, R. S., Braff, D. L., & Mintz, J. (2000). Neurocognitive deficits and functional outcome in schizophrenia: Are we measuring the "right stuff"? *Schizophrenia Bulletin, 26,* 119–136.

Harvey, P. D., Davidson, M., Mueser, K. T., Parrella, M., White, L., & Powchik, P. (1997). Social-Adaptive Functioning Evaluation (SAFE): A rating scale for geriatric psychiatric patients. *Schizophrenia Bulletin, 23,* 131–145.

Heinssen, R. K., Liberman, R. P., & Kopelowicz, A. (2000). Psychosocial skills training for schizophrenia: Lessons from the laboratory. *Schizophrenia Bulletin, 26,* 21–46.

Herz, M. I. (1996). Psychosocial treatment. *Psychiatric Annals, 26,* 531–535.

Johnstone, E. C., MacMillan, J. F., Frith, C. D., Benn, D. K., & Crow, T. J. (1990). Further investigation of the predictors of outcome following first schizophrenic episodes. *British Journal of Psychiatry, 157,* 182–189.

Katz, M. M., & Lyerly, S. B. (1963). Methods for measuring adjustment and social behavior in the community: 1. Rationale, description, descriminative validity and scale development. *Psychological Reports, 13,* 503–535.

Kern, R. S., Green, M. F., & Satz, P. (1992). Neuropsychological predictors of skills training for chronic psychiatric patients. *Psychiatry Research, 43,* 223–230.

Kopelowicz, A., Liberman, R. P., Mintz, J., & Zarate, R. (1997). Comparison of efficacy of social skills training for deficit and nondeficit negative symptoms in schizophrenia. *American Journal of Psychiatry, 154,* 424–425.

Liberman, R. P. (1998). International perspectives on skills training for the mentally disabled. *International Review of Psychiatry, 10,* 5–8.

Liberman, R. P., DeRisi, W. J., & Mueser, K. T. (1989). *Social skills training for psychiatric patients.* New York: Pergamon Press.

Liberman, R. P., Mueser, K., Wallace, C. J., Jacobs, H. E., Eckman, T., & Massel, H. K. (1986). Training skills in the psychiatrically disabled: Learning coping and competence. *Schizophrenia Bulletin, 12,* 631–647.

Liberman, R. P., Wallace, C. J., Blackwell, G., Kopelowicz, A., Vaccaro, J. V., & Mintz, J. (1998). Skills training versus psychosocial occupational therapy for persons with persistent schizophrenia. *American Journal of Psychiatry, 155,* 1087–1091.

Liberman, R. P., Wallace, C. J., Blackwell, G., MacKain, S., & Eckman, T. A. (1992). Training social and independent living skills: Applications and impact in chronic schizophrenia. In J. Cottraux, P. Legeron, & E. Mollard (Eds.), *Which psychotherapies in year 2000?* (pp. 65–90). Amsterdam: Swets & Zeitlinger.

Marder, S. R., Wirshing, W. C., Mintz, J., McKenzie, J., Johnston, K., Eckman, T. A., Lebell, M., Zimmerman, K., & Liberman, R. P. (1996). Two-year outcome of social skills training and group psychotherapy for outpatients with schizophrenia. *American Journal of Psychiatry, 153,* 1585–1592.

Martin, G., & Pear, J. (1996). *Behavior modification: What it is and how to do it* (5th ed.). Upper Saddle River, NJ: Prentice-Hall.

Matousek, N., Edwards, J., Jackson, H. J., Rudd, R. P., & McMurry, N. E. (1992). Social skills training and negative symptoms. *Behavior Modification, 16,* 39–63.

McEvoy, J. P., Hartman, M., Gottlieb, D., Godwin, S., Apperson, L. J., & Wilson, W. (1996). Common sense, insight, and neuropsychological test performance in schizophrenia patients. *Schizophrenia Bulletin, 22,* 635–641.

Mueser, K. T. (1998). Social skill and problem solving. In A. S. Bellack & M. Hersen (Eds.), *Comprehensive clinical psychology* (Vol. 6, pp. 183–201). New York: Pergamon Press.

Mueser, K. T., & Bellack, A. S. (1998). Social skills and social functioning. In K. T. Mueser & N. Tarrier (Eds.), *Handbook of social functioning in schizophrenia* (pp. 79–98). Boston: Allyn & Bacon.

Mueser, K. T., Bellack, A. S., Douglas, M. S., & Wade, J. H. (1991). Prediction of social skill acquisition in schizophrenic and major affective disorder patients from memory and symptomatology. *Psychiatry Research, 37,* 281–296.

Mueser, K. T., Bellack, A. S., Morrison, R. L., & Wixted, J. T. (1990). Social competence in schizophrenia: Premorbid adjustment, social skill, and domains of functioning. *Journal of Psychiatric Research, 24,* 51–63.

Mueser, K. T., Blanchard, J. J., & Bellack, A. S. (1995). Memory and social skill in schizophrenia: The role of gender. *Psychiatry Research, 57,* 141–153.

Mueser, K. T., & Bond, G. R. (2000). Psychosocial treatment approaches for schizophrenia. *Current Opinion in Psychiatry, 13,* 27–35.

Mueser, K. T., Doonan, R., Penn, D. L., Blanchard, J. J., Bellack, A. S., Nishith, P., & DeLeon, J. (1996). Emotion recognition and social competence in chronic schizophrenia. *Journal of Abnormal Psychology, 105,* 271–275.

Mueser, K. T., Kosmidis, M. H., & Sayers, M. D. (1992). Symptomatology and the prediction of social skills acquisition in schizophrenia. *Schizophrenia Research, 8,* 59–68.

Mueser, K. T., Levine, S., Bellack, A. S., Douglas, M. S., & Brady, E. U. (1990). Social skills training for acute psychiatric patients. *Hospital and Community Psychiatry, 41,* 1249–1251.

Mueser, K. T., & Sayers, M. D. (1992). Social skills assessment. In D. J. Kavanagh (Ed.), *Schizophrenia: An overview and practical handbook* (pp. 182–205). New York: Chapman & Hall.

Penn, D. L., & Mueser, K. T. (1996). Research update on the psychosocial treatment of schizophrenia. *American Journal of Psychiatry, 153,* 607–617.

Penn, D. L., Mueser, K. T., Spaulding, W., Hope, D. A., & Reed, D. (1995). Information processing and social competence in chronic schizophrenia. *Schizophrenia Bulletin, 21,* 269–281.

Perlick, D. Stastny, P., Mattis, S., & Teresi, J. (1992). Contribution of family, cognitive, and clinical dimensions to long-term outcome in schizophrenia. *Schizophrenia Research, 6,* 257–265.

Rosen, A., Hadzi-Pavlovic, D., & Parker, G. (1989). The Life Skills Profile: A measure assessing function and disability in schizophrenia. *Schizophrenia Bulletin, 15,* 325–337.

Sayers, M. D., Bellack, A. S., Wade, J. H., Bennett, M. E., & Fong, P. (1995). An empirical method for assessing social problem solving in schizophrenia. *Behavior Modification, 19,* 267–289.

Schaub, A., Behrendt, B., & Brenner, H. D. (1998). A multi-hospital evaluation of the Medication and Symptom Management Modules in Germany and Switzerland. *International Review of Psychiatry, 10,* 42–46.

Schaub, A., Behrendt, B., Brenner, H. D., Mueser, K. T., & Liberman, R. P. (1998). Training schizophrenic patients to manage their symptoms: Predictors of treatment response to the German Version of the Symptom Management Module. *Schizophrenia Research, 31,* 121–130.

Schooler, N., Hogarty, G., & Weissman, M. (1979). Social Adjustment Scale II (SAS-II). In W. A. Hargreaves, C. C. Atkisson, & J. E. Sorenson (Eds.), *Resource materials for community mental health program evaluations* (DHEW Publication No. [ADM] 79–328, pp. 290–303). Rockville, MD: National Institute of Mental Health.

Scott, J. E., & Lehman, A. F. (1998). Social functioning in the community. In K. T. Mueser & N. Tarrier (Eds.), *Handbook of social functioning in schizophrenia* (pp. 1–19). Boston: Allyn & Bacon.

Silverstein, S. M., Schenkel, L. S., Valone, C., & Nuernberger, S. W. (1998). Cognitive deficits and psychiatric rehabilitation outcomes in schizophrenia. *Psychiatric Quarterly, 69,* 169–191.

Skinner, B. F. (1953). *Science and human behavior.* New York: Macmillan.

Smith, T. E., Bellack, A. S., & Liberman, R. P. (1996). Social skills training for schizophrenia: Review and future directions. *Clinical Psychology Review, 16,* 599–617.

Smith, T. E., Hull, J. W., Romanelli, S., Fertuck, E., & Weiss, K. A. (1999). Symptoms and neurocognition as rate limiters in skills training for psychotic patients. *American Journal of Psychiatry, 156,* 1817–1818.

Spaulding, W. D., Reed, D., Sullivan, M., Richardson, C., & Weiler, M. (1999). Effects of cognitive treatment in psychiatric rehabilitation. *Schizophrenia Bulletin, 25,* 657–676.

Sullivan, G., Marder, S. R., Liberman, R. P., Donahoe, C. P., & Mintz, J. (1990). Social skills and relapse history in outpatient schizophrenics. *Psychiatry, 53,* 340–345.

Tauber, R., Wallace, C. J., & Lecompte, T. (2000). Enlisting indigenous community supporters in skills training programs for persons with severe mental illness. *Psychiatric Services, 51,* 1428–1432.

Wallace, C. J., Liberman, R. P., MacKain, S. J., Blackwell, G., & Eckman, T. A. (1992). Effectiveness and replicability of modules for teaching social and instrumental skills to the severely mentally ill. *American Journal of Psychiatry, 149*, 654–658.

Wallace, C. J., Liberman, R. P., Tauber, R., & Wallace, J. (2000). The Independent Living Skills Survey: A comprehensive measure of the community functioning of severely and persistently mentally ill individuals. *Schizophrenia Bulletin, 26*, 631–658.

Wykes, T., & Sturt, E. (1986). The measurement of social behaviour in psychiatric patients: An assessment of the reliability and validity of the S.S. schedule. *British Journal of Psychiatry, 148*, 1–11.

Zubin, J., & Spring, B. (1977). Vulnerability: A new view of schizophrenia. *Journal of Abnormal Psychology, 86*, 103–126.

3

Personal Therapy

A Practical Psychotherapy for the Stabilization of Schizophrenia

Gerard E. Hogarty

While psychotherapy continues to be the "cornerstone" of nonsomatic treatment for schizophrenia, little data had supported its efficacy until recently (Fenton, 2000). Decades of negative findings had in fact led to a recommended "moratorium" on dynamic forms of therapy (Mueser & Berenbaum, 1990), variously described as investigative, uncovering, analytical, or insight-oriented in nature. However, these uninspiring results could often be traced to various problems in the design of psychotherapy studies rather than to a lack of efficacy. Problems included the choice of controls, high attrition, therapist experience, equivocal diagnoses, small samples, a failure to access entitlements or control for medication, and more importantly, the conceptual relevance of the studied therapy to schizophrenia. Forms of brief therapy for an often chronic illness had tended to focus on the "crisis of the day" that typically characterized the early stages of recovery from an episode but were less relevant to the resumption of life roles.

In the modern era of psychopharmacology, only social skills training and a version of cognitive-behavioral therapy for schizophrenia have held evidence-based credibility as individual psychosocial approaches for the patient with schizophrenia. While the advantages of these interventions are well described elsewhere in this volume, they tend by design to be problem-focused, usually on specific social deficits in the case of social skills training, or on medication refractory symptoms in the practice of cognitive-behavioral therapy. The patient populations most often targeted have been more seriously impaired, if not hospitalized. In all but a few studies, treatment exposure has been 9 months or less. Personal therapy (PT) incorporates selected social skills training techniques that were found useful in an earlier study (Hogarty et al., 1986), but it has had little success with patients who remain medication refractory, thus indicating an important, abiding role for cognitive-behavioral therapy. Today, the newer, atypical antipsychotic medications allow a majority of patients to achieve a better remission of positive symptoms than earlier medications. The need to maintain clinical stability, accomplish important life goals, and develop a management mastery of one's illness would likely fall to a longer term psychotherapeutic approach that could accommodate the spectrum of residual psychological, social, and neurobiological constraints imposed by schizophrenia.

In response to these issues, PT was conceived as a disorder-relevant intervention and tested between 1986 and 1995 in two, long-term (3-year) controlled trials involving 97 patients who lived with family, and 54 patients who lived on their own. Relapse was reduced to its practical limits among patients who lived with their families (13% relapsed on PT alone over 3 years), and the social adjustment of both PT cohorts greatly surpassed those of our previously tested interventions, including our popular family psychoeducation approach (Hogarty, Greenwald, et al., 1997; Hogarty, Kornblith, et al., 1997). In the era of managed care and decreasing lengths of hospitalization for acute exacerbations of symptoms, the need for a more efficacious, comprehensive, and durable approach to the maintenance of clinical stability and recovery of interpersonal and instrumental role performance was addressed by PT.

OVERVIEW

PT seeks to achieve and maintain clinical stability using both appropriate pharmacotherapy and incremental acquisition of adaptive, self-regulating strategies. The latter are designed to counter the stress-induced, affective dysregulation that frequently precipitates an episode of psychosis. Given the well-established vulnerability of patients with schizophrenia to environmental stress, PT is intended to be applied in three distinct phases that accommodate the various stages of clinical recovery and reintegration following a psychotic episode. It is a collaborative intervention that utilizes the patient's own self-protective strategies, as well as a repertoire of well-tested techniques for prodromal management and the mastery of environmental stress.

In this brief chapter, only a summation of PT practice principles will be possible; the working manual itself is provided elsewhere (Hogarty, in press). The clinician will find that the manual is not a "cookbook" of clinical recipes that narrowly focus on a specific problem. Rather, it offers a number of flexible clinical approaches to the multiple problems that inevitably characterize individual patients. Patients learn to gain control over their schizophrenia and improve their quality of life in the context of potentially provocative interpersonal and vocational environments. When a patient appears not to profit from a specific technique, the systemic nature of PT offers a range of options within and across the three treatment phases that help to counter the therapeutic stalemate. In the following pages, I focus on describing the core principles themselves as they evolve across the various phases rather than a serial description of each PT phase, as is offered in the manual. With this change of emphasis, I hope the incremental nature of the core strategies can become better appreciated as a seamless set of exercises that accommodate patients' clinical state, strengths, and vulnerabilities as they recover from an episode and seek to maintain stability. Case material is not presented for many reasons, including the issues of confidentiality and the need to avoid inappropriate expectations for recovery (see Hogarty, in press, Chap. 1).

PREPARING FOR PERSONAL THERAPY

PT proceeds on the assumption that no psychosocial treatment can attain optimal efficacy unless the fundamentals of good care are firmly established. Foremost is the need for a very effective psychopharmacological regimen. While seemingly self-evident, no more than 29% of patients with schizophrenia are believed to be appropriately medicated (Lehman & Steinwachs, 1998). It has been my experience that many providers have an inappropriately high threshold for persistent symptoms. As PT and my former studies have shown, a high-contact, flexible, and persistent approach to medication management can achieve an optimal remission of symptoms for the vast majority of patients (Hogarty, in press). PT does not presume to address the cognitive or affective problems that are more appropriately and effectively managed with medication. Contemporary "atypical" antipsychotic medications now provide a better foundation for an optimal psychosocial treatment response. These medications, for example, rarely disable patients with extrapyramidal symptoms (particularly an assault on affect and volition), most often preclude the need for antiparkinsonian medications, thus minimizing the well-known anticholinergic effect on short-term verbal memory, and generally manifest a better therapeutic profile across cognitive and affective symptoms.

In the context of rational pharmacotherapy, PT also relies on the established principles of psychological and material support. The former permeate each PT session and include attending to, observing, listening, and responding to the patient's personal accounts and descriptions of subjective state; a correct empathy; and the reinforcement, as well as encouragement, of the patient's own health-promoting efforts. The theoretical basis of this support is more interpersonal than intrapsychic or interpretive. Perhaps more troublesome to providers who remain ambivalent about the potential for dependency, PT nevertheless assumes an active role in assisting patients to access entitlement benefits for which they are eligible, primarily those administered by the Social Security Administration (Social Security disability insurance and supplemental security income) or the public welfare department. Otherwise, the case-management component of PT extends to facilitating the acquisition of needed (public) health insurance for the patient, supported housing, when indicated, and, as recovery improves, supported education and/or employment opportunities that are often administered through local rehabilitation agencies. The need to engage essential human services is paramount for patients who no longer have the support or resources of an available family. In fact, initiating the learning-based strategies of PT among such patients before residential stability, food, and clothing are secure has been shown to increase relapse in this vulnerable group of patients (Hogarty, Kornblith, et al., 1997), as I discuss later. The fundamentals of medication management, as well as psychological and material support, are described in detail in the working manual (Hogarty, in press, Chap. 3).

Insights gained from our study of *integrated* medication and psychosocial treatment over the previous 25 years also served to guide the application of PT. Among the more relevant insights was the reality that patients who suffered a relapse but were unequivocally faithful in taking medication almost always had experienced a severe and independent life event—an observation that held clear potential for prevention. Similarly, patients who remained withdrawn, disorganized, overly aroused, or who had little insight, could easily become dysregulated by a prematurely ambitious treatment plan. Otherwise, minor exacerbations could often be traced to environmental stress that could be negotiated by the therapist, rather than embark on a *permanent* increase in medication dose or type. (Often a *short-term* supplemental dose is helpful while attempts at environmental manipulation are being made.) It was also found that coping and other learned strategies should be introduced *slowly*, following the achievement of a stable dose of medication. The resolution of psychotic symptoms takes time, and patients often pass through months of inactivity, amotivation, and increased sleep before finding the energy to take on initiatives that could improve their quality of life. Once the treatment plan was initiated, we learned that one change at a time was also crucial. If a stable patient were beginning a job, finding a new residence, reestablishing or forming a new relationship, for example, this was not the time to change the medication dosage or try a new medication. (If the patient were to decompensate, one would never know what the precipitant might have been in the face of multiple changes.)

Regarding noncompliance, we also observed that patients should not be misled by the apparent "improvement" that follows discontinuation of antipsychotic medication. Side-effect reduction is most responsible for the increased feelings of well-being. Depolarization or receptor blockade can continue for days or weeks, depending on the medication, and when symptoms eventually reappear, the relationship between noncompliance and relapse is often lost on the patient. Most important, low dose does not mean "no dose." Many patients do well on a low doses of certain antipsychotic medications (such as the typical neuroleptic medications), but the majority of these better functioning patients will quickly decompensate if medication is discontinued (Hogarty, Ulrich, & Mussare, 1976). Once patients functionally recover, they might not need the intensity of weekly or biweekly sessions, but they do need the "safety net" of regular, often monthly, checkups. Booster sessions of the preferred psychosocial treatment are particularly necessary for stable patients, since these patients are most likely to initiate attempts to acquire or enhance social and vocational roles. While the interests and priorities of nonphysician therapists might understandably be focused on psychosocial issues, they need always to remain sensitive to potential medication problems as well. One cannot become passive about the question of treatment specificity for behavioral problems (i.e., whether the issue is better addressed by medication or psychosocial treatment). Finally, we learned that the therapist must be ever-vigilant about strongly held but potentially false assumptions, including the following incorrect beliefs: Persistent symptoms are an inevitable part of schizophrenia; supplemental medication will not work; one can "predict" how a patient will respond to an untried medication (e.g., with weight gain or other side effects); the diagnosis of early schizophrenia should be avoided (but at the price of mistreatment); one's knowledge of the patient is complete and further information from the patient, family, or a past provider is unnecessary. (Many patients will not spontaneously volunteer information on side effects, subjective state, or interpersonal problems in the absence of regular probing.)

Finally, in preparing for PT, compliance and success will depend a great deal on the strength of the therapeutic alliance. The task can be difficult when the clinician is faced with the fear, anxiety, blame, or denial that often accompany the first episode of schizophrenia, or with the demoralization and despair frequently associated with a recurrence of symptoms. PT strategies and goals can be presented as an opportunity for a more hopeful "new beginning," namely, that life stressors that might lead to a new episode can be identified, reduced, and controlled. In time, the patient's own social and vocational objectives can be increasingly pursued with confidence and safety. The treatment plan represents the blueprint for reaching these objectives and is driven by careful assessment of the patient's needs, strengths, personal goals, and coping strategies (particularly regarding the characteristic prodromes of a new episode), as well as existing supports and liabilities. "Therapy" is described for the patient as a series of progressive steps needed to maintain survival without psychosis; develop awareness and foresight regarding the relationship between relapse and the subjective cues of distress that arise internally or externally; acquire adaptive strategies designed to manage the sources of stress; and gradually resume expressive and instrumental roles. The plan also represents a collaborative agreement to work together to reach these goals. A time frame for treatment is established (e.g., up to 24 months for a symptomatically stable patient, but as long as 3 years for a recently hospitalized patient). Initially, weekly sessions will vary in length from 15 to 45 minutes, depending on the patient's ability to concentrate and tolerate discussions. Once stabilization is secure, sessions are typically reduced to two or three per month. For clinicians who work in mental health systems, PT can be easily integrated into the service mission of their agency. For private practitioners, the PT manual (Hogarty, in press) provides a guideline for working safely and effectively with the patient with schizophrenia.

CORE PRINCIPLES OF PERSONAL THERAPY

Psychoeducation

Likely inspired by the family psychoeducation movement, patient psychoeducation has also become a central component of direct care in recent years (Sullwold & Herrlich, 1992). For many patients, schizophrenia has been little more than a chaotic, frightening, and inexplicable alteration of beliefs, perceptions, and emotions. Education can help to make sense of the psychotic experience and represents the beginning of cognitive mastery over the illness itself. Throughout all phases of PT, education is an integral component of most sessions, the content of which will vary in depth depending on the patient's level of symptom remission and cognitive capacities available to process information. (Attention, memory, and problem-solving deficits have a strong influence on the method and process of applying each PT strategy.)

In the basic phase, which typically occurs in the first 6–9 months following a psychotic episode, a psychoeducation summary can be offered in small groups of 8 to 10 patients, particularly in agency-based practice. This format is not only economically feasible but also serves to establish the expertise of the therapist. Patients have the opportunity for increased peer support as well as interpersonal comfort and often come to appreciate that their own experiences have also been shared by others. Information on the nature of schizophrenia, its subjective and public presentation, the relationship between stress and the prodromes of psychosis, and how medication and psychosocial treatment work together to control symptoms, represent the basic content of this phase. Specific information can be found in the earlier text on family psychoeducation (Anderson, Reiss, & Hogarty, 1986) that has been updated in the PT manual (Hogarty, in press). A greater elaboration of the developmental basis of schizophrenia is offered, including the origins of neuro- *and* social-cognitive deficits. Theories that describe a possible biochemically mediated hypersensitivity to life experiences are reviewed. Information regarding schizophrenia continues to evolve and carries with it the clinician's responsibility to remain familiar with relevant and current literature. However, no matter what information is shared, the metacommunications of the basic phase are constant: (1) Schizophrenia is a no-fault brain disorder and not a willful or learned set of behaviors that imply moral or character failure; (2) schizophrenia has an increasingly clear pathophysiology that has been determined from extensive scientific studies; (3) this pathophysiology leaves the brain exquisitely sensitive (or hyperreactive) to life experiences that need to be wisely negotiated; and (4) greater symptom stability and recovery are increasingly possible as newly developed treatments (both medication and psychosocial forms) more closely reflect this pathophysiology.

Once patients have gained some distance from their acute symptoms, the content of psychoeducation in the intermediate phase (a 9- to 12-month treatment period) begins to tailor broadly the themes of schizophrenia symptoms, vulnerability, and treatment to individual circumstances. The coping strategies that will be learned in the intermediate phase essentially constitute this integrative educational approach. Information is provided in the form of an "overview" of forthcoming PT principles, again using the small-group format, if desired. The content of these themes includes a description of the initial cues of distress that often precede formal prodromes, as well as the associated strategies that can help the patient to control these affective, cognitive, physiological, or behavioral signs of dysregulation. Simple relaxation techniques and social perception training are key strategies to be learned. Emphasis is placed on the more common impairments of schizophrenia and their residual disabilities and social handicaps. A process for accommodating or "accepting" disability is provided, and patients learn that it is possible to pursue forms of remediation and compensation. Psychoeducation also includes a description of the rationales for learning each of the proposed coping strategies.

In the advanced phase (that extends from 9 to 15 months), education moves from broad information regarding schizophrenia, its treatment, and common disabilities and handicaps, to a greater specification of the patient's own residual deficits that might impact upon an optimal resumption of social and vocational roles outside the home. Such deficits frequently include problems with motivation, mental stamina, social comfort, cognitive organization, and information processing. This review serves to guide the timing of new initiatives and temper the expectations for performance held by the patient, significant others, or the therapist. The pattern of the patient's subjective cues of distress related to prior social and vocational roles is reviewed, and reassurance is offered about past and recent success at personal management. Psychoeducation concludes with an overview of the remaining strategies, their rationales, and relevance to the patient that will help him or her to negotiate new excursions into the community (e.g., progressive relaxation, guided imagery, criticism management, and conflict resolution).

Internal Coping

Internal coping is the centerpiece of PT, a process from which most adaptive strategies logically flow. In the basic phase, it attempts historically to draw the association between personally perceived stress and its consequences, particularly the manifestation of prodromal signs of relapse. Patient recognition of early signs and symptoms has a long clinical tradition, but the challenge to apply this awareness autonomously remains formidable. Disorganized or affectively labile patients, for example, will often struggle with the task of conceptually organizing their highly individual response to stress; those with persistent symptoms will require assistance in differentiating the precursors of greater symptom exacerbation from abiding symptoms; and the patient with negative symptoms will often need help in simply articulating a subjective response to stress. Internal coping begins with a determination of the patient's own, often idiosyncratic, definition of stress. Therapy then moves to the identification of the interpersonal contexts and life events that the patient associates with these feelings of distress. Equipped with a knowledge of prior precursors to psychotic episodes (determined during the earlier assessment period), the therapist can now begin to identify these potential prodromes in the context of environmental stress and subjective response. Self-protective strategies used successfully by the patient in the past are identified, and their utility is reinforced.

Capitalizing on the acquired ability to scan broadly for stressful events and their prodromal consequences, internal coping in the intermediate phase moves to an elaboration of what is often a progressive "march of symptoms" that frequently precedes formal prodromal signs or an episode. As medication becomes more fine-tuned and symptoms are better managed, patients come to appreciate that the process typically begins with internal or external stimuli (and arousal), progresses to minor behavioral changes (weak signs), major behavioral changes (strong prodromal signs), minor psychotic exacerbations (symptoms of a miniepisode) and, if unaddressed, to a major psychotic episode (a clear syndrome). Patients are assured that disrupting this process *as early as possible* is at the heart of successful self-management. Even though many clear prodromes and minor exacerbations do *not* lead to a full psychotic episode (perhaps as many as 50%), these symptom experiences can nonetheless destabilize the patient, disrupt the resumption of important roles, and contribute greatly to the demoralization of the patient and loved ones. A formal didactic regarding the emotional, cognitive, behavioral, and physical "early cues of distress" is provided, and, with therapist assistance, patients come to identify their own individual signs. For patients who have difficulty conceptualizing or verbalizing the earliest subjective cues of distress, an extensive list is provided from which they can choose relevant cues (see Hogarty, in press, Chap. 5). The "autoprotective strategies" described in the basic phase are further enhanced to include deep breathing and the simple "relaxation response" of Benson (1996).

In the advanced phase, the appreciation of subjective cues and their signal value and success in achieving personal comfort in the home or clinic are challenged by the need to apply these coping strategies spontaneously in novel and potentially more disruptive community settings. The community becomes something of a laboratory for testing old and new strategies, where more autonomously selected adaptive techniques can be applied. The key to a successful integration of skills and stressful encounters will depend on the patient's developing a sense of behavioral reciprocity (i.e., how one's coping strategies and associated mood and behavior impact upon other people). This "reflective consideration" (Hollis, 1964) is crucial to the patient's ability to interpret correctly the verbal and nonverbal cues that indicate another person's thoughts, feelings, and likely response. Through reflection, patients will often come to appreciate better the positive and negative consequences of their own behavior, and to increasingly ensure the acceptance and approval of others. In the process, they develop a better chance to advance their own self-interests. For those whose symptom stability has been well established, the techniques of deep breathing and simple relaxation can be expanded to include various components of progressive relaxation and guided imagery. The goal, rather than having the patient acquire a rarely used repertoire of relaxation techniques, is to select carefully and tailor one or two strategies that the patient finds meaningful and useful, and then to develop their utility and efficacy.

Social Skills Training

As is the case with most PT strategies, the choice of specific social skills techniques can be highly individualized in deference to the patient's needs, preferences, and ability. For example, many ambulatory patients today do not suffer profound problems with topographical behaviors such as eye contact, speech latency, or other paralinguistic defects. While all will profit from the advanced skills of criticism management and conflict resolution, many will not need or desire the formal induction process that includes modeling, role play, rehearsal, and feedback with a therapist. The basic phase skills training techniques of PT, as mentioned earlier, were preserved from the successful first-year outcomes of our earlier skills training study (Hogarty et al., 1986).

In achieving the basic phase goals of symptom remission and stability, skills training is introduced as a way most easily to negotiate the potential sources of serious environmental provocation frequently found in the immediate or extended family. In the course of discussion about prodromal identification and management, three skills are introduced. The first involves role structuring that typically discourages patients from taking on the challenges of work or school until symptoms are stabilized. If such counsel fails, patients are encouraged to reduce their "social load," such as the number of hours worked, classes taken, or social activities pursued. The second "skill" seeks to modify specific behaviors that provoke negative feedback, such as swearing or playing the television or stereo too loud. Otherwise, patients are simply encouraged to leave tactfully the stressful situations that could prove overwhelming, or that might escalate the stress itself. Third, patients are encouraged to interact more positively with significant others, such as giving compliments, showing concern or interest, and expressing appreciation. These are fundamental skills that often become dormant during a psychotic episode and its aftermath. Such training in negative and positive assertion provides the rationale for maintaining and building other relationships in later phases.

Social skills training in the intermediate phase builds upon the elementary approaches of the basic phase (avoidance and prosocial response) and expands to include social perception skills and a more refined ability to assert oneself in a manner that would decrease potentially distressing interactions. The social skills of the intermediate phase are introduced with the intent of applying them initially in the least conflicted and minimally stressful interpersonal encounters. With success, they ultimately are applied more broadly in confrontational and disruptive interpersonal relationships that often accompany community initiatives. Social perception is presented as a way to take the "emotional temperature" of another person. A schedule to assess the other person's behavioral cues is provided and reviewed. Suggested self-instructions serve to guide the "approachability" of a key person, as well as how to "time" an interaction or make a request.

As mastery improves, skills training in the advanced phase extends to the social and vocational challenges of community life. The more sophisticated skills of criticism management and conflict resolution are introduced. Criticism, for example, is one of the best documented predictors of schizophrenia symptoms (Kavanagh, 1992). Patients are trained to assess and respond to criticism by first estimating the voice tone of the critic, briefly assessing the critic's perspective, determining whether the criticism itself is valid, and generating an appropriate response. Relaxation and self-instruction skills are integrated as methods for remaining calm and in control during a conflictual encounter. Patients are counseled not to misinterpret the criticism, to employ appropriately negative assertions (such as "I statements"), to listen empathetically, to request information, to reframe the criticism cognitively, and ultimately, to set limits.

Resumption of Responsibility

An acute episode of schizophrenia will often lead to the neglect of previous roles, including those related to personal hygiene and nutrition. In the basic phase, the therapist will first look for some evidence that symptoms are beginning to stabilize prior to encouraging a resumption of role obligations. These indicators might variably include a decrease in mood lability, hallucinations, or the strength of delusions; a normalization of sleep, energy, or concentration; or a renewed interest in the world or in the welfare of friends and family. The plan begins with reasonable tasks that convey a sense of satisfaction and can be accomplished in small steps. An assigned task is reviewed in the following PT session. The patient is encouraged to appreciate that establishing a routine, no matter how boring, builds the tolerance and stamina that eventually will be needed for important social and vocational roles outside the home. Tasks in the basic phase might include the negotiation of a regular shower or maintenance of a simple but nutritious diet. In the intermediate phase, these activities will expand to include interpersonal (or shared) tasks within the home. Later, in the advanced phase, the resumption of social, recreational, and vocational roles will represent finely orchestrated initiatives that integrate the acquired strategies that have proven helpful in controlling stress and its effects.

Two extremes of patient behavior present particular challenges. The first represents the undermotivated patient. A psychotic episode will often rob a patient of the stamina and energy needed to resume even basic functions. For patients who can become easily overwhelmed or fear that task failure will evoke further criticism, the plan is to become motivated to "work on getting motivated." The sequencing of incremental tasks and the associated success can often provide the beginning of a personal reward system. Allowing greater patient choices in the tasks assigned can also be facilitative.

Often the overmotivated patient is more difficult to treat, the one who by choice or necessity feels compelled to resume vocational or academic roles quickly. Here, the task is temporarily to limit demands as much as possible, either through part-time employment, flexible hours, or a reduction in the number and complexity of academic courses. This counsel is integrated with the psychoeducation theme of "stress and vulnerability," principally with regard to residual but less noticeable cognitive deficits. These patients are often willing to limit temporarily the amount of social stimulation outside the vocational role. At times, other family members will be willing to assume traditional household tasks for patients who feel the need to resume full-time vocational roles prior to attaining an optimal remission of symptoms.

Pursuit of Social and Vocational Goals

PT attempts the fullest integration of acquired coping skills and social or vocational objectives in the advanced phase. Therapist, patient, and family expectations for performance are tempered by a review of the cognitive demands associated with even the most elementary job, and by the patient's specific residual deficits. A recent study, for example, has shown that problems with working memory load can lead to symptom exacerbation in the context of a stressful (critical) interpersonal encounter (Rosenfarb, Nuechterlein, Goldstein, & Subotnik, 2000). Nearly all patients, including those with the greatest clinical stability, will harbor fears about community reintegration. Assurances are offered that there will be a review of past social and vocational experiences, including an assessment of the coping strategies that did and did not work; a reappraisal of the patient's "subjective cues" of distress in social and vocational contexts, and through practice simulations; the selection of one or more newly acquired PT strategies that can be applied in lieu of previous approaches that proved unsuccessful. Much of this reintegration is a slow, trial-and-error process that will ultimately identify the patient's functional strengths and liabilities, including which social and vocational goals can be pursued, and which need to be avoided or approached differently. The objective is to make PT coping strategies spontaneous and portable in the unpredictable community ventures that could prove to be dysregulating.

Otherwise, PT assists patients in accounting for the gaps in social and vocational history, a major concern for those whose illness had led to a prolonged period of inactivity. Patients are counseled how to "finesse" questions about their illness or interim work history. They are prepared to "put their best foot forward," trained in the messages they want to communicate, and provided practical skills in redirecting questions, listening, taking perspectives, and being supportive. Opportunities for *in vivo*, real-world experiences that can be created by most PT clinicians are described in the manual, and the reciprocal feedback between clinician and work supervisors is addressed (Hogarty, in press, Chap. 6). Patients are also provided with practical suggestions regarding the establishment of new or old relationships, how to explain their illness, and the fundamentals of relationship maintenance.

Finally, PT has had unexpected success in facilitating the sobriety and outcome of comorbid patients who misuse alcohol and/or cannabis (Hogarty, in press, Chap. 2). While the substance-misusing patients (20%) who received PT in our formal studies did significantly better than misusing patients who received family psychoeducation or supportive therapy alone, they were not fully representative of the larger population of comorbid patients. (Patients for whom substance abuse *seriously* compromised adjustment were ruled out at baseline.) We plan to tailor further PT strategies to the temperaments of patients, dimensions of personality that are thought to precipitate substance abuse, such as those inclined toward negative affectivity or disinhibition and impulsivity (Blanchard, Brown, Horan, & Sherwood, 2000). These authors provide convincing evidence of a shared pathophysiology among patients with schizophrenia and substance abusers. Many existing PT strategies seem intuitively relevant for addressing poor coping responses to stress (such as drug and alcohol use) and likely account for the PT success that has been achieved to date. Basic phase techniques that depict stress as a "trigger" of symptoms (or substance abuse) are relevant, as are avoidance and positive assertion skills. The identification of subjective cues, social perception training, enhanced positive assertion when negotiating requests to drink or use illicit substances, and simple relaxation skills also appear to be relevant intermediate phase techniques. Selected advanced phase strategies that might further serve to circumvent substance misuse include reflective awareness of one's behavior, an advanced form of relaxation, and skills related to conflict resolution or the negotiation of criticism.

CRITERIA FOR PHASE TRANSITIONS

Given the documented vulnerability to expectations (therapeutic and otherwise) that might exceed cognitive capacity of patients with schizophrenia (Hogarty, in press, Chap. 1), entry into each of the three PT phases is determined by a set of operational, behavioral criteria offered as guidelines rather than as a rigidly enforced set of rules. A failure to satisfy one or more criteria, however, would indicate that the clinician should proceed cautiously if a decision is made to advance to the next phase. At least, the patient should be closely monitored for signs of therapeutic overload.

While explicit criteria served to guide the transitions to the intermediate and advanced phases prior to the PT studies, we neglected to specify criteria for the application of the basic phase strategies themselves, beyond support, medication, and case management. As a result, PT recipients who lived without the resources of an available family experienced significantly more psychotic episodes than patients who received supportive therapy and medication. These PT recipients were faced with problems in securing food, clothing, and, most importantly, a stable residence when they relapsed. In retrospect, it is not difficult to appreciate the negative consequences of a psychotherapeutic approach that contained cognitive demands that might have exceeded the capacity of patients preoccupied with whether they might be shortly "on the street." We have speculated that similar circumstances might also have contributed to the negative effects of prior psychotherapy studies among ambulatory patients with schizophrenia. Thus, we now recommend that the following criteria be used *prior to* the application of many basic phase strategies: *For residentially unstable patients who struggle with the challenges of meeting basic needs, PT should be limited to the principles of joining, support, medication, and case management until safe and predictable housing and other basic necessities are secured* (Hogarty, in press, Chap. 4). Once these assurances are met, relapse clearly declines.

For patients who are able to move through the basic phase, the following conditions should be reasonably satisfied before proceeding to the intermediate phase. The first criterion represents symptom status. Positive symptoms should be in remission, or if persistent at a low level, they should be stable and not have a significant influence on behavior (e.g., responding to hallucinations or delusions). Nor should symptoms interfere with clinic attendance. In this regard, a relatively constant maintenance dose of antipsychotic medication should have been achieved. Patients should have attended at least one-half of scheduled PT sessions such that requisite assessments of clinical state and role performance could be made. Residential stability should continue to be assured. Cognitively, the patient should be able to maintain a span of attention sufficient for a 30-minute discussion of clinical state, social problems, and basic coping skills. Schizophrenia should be understood as an illness that often has its own individual prodromes for which treatment is indicated. Finally, the clinician should have some evidence that the patient can make appropriate use of positive comments or demonstrate some ability to reduce stress by avoiding conflictual situations.

In cases where patients (or the therapist) are uncomfortable with mastering intermediate or advanced phase techniques, they can be assured that the practice principles of the basic phase, coupled with the fundamentals of support, medication, and case management, constitute a very effective form of care in its own right. (Our ongoing study that uses these principles as a "control" condition for the test of a new cognitive enhancement therapy has shown significant effects on personal and social adjustment [see Hogarty & Flesher, 1999, for an introduction]). Of our study patients, 93% completed the basic phase and graduated to the intermediate phase, and over 50% ultimately proceeded to the advanced phase, a number constrained by the time limitations of the study. These observations challenge the belief that patients with schizophrenia cannot learn and apply motivational change strategies.

For those who progress to the advanced phase of PT, the following transitional criteria can better be used to assure a safe and effective exposure to these latter techniques. Of primary importance, such patients should have continued to meet the criteria for entry into the intermediate phase itself. In addition, patients should have a basic understanding of the more common forms of disability, the effects of stress on personal vulnerability, and the possible consequences of the "march of symptoms." In this regard, patients should be able to articulate the experience of stress and at least one physical, affective, behavioral, or cognitive analogue (a "subjective cue"). Evidence of social perception in vulnerable situations, and effective listening and assertiveness, including the ability to express preferences, requests, and dislikes appropriately, as well as to refuse unreasonable demands, are highly desirable. Finally, the patient should be able to reduce personal feelings of distress below baseline levels using diaphragmatic breathing or basic relaxation techniques. For those who might prefer to quantify and periodically rate these transitional criteria, the manual provides a process rating scale (Hogarty, in press, Appendix B).

THE EVIDENCE BASE FOR PERSONAL THERAPY

The two 3-year studies of PT represent the longest controlled trials of a psychosocial treatment among patients with schizophrenia that have been published. They provide a unique opportunity to examine prospectively the longitudinal effects of a disorder-relevant psychotherapy. All patients, in both trials, received the minimum effective dose of an antipsychotic medication (Hogarty et al., 1988), usually fluphenazine decanoate, thus assuring that PT effects were not due to differences in medication compliance. There were no differences in drug type, dose, or route of administration that could explain the differential effects of the investigated psychosocial treatments. In the study of 97 patients with schizophrenia or schizoaffective disorder (Trial 1) randomly assigned to PT alone, supportive therapy alone (ST), family psychoeducation alone (FT), and the combination of PT and FT, there were significant effects on relapse reduction that favored PT. However, the "control" patients in the PT studies did so much better than the control subjects in prior studies that the magnitude of the relapse difference was reduced. For example, only 22% of the ST subjects experienced a schizophrenia relapse over 3 years, a rate considerably lower than the 68% relapse rate found at 2-year follow-up in our own and other previous investigations (e.g., Hogarty et al., 1991). This has been a more common observation in modern "efficacy" studies that are required to provide quality of care to control subjects that often exceeds that available in nonresearch settings. However, in the so-called "real-world" effectiveness studies, the differences between standard care and a psychosocial treatment remain striking (e.g., see Dixon, Adams, & Lucksted, 2000). However, among the 54 patients who lived alone (Trial 2), relapse was much greater for PT recipients than for those who received ST, for the reasons described earlier.

Independent of relapse effects, differential treatment effects on social adjustment favoring PT were both comprehensive and consistent in both trials. Patients were assessed at baseline and again every 6 months for 3 years. In order to be considered "significant," an effect had to be observed across the six rating periods overall, as well as at two of the six specific assessment periods. (In fact, PT effects typically occurred at four of these six assessments, and "p values" most often exceeded the .01 level [see Hogarty, Greenwald, et al., 1997].) Significance tests of individual outcomes (derived from regression analyses) were "protected" by significant effects on various multivariate indices. (Unlike the traditional psychotherapy text, the PT manual also offers a "statistical primer" for clinicians that is designed to foster a better understanding of both PT results and the findings from other clinical studies [Hogarty, in press, Appendix A].)

The first observation of note was that nearly all adjustment effects occurred between 18 and 36 months, and not before. Most striking were the effects of PT on a summary measure that indicated a decrease in patient sensitivity, loneliness, self-abasement, worry, guilt, and feelings of being wronged in social relationships. Improved self-care and a decrease in conflict, communication difficulty, and friction associated with interpersonal relationships were also shown to favor PT. Improved work performance further characterized PT recipients. For example, at 3 years, 43% of the PT-alone recipients across both trials were working full- or part-time in the open labor market compared to only 20% of the ST-alone groups. The effects of FT in the first trial were also interesting, if

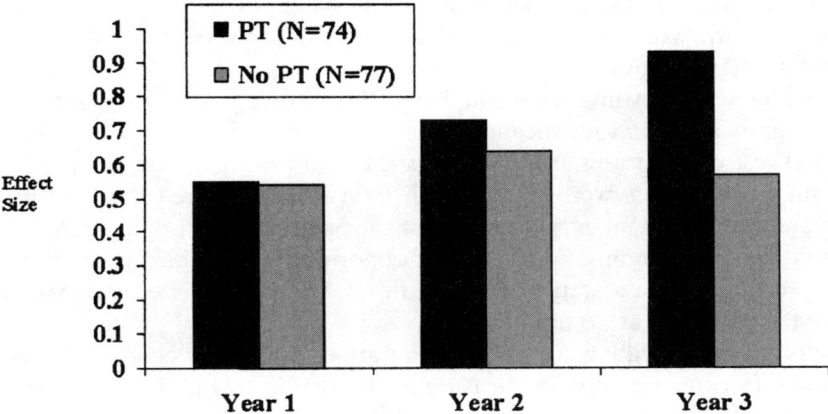

FIGURE 3.1. Cumulative effects of personal therapy on 11 symptom outcomes. Data from Hogarty, Greenwald, Ulrich, et al. (1997).

not provocative. FT improved the personal comfort (primarily affective symptoms) of patients, particularly *female* subjects, but it had no appreciable effect on social adjustment. PT, on the other hand, showed highly significant effects on social adjustment but fewer effects on personal comfort. (Expectations for performance were higher in PT than in FT.) In fact, PT recipients were shown to be more "anxious," which was not so much a "disorder" as an increase in arousal needed to assume life roles. Furthermore, these improved PT outcomes were most often applicable to *male* patients. Predictors of improvement and the characteristics of the more likely responders to the PT and no-PT conditions are described elsewhere (Hogarty, in press, Chapter 2).

In order to appreciate better the overall effects of a long-term psychotherapy on symptoms and social adjustment, this description of PT concludes with a summary of "within-treatment" longitudinal effects over 3 years that complement the cross-sectional semiannual effects described earlier. The analyzed summary measures were standardized (Z) scores from the composite indices of symptoms and social adjustment. Figures 3.1 and 3.2 illustrate longitudinal improvement over 3 years in terms of "effect sizes." Ex-

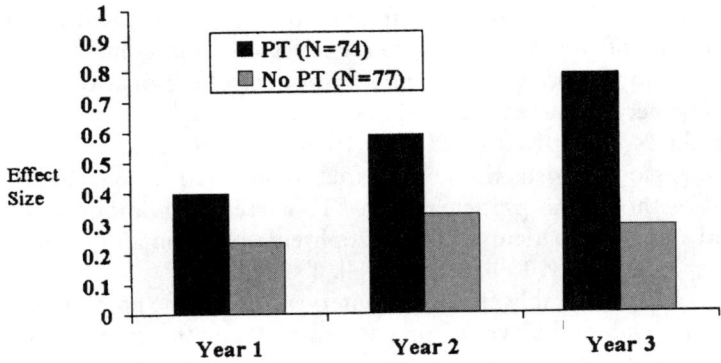

FIGURE 3.2. Cumulative effects of personal therapy on 12 social adjustment outcomes. Data from Hogarty, Greenwald, Ulrich, et al. (1997).

pressed in standard deviation units, a pre–post change of one-half standard deviation (effect size = 0.50), would be clinically significant and an effect size of 0.75 would be both significant and compelling.

Regarding symptom improvement, Figure 3.1 shows that both groups of patients improved significantly *and* identically in the first year, with similar outcomes observed at 2 years. These observations are characteristic of our prior psychosocial treatment trials as well, since all patients were treated with individually tailored doses of medication. Furthermore, there were no expectations that the principal effect of a psychosocial treatment would be on symptoms. With the rare opportunity for a third year of observation, however, we do observe a statistically significant, differential effect on symptoms that favors the PT condition at 36 months.

Results are more striking and policy implications are clearly contained in Figure 3.2. Differential effects on a composite measure of social adjustment (12 outcomes) favor PT at 1 year, but are, again, not statistically different, a rather common observation in longitudinal trials that measure outcomes other than relapse. However, much like our earlier trials (e.g., Hogarty, Goldberg, & Schooler, 1974; Hogarty et al., 1991), differentially significant social adjustment effects again favor PT at 24 months. It is the unprecedented observations provided by 3-year assessments that indicate a dramatic and increasingly significant effect of PT.

Both figures show that with ST and/or FT alone, most improvement occurs in the *first year* following a psychotic episode, but then effects essentially "plateau," without noticeable improvement thereafter. PT improvement, on the other hand, continues to increase over time, with no evidence at the end of 3 years that these effects have plateaued. (Only a longer period of controlled observation could determine when the effects of PT might level off.) From a policy perspective, mental health systems that either ration or fail to use a definitive psychosocial treatment, or that rely primarily on supportive approaches and "warm" medication, can look forward to an adequate stabilization of symptoms after 1 year of treatment, but only modest improvement in social functioning. This symptomatic and role performance "recovery" essentially does not change after 1 year. However, with a disorder-relevant approach such as PT, improvement regarding personal and social adjustment continues to increase significantly for at least 3 years, if not longer. Sooner or later, the price of not treating schizophrenia adequately must be factored into the "cost–benefit" equation.

In conclusion, some clinicians might argue that they observe the effects of their own psychotherapeutic intervention much sooner than 18 months. Such was the case in the studies of PT as well. Patients in all treatment conditions improved significantly in the first 12–18 months of treatment. However, the lesson from controlled clinical trials is that it takes time for a specific *differential* treatment effect of a relevant psychosocial intervention to emerge. But emerge it does, much to the relief and quality of life of patients. Two-thirds of patients rated their PT-alone experience as "very helpful" (the highest level of personal satisfaction), compared to only half the ST-alone recipients, and only one-third of those who participated in FT. These observations serve to remind us of the personal value that patients with schizophrenia place on an individual psychotherapeutic experience (Coursey, Keller, & Farrell, 1995).

Thus, PT is a demonstrably efficacious intervention for the postacute, "stabilization" phase of schizophrenia and serves to prepare patients for the contemporary "recovery" phase, cognitive rehabilitation approaches that are under development (see Hogarty & Flesher, 1999). PT's potential place in the armamentarium of psychosocial treatment is illustrated elsewhere in a proposed psychosocial treatment algorithm for schizophrenia and related disorders (Hogarty, in press, Chap. 7). Depending on the patient's level of disability, the relevance of various PT phases is identified, and the practice principles of other cognitive and behavioral rehabilitation approaches that can be used interchangeably are described.

REFERENCES

Anderson, C. M., Reiss, D. J., & Hogarty, G. E. (1986). *Schizophrenia and the family: A practitioners guide to psychoeducation and management.* New York: Guilford Press.

Benson, H. (1996). *Timeless healing.* New York: Scribner.

Blanchard, J. J., Brown, S. A., Horan, W. P., & Sherwood, A. R. (2000). Substance use disorders in schizophrenia: Review, integration and a proposed model. *Clinical Psychology Review, 20,* 207–234.

Coursey, R. D., Keller, A. B., & Farrell, E. W. (1995). Individual psychotherapy and persons with serious mental illness: The client's perspective. *Schizophrenia Bulletin, 21,* 283–301.

Dixon, L., Adams, C., & Lucksted, A. (2000). Update on family psychoeducation for schizophrenia. *Schizophrenia Bulletin, 21,* 631–643.

Fenton, W. S. (2000). Evolving perspectives on individual psychotherapy for schizophrenia. *Schizophrenia Bulletin, 26,* 47–72.

Hogarty, G. E. (in press). *Personal therapy: A guide to the individual treatment of schizophrenia and related disorders.* New York: Guilford Press.

Hogarty, G. E., Anderson, C. M., Reiss, D. J., Kornblith, S. J., Greenwald, D. P., Javna, C. D., & Madonia, M. J. (1986). Family psychoeducation, social skills training, and maintenance chemotherapy in the aftercare treatment of schizophrenia: I. One-year effects of a controlled study on relapse and expressed emotion. *Archives of General Psychiatry, 43,* 633–642.

Hogarty, G. E., Anderson, C. M., Reiss, D. J., Kornblith, S. J., Greenwald, D. P., Ulrich, R. F., & Carter, M. (1991). Family psychoeducation, social skills training, and maintenance chemotherapy in the aftercare treatment of schizophrenia: II. Two-year effects of a controlled study on relapse and adjustment. *Archives of General Psychiatry, 48,* 340–347.

Hogarty, G. E., & Flesher, S. (1999). Practice principles of cognitive enhancement therapy for schizophrenia. *Schizophrenia Bulletin, 25,* 693–708.

Hogarty, G. E., Goldberg, S. C., & Schooler, N. R. (1974). Drug and sociotherapy in the aftercare of schizophrenic patients: III. Adjustment of nonrelapsed patients. *Archives of General Psychiatry, 31,* 797–805.

Hogarty, G. E., Greenwald, D., Ulrich, R. F., Kornblith, S. J., DiBarry, A. L., Cooley, S., Carter, M., & Flesher, S. (1997). Three-year trials of personal therapy among schizophrenic patients living with or independent of family: II. Effects on adjustment of patients. *American Journal of Psychiatry, 154*(11), 1514–1524.

Hogarty, G. E., Kornblith, S. J., Greenwald, D., DiBarry, A. L., Cooley, S., Ulrich, R., Carter, M., & Flesher, S. (1997). Three-year trials of personal therapy among schizophrenic patients living with or independent of family: I. Description of study and effects on relapse rates. *American Journal of Psychiatry, 154*(11), 1504–1513.

Hogarty, G. E., McEvoy, J. P., Munetz, M., DiBarry, A. L., Bartone, P., Cather, R., Cooley, S. J., Ulrich, R. F., Carter, M., & Madonia, M. J. (1988). Dose of fluphenazine, familial expressed emotion, and outcome in schizophrenia: Results of a two-year controlled study. *Archives of General Psychiatry, 45,* 797–805.

Hogarty, G. E., Ulrich, R. F., & Mussare, F. (1976). Drug discontinuation among long term successfully treated schizophrenic outpatients. *Diseases of the Nervous System, 57,* 494–500.

Hollis, F. (1964). *Casework: A psychosocial therapy.* New York: Random House.

Kavanagh, D. J. (1992). Recent developments in expressed emotion and schizophrenia. *British Journal of Psychiatry, 160,* 601–620.

Lehman, A. F., & Steinwachs, D. M. (1998). Patterns of usual care for schizophrenia: Initial results from the schizophrenia Patient Outcomes Research Team (PORT) client survey. *Schizophrenia Bulletin, 24,* 11–20.

Mueser, K. T., & Berenbaum, H. (1990). Psychodynamic treatment of schizophrenia: Is there a future? *Psychological Medicine, 20,* 253–262.

Rosenfarb, I. S., Nuechterlein, K. H., Goldstein, M. J., & Subotnik, K. L. (2000). Neurocognitive vulnerability, interpersonal criticism, and the emergence of unusual thinking by schizophrenic patients during family transitions. *Archives of General Psychiatry, 57,* 1174–1179.

Sullwold, L., & Herrlich, J. (1992). Providing schizophrenic patients with a concept of illness: An essential element of therapy. *British Journal of Psychiatry, 161*(Suppl. 18), 129–132.

4

Cognitive-Behavioral Therapy for Schizophrenia

A Case Formulation Approach

NICHOLAS TARRIER
GILLIAN HADDOCK

There have been published accounts of case studies of psychotic symptoms using structured psychological treatments for many years (see Haddock, Tarrier, et al., 1998, for a review). In fact, one early case study of cognitive therapy was published by Beck (1952) prior to developing his work on the treatment of depression. However, it is only recently that the interest in developing cognitive-behavioral therapy (CBT) for schizophrenia has become more widespread and robust clinical trials have been carried out. A number of centers, mainly in the United Kingdom, have developed these methods using a broad array of cognitive and behavioral techniques. The impact of this work has been such that the British Psychological Society (1999) has recently published a position paper on psychosis and its treatment supporting such nondrug treatments. There has also been a recent joint report by the British Psychological Society and the Royal College of Psychiatrists on the psychosocial management of schizophrenia (Joint British Psychological Society and Royal College of Psychiatrists Schizophrenia Guideline Development Group, 2001). Systematic reviews have concluded that CBT "may decrease relapse/readmission rates and may improve the patient's mental state" (Adams, 2000, p. 6), and psychological treatments have been included within the National Service Framework, a U.K. government-produced guideline for quality mental health services (Department of Health, 2000). Thus, CBT as a treatment for psychotic disorders has become an established mainstream intervention, at least in the United Kingdom.

THEORETICAL BACKGROUND

Although different centers have developed different approaches to CBT, there has been much overlap with psychosis (Tarrier, 1995). However, treatments have usually not been strongly influenced by any particular theoretical model of schizophrenia, and numerous factors, both historical and practical, have been responsible for the sudden upsurge of interest in CBT for schizophrenia. Not the least of these has been the widespread adoption of CBT to treat a whole range of mental disorders, especially affective disorders (cf. Hawton, Salkovskis, Kirk, & Clark, 1989), and the attention to promoting evidence-based practice (Drake et al., 2001; Geddes, Reynolds, Streiner, Szatmari, & Haynes, 1998).

Some of the initial influences on the development of CBT for psychosis were based on theoretical mechanisms thought to underpin the use of coping strategies (Tarrier, 2001). Central to the idea of coping is the process of appraisal whereby the person evaluates a set of circumstances or experiences as a problem, attempts to cope with these, and subsequently evaluates the relative success of these attempts. Patients' beliefs about their symptoms and appraisal have been shown to be important factors in determining how well they cope and whether they persist in these attempts (Kinney, 2000). It has long been recognized that the use of personal resources such as coping strategies are important in buffering against psychotic decompensation leading to exacerbations or relapse of positive psychotic symptoms. For example, in Nuechterlein's (1987) model of stress–vulnerability of psychosis, coping and self-efficacy are cited as important personal protective factors. Moreover, there have been consistent findings that patients with schizophrenia do make effortful attempts to overcome or cope with persistent positive psychotic symptoms, with at least some success (e.g., Breier & Strauss, 1983; Brenner, Boker, Muller, Spichtig, & Wurgler, 1987; Carr, 1988; Cohen & Berk, 1985; Falloon & Talbot, 1981; Kinney, 2000; Romme & Escher, 1989; Tarrier, 1987). It was reasoned that since many patients used coping strategies naturally, they would further benefit from systematic training in coping skills combined with an awareness of the antecedents and context of their symptoms.

Other attempts to understand individual psychotic symptoms, such as hallucinations and delusions, have suggested promising candidate intervention methods. For example, the similarity between delusional and normal belief processes has been noted. Maher (1988) suggested that delusions are the result of normal reasoning processes applied to, and secondary to, unusual or abnormal perceptual experiences. Whereas Bentall, Haddock, and Slade (1994) have hypothesized that although delusional beliefs may share important characteristics with normal beliefs, deluded patients exhibit abnormal biases in their reasoning processes. Both perspectives suggest that therapeutic interventions designed to modify reasoning processes and strategies that enhance cognitive or other coping strategies will be effective at reducing the severity of delusional beliefs. This has resulted in belief modification strategies that form an important part of CBT treatment for psychosis.

Similarly, there have been attempts to understand the processes underlying auditory hallucinations. While it has been assumed that auditory hallucinations result from some sort of misattribution to external sources of inner speech, accounts of the type of deficit or bias that may bring about this misattribution have varied considerably. For example, Hoffman (1986) assumed that auditory hallucinations occur from random firing of speech-processing mechanisms, resulting in "parasitic memories" being brought into consciousness. As these are unexpected and unplanned, the patient perceives them as being alien and attributable to an external source. David (1994) also accounted for auditory hallucinations in terms of a deficit in the speech-processing mechanisms. The location of the deficit in the speech-processing pathway resulted in different types of auditory experiences, such as hallucinations, thought echo, or thought broadcast. Frith (1992) proposed that the actual inner speech of hallucinators is normal, but that the fault lies in the internal monitor of speech, resulting in speech perceived as originating from an external source. Finally, Bentall (1990) suggested that the speech processing pathways perform normally in hallucinators but that biases resulting from their specific beliefs and attitudes determine their interpretation of inner speech. Although there is not sufficient evidence to account totally for auditory hallucinations by any of these deficits alone, there is some evidence to support all of them and, as with delusions, the accounts are not mutually exclusive, and all mechanisms may be implicated. There may be an underlying neuropsychological deficit that leads to a vulnerability to develop psychosis, upon which cognitive factors such as monitoring, beliefs, and attributions act to determine their occurrence, interpretation, and effect on the individual. Further research is required to elucidate the actual mechanisms involved and the relative contribution of each so as to further inform treatment (Nuechterlein & Subotnik, 1998).

CLINICAL TRIALS

A number of randomized controlled trials of CBT have now been carried out (see Table 4.1). These trials have addressed two major topics: (1) whether CBT in combination with routine care would reduce persistent drug-resistant psychotic symptoms in chronic patients with schizophrenia, and (2) whether CBT would effectively speed recovery and buffer against later deterioration in acutely ill patients. With respect to chronic patients, there is good evidence that CBT in combination with routine care (usually involving medication and case management) is superior to routine care alone in reducing positive symptoms over the treatment period (Kuipers et al., 1997; Tarrier, Yusupoff, Kinney, et al., 1998). There is also evidence that treatment gains are maintained over the first year (Kuipers et al., 1998; Sensky et al., 2000; Tarrier, Wittkowski, et al., 1999) and up to 2 years after the termination of treatment (Tarrier et al., 2000). Comparisons between CBT and nonspecific treatments, such as supportive counseling and befriending, have been less clear-cut in their findings. Tarrier and colleagues (2000) reported a convergence over time between CBT and supportive counseling in their effect on both positive and negative symptoms. Supportive counseling, although achieving good results with delusions, performed poorly in treating hallucinations, with those patients receiving CBT showing significant benefits over those receiving supportive counseling. Conversely, Sensky and colleagues (2000) reported a divergence between CBT and befriending, with no apparent difference between the two at posttreatment, but with a deterioration in the befriending group 9 months later, indicating the superiority of CBT. CBT has also been used successfully in combination with motivational interviewing and family intervention to reduce psychopathology and substance abuse in dual-diagnosis patients with chronic schizophrenia and substance and/or alcohol abuse (Barrowclough et al., 2001) following a 9-month intervention package. Gains on negative symptoms and overall functioning were maintained over an 18-month follow-up period (Haddock et al., 2002).

There has been less research on the efficacy of cognitive-behavioral therapy in acutely ill patients. Preliminary studies suggested that cognitive-behavioral therapy speeded recovery by between 25% and 50%, with a 50% reduction in the time spent in the hospital (Drury, Birchwood, Cochrane, & MacMillan, 1996a, 1996b). Although extremely innovative, this study had a number of methodological shortcomings, including lack of independent and blind assessors, and utilization of a range of psychosocial interventions, of which CBT was just one. Another small study that used only CBT

TABLE 4.1. Randomized Controlled Trials of CBT with Schizophrenia

Study	Treatment condition	Patients	n	Frequency and duration of treatment	Follow-up assessments	Results
Tarrier et al. (1993)	1. CBT + RC 2. PS + RC 3. 50% wait-list control	Chronic schizophrenia, persistent symptoms	27	10 sessions; 2 per week for 5 weeks	Posttreatment; 6-month FU	CBT and PS showed significant improvements in positive symptoms compared to wait list.
Haddock, Slade, et al. (1998)	1. Distraction 2. Focusing	Chronic schizophrenia, persistent auditory hallucinations	33	18–20 sessions; weekly treatment of hallucinations only	Posttreatment; 24-month FU	Both groups showed a reduction in hallucinations at posttreatment, which was not maintained at FU.
London–East Anglia Study: Kuipers et al. (1997, 1998)	1. CBT + RC 2. RC	Chronic schizophrenia, persistent symptoms	60 initially; 47 at FU	Mean 19 sessions (0–50) over 9 months; initially weekly, then fortnightly	Posttreatment; 9-month FU	CBT significantly improved on the BPRS rating score, maintained at FU.
Manchester Study: Tarrier, Yusupoff, Kinney, et al. (1998); Tarrier, Wittkowski, et al. (1999); Tarrier et al. (2000, 2001)	1. CBT + RC 2. SC + RC 3. RC	Chronic schizophrenia, persistent symptoms	87 initially; 70 at 12 months; 61 at 24 months	20 sessions over 3 months; 2 per week + 4 monthly boosters	Posttreatment; 12- and 24-month FU	CBT significantly improved on positive and negative symptoms compared to RC and in hallucination compared to SC. At 12- and 18-month FU, CBT and SC significantly improved compared to RC.
Sensky et al. (2000)	1. CBT + RC 2. Befriending	Chronic schizophrenia, persistent symptoms	90 at posttreatment and FU	Flexible mean 19 sessions (2–33) over 9 months	Posttreatment; 9-month FU	Improvements in both groups at posttreatment but no group differences at FU. CBT significantly improved compared to befriending.

Study	Conditions	Population	N	Sessions	Assessments	Outcomes
Barrowclough et al. (2001)	1. CBT + FI + MI + family support + RC 2. RC + family support	Dual diagnosis (schizophrenia + substance abuse) with close family contact	36	MI: 5 sessions; CBT: 24 sessions weekly, then fortnightly; FI: 10–16 sessions	Posttreatment; 12-month FU	Significant improvement in positive symptoms and functioning, reduced relapse, and decreased substance abuse in CBT and FI group.
Drury et al. (1996a, 1996b)	1. CBT (individual + group + family engagement) + RC 2. Semistructured recreation and support activities + TAU	Acutely ill hospitalized with schizophrenia	40	Flexible 8 hours per week for a maximum of 6 months	Posttreatment; 3-month FU	Greater and faster (25–50%) reduction in symptoms in the CBT group.
Haddock, Tarrier, et al. (1999)	1. CBT + RC 2. SC + RC	Acutely ill hospitalized with schizophrenia, illness detection greater than 5 years	21	Flexible mean 10 sessions over 5 weeks postadmission + 4 monthly boosters	Posttreatment; 24-month FU	Improvement in both groups on group differences at posttreatment, not significantly fewer releases in CBT over FU.
SOCRATES Study: Lewis et al. (2001)	1. CBT + RC 2. SC + RC 3. RC	Acutely ill recent-onset (80% first episode, 20% second episode) hospitalized with schizophrenia	309	Flexible up to 20 hours over 5 weeks postadmission; mean = 16 sessions; mean duration of session = 40 minutes + 4 booster sessions	Posttreatment; 18-month FU	CBT shows significantly faster improvement compared to other groups.

Note. BPRS, Brief Psychiatric Rating Scale; CBT, cognitive-behavioral therapy; FI, family intervention; FU, follow-up (follow-up assessments are dated from the posttreatment assessment); MI, motivational interviewing; PS, problem solving; RC, routine care; SC, supportive counseling; TAU, treatment as usual.

during an inpatient stay for an acute episode found lower relapse rates and much longer time to first psychotic relapse over a 2-year follow-up in patients who had received CBT, although these differences did not reach significance (Haddock, Tarrier, et al., 1999). In the largest trial to date, the SOCRATES Trial, 318 patients with recent-onset schizophrenia (80% first episodes) were randomly allocated to cognitive-behavioral therapy plus routine care, supportive counseling and routine care, or routine care alone. Recruitment occurred within 10 days of hospital admission for a psychotic episode, and treatment took place over 5 weeks. Analysis of the treatment phase demonstrated that cognitive-behavioral therapy significantly speeded recovery, with significant differences appearing at 3 and 4 weeks (Lewis et al., in press). Similar to the results reported previously in chronic patients (Tarrier et al., 2001), supportive counseling performed well with delusions but significantly worse than CBT with hallucinations.

TREATMENT MODEL AND CASE FORMULATION

Optimally, treatment or intervention for a clinical disorder should be based on a testable theoretical position. As discussed earlier, there are no unifying theories of schizophrenia or understanding of the psychological processes that would direct therapy, as in desensitization formulated from learning theory (e.g., Wolpe, 1958). We have attempted to produce an explanation of psychotic symptoms drawn from a number of theoretical and pragmatic sources as a clinical heuristic to guide CBT interventions (Haddock & Tarrier, 1998). This is represented in Figure 4.1. The process of case formulation is to identify important clinical problems and their determinants, thus leading to intervention strategies that produce the optimum clinical benefit (see Persons, 1989; Tarrier & Calam, in press; Tarrier, Wells, & Haddock, 1998). This clinical heuristic serves as a guide to case formulation in the treatment of the psychotic patient.

It was speculated that psychotic experience could be a response to a combination of internal or environmental antecedents that may operate on cognitive functioning through a common mediating pathway, such as a dysfunction in the arousal system or its regulation (Tarrier & Turpin, 1992). These internal factors could be biological or psychological and inherent or acquired. An example of an inherent biological factor would be the transmission of genetic heritability; acquired factors would be brain damage resulting from birth trauma or infection. Examples of inherent psychological factors would be cognitive deficits; and acquired factors would be cognitive biases or schematic representations. This is basically a threshold model in which interacting internal vulnerabilities and external stresses culminate in precipitating, and possibly maintaining, psychotic symptoms. It is proposed that the experience of hallucinations and delusions has its consequences. Such psychotic experiences may well evoke a range of emotions that may be perplexing or frightening, disgusting or annoying, and so on. Furthermore, psychotic experience will almost inevitably have cognitive and behavioral consequences as persons react to, or attempt to explain or understand what is happening to them. Various attributions about the origins or nature of the voices or ideas have important implications in maintaining psychopathology (e.g., Chadwick & Birchwood, 1994; Morrison & Baker, 2000) and depression (Birchwood & Iqbal, 1998).

Symptoms can be maintained by the activation of feedback loops. Thus, emotional responses to the psychotic experience, such as anxiety, fear, or anger, would initiate a feedback loop and increase the severity of psychotic symptoms by contributing via in-

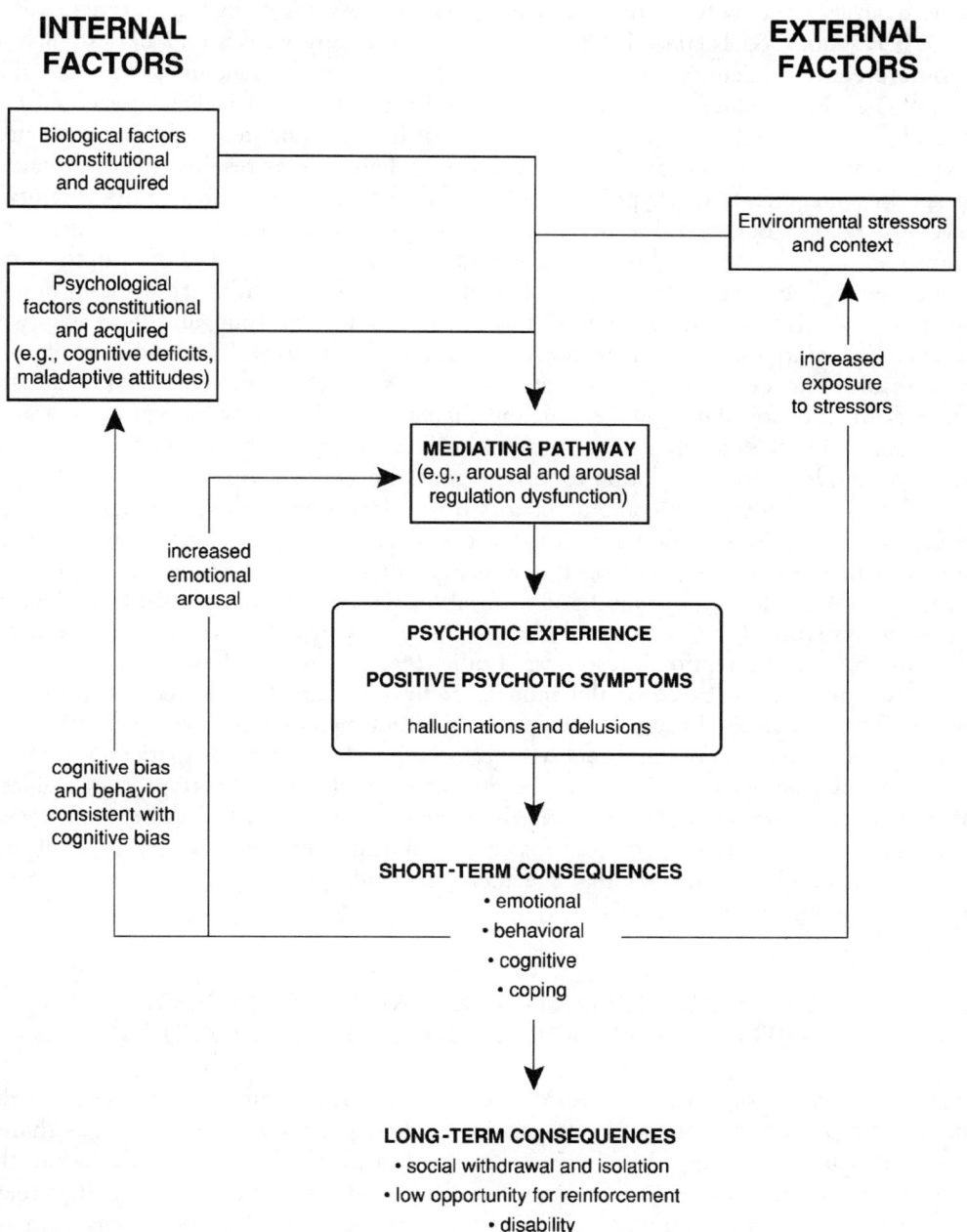

FIGURE 4.1. Clinical heuristic of psychotic symptoms.

creased levels of activity within the arousal system (Barrowclough & Tarrier, 1992, p. 161; Haddock & Tarrier, 1998). Similarly, cognitive responses and biases, such as misinterpretation, attention to perceived threat, selective attribution, and failure to reality test, would also produce emotional sequelae and activate feedback. Behavior could further serve to reinforce these cognitive responses if it were consistent with cognitive process or content, so that behavior congruent with beliefs or that resulted in confirmation of specific interpretations (hypothesis protection) would likely reinforce and maintain psychopathology. Behavioral responses could increase patients' exposure to various environmental antecedents or stressors that would increase the probability of symptoms occurring, including the potential for patients' increased conflict with their social group or families. The effects of the psychotic disorder will change over time, and there may well be a buildup of long-term consequences, such as social withdrawal, isolation, and loneliness, resulting in decreased opportunities for reward, ineffectual social skills, and the chronic effects of social marginalization and stigma. These in turn will perpetuate disability by restricting the patient's social networks, decreasing the opportunity for purposeful behavior and lowering motivation to initiate goal-directed behavior.

The model attempts to combine factors from general psychological models with an understanding of the specific nature of schizophrenia and psychotic symptoms. In addition, specific pathological processes that appear central to schizophrenia are also considered, such as the nature of arousal and arousal regulation dysfunction (Dawson, Nuechterlein, & Adams, 1989) or cognitive deficits, deficits in executive function, and the inability to control attentional resources (Frith, 1994; Hemsley, 1994).

The aims of CBT, based on this model, are to influence the occurrence and maintenance of the psychosis through a number of different methods, for example, enhancing coping, belief modification, and reality monitoring, and changing the patient's behavior and interpretation of events. However, because of the multiple effects of psychotic illness, we would anticipate that the many needs of patients would also require multiagency case management or similar, comprehensive mental health service involvement. Table 4.2 illustrates a number of factors that the therapist needs to be aware of that affect the procedure and process of therapy.

ENGAGEMENT AND GENERAL PRINCIPLES OF COGNITIVE-BEHAVIORAL THERAPY FOR PSYCHOSIS

Due to the nature of psychotic disorder, engagement forms an important part of the therapeutic process to enhance collaboration and to promote agreement on a shared problem focus for therapy. Rigidly persisting with a highly structured style before the patient has become engaged in the approach is not advisable, which means that there may need to be flexibility regarding the number of sessions necessary for engagement, assessment, and building motivation. There is little point in progressing until this process has been completed effectively; otherwise, there is a risk of the patient dropping out of treatment. Furthermore, the absence of a positive relationship between therapist and patient has been shown to predict poor clinical outcome in patients with chronic schizophrenia (Tattan & Tarrier, 2000). The aim of the engagement phase, which can often last between one and five sessions, is to explain the nature of CBT, to agree that the approach is a collaborative venture, and to establish a working agreement between the patient and therapist on the key problems. The use of handouts to explain the nature of CBT can be useful. In addition, it is not unusual for engagement sessions to include some

TABLE 4.2. Associated Features That Need to Be Assessed and Possibly Taken into Consideration in CBT for Psychotic Patients

Psychological	Psychosocial	Social
• Interference, disrupted or slowed thought processes • Difficulty discriminating signal from noise • Restricted attention • Hypersensitivity to social stressors and social interactions • Difficulty processing social stimuli and acting appropriately • Flat and restricted affect • Elevated arousal or dysfunctional arousal regulation • Hypersensitivity to stress and life events • High risk of suicide • Stigmatization • Risk of depression and hopelessness • High risk of substance abuse • Onset in late adolescence/ early adulthood interfered with normal developmental processes	• Hypersensitivity to family environments and social relationships • Risk of perpetrating, or being the victim of, violence • Integration of CBT with other interventions (e.g., family interventions)	• Conditions of social deprivation • Poor housing • Downward social drift • Unemployment and difficulty competing in the job market • Restricted social network • Psychiatric career interferes with utilization of other social resources

discussion of the nature of the diagnosis. Patients who disagree with their diagnosis may need the opportunity to discuss issues relating to diagnosis and treatment during this phase. Our experience suggests that to insist on a diagnoses when the patient is unsure or disagrees is counterproductive, and that engagement can be enhanced by therapists who agree to assist patients to explore the correctness (or not) of their diagnostic status.

It is also important for therapists to be sensitive and aware that the psychopathology may be contributing to their interactions with the patient. It is appropriate to reflect concerns about this back to patients and to encourage them to elaborate on this where appropriate. The CBT approach acknowledges that patients may be ambivalent about making changes in their behavior and cognitions in regard to some key areas, including psychotic symptoms, compliance with treatment, or aspects of functioning. It is of particular value with patients who are ambivalent about using motivational interviewing strategies to facilitate increased motivation for change (Handmaker & Walters, Chapter 11, this volume; Miller & Rollnick, 1995, 2002) in order to facilitate engagement. However, patients suffering from psychoses can be difficult to engage and maintain in treatment, and it is helpful for the therapist to be forewarned about any characteristics that might predict such attrition. Patients who refuse, or who drop out of treatment, tend to be male, unemployed, unskilled, and single, with a low level of educational attainment and low premorbid IQ. They have a long duration of illness and frequently suffer both delusions and hallucinations but do not tend to be severely ill at the time of dropout. Often paranoid and suspicious, although not necessarily toward the therapist, they usually feel depressed and hopeless (Tarrier, Yusupoff, McCarthy, et al., 1998).

ASSESSMENT AND FORMULATION

As with engagement, there is no set number of sessions during which a thorough and comprehensive assessment can be carried out. This phase is dependent on the ability of the therapist and patient to explore collaboratively the key problem areas and to agree on a working cognitive-behavioral formulation of factors that have contributed to the development and maintenance of patient difficulties (see Kinderman & Lobban, 2000). Proceeding to interventions before this process is complete is usually counterproductive, except when a patient may be suffering from extreme distress or discomfort resulting from problems that interfere with the ability to take part in assessment. This may mean that the therapist will have to help the patient apply anxiety reduction or coping techniques to allow the therapy to proceed. In other cases, the patient may be so disturbed or suffer so severely from cognitive deficits that a detailed collaborative case formulation is not feasible. A more detailed description of the various levels of engagement and therapeutic aims is given later in the chapter.

THE ANTECEDENT AND COPING INTERVIEW

The Antecedent and Coping Interview (ACI) is a semistructured interview (Tarrier, 1992a, 1992b, 2001) that provides adequate information for use as a basis for intervention. Based on the model outlined earlier and in Table 4.1, it assumes therapist knowledge and skill in being able to elicit psychotic symptoms and to conduct a cognitive-behavioral analysis and case formulation. The ACI consists of the following stages.

The Nature and Variation of Psychotic Symptoms

Each psychotic symptom needs to be elicited (the Present State Examination [Wing, Cooper, & Sartorius, 1974] interview schedule is a useful tool and gives very good examples of questions that can be used). The interviewer needs to inquire about all psychotic experience, for example, the types and nature of hallucinations, the types of delusions, and the nature of any interference with thought processes. Once each symptom has been identified, the interviewer should elicit the frequency of the symptom by starting with general questions such as "How often do you hear the voices?" and then being more specific: "How often did you hear them yesterday?" The interviewer needs to elicit the various dimensions of each symptom, such as severity or intensity of hallucinations or delusional thought, physical characteristics of the voices, and so on. Specialist assessment methods (such as psychiatric symptom rating scales [PSYRATS; Haddock, McCarron, & Tarrier, 1999]; the Maudsley Assessment of Delusions [Buchanan et al., 1993]; and the Beliefs about Voices Questionnaire [Chadwick & Birchwood, 1996]) provide scales for rating these various dimensions. Additional techniques such as experience sampling (Delespaul, 1995), concurrent monitoring or focusing (Haddock, Slade, et al., 1998), shadowing, symptom simulation, and diaries can be used in the collection of data relating to the subjective experience of the psychosis.

The interviewer should be particularly alert to variations and patterns in the experience of the symptoms. If patients hear voices, it is important to know to whom or what they attribute them, and where they think the voices are coming from, their level of power and control, and whether the voices are positive or negative, supportive, neutral, or hostile. For example, Birchwood and Iqbal (1998) reported that patients experiencing "powerful" voices were twice as likely to be depressed as those with less powerful voices.

The Emotions That Accompany Each Psychotic Symptom

For each symptom or psychotic experience, the interviewer should elicit the patient's emotional reaction that accompanies the symptom, starting with general questions such as "How do you feel when this happens?" and "How does this affect you?" and then move on to probe for more specific emotions: "Do you feel frightened/nervous/angry/sad/fed up/guilty/ashamed/down . . . ?" It is often a good idea to use a number of different descriptors for the same emotion (e.g., sad, down, fed up, moody, etc.). Once the interviewer has elicited the emotional reactions to the symptom in global terms, he or she should attempt to break down the emotion into three systems, that is, cognition (subjective experience), behavior, and physiological reaction (self-report). Thus, detailed questions should be asked about a specific emotion; for example, "When you feel angry about the voices, what type of thoughts go through your head?" Simulation exercises can assist this questioning, such as saying to the patient: "Imagine you were hearing the voices now and you are getting angry. What would be on your mind? What thoughts would you be having?" Similarly, the therapist can ask about the behavioral components of the emotion—"What do you do when you feel anxious?"—and physiological reactions—"How do you feel inside, in your body?" Here, probe questions about the type of physical reactions can be used, such as probes about increased heart rate, sweating, muscle tension, and so on. At the end of this section of the interview, the therapist should have a good picture of the psychotic symptoms and the emotions they elicit.

Antecedent Stimuli and Context

The interviewer is searching for triggers or precipitators that determine the context for the symptoms. Patients may be very aware of these; sometimes they are unaware of any pattern, but one does unfold with questioning; other patients, even with detailed questioning, are unable to identify any obvious context to their symptoms. Patients can be asked to monitor their symptoms and keep diaries to establish cues and patterns. It is helpful initially to obtain a time budget from patients about how they spend a typical day and week. This can alert the interviewer to any aspects of the patients' lifestyles or schedules that may be important and need further inquiry. For example, if a patient sleeps during the day and is up at night, there will be less to keep him or her occupied or distracted. The interviewer should ask about each symptom in turn and question whether there are any triggers, or whether the symptom occurs in certain circumstances, for example, asking whether the patient knows in what circumstances a symptom is going to "come on." Sometimes this can be asked in a different way; for example, "Are there any situations in which you always hear the voices?" Besides locations and circumstances, the interviewer should inquire about situations such as the time of day and, especially, social contexts.

Once the interviewer has asked about potential external stimuli, he or she should then ask about internal stimuli, such as internal feelings or specific thought patterns. The interviewer should also inquire about potential links between internal and external stimuli. For example, being with people may make patients aware of feeling tense and of a throbbing sensation in the head that makes them think that something has been implanted in their heads. A patient can be asked "Have you noticed that your head throbs at any particular time, or when you are doing anything in particular, or are in a specific place? Does it happen to you when you are with others and finding talking difficult? Does it happen when you feel you're under a lot of pressure or when demands are being made of you?" As a general rule, it is best to start with general questions and then probe for more specific examples.

Particular attention should be paid to chains of stimuli and responses, especially as these relate to misidentifications or misattribution (e.g., misattribution of physical sensations or misidentification of noises or olfactory cues). For example, one patient heard voices and attributed these to a gang of Hell's Angels that was going to attack him. This then generalized to attributing other noises, which were quite real, to evidence of the gang's imminent attack. Also, situations that patients find stressful need to be probed, including situations characterized by deficits or absence of purposeful behavior, such as periods of inactivity or insomnia. In these examples, the patient can be asked, "Do you find that there are particular times of the day or week when you have nothing to do or feel bored? Do you notice that these feelings or these experiences [psychotic symptoms] are especially strong at this time?"

Consequences

The interviewer should inquire about consequences of the symptoms. These can apply to a number of areas of long-term behavioral changes, such as severe avoidance and social withdrawal, isolation and loneliness, and also the consequence of persistent symptoms and psychotic disability, such as poor employment prospects, restricted social networks, and deprivation. The patient can be asked questions such as "How have these problems [voices/fears/illness] affected you/your life?" "How would things be different if these problems hadn't happened?" "How would you like to change things in your life/daily routine/circumstances?" and similar questions that investigate the effect of schizophrenia. Inquiry should also be made about behavior that protects or encourages particular types of thought or attitudes, such as those that reinforce delusional thinking or cause the patient to act in a way that sustains negative self-esteem. For example, the paranoid patient who accuses complete strangers of looking at him in a "funny way" finds that these actions attract attention.

Besides these overt consequences of symptoms and psychosis, there are also opportunities to establish reactions to the psychotic experience that may serve as feedback and maintain the psychosis. This line of inquiry is particularly important and can include behavior change that further exposes the patient to stressful or difficult situations, such as exposure to arguments or hostile social situations, increased inactivity or disengagement, and thought patterns about the experience. Here, it is useful to ask how patients interpret their experience and why it has happened, what they make of the voices, or how they think about themselves, particularly in terms of their own self-worth.

Coping

Having established a comprehensive picture of what patients experience and how it affects them, it is now important to find out how they deal with it. Patients can be asked about how they manage each symptom or particular experience: "How do you cope with that?" "Is there anything you can do to make that better or easier (or does anything make it worse)?" "What do you do when that happens, or when you feel like that?" It is also useful to evaluate how successfully the patient copes. By ranking the coping strategy on a 3-point scale, with 0 = "No or little use or moderately effective for a very short time"; 1 = "Moderately effective for a reasonable time, or very effective for a short time"; 2 = "Very effective for an extended period of time."

Many of these sections in the ACI will overlap, and a breakdown of some areas that are artificially divided provides a comprehensive and overinclusive structure for obtaining information about the experience of psychotic symptoms, their effects, and how patients react.

Once a comprehensive picture of the patient's psychotic experience has been built up, the interviewer should prepare a formulation of the patient's difficulties. The interviewer can discuss this formulation with the patient and outline the rationale for intervention. This process is assisted by the fact that the ACI will already have generated examples of the patient's coping ability. The patient will usually find it helpful if the interviewer emphasizes the natural and normal aspect of coping. For example, the interviewer can say:

"We all experience difficulties and unpleasant experiences in our life, and it is normal to attempt to cope and reduce the impact of such experiences. The experience of psychosis is no different in this respect. We have already talked at some length about how these experiences affect you. What we want to do now is to build systematically on your coping abilities and see if we can work together to reduce the experience and impact of the psychosis."

Discussing formulations is usually most successful if carried out collaboratively, with the patient playing an active part in identifying the factors that have contributed to his or her difficulties. Initial formulations may often just attempt to describe the cognitive, behavioral, and physiological/emotional factors contributing to the maintenance of the problems. The interviewer can then elaborate, highlighting possible explanatory and developmental factors, if necessary.

INTERVENTIONS

Cognitive-behavioral interventions tend to fall into three main areas: (1) those that emphasize coping and compensation, (2) those that emphasize changing reality monitoring skills, and (3) those that emphasize belief and attributional change. Intervention based upon the detailed and comprehensive information provided by the assessment and formulation should produce an overall intervention strategy, which includes a number of possible tactics for reducing dimensions of symptoms and distress. A range of intervention techniques has been developed through clinical experience and clinical trials, and this is outlined briefly under the three headings described.

Coping Enhancement and Compensation Strategies

The following general characteristics of coping training act as guiding principles; it is worth both discussing these with the patient at the start of treatment and using them to guide the therapy:

1. In the emphasis on the normal and general process of dealing with adversity, coping with a psychosis is an example.
2. Coping training is to be carried out systematically through overlearning, simulation, and role play.
3. Coping skills are additive in that different strategies can be added together in a sequence that progresses to *in vivo* implementation.

4. Intervention is based upon providing a new response set; this is a method of coping with an ongoing problem rather than being curative.
5. Learning cognitive coping skills is often through a process of external verbalization, which is slowly diminished until the required procedure is internalized and under covert control.
6. Learning behavioral coping skills is usually through a process of graded practice or rehearsal.

Examples of strategies that generally fall under this heading follow.

Attention Switching

This process whereby patients actively change the focus of their attention from one subject or experience to another involves inhibiting an ongoing response and initiating an alternative response. There is evidence that switching attention is a specific deficit found in patients with schizophrenia (Smith et al., 1998); hence, training in this task may be particularly helpful. Patients are trained to switch attention on cue through rehearsal, often to a set of positive images, within the session. For example, patients can be trained in eliciting a visual image of a pleasant experience from their past, until they are able to produce a strong, vivid image at will. They can then be trained to be aware of a type of thought or hallucination and use this to cue their positive visual image as a distraction. This can be practiced in the therapy session, with the therapist simulating the delusional thought or voice by speaking it out loud, while the patient activates the attention-switching strategies. This method works best when it is overlearned.

Attention Narrowing

This is a process whereby patients restrict the range and content of their attention. Many patients talk about "blanking" their mind or focusing their attention as a method of coping. Evidence suggests that one problem faced by patients with schizophrenia is an inability to filter information input adequately, to distinguish signal from noise (Shakow, 1962). Training in response inhibition and being able to focus and improve attentional control may assist patients in overcoming this difficulty.

Increased Activity Levels

Many patients appear vulnerable to delusional thoughts or hallucinations during periods of inactivity, a problem to which patients with schizophrenia appear particularly prone. They also report that finding something to do and engaging in activities is helpful (Tarrier, 1987). Thus, simple activity scheduling can be a powerful coping strategy, especially if implemented at the onset of the symptom, thus creating a dual-task competing for attentional resources.

Social Engagement and Disengagement

Although many patients tolerate social interactions poorly, surprisingly, many also find social engagement a useful method of coping. It is advisable to balance the amount of social stimulation involved in any interaction with the patient's tolerance level and teach the patient that there are levels of social disengagement that can be used to help develop tolerance of social stimulation. Social withdrawal and avoidance are common responses to experiencing overstimulation due to social interaction. However, patients can learn less drastic methods of disengagement, such as leaving the room for a short period and then returning, or temporarily moving away from the social group and functionally disengaging by not conversing for short periods or lowering their gaze. By using these methods, patients can control and tolerate social stimulation, and learn that their beliefs about the unpleasant or threatening nature of social interaction are excessive and open to disconfirmation. Patients may also feel more confident to initiate social interaction as a coping method to reduce the impact of their symptoms and to reinforce the belief that they have control over their circumstances. Simple training in specific skills for interaction and role plays can facilitate this learning.

Modified Self-Statements and Internal Dialogue

Patients' use of internal dialogue to direct behavior can be incorporated successfully into intervention (e.g., Meichenbaum & Cameron, 1973). The use of self-statements and internal dialogue can serve a number of functions: in emotion control, such as teaching patients to overcome negative emotions associated with their voices; in cueing goal-directed behavior; and in cueing and directing reality testing. In each case, the patient is taught statements that direct an appropriate response such as "I don't need to be afraid," "I need to keep going and walk down the street," or "Why do I think that woman is looking at me when I've never seen her before?" During the treatment session, the patient is first asked to repeat the set of statements out loud when given the appropriate cue, with the appropriate statements written down on cue cards. The verbalized statements are then gradually reduced in loudness until they are internalized. Patients then practice these in simulated situations within the session.

Dearousing Techniques

Since high levels of arousal have been implicated in the psychopathology of schizophrenia (Dawson et al., 1989) and frequently occur as both antecedents (Slade, 1972) and responses to psychotic experience (Tarrier & Turpin, 1992), teaching patients to cope with this arousal is important. These coping strategies can be simple, passive behaviors to avoid agitation, such as sitting quietly instead of pacing up and down, or they can be more active methods of arousal control, such as breathing exercises or quick relaxation.

Increasing Reality or Source Monitoring

Increasing patients' ability to source-monitor correctly (particularly in relation to monitoring the source of hallucinations) can be achieved using a number of strategies. The aim is to help individuals to examine their experience in more detail, with the assumption that this will help them to identify the source of the experience more accurately. Strategies include the following.

Awareness Training

Patients are taught to be aware of and monitor the onset and cessation of their positive symptoms. There are similarities here with self-monitoring in the self-regulation processes described by Karoly and Kanfer (1982), and multiple ways in which the individual can achieve this. For example, during sessions, patients can be encouraged to indicate the onset and cessation to the therapist and to explore the factors that may contribute to positive symptoms. Between sessions, patients can use diaries and other self-report strategies to increase awareness.

Focusing and Self-Monitoring

Focusing strategies to increase patients' source-monitoring skills and prepare them to engage in belief-modification strategies have been described in detail by Haddock and colleagues in the treatment of auditory hallucinations (Haddock, Bentall, & Slade, 1996; Haddock, Slade, et al., 1998). This approach encourages patients to concentrate on their hallucinatory experience, attending to the physical characteristics, the content, and the origin and beliefs about their voices. This involves encouraging patients to record the characteristics of their voices and use these records during the treatment sessions to examine beliefs about their experiences. Belief modification techniques (see below) can then be used to modify the experience. This type of approach has also been described by Persaud and Marks (1995), who emphasized focusing on the hallucinatory experience in order to expose individuals to the anxiety associated with their symptoms.

Belief and Attribution Modification

Identifying and helping patients examine their beliefs about their psychotic symptoms is an important aspect of intervention. During the assessment phase, a historical consideration of how these beliefs have changed over time can provide important information about how and why individuals have developed their beliefs. It is often possible to see that even bizarre delusional beliefs can be understandable in the light of the contextual circumstances that led to their formation. The following techniques can be useful in belief change.

Examination of Beliefs and Reattribution

Patients are asked to generate an alternative explanation for an experience and then practice a reattributional statement when it occurs. For example, patients can reattribute a voice that appears to come from an external source to an internal one, such as their own thoughts. They can be taught to reattribute the actions and motives of others from the sinister and personal to the more mundane and ordinary, thus removing the threatening aspects. These reattributions can be learned systematically through self-statements as part of the internal dialogue. Once patients make changes that increase their control over their symptoms or circumstances, their attention can be drawn to these self-statements as evidence for a change in belief about the nature of their symptoms or their ability to exert control. In this way, attributions relating to the dimensions of internal–external, personal–general, controllable–uncontrollable, and stable–unstable to explain events and experience can be changed.

Belief Modification

Patients can learn to examine and challenge inappropriate beliefs by examining the evidence and generating alternative explanations. Many patients do this to some extent already, but the level of arousal, or the level of isolation and avoidance experienced can make these attempts largely unsuccessful. These methods are very similar to those used in traditional cognitive therapy except that the patient may need more prompting and the goal is to incorporate the skills of belief modification into a self-regulatory process. Patients can be encouraged to question their beliefs as they occur: "What would be the purpose of someone spying on them? How much effort and cost would it take? How would this be resourced and organized, and for what gain?" Similarly, patients can be encouraged to investigate inconsistencies in their thinking and to use these to make challenges. For example, one patient who was involved in a fight 15 years earlier still avoided young men because he feared that the same group of young men was out to get revenge. He was asked to consider the fact that the members of the gang would now be in their mid- to late 30s and that he has been vigilant for the wrong age group. This can be used to challenge the fear that he needs to be vigilant in order to stay safe, because, over recent years, he has been concentrating on the wrong characteristics of these men. Patients can also learn to examine evidence to challenge their beliefs about their voices. Whereas they have perceived the voices as omnipotent and truthful, they can investigate the evidence to see if they have been incorrect at any time. Identifying such errors can be used as evidence that the voices have been wrong on occasions and are hence fallible. For example, one patient who heard voices telling him that he had committed a murder and rape was convinced the voices were true because he thought they were omnipotent, and because he could not remember *not* committing the crime. The voices also told him he was "Russian"; of this he was less convinced. Encouraged to examine the evidence for his being "Russian," he was able to conclude that he was not, and that the voices were incorrect. This allowed the therapist to challenge the truth of the voices accusing him of crimes. The patient was also encouraged to examine whether his use of "evidence" in concluding that he must have committed the crime, because he could not remember *not* doing so, was the best way to evaluate the situation. He was asked instead to elicit what objective evidence there would have been if the crime had been committed, such as a police investigation, and then to evaluate the facts as he knew them against the presence or absence of this more objective evidence.

Reality Testing and Behavioral Experiments

Probably the strongest way of testing a belief is to test it out in reality by taking some type of action, behavior change being likely the best way to produce cognitive change. Patients sometimes do this naturally, although a tendency toward biased interpretation and hypothesis protection can lead them to erroneous conclusions. Patients can learn to identify specific beliefs and generate competing predictions that can be tested. The failure to do this in real life usually leads to patterns of avoidance, which can be reversed to challenge the beliefs upon which they are underpinned. For example, a patient who believes that he cannot travel on a particular bus route because all the passengers know he is gay can be asked to specify how he would predict the other passengers will act. He is then asked to travel a short distance on the bus to test this out, followed by increasingly longer journeys to confirm the test. Patients can also use strategies such as attention switching to test the belief that hallucinations are uncontrollable. If the hallucinatory effect is diminished, even briefly, then this belief has been disproved.

Another useful experiment to demonstrate that voices may be interpreted as internal speech or thought that is not correctly identified, is as follows: First is the given possibility of hallucinations being internal, and unrecognized as such, as an alternative to being external and real. Patients are then asked to help in a short experiment by closing their eyes and raising their right hand above their shoulder. They are then asked to keep their eyes shut and say where their arms are located. Of course, they are able to do this correctly. Patients are then asked how they knew where their arm was, since they did not see it move. If unable to provide an answer, patients can be told that there is a feedback mechanism inside their body that allows their brain to know where their arm, or any other part of their body, is at all times. They can then be asked what would happen if this feedback mechanism went wrong and they saw their arm moving but no longer realized that they themselves were moving it. They could be asked, "Would it seem as though some external force was moving your arm?" Patients will usually agree with this. (This is very similar to Frith's [1987] explanation of passivity.) It can then be suggested that perhaps something similar is happening with their voices and thoughts. The process by which the brain is able to identify thoughts as their own is malfunctioning, so what might be the result of this? The conclusion is that thoughts and subvocal speech might be explained as originating from an external source. This is normally how an auditory hallucination is perceived, as though it were emanating from a real and external entity. The outcome of the experiment is that the therapist and patient have come to a plausible alternative explanation for the patient's experience of hearing voices.

DECIDING ON THE BEST WAY TO INTERVENE

Patients' strategies to deal with their symptoms have usually developed over time and vary in complexity from simple and direct attempts to control cognitive processes, such as attention switching or distraction, to more complex, self-directed methods that modify cognitive content and inference. Frequently, combinations of different strategies can be built up during treatment, for example, the use of attention-switching and dearousing techniques to help reduce the emotional impact of a delusion, so that reality testing can be implemented. Without these initial coping methods, patients are sometimes not able to undergo reality testing or belief modification approaches. Furthermore, some initial coping strategies can be used to challenge the strength of the delusion of omnipotence of the voices and provide an increase in self-efficacy. Questions can be asked such as "You've used these attention-switching methods to cope effectively with your voices. What does that tell you about them being all powerful and you being helpless?" Patients may well make statements that indicate the voices have been demonstrated as fallible, and that they had some control over the situation, which can then be used as self-statements or a modified internal dialogue to enhance further self-efficacy and coping.

It is also anticipated that practice in the selection, inhibition, and generation of responses will result in improvements of executive control and compensate for deficits in this function.

Providing an alternative framework in which to understand patients' experience is important. Simply trying to persuade them that they have an illness, and that all their experiences are due to this, is seldom effective and has usually been tried before, often by the treating psychiatrist. The "You are ill" explanation goes against patients' own experience, and they are usually well versed in being able to reject this as a credible explanation. Providing alternative psychological explanations for patients' symptoms and experience helps to set the scene for active intervention. Showing patients that they have some control over their symptom through a behavioral experiment begins to erode their belief that the voices are omnipotent and all powerful. This may be a gradual erosion of belief that has to be repeated many times given that such delusional beliefs are often very strong and impervious to challenge.

DIFFICULT CLINICAL ISSUES

There may well be cases in which patients are so convinced in the reality of their delusions that attempting to weaken them by belief modification and reality testing is counterproductive. This may be easier to understand when one has explored the possible functional nature of delusional belief. This may be obvious when a person has a grandiose delusional belief; however, many psychotic experiences commonly have important maintaining factors. Strategies to improve low self-esteem, depression, and suicidal ideation may be necessary before embarking on specific strategies designed to reduce the severity of psychotic symptoms. This should be apparent from the formulation. In these cases, maintaining the engagement of the patient in treatment and identification of a commonly agreed-upon treatment goal are important. Thus, it is advisable to identify the patient's distress rather than immediately target the delusions or hallucinations. It may well be that once the patient's level of arousal has been reduced, then attending to the symptoms themselves may be more acceptable and productive.

In addition to the complex issues that may arise when working with patients with only one diagnosis, mental health services are increasingly being challenged with patients who meet criteria for more than one disorder. For example, large numbers of patients may have coexisting substance misuse problems, personality disorder, learning disability, or problems relating to treatment adherence, poor engagement with services, and aggressive or violent behavior problems. Although very little evaluation of CBT as applied to these more complex groups has been carried out, these issues are increasingly presented to therapists. Recent research has indicated that combining CBT approaches to different disorders can be effective. For example, a recent, small, randomized trial has shown that integrating CBT for psychosis and motivation interviewing for substance use problems can result in significantly better outcomes than enhanced treatment as usual (Barrowclough et al., 2001; Haddock et al., 2002). In addition, case series evidence suggests that combining CBT approaches for psychosis and anger can be effective at reducing the severity of these problems (Lowens, Haddock, Barrowclough, Brosnan, & Novaco, 2001).

Ideally, the therapist will be able to engage the patients and they will work together to arrive at an agreed-upon formulation that allows the initiation of a strategic intervention to resolve the patient's difficulties. The increasing complexity and commitment from both the patient and therapist are presented diagrammatically by the pyramid in Figure 4.2. Because schizophrenia is such a severe disorder, it may not be possible to achieve this ideal with all patients, or it may take considerable time. With some patients, especially those who are very suspicious and noncompliant, or who abuse substances or are violent, engagement may be a difficult process. Even when engagement is achieved, the therapist may have to adopt a symptom-relief approach, because the patient may be unwilling or unable to undergo a more detailed case formulation assessment.

CASE EXAMPLE

The following case example illustrates the typical presentation of a CBT-treated patient with chronic psychosis.

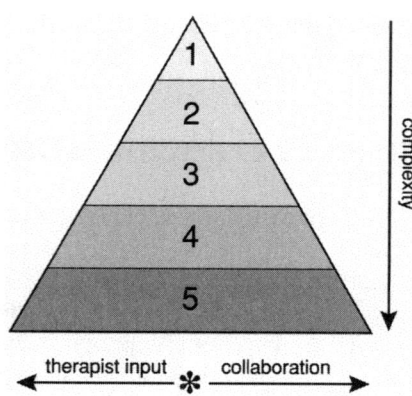

FIGURE 4.2. Levels of intervention. Level 1, engagement; level 2, pragmatic intervention (formulation not possible); level 3, problem identification and collaborative formulation; level 4, formulation-based strategic intervention; level 5, schematic intervention.

James, a 32-year-old man with a 12-year history of schizophrenia, lived in supported accommodation, where he was responsible for his own care but had staff on call at all times, if needed. He saw his mother, who lived nearby, one to two times per month. James also had a brother, whom he saw approximately once a year. He experienced a range of psychotic symptoms, including auditory hallucinations, paranoid delusions, occasional thought disorder, and negative symptoms. He was referred for CBT by his caseworker, who was concerned that James's auditory hallucinations and paranoia were having a severely negative effect on his mood. These symptoms had persisted despite optimum doses of neuroleptic medication.

Engagement and Initial Assessment

Initially, James was slightly hostile when approached by the therapist. He felt that his caseworker and psychiatrist were not helpful, since they attributed all his problems to his "schizophrenia" and did not acknowledge that people were trying to do him harm. Hence, initial engagement sessions focused on trying to establish whether there were concerns with which the therapist could help James. This was initially hampered by James's wish that the therapist would try to persuade the psychiatrist that his experiences were "real" and to ask that his medication be discontinued. The therapist empathized with his worries and suggested that if it were possible for James to explore and describe his experiences, this would help illustrate to all involved the true origin of his experiences. Psychological treatment was presented as a possible "independent" help to resolve the disagreement between James and the mental health service. The nature of weekly sessions and the role of the therapist were described to highlight the key features of the CBT approach. Also discussed was a handout that described the nature of CBT in terms of its key features, that is, its focus on problems rather than diagnoses; its collaborative, practical, and goal-oriented nature; and its focus on thoughts and feelings, and their links with key problems. James was skeptical about the approach at first but agreed to give it a try. After four sessions, it was possible for James and the therapist to agree as to the nature of the key problems:

1. Frustration with his mental health care and the belief that his illness was really depression, not schizophrenia.
2. Constant worry that a government intelligence agency (MI5) was tracking and monitoring his actions.
3. Being bothered almost constantly by MI5 transmitting messages to him (which he experienced as voices in his head).
4. Depression and thoughts of suicide.

Because it was causing him some considerable distress, James and the therapist agreed that problem 1 would be an initial target for possible resolution before proceeding to explore the other areas of concern. As a result, it was agreed that the therapist would spend some time gaining a clear idea of James's experience and compare this to the diagnostic criteria for schizophrenia and depression by getting written information on the nature of schizophrenia and depression, and working through this over the next two sessions. James previously had not seen this type of information, and it became apparent that his beliefs about schizophrenia were based on inaccurate impressions that were akin to "Hollywood" ideas of mental illness. This was despite his having received information leaflets in the past, which James had dismissed, because he did not feel they applied to him. However, this information did not result in James's acceptance that he suffered from schizophrenia. He was able to acknowledge that some of his experiences were very similar to those found in schizophrenia. However, he felt that, for him, the difference was that his experiences were "real," whereas the experiences of people who suffered from schizophrenia were not. James felt it was possible that he had had schizophrenia in the past, since he had previously heard voices that he believed came from the devil. He thought these types of voices were typical of schizophrenia and was able to acknowledge that medication may have been helpful in reducing these experiences. This shift in thinking marked a change in James's willingness to engage in further sessions of CBT, and he expressed a desire to look in more detail at ways that could help with his current "nonschizophrenic" difficulties.

The next phase of assessment focused on the three latter problems on James's problem list. In order to facilitate a detailed cognitive-behavioral analysis of James's key symptoms, the therapist provided a rationale that exploring these areas might help James to develop ways of coping and improve his feelings of hopelessness and depression. He also conducted a detailed historical review to examine the onset and course of James's symptom development, which revealed some salient points to use as a focus of therapy:

1. The onset of his illness coincided with an extremely stressful time in James's life, coupled with experimentation with a range of street drugs. This had been preceded by a gradual deterioration in his social and academic functioning.
2. He had been given a range of antipsychotic medication since the onset of his problems.
3. James had limited social contacts and had had few opportunities to pursue "normal" life experiences, which saddened him. His main wish was to have an ordinary job, his own flat, a car, and a girlfriend. He thought that MI5 was preventing him from doing these things.
4. His beliefs about MI5 began at the onset of his illness. However, the voices he experienced did not begin until a couple of years after his first hospital admission. James believed that MI5 was targeting him for special attention because he had special knowledge about scientific issues to which it wanted access. James felt that, over recent years,

the government had used many of his ideas. James was proud of his ideas but wished that the harassment from MI5 would stop.

5. The content of his voices was usually derogatory and consisted of comments suggesting that he was stupid, a waste of time, would never amount to anything, and would never have a job, a girlfriend, or be normal. James believed that these voices originating from MI5 were to prevent him from getting on with his life and receiving recognition for his ideas. As a result, he felt depressed and hopeless. Occasionally, a voice said positive things, such as "You'll be okay, don't worry." He found this voice supportive and enjoyed it, but James was unclear as to its origin. Sometimes he thought it was MI5 trying to lull him into a false sense of security.

Formulation and Intervention

Initially, a basic maintenance formulation proposed to James involved translating this information into a structure that allowed him to view how thoughts, feelings, and behavior interact to exacerbate problems. This focused on the voices, since they appeared to be key factors contributing to James's low mood.

It was hypothesized that the occurrence of the voices triggered thoughts such as "They are right; I'm never going to get a job; no one will every fancy me." This triggered intense feelings of hopelessness, frustration, and sometimes anger. Often, it resulted in James's withdrawing from other people and his occasional hostility or aggression toward people around him. Having fewer positive social contacts increased James's sensitivity to voice content with similar themes. He was encouraged to explore the idea that a key feature of this experience was that he usually agreed with the voice content, and that it was possible that if he thought the voices were wrong, he might be less upset when he heard them. These observations then led to explorations of whether the voices were true, the evidence for this, and tests of some of the things the voices were saying. For example, James believed that the voices were trying to put him down, to stop his getting a job, and a girlfriend, and so on. However, when the practical problems that prevented him from achieving these goals were explored, a number of non-voice-related hurdles were discovered. Therapy then focused on overcoming these hurdles to demonstrate that the voices had little control over James's potential achievements. He accepted this rationale, and it was possible for him to set targets associated with daytime occupation and increasing his social contact. These targets and the disconfirmation of the perceived control of the voices over his behavior then became the main focus of therapy.

James was also instructed in attention-switching techniques to elicit a vivid mental image of a pleasant experience. He was then instructed to be aware of the onset of his voices; this was practiced in training sessions, with the therapist simulating James's auditory hallucination. James then was trained to switch his attention away from the content of his auditory hallucinations to his positive mental images as quickly as he could, after the onset of the voices. His ability to do this was another example of James's exerting control over his voices. This also gave him a powerful coping strategy to deal with the voices when they became distressing and intrusive. He was also able to use this technique to cope with delusional paranoid thoughts.

The therapist also discussed the role of depression in the formulation and a CBT explanation of this was incorporated into James's training. Education about the nature of depression and its components was included as part of the intervention program, and strategies to manage depression were explored. Activity scheduling and work on management of negative thoughts were particularly relevant for James, and he was able to adopt the strategies into his life.

Discussion and Outcome

Over 20 sessions, a number of positive developments had occurred. James felt that his diagnosis was probably correct, although he still felt his depression was a key feature. He continued to experience voices, but these were much reduced in frequency and impact. James had a range of strategies to deal with these and was making some inroads into increasing his social and recreational contacts. The belief that MI5 had targeted James was never a main focus of therapy. It was hypothesized that this belief was extremely functional for him, providing him with a great deal of positive esteem, which he had not gained from other sources; hence, the therapy aim was to increase self-esteem rather than to engage in belief modification procedures directly. This procedure was appropriate, and James reported a decrease in the degree to which he was bothered by MI5 over the remaining weeks of therapy. Although his belief that this was happening did not change, the evidence that MI5 was able to control his life was clearly weakened. A detailed "staying well" plan developed by the therapist included handouts used during therapy, copies of formulations compiled in therapy, a detailed account of the most helpful strategies James had discovered, and an action plan for keeping well. This was a detailed description of strategies he could use to maintain his current status, of an action plan to use should his problems start to become more troublesome, and of a strategy to use if James felt he needed emergency help. This was written in terms of not only things that James could do in these situations but also what mental health services would provide for him. This was agreed collaboratively between James and his caseworker, who agreed to monitor and implement this plan.

CONCLUSIONS

There is now significant evidence to establish the efficacy of CBT with chronic psychotic patients and encouraging data indicate that acute patients may also benefit, although the lack of trained therapists may limit the availability of such treatment at the present time (Adams, 2000). In the United Kingdom, efforts over the last decade to train the mental health professional workforce in the methods described in this chapter have met with varying degrees of success (Tarrier, Barrowclough, Haddock, & McGovern, 1999). In 1992, two training centers were funded in England, one at the Institute of Psychiatry in London and the other in Manchester, to train community psychiatric nurses in psychosocial interventions. The training course was for 1 year, part-time, and consisted of three modules: (1) case management, which included a psychiatric assessment and service organization; (2) family intervention, which consisted of family functioning assessment and behavioral family management (see Barrowclough & Tarrier, 1992, for details of this intervention); and (3) CBT, which has been described in this chapter. Considerable emphasis was placed on clinical supervision and, in addition to the academic teaching, trainees had to recruit two individual patients and two families to treat for the duration of the course. Trainees were required to obtain a satisfactory standard in this clinical work, which was assessed through the rating of audiotaped clinical sessions. The Thorn Nurse Training Project, so named because the initial funding came from the Sir Jules Thorn Charitable Trust, was evaluated from its inception. The results demonstrated that trainees increased their knowledge and skills during training, and patient outcomes for those who received individual and family interventions showed improvements (Lancashire et al., 1996). Thus, there appeared to be empirical evidence that these psychosocial interventions could be effectively applied within standard mental health services. The Manchester center now receives funding from the National Health Service (the Collaboration of Psychosocial Education—COPE—Initiative). Training is multidisciplinary, and as well as nurses, occupational therapist, psychiatrists, and clinical psychologists have also been trained. The structure of the original project course has been retained, with an additional focus on mental health teamwork in the case management module. Satellite courses are now running under contract at other centers throughout the country, and it is anticipated that this method of dissemination will make these innovative psychological treatments much more widely available throughout the U.K. National Health Services.

REFERENCES

Adams, C. (2000). Psychosocial interventions for schizophrenia. *Effective Health Care, 6,* 1–8.

Barrowclough, C., Haddock, G., Tarrier, N., Lewis, S., Moring, J., O'Brien, R., Schofield, N., & McGovern, J. (2001). Randomized controlled trial of integrated cognitive behavior therapy and motivational intervention for people with schizophrenia and substance misuse. *American Journal of Psychiatry, 158,* 1706–1713.

Barrowclough, C., & Tarrier, N. (1992). *Families of schizophrenic patients: A cognitive-behavioural intervention.* London: Chapman & Hall.

Beck, A. T. (1952). Successful outpatient psychotherapy of a chronic schizophrenic with a delusion based on borrowed guilt. *Psychiatry, 15,* 305–312.

Bentall, R. P. (1990). The illusion of reality: A review and integration of psychological research on hallucinations. *Psychological Bulletin, 107,* 82–95.

Bentall, R. P., Haddock, G., & Slade, P. (1994). Psychological treatment of auditory hallucinations: From theory to therapy. *Behavior Therapy, 25,* 51–66.

Birchwood, M., & Iqbal, Z. (1998). Depression and suicidal thinking in psychosis: A cognitive approach. In T. Wykes, N. Tarrier, & S. Lewis (Eds.), *Outcome and innovation in psychological treatment of schizophrenia* (pp. 81–100). Chichester, UK: Wiley.

Breier, A., & Strauss, J. S. (1983). Self-control in psychotic disorders. *Archives of General Psychiatry, 40,* 1141–1145.

Brenner, H. D., Boker, W., Muller, J., Spichtig, L., & Wurgler, S. (1987). Autoprotective efforts among schizophrenics, neurotics and controls. *Acta Psychiatrica Scandinavica, 75,* 405–414.

British Psychological Society. (1999). *Recent advances in understanding mental illness and psychotic experience: A report by the British Psychological Society.* Leicester, UK: Author.

Buchanan, A., Reed, A., Wessely, S., Garety, P., Taylor, P., Grubin, D., & Dunn, G. (1993). Acting on delusions: II. The phenomenological correlates of acting on delusions. *British Journal of Psychiatry, 163,* 77–81.

Carr, V. (1988). Patients' techniques for coping with schizophrenia: An exploratory study. *British Journal of Medical Psychology, 61,* 339–352.

Chadwick, P., & Birchwood, M. (1994). The omnipotence of voices: I. A cognitive approach to auditory hallucinations. *British Journal of Psychiatry, 164,* 190–201.

Chadwick, P., & Birchwood, M. (1996). The omnipotence of voices: II. The Belief about Voices Questionnaire (BAVQ). *British Journal of Psychiatry, 166,* 773–776.

Cohen, C. I., & Berk, B. S. (1985). Personal coping styles in schizophrenic out patients. *Hospital and Community Psychiatry, 36,* 407–410.

David, A. (1994). The neuropsychological origin of auditory hallucinations. In A. David & J. Cutting (Eds.), *The neuropsychology of schizophrenia* (pp. 269–316). Hove, UK: Erlbaum.

Dawson, M. E., Nuechterlein, K. H., & Adams, R. M. (1989). Schizophrenic disorders. In G. Turpin (Ed.), *Handbook of clinical psychophysiology* (pp. 393–418). Chichester, UK: Wiley.

Delespaul, A. E. G. (1994). *Assessing schizophrenia in daily life: The experience sampling method.* Maastricht, Netherlands: Universitaire Pers Maastricht.

Department of Health. (2000). *The National Service Framework for mental health: Modern standards and service models.* London: Author.

Drake, R. E., Goldman, H. H., Leff, H. S., Lehman, A. F., Dixon, L., Mueser, K. T., & Torrey, W. C. (2001). Implementing evidence-based practises in routine mental health service settings. *Psychiatric Services, 52,* 179–182.

Drury, V., Birchwood, M., Cochrane, R., & MacMillan, F. (1996a). Cognitive therapy and recovery from acute psychosis: A controlled trial: I. Impact on psychotic symptoms. *British Journal of Psychiatry, 169,* 593–601.

Drury, V., Birchwood, M., Cochrane, R., & MacMillan, F. (1996b). Cognitive therapy and recovery from acute psychosis: A controlled trial: II. Impact on recovery time. *British Journal of Psychiatry, 169,* 601–607.

Falloon, I. R. H., & Talbot, R. E. (1981). Persistent auditory hallucinations: Coping mechanisms and implications for management. *Psychological Medicine, 11,* 329–339.

Frith, C. (1987). The positive and negative symptoms of schizophrenia reflect impairment in the perception and initiation of action. *Psychological Medicine, 17,* 631–648.

Frith, C. (1992). *The cognitive neuropsychology of schizophrenia.* Hove, UK: Erlbaum.

Frith, C. (1994). Theory of mind in schizophrenia. In A. S. David & J. C. Cutting (Eds.), *The neuropsychology of schizophrenia* (pp. 147–162). Hove, UK: Erlbaum.

Geddes, J., Reynolds, S., Streiner, D., Szatmari, P., & Haynes, B. (1998). Evidence-based practice in mental health. *Evidence-Based Mental Health, 1,* 4–5.

Haddock, G., Barrowclough, C., Tarrier, N., Lewis, S., Moring, J., Schofield, N., Quinn, J., Lowens, I., Davies, L., & Palmer, L. (2002). *Randomised controlled trial of integrated cognitive behaviour therapy and motivational intervention for people with schizophrenia and substance misuse: 18 month follow-up and service outcomes.* Manuscript submitted for publication.

Haddock, G., Bentall, R., & Slade, P. D. (1996). Psychological treatment of auditory hallucinations: Focussing or distraction. In G. Haddock & P. D. Slade (Eds.), *Cognitive-behavioural interventions with psychotic disorders* (pp. 45–70). London: Routledge.

Haddock, G., McCarron, J., & Tarrier, N. (1999). Scales to measure dimensions of hallucinations and delusions: The psychotic symptom rating scales (PSYRATS). *Psychological Medicine, 29,* 879–889.

Haddock, G., Slade, P., Bentall, R. P., Reid, D., & Faragher, E. B. (1998). A trial examining the long-term effectiveness of focussing and distraction in the management of auditory hallucinations. *British Journal of Medical Psychology, 71,* 339–349.

Haddock, G., & Tarrier, N. (1998). Assessment and formulation in the cognitive behavioral treatment of psychosis. In N. Tarrier, A. Wells, & G. Haddock (Eds.), *Treating complex cases: The cognitive behavioural therapy approach* (pp. 155–175). Chichester, UK: Wiley.

Haddock, G., Tarrier, N., Morrison, A. P., Hopkins, R., Drake, R., & Lewis, S. (1999). A pilot study evaluating the effectiveness of individual inpatient cognitive-behavioural therapy in early psychosis. *Social Psychiatry and Psychiatric Epidemiology, 34,* 254–258.

Haddock, G., Tarrier, N., Spaulding, W., Yusupoff, L., Kinney, C., & McCarthy, E. (1998). Individual cognitive-behavior therapy in the treatment of schizophrenia: A review. *Clinical Psychology Review, 18,* 821–838.

Hawton, K., Salkovskis, P., Kirk, J., & Clark, D. M. (1989). *Cognitive behaviour therapy for psychiatric problems.* Oxford, UK: Oxford University Press.

Hemsley, D. (1994). Perceptual and cognitive abnormalities as the bases for schizophrenic symptoms. In A. S. David & J. C. Cutting (Eds.), *The neuropsychology of schizophrenia* (pp. 97–118). Hove, UK: Erlbaum.

Hoffman, R. E. (1986). Verbal hallucinations and language production processes in schizophrenia. *Behavioural and Brain Sciences, 9,* 503–548.

Joint British Psychological Society and Royal College of Psychiatrists Schizophrenia Guideline Development Group. (2001). *The psychosocial management of schizophrenia*. London: Department of Health.

Karoly, P., & Kanfer, F. H. (1982). *Self-management and behavior change: From theory to practice*. New York: Pergamon Press.

Kinderman, P., & Lobban, F. (2000). Evolving formulations: Sharing complex information with clients. *Behavioural and Cognitive Psychotherapy, 28*, 307–310.

Kinney, C. F. (2000). *Coping with schizophrenia: The significance of appraisal*. Unpublished PhD thesis, Faculty of Medicine, University of Manchester, Manchester, UK.

Kuipers, E., Garety, P., Fowler, D., Chisholm, D., Freeman, D., Dunn, G., Bebbington, P., & Hadley, C. (1998). London–East Anglia randomised controlled trial of cognitive-behavioural therapy for psychosis: III. Follow-up and economic evaluation at 18 months. *British Journal of Psychiatry, 173*, 61–68.

Kuipers, E., Garety, P., Fowler, D., Dunn, G., Bebbington, P., Freeman, D., & Hadley, C. (1997). London–East Anglia randomised controlled trial of cognitive-behavioural therapy for psychosis: I. Effects of the treatment phase. *British Journal of Psychiatry, 171*, 319–327.

Lancashire, S., Haddock, G., Tarrier, N., Baguley, I., Butterworth, C. A., & Brooker, C. (1996). The impact of training community psychiatric nurses to use psychosocial interventions with people who have serious mental health problems: The Thorn Nurse Training Project. *Psychiatric Services, 48*, 39–41.

Lewis, S., Tarrier, N., Haddock, G., Bentall, R., Kinderman, P., Kingdon, P., & the SOCRATES Group. (in press). A randomised trial of cognitive-behaviour therapy in early schizophrenia and related disorders. *British Journal of Psychiatry*.

Lowens, I., Haddock, G., Barrowclough, C., Brosnan, N., & Novaco, R. W. (2001). *Cognitive-behaviour therapy for inpatients with psychosis and anger problems within a low secure environment*. Manuscript submitted for publication.

Maher, B. A. (1988). Anomalous experience and delusional thinking: The logic of explanation. In T. F. Oltmans & B. A. Maher (Eds.), *Delusional beliefs* (pp. 15–33). New York: Wiley.

Meichenbaum, D., & Cameron, R. (1973). Training schizophrenics to talk to themselves: A means of developing attentional control. *Behavior Therapy, 4*, 515–534.

Miller, W. R., & Rollnick, S. (1995). What is motivational interviewing? *Behavioural and Cognitive Psychotherapy, 23*, 325–334.

Miller, W. R., & Rollnick, S. (2002). *Motivational interviewing: Preparing people for change* (2nd ed.). New York: Guilford Press.

Morrison, A. P., & Baker, C. A. (2000). Intrusive thoughts and auditory hallucinations: A comparative study of intrusions in psychosis. *Behaviour Research and Therapy, 38*, 1097–1106.

Nuechterlein, K. H. (1987). Vulnerability models for schizophrenia: State of the art. In H. Hafner, W. F. Gattaz, & W. Janzarik (Eds.), *Search for the cause of schizophrenia* (pp. 297–316). Heidelberg: Springer-Verlag.

Nuechterlein, K. H., & Subotnik, K. L. (1998). The cognitive origins of schizophrenia and prospects for intervention. In T. Wykes, N. Tarrier, & S. Lewis (Eds.), *Outcome and innovation in psychological treatment of schizophrenia* (pp. 18–41). Chichester, UK: Wiley.

Persaud, R., & Marks, I. (1995). A pilot study of exposure control of auditory hallucinations in schizophrenia. *British Journal of Psychiatry, 167*, 45–50.

Persons, J. B. (1989). *Cognitive therapy in practice: A case formulation approach*. New York: Norton.

Romme, M. A. J., & Escher, A. D. (1989). Hearing voices. *Schizophrenia Bulletin, 15*, 209–216.

Sensky, T., Turkington, D., Kingdon, D., Scott, J. L., Scott, J., Siddle, R., O'Carroll, M., & Barnes, T. R. E. (2000). A randomised controlled trial of cognitive behavioural therapy for persistent symptoms in schizophrenia resistant to medication. *Archives of General Psychiatry, 57*, 165–172.

Shakow, D. (1962). Segmental set: A theory of the formal psychological deficits in schizophrenia. *Archives of General Psychiatry, 6*, 600–612.

Slade, P. D. (1972). The effects of systematic desensitisation on auditory hallucinations. *Behaviour Research and Therapy, 10*, 85–91.

Smith, G. L., Large, M. M., Kavanagh, D. J., Karayanidis, F., Barrett, N. A., Michie, P. T., & O'Sullivan, B. T. (1998). Further evidence for a deficit in switching attention in schizophrenia. *Journal of Abnormal Psychology, 107,* 390–398.

Tarrier, N. (1987). An investigation of residual psychotic symptoms in discharged schizophrenic patients. *British Journal of Clinical Psychology, 26,* 141–143.

Tarrier, N. (1992a). Psychological treatment of positive schizophrenic symptoms. In D. J. Kavanagh (Ed.), *Schizophrenia: An overview and practical handbook* (pp. 356–373). London: Chapman & Hall.

Tarrier, N. (1992b). Management and modification of residual positive psychotic symptoms. In M. Birchwood & N. Tarrier (Eds.), *Innovation in the psychological management of schizophrenia* (pp. 147–170). Chichester, UK: Wiley.

Tarrier, N. (1995, September 28–29). *Coping skills and psychotic symptoms.* Paper presented at the First International Conference on Psychological Treatments for Schizophrenia, Cambridge, UK.

Tarrier, N. (2001). The use of coping strategies and self-regulation in the treatment of psychosis. In A. Morrison (Ed.), *A casebook of cognitive therapy for psychosis* (pp. 79–107). Cambridge, UK: Cambridge University Press.

Tarrier, N., Barrowclough, C., Haddock, G., & McGovern, J. (1999). The dissemination of innovative cognitive-behavioural psychosocial treatments for schizophrenia. *Journal of Mental Health, 8,* 569–582.

Tarrier, N., Beckett, R., Harwood, S., Baker, A., Yusupoff, L., & Ugarteburu, I. (1993). A controlled trial of two cognitive behavioural methods of treating drug-resistant residual psychotic symptoms in schizophrenic patients: I. Outcome. *British Journal of Psychiatry, 162,* 524–532.

Tarrier, N., & Calam, R. (in press). New developments in Cognitive-Behavioural care formulation. Epidemiological, systemic and social context: An integrative approach. *Behavioural and Cognitive Psychotherapy.*

Tarrier, N., Kinney, C., McCarthy, E., Humphreys, L., Wittowski, A., & Morris, J. (2000). Two year follow-up of cognitive behaviour therapy and supportive counselling in the treatment of persistent symptoms in chronic schizophrenia. *Journal of Consulting and Clinical Psychology, 68,* 917–922.

Tarrier, N., Kinney, C., McCarthy, E., Wittkowski, A., Yusupoff, Y., Gledhill, A., Morris, J., & Humphreys, L. (2001). The cognitive-behavioural treatment of persistent symptoms in chronic schizophrenia: Are some types of psychotic symptoms more responsive to cognitive-behaviour therapy? *Behavioural and Cognitive Psychotherapy, 29,* 45–56.

Tarrier, N., & Turpin, G. (1992). Psychosocial factors, arousal and schizophrenic relapse. The psychophysiological data. *British Journal of Psychiatry, 161,* 3–11.

Tarrier, N., Wells, A., & Haddock, G. (1998). *Treating complex cases: The cognitive behavioural therapy approach.* Chichester, UK: Wiley.

Tarrier, N., Wittkowski, A., Kinney, C., McCarthy, E., Morris, J., & Humphreys, L. (1999). The durability of the effects of cognitive behaviour therapy in the treatment of chronic schizophrenia: Twelve months follow-up. *British Journal of Psychiatry, 174,* 500–504.

Tarrier, N., Yusupoff, L., Kinney, C., McCarthy, E., Gledhill, A., Haddock, G., & Morris, J. (1998). A randomised controlled trial of intensive cognitive behaviour therapy for chronic schizophrenia. *British Medical Journal, 317,* 303–307.

Tarrier, N., Yusupoff, L., McCarthy, E., Kinney, C., & Wittkowski, A. (1998). Some reason why patients suffering from chronic schizophrenia fail to continue in psychological treatment. *Behavioural and Cognitive Psychotherapy, 26,* 177–181.

Tattan, T., & Tarrier, N. (2000). The expressed emotion of case managers of the seriously mentally ill: The influence of EE and the quality of the relationship on clinical outcomes. *Psychological Medicine, 30,* 195–204.

Wing, J., Cooper, J., & Sartorius, N. (1974). *Measurement and classification of psychiatric symptoms.* Cambridge, UK: Cambridge University Press.

Wolpe, J. (1958). *Psychotherapy by reciprocal inhibition.* Stanford, CA: Stanford University Press.

II

Psychological Treatments for Mood Disorders

Although the term "mood disorders" refers to a disturbance in mood or affect, these conditions involve multiple dysfunctions in mood, attention, cognition, physical health, and interpersonal relationships. Major depressive episodes are characterized by dysphoric mood, diminished pleasure or interest in activities, changes in appetite, disturbances in sleep, psychomotor disturbances, fatigue, feelings of worthlessness and guilt, diminished capacity for thinking and concentrating, and suicidality (American Psychiatric Association, 1994, p. 327). Manic episodes are characterized by inflated self-esteem and grandiosity, decreased need for sleep, increased talkativeness and/or pressured speech, flight of ideas, distractibility, increases in goal-directed behavior, and excessive risk taking (American Psychiatric Association, 1994, p. 332).

Studies of both the epidemiology and course of mood disorders underscore the importance of effective interventions for these significant public health problems. First, mood disorders are very common. Recent epidemiological data suggest a 1-year prevalence of 10% for unipolar depression (including major depressive and dysthmic disorders). Thus, a substantial proportion of individuals will experience a mood disorder at some point. Second, longitudinal studies of course and outcome have repeatedly demonstrated that both major depressive disorder and bipolar disorder are frequently chronic, severe, characterized by high levels of impairment and disability, and associated with increased risk of suicide. Although dysthymic and hypomanic episodes present with fewer and less severe symptoms of mood disorder, recent data indicate the severe dysfunction often associated with these "lesser" mood disturbances. Given the frequently chronic and/or recurrent nature of these problems, effective treatments need to focus not only on the amelioration of current difficulties but also on the prevention of future episodes and impairment. In summary, both prevalence and course of the mood disorders are strong reasons for developing effective treatments strategies.

These six chapters represent the best of what is known about psychological treatment of mood disorders. First, cognitive approaches for the treatment of depression are among the most thoroughly studied psychotherapeutic strategies, and numerous clinical trials have demonstrated their efficacy. More recently, clinical researchers have applied these approaches to the treatment of bipolar disorder. Kate Hamilton and Keith Dobson

(Chapter 5) describe the application of cognitive therapy to depression, and Michael Otto and Noreen Reilly-Harrington (Chapter 6) discuss the modification of cognitive therapy for treatment of bipolar disorders. Second, recent research in the processes underlying depression have emphasized the critical role of interpersonal relationships in the development and maintenance of mood disorders (for a review, see Joiner & Coyne, 1999). Chapters 7 through 10 all describe intervention strategies that focus on the important interpersonal world. In Chapter 7, Holly Swartz, John Markowitz, and Ellen Frank describe interpersonal therapy for the treatment of both depression and mania. This treatment helps individuals identify interpersonal factors that contribute to their mood problems and develop strategies for improving relationship functioning. David Miklowitz (Chapter 8) describes a family-focused treatment approach for patients who have recently experienced a manic episode. This exciting intervention has been shown to reduce both relapse and hospitalization for patients with bipolar disorders. Daniel O'Leary (Chapter 9) discusses couple therapy for addressing depression. In cases where depression and marital discord coexist, these couple-based strategies have particular power for addressing both problems. Finally, Mary Jane Rotheram-Borus, Alison Goldstein, and Amy Elkavich (Chapter 10) describe a family-based treatment approach for suicidal behavior in adolescents. Given the frequent co-occurrence of depression and suicidality, specific approaches for dealing with suicidal behavior have an important role to play in depression treatment.

REFERENCES

American Psychiatric Association. (1994). *Diagnostic and statistical manual of mental disorders* (4th ed.). Washington, DC: Author.

Joiner, T., & Coyne, J. C. (1999). *The interactional nature of depression.* Washington, DC: American Psychological Association Press.

Regier, D. A., & Kaelber, C. T. (1995). The Epidemiologic Catchment Area (ECA) program: Studying the prevalence and incidence of psychopathology. In M. T. Tsuang, M. Tohen, & G. E. P. Zahner (Eds.), *Textbook in psychiatric epidemiology.* New York: Wiley.

5

Cognitive-Behavioral Therapy for Depression

KATE E. HAMILTON
KEITH S. DOBSON

The pervasive nature of major depression, its devastating impact on interpersonal and occupational functioning, and its profound monetary liability, have prompted the generation of diverse theoretical models for the disorder. Etiological models derived from psychodynamic, behavioral, interpersonal, biological, and cognitive orientations have enjoyed a history of empirical support (Beckham & Leber, 1995; Gotlib & Hammen, 1992; Paykel, 1992). The cognitive model of depression has achieved considerable notoriety within psychology.

Cognitive therapy for depression, as formulated by Aaron Beck in the 1960s, is a short-term, goal-oriented, present-focused therapy designed to modify dysfunctional thinking and the emotion and behavior it is thought to influence. A wealth of empirical data derived from randomized, controlled treatment outcome studies supports the efficacy of cognitive therapy for depression (Dobson, 1989; Gloaguen, Cottraux, Cucherat, & Blackburn, 1998). A growing body of empirical research suggests that cognitive-behavioral therapy for depression is indicated for a variety of populations (Jarrett, Eaves, Brannemann, & Rush, 1991).

THE COGNITIVE MODEL OF DEPRESSION

Cognitive-behavioral therapy for depression is derived from Beck's original cognitive model of depression (Beck, Rush, Shaw, & Emery, 1979). The model postulates that dysfunctional cognitive processing mediates the relationship between stressful life events and depression. How an individual perceives and interprets his or her life experiences critically influences his or her physiological, affective, and behavioral response (Beck, 1964).

The cognitive triad (Beck et al., 1979) is conceived as a central component of depression. Individuals vulnerable to depression tend to view themselves, the world, and the future in a negatively biased manner. For example, an individual may perceive him- or herself to be inadequate despite contrary evidence. This view of the world is a harsh and demanding one. Furthermore, he or she may believe that the future is bleak and hopeless.

This negative cognitive set is a product of enduring, negative, and self-referent core beliefs that are based on past experience—commonly referred to as schemata (Beck, 1963, 1967, 1976, 1987). These rigid, global schemas are assumed to be the critical architectural foundation upon which information is meaningfully organized. The schematic template actively filters, categorizes, and evaluates incoming stimuli. A critical assumption of the cognitive model is that these maladaptive cognitive structures remain dormant until activated by stressful life events. When activated, these schemas are thought to provide access to an intricate network of depression-related themes and to instigate a corresponding pattern of negative, self-focused information processing (Ingram, Miranda, & Segal, 1998; Segal & Ingram, 1994).

At an intermediate level, attitudes, rules, and assumptions characterize this self-focused information processing. For example, an individual assumes that it is unacceptable to fail, and that he or she must perform optimally in every situation. This intermediate level gives rise to a superficial level of cognitive processing characterized by automatic thoughts. Automatic thoughts are brief, transient images or thoughts that rapidly materialize but have consequences for the feelings and behavior the person then experiences. These automatic thoughts frequently go unrecognized; rather, it is often the consequent mood that is brought to awareness (J. Beck, 1995).

In summary, underlying schemas influence perception and manifest as automatic thoughts. Enduring maladaptive core beliefs generate distorted assumptions or expectations and produce situation-specific negative automatic thoughts, which consequently induce depressive affect and behavior in response to typical, but stressful, life events. The causal relationship between cognition, affect, and behavior remains controversial (DeRubeis & Feeley, 1990).

THE PROCESS OF COGNITIVE-BEHAVIORAL THERAPY FOR DEPRESSION

Cognitive-behavioral therapy for depression is a collaborative, goal-oriented, time-limited, and present-focused psychoeducational approach that adheres to three fundamental principles based on the cognitive model of depression. The critical, first assumption is that depressive affect and behavior are influenced by cognitive interpretation of situational experiences. The second assumption presumes that, with practice, cognitions can be identified, monitored, and evaluated. Finally, it is assumed that modifying distorted cognitions influences affect and behavior (Beck et al., 1979; Sacco & Beck, 1995).

The first phase of therapy focuses on identifying and monitoring dysfunctional automatic thoughts and recognizing the link among cognition, mood, and behavior. The second phase of therapy involves evaluating, modifying, and ultimately replacing dysfunctional automatic thoughts, intermediate assumptions, and core beliefs with more reasonable interpretations. The final phase of therapy focuses on termination and relapse prevention. Each phase is here discussed in turn.

Case Conceptualization and Early Therapy Strategies

The initial phase of therapy includes malleable cognitive conceptualization of the client and provides a framework for therapy. With the cognitive model in mind, the therapist strives to identify the relationship between the client's cognitions, affect, and behavior. Hypotheses are generated regarding etiology, the significance of life events, and potential precipitating and maintaining cognitive factors. Cognitive conceptualization is a fluid process subject to modification in response to ongoing hypothesis testing.

Efforts toward achieving a sound therapeutic alliance are initiated in the first session and maintained throughout therapy. Empathy and accurate reflection of the client's concerns facilitate rapport. The therapist must instill hope and communicate that he or she does not view the client's concerns as overwhelming. Overall, a questioning attitude and a desire to find out what is really happening in the client's life characterize the therapist's attitude, in what has been termed a "collaborative empiricist" relationship (Beck et al., 1979).

Therapy sessions follow a psychoeducational approach and attempt to socialize the client into the structured nature of cognitive-behavioral therapy. The rationale for setting an agenda at the beginning of each session is presented—specifically, to demystify the process and maximize the time devoted to critical issues. A mood check is conducted at the outset and the end of each therapy session to monitor progress. The therapist reviews the client's presenting problem, identifies principal concerns, and translates these into therapy goals. The cognitive model of depression (Beck et al., 1979) and the rationale for therapy are presented, most commonly, in the first treatment session. Ultimately, the client is taught to become his or her own therapist; hence, it is critical that the client both comprehend and embrace the model as the responsibility for setting the session's agenda gradually shifts to him or her. The client is given information on the nature of the disorder, and expectations and estimated therapy time frame are discussed. The therapist or client summarizes the session, and any assignments that have emanated from the treatment session are reviewed (e.g., bibliotherapy, monitoring mood and automatic thoughts, activity scheduling). Assignments, or homework, are an integral component of therapy. The therapist must ensure that the assignments are appropriate and manageable, particularly during the initial stages of therapy. Finally, for clarification and rapport building purposes, the therapist requests feedback from the client regarding his or her impressions of the session.

A standard format is recommended for all subsequent sessions, with the exception of the final phase termination and relapse prevention sessions. Each therapy session begins with a brief update and mood check. Objective measures, such as the Beck Depression Inventory (BDI; Beck, Steer, & Brown, 1996; Beck, Ward, Mendelson, Mock, & Erbaugh, 1961), may be used to monitor symptom change (e.g., suicidal ideation, hopelessness). The therapist bridges each session with the previous one; the client is asked to reiterate salient issues addressed in the previous session. This exercise fosters client responsibility in terms of understanding and reviewing therapy content. Reviewing homework each session also reinforces the value of independent work and increases the likelihood of future compliance. Regular homework is associated with superior outcome in cognitive-behavioral therapy (Persons, Burns, & Perloff, 1988).

Once the bridging, mood check, and review of homework are completed, an agenda for the session is set. Items on the agenda are addressed in order of perceived importance to the client. The therapist accomplishes many tasks while discussing each item on the agenda. He or she skillfully teaches the client to recognize dysfunctional thoughts, draws the connection between these thoughts and consequent mood and behavior, and collaboratively generates appropriate homework assignments. Finally, the session is summarized and feedback is elicited from the client. Eventually, the client assumes full responsibility for setting the agenda, generating homework assignments, and summarizing sessions.

Various cognitive techniques are used to achieve goals during the initial phase of therapy. Objectives include reviewing and reinforcing the cognitive model, selecting a problem focus, identifying and monitoring automatic thoughts, and recognizing the link between mood, behavior, and thought. The concept of automatic thoughts and their influence on mood and behavior is best illustrated by having the client recall a recent experience that made him or her feel sad. The client is asked to identify what was going through his or her mind just prior to the onset of the negative mood. Within-session mood shifts provide an ideal opportunity for illustrating the role of automatic thoughts in depressive affect. In some instances, hypothetical or imagined situations can be profitably used to examine the type of thinking that the client believes he or she would employ.

Assessing and Modifying Negative Automatic Thoughts and Beliefs

When the client has grasped the concept of cognitive therapy, the Dysfunctional Thought Record (DTR; Beck et al., 1979; J. Beck, 1995; see Figure 5.1, top part) may be introduced as a tool for monitoring automatic thoughts. The record is organized into the five labeled columns: situation, emotion, automatic thought, rational response, and outcome. At this initial stage of therapy, only the first three columns are relevant. When the client experiences a negative emotion, he or she notes the situation/event in which it was instigated and then records the automatic thought that preceded the emotion. The DTR is an ideal homework exercise and typically promotes awareness of the association between thoughts, mood, and behavior. These automatic thoughts can be reviewed in therapy sessions or by the client, until he or she achieves some facility with recording these processes.

Using the standard session format, therapy progresses into its second phase, whereby dysfunctional automatic thoughts, intermediate assumptions, and core beliefs are evaluated, modified, and replaced with more adaptive alternatives. The client is encouraged to evaluate his or her thoughts in a more objective and realistic manner. Hypotheses that the automatic thoughts are illogical, inaccurate, or maladaptive are examined with respect to the available evidence. It is critical that the client learn to think as a scientist; specifically, the client is taught to view his or her thoughts as tentative hypotheses subject to empirical investigation.

A number of data-gathering techniques are employed to test the validity of dysfunctional thoughts. Questioning to evaluate the automatic thoughts is a fundamental component of cognitive-behavioral therapy for depression (J. Beck, 1995). First, the client learns to ask him- or herself, "What is the evidence for and against this idea?" The therapist uses Socratic questioning to investigate the accuracy of the automatic thought. The therapist does not directly challenge the automatic thought; instead he or she adopts the role of an empirical scientist to test the validity of the premises or logic upon which the client's conclusions are based. In addition, behavioral experiments are designed to gather data and test the validity of the client's automatic thoughts.

The client learns to ask him- or herself a second critical question: "Are there alternative explanations of the situation or event?" Depressed individuals tend to interpret ambiguous situations or events in a negative light. The therapist teaches the client to brainstorm for possible alternative conclusions. In this way, the client keeps an open mind in terms of testable hypotheses. The generation of plausible, alternative explanations also naturally encourages assignments that test out the validity of the various possible interpretations of situations, which, in and of themselves, engage the patient more fully in his or her life and generally encourage an active problem-solving orientation to issues he or she faces.

A third question that is sometimes employed in the cognitive-behavioral therapy of depression addresses the accuracy of the client's attributions: "Is my explanation of the causes of this negative event accurate?" Depressed individuals tend to attribute negative events to internal, stable, and global factors as opposed to external, variable, and situation-specific factors. A depressed individual may interpret a social slight in terms of global, stable, and internal factors (e.g., "Everyone thinks I am boring," "I am always excluded"), whereas the nondepressed individual may interpret the same slight as an oversight. After reviewing the evidence associated with automatic thoughts, it is sometimes beneficial to draw specifically negative attributions to the client's attention. Another technique for obtaining more objective attributions is to have the client reinterpret a negative event from another individual's perspective. These reattributions tend to be more favorable and serve as an excellent referencing point.

Finally, and particularly if the client is prone to make negative predictions for the future, he or she may be taught to ask the following questions: "What is the worst that could happen?", "What is the best that could happen?", and "What is most likely to happen?" This technique helps depressed clients to adopt a more realistic perspective and to realize that they are capable of coping with negative outcomes.

A number of additional techniques are available to evaluate dysfunctional thoughts. It is often useful to present clients with a list of typical cognitive distortions (Beck, 1976) and have them label their own distortion tendencies (e.g., overgeneralization, mind reading, catastrophizing, all-or-nothing thinking, labeling, etc.). In addition, clients may benefit from examining the value of their automatic thoughts. A client can be taught to ask him- or herself, "What is the effect of my believing the automatic thought?" and "What could be the effect of changing my thinking?" Exploring the advantages and disadvantages of holding a dysfunctional thought requires that the client examine its utility (J. Beck, 1995).

Replacing dysfunctional automatic thoughts with more reasonable interpretations directly follows from their identification and evaluation. The last two columns of the DTR (e.g., adaptive response and outcome) are introduced as a tool for responding to dysfunctional cognitions. Having developed the skills to complete the first portion of the DTR, the client is instructed to generate an adaptive or "rational" response based on the techniques learned. He or she not only identifies the cognitive distortion, evaluates the evidence for and against the thought, generates alternative interpretations, contemplates the worst outcome, assesses the value of maintaining this distorted thought, and produces a more adaptive interpretation, but also indicates the degree to which he or she endorses the new interpretation. It is critical that the client genuinely endorse the rational response. Reluctance can take the form of additional dysfunctional automatic thoughts to counter the rational response (J. Beck, 1995). These automatic thoughts must be identified, evaluated, and modified until the client endorses rational response. Written completion of the DTR is recommended. Eventually, the client can learn to respond adaptively to dysfunctional thoughts without using the DTR. Finally, the client completes the outcome column, which serves as an index of the extent to which evidence-based and reasonable thinking in the situation is associated with less emotional distress.

At some point during the second phase of therapy, the focus shifts from dysfunctional automatic thoughts to intermediate assumptions and underlying core beliefs. Therapist goals include identifying and modifying underlying assumptions and core beliefs that predispose the client to develop depression. Underlying assumptions are ingrained rules, premises, and expectations that negatively bias the client's interpretation of events, whereas core beliefs are enduring, rigid ideas concerning oneself, the world, and the future. The client is often unaware of these underlying assumptions and core beliefs. Common underlying assumptions include "If I am unloved, life is meaningless," "To be happy, everyone must like me," and "To be happy, I must be successful in every aspect of my life." Core beliefs include "I am inadequate," "I am unlovable," and "I am stupid" (Ingram, Miranda, & Segal, 1998). Intermediate assumptions are less malleable than automatic thoughts, yet more pliable than core beliefs.

The identification of underlying assumptions and core beliefs follows directly from the examination of automatic thoughts. Typically, the identified automatic thoughts derive from one or more underlying themes. The Dysfunctional Attitudes Scale (Weissman, 1979) represents one tool for uncovering typical assumptions and facilitates ongoing cognitive conceptualization of the client. The downward arrow technique investigates the meaning attached to automatic thoughts to uncover important beliefs (J. Beck, 1995). The following line of questioning is used: "If the automatic thought is true, so what?", "What is so bad about the automatic thought?", "What is the worst part about the automatic thought?", and "What does that mean about you?" The first three questions tend to elicit underlying assumptions, rules, and expectations, whereas the fourth question tends to elicit clients' core beliefs about themselves. J. Beck's (1995) cognitive conceptualization diagram is an excellent data-gathering tool for piecing together a cognitive conceptualization of the client.

The modification of underlying assumptions and core beliefs is the next step in the treatment of depression. First, the therapist makes the existing underlying assumptions and core beliefs explicit to the client. Where possible, rules are converted into assumption form to facilitate their malleability. A new, more adaptive belief is formulated, and the following belief modification techniques are employed (J. Beck, 1995): Socratic questioning is used to evaluate the evidence for and against the existing belief; the advantages and disadvantages of maintaining the belief are examined. The therapist emphasizes the disadvantages of existing beliefs, while encouraging consideration of the advantages of alternative, more adaptive beliefs. He or she adopts a more persuasive stance as compared to the Socratic questioning used to modify automatic thoughts. Behavior experiments designed to test the validity of a belief or assumption are particularly effective. The cognitive continuum technique helps to alleviate all-or-nothing thinking. Developing a cognitive continuum for an idea gives the client perspective in terms of recognizing middle ground. In rational–emotional role play, therapist and client alternate playing the roles of the client's emotional and rational mind. This technique is particularly useful when the client indicates that he or she can intellectually understand that the belief is dysfunctional but feels that it is emotionally valid. Using other individuals as reference points is an effective method for gaining perspective and objectivity. Finally, the "acting as if" technique rests on the principle that cognition affects behavior and behavior affects cognition. The client is instructed to act as if he or she does not believe the dysfunctional idea, but to experiment with the consequences of acting "as if" he or she had adopted a more adaptive belief.

Several techniques are particularly salient for modifying core beliefs and strengthening new beliefs. The Core Belief Worksheet (J. Beck, 1995) can be introduced as a tool for recording empirical evidence for and against old core beliefs and new beliefs. Using extreme contrasts and metaphors to modify core beliefs may benefit the client who does not view his or her situation objectively. Historical tests of core beliefs may facilitate their modification by restructuring the meaning of depression-related events. Additional cognitive-behavioral techniques include problem solving, activity monitoring and scheduling, distraction and refocusing, relaxation, and graded exposure (see J. Beck, 1995, for a review).

Termination and Relapse Prevention

The final phase of therapy focuses on termination and relapse prevention. Preparing the client for termination begins during the very first session. The therapist identifies client expectations and clearly specifies the estimated time course of therapy. Throughout therapy, client self-efficacy is promoted by attributing progress to his or her efforts and not to the therapist or external factors (e.g., medication, situational change); the therapist emphasizes that the techniques are lifelong skills for managing depression. When symptom reduction is achieved, the therapist prepares the client to cope with potential setbacks by viewing them as transient lapses, not failures. Toward the end, therapy can be tapered into biweekly, and eventually monthly, sessions to prepare the client for termination. We have recently experimented with the use of "self-sessions," in which the client makes an appointment with him- or herself, in order to conduct an analogue of a therapy session. Self-sessions include setting an agenda, doing a mood check, thinking about current problems, and developing assignments as a way to prepare the client for the time when the therapist is not immediately available. It is critical that the client's automatic thoughts and feelings concerning termination be investigated and dealt with appropriately.

A prevention of depression plan tailored to the client's individual needs is generated, and strategies for maintaining this plan are discussed. Finally, booster sessions at 3, 6, and 12 months posttermination are scheduled. The goal of these booster sessions is to monitor progress, problem-solve, if necessary, and plan for continued maintenance. Pride in the client's achievements and optimism regarding the future are conveyed by the therapist and, we hope, adopted by the client.

EMPIRICAL VALIDITY

Cognitive therapy for depression is recognized by the Division 12 Task Force of the American Psychological Association as a "well-established treatment" for depression (Chambless et al., 1996). The relative efficacy of cognitive therapy for depression is well documented. Dobson's (1989) meta-analysis indicates superior efficacy for cognitive therapy relative to a wait-list control, as well as to alternative treatments, including pharmacotherapy, behavior therapy, and other psychotherapies. A more recent meta-analysis (Gloaguen et al., 1998) confirmed these results with respect to cognitive therapy's superiority to control conditions, medications, and other psychotherapies, but not with respect to behavior therapy, which was found to be as effective as cognitive therapy. A number of other reviews have yielded nonsignificant treatment differences among cognitive therapy, behavior therapy, and interpersonal therapy (Barlow, 1994; Elkin et al., 1989; Shapiro et al., 1994). Collectively, these treatments are found to be superior to a wait-list control or placebo condition.

POPULATION CONSIDERATIONS

Cognitive-behavioral therapy is an effective treatment for unipolar, nonpsychotic, major depressive disorder. Standard cognitive-behavioral therapy has been adapted to benefit geriatric and child–adolescent populations. Collectively, a number of empirical studies suggest that age, gender, education, and socioeconomic status are not meaningful predictors of outcome in cognitive-behavioral therapy for depression (Abraham, Neudorfer, & Currie, 1992; Dobson, 1989; Futterman, Thompson, Gallagher-Thomson, & Ferris, 1995; Jarrett et al., 1991; Speier, Sherak, Hirsch, & Cantwell, 1995; Thase et al., 1994). Marital status, however, has been found to be a meaningful predictor of response, in that married clients respond better to cognitive-behavioral therapy than nonmarried clients (Jarrett et al., 1991; Thase et al., 1992).

There is a paucity of empirical literature examining the efficacy of cognitive-behavioral therapy for depression among ethnic minorities (Doyle, 1998). For depression, for example, it has been demonstrated to be effective for Puerto Rican women (Comas-Diaz, 1981). Future research must determine the degree to which standard cognitive-behavioral therapeutic efficacy generalizes to diverse ethnic populations.

Controversy surrounds the relative efficacy of cognitive therapy for severely depressed outpatients (Hollon, 1996; Garvey, Hollon, & DeRubeis, 1994; Jacobson & Hollon, 1996). Recently, DeRubeis, Gelfand, Tang, and Simons (1999) conducted a mega-analysis of four randomized trials comparing pharmacotherapy and cognitive-behavioral therapy for depression, in which they obtained the raw data and pooled the information across studies. Results suggest that overall effect sizes favor cognitive-behavioral therapy over medication; however, the two modalities did not differ statistically in terms of overall therapeutic advantage. Furthermore, initial depression severity did not mediate the effectiveness of these two therapies. The authors conclude that cognitive-behavioral therapy is an empirically sound approach for the acute treatment of both moderately and severely depressed clients.

CASE EXAMPLE

Bernice Andrews, a 37-year-old single woman, was referred for therapy due a recurrence of depression. On examination, it was learned that she was suffering from recurrent major depressive disorder; she had experienced two previous episode of depression. Several aspects of Bernice's history appeared relevant to the depression she was experiencing. She had grown up as the only child of rather unhappily married parents, who, still married, lived together in Milwaukee. Bernice's mother in particular seemed to be a dour influence on Bernice. Born of German stock, she reportedly had a rather mirthless and instrumental approach to life. Her house was bound by rules that she applied without exception. In contrast, Bernice's father, who was of British extraction and perceived as a rather ineffectual but affable man, had worked in the same company for decades without any particular advancement.

A bright girl, Bernice had always excelled at school, although she had never been particularly praised or rewarded for her performance. She had one close friend, Paula, and the two girls were inseparable for many years. The loss of Paula, when her parents moved away, was a serious blow to Bernice, and she never really entered into another deep friendship. Rather, the pattern throughout the rest of her life has been to have a number of more casual acquaintances, work associates with whom she socializes, and occasional ventures into problematical relationships.

On completing high school, Bernice went directly into college in Madison, Wisconsin. She obtained her nursing degree with ease, due in part to her intelligence and in part to the way that she threw herself into her studies. Although she rarely partied with her classmates, she did get somewhat involved in student life by serving as a student representative on her nursing program's training committee. Praised by her instructors for her exacting preparedness and excellent work, Bernice felt somewhat "above" and emotionally removed from her colleagues.

Bernice had limited dating experience prior to meeting her first significant partner. She had been invited to some high school functions and social activities in college, and despite the efforts of men she dated, Bernice never let any relationship get serious. In her fourth year of nursing, however, at age 22, she met a somewhat older man named Marshall, who worked in an administrative position in the hospital where she was training. Marshall pursued Bernice with a quiet determination, never advancing too rapidly or making her apprehensive. Slowly, they began to spend lunchtimes together, and then occasional afternoons on the weekend. Bernice realized she was falling in love with Marshall, but kept these feelings to herself. About 6 months after they met, Marshall professed his love to Bernice and confessed his marriage to another woman.

Devastated by this news, Bernice broke off the relationship but ruminated about it excessively. She often fantasized about phoning Marshall and convincing him to leave his wife. She even obtained his address and went by the house to see if she could see him. Eventually, Bernice began to become self-critical for making herself vulnerable in this way, and her mood started to slip. Attendant to these problems was the fact that Bernice could not concentrate and her grades took a dip. Two of Bernice's instructors took her aside and expressed concern about the impaired work that they saw, which she took as criticism. She withdrew even more from social activities, did some self-help reading, and tried to focus on her schoolwork. Eventually, although it was difficult, she began to think less of Marshall; her ability to perform increased, and this first depressive episode passed. Within 2 months of the separation, she was more or less "back to normal."

Bernice's second depression occurred when she was 32 and working in Chicago as an emergency room nurse, a position she found challenging but rewarding. Two years earlier, she had met an average-looking and apparently hardworking medical supply salesperson named Mike, who asked her out four times before she finally agreed to go. Although initially very wary of him, she found that he was well mannered, if a bit diffident or even shy in how he related to her. Eventually, they began to date more. When he asked her to marry him after only 4 months of dating, Bernice found herself relieved: The "need" to date was over, and she could get married like most of her coworkers.

The marriage with Mike was not successful. Bernice found that she wanted to maintain her demanding work schedule, and Mike was often petulant when she did so. Over time, she found Mike to be increasingly needy of her. If she had to work in the evening, he often did little but watch television and drink. She became increasingly critical of him, which seemed to drive a wedge further between them. Bernice also became somewhat dissatisfied at work, thinking that she could do better. At 30, she resolved to return to school to obtain an MBA in hospital administration. To support her education, she often worked evening or weekend shifts at the hospital, but this reduction in salary led to some bitterness between herself and Mike. Never fully comfortable with physical intimacy, Bernice was actually relieved when they stopped having intercourse. In retrospect, she believes it was this step that eventually led Mike to have an affair, which precipitated their separation, as well as her second depression.

On interview, Bernice was found to meet diagnostic criteria for major depressive disorder. Her depression was supported by a BDI score of 34, which indicates moderate to severe depression. Her primary symptoms included sadness, loss of interest, reduced energy, self-depreciation, loss of appetite, sleep disturbance (early morning awakening), problems in concentration, and thoughts (but no plan) of suicide. Other significant, possibly comorbid problems (e.g., alcohol or substance abuse, anxiety disorders, psychotic processes) were evaluated but found not to be present.

Bernice was told about the cognitive model of depression, with which she was already somewhat familiar, having done some self-help reading when previously depressed. She accepted the treatment model and the need for therapeutic assistance, because she saw the pattern of getting depressed after breakups and wanted to "understand why I pick bad men and end up getting hurt." A list of treatment goals was established, including (1) eliminating Bernice's depression, (2) restoring her previous level of occupational and school functioning, (3) helping her to plan for the pending divorce proceedings, and (4) understanding her pattern of relationships and depressions, with a view toward preventing the recurrence of problems in the future.

From the outset, the therapist tried to develop a case conceptualization to guide the treatment (J. Beck, 1995). In this case, the therapist hypothesized that there were actually two core schemas related to Bernice's problems and depressions. First, she had a core belief of herself as inadequate, based on her early childhood experiences and the way that she responded to teachers and others in authority with extreme efforts to please them. Consistent with this core belief was her way of speaking and acting: If only she could do enough (get high grades, achieve at work, etc.), she would be accepted. Related to the first belief, but somewhat distinct, was another core belief: that of being unlovable. Again, the therapist hypothesized that this belief emanated from a cold, non-nurturing family but was maintained by her style of withdrawing from opportunities for intimate relationships, or else being "injured" when she risked these involvements.

The therapist began by assessing Bernice's daily routines, using a daily activity schedule. Although she was maintaining her work schedule, Bernice's schoolwork and social life had largely fallen away. Furthermore, her current apartment (she had moved out after finding out about Mike's affair) was by her own account "a mess." Working together, the therapist and Bernice prioritized these problem areas for intervention. Consistent with the tentative case formulation, Bernice targeted work and school as her first priorities. Although the therapist was aware that helping her to be more competent in these domains might contribute to Bernice's need to maintain a sense of being "good" enough, these goals were agreed upon. By a process of setting realistic targets and graded task assignment over the next 4 weeks, Bernice got her studying "under control" and worked to make her apartment feel more like a "home," even if it was only temporary. Furthermore, although the therapist promoted this idea more than Bernice, she added some relaxation and fun to her schedule, including socializing some with work acquaintances and limited exercise (e.g., walks).

With Bernice's gradual restoration of functioning, the focus of therapy shifted to examining her thoughts more systematically. In the course of doing the above work, the therapist discovered that Bernice tended to have high and fairly rigid standards for herself, and that if she did not fully meet her own expectations, she labeled herself and became self-critical and depressed. The following dialogue illustrates the downward arrow technique for uncovering silent assumptions:

CLIENT: I always make mistakes at work. [Overgeneralization]

THERAPIST: If this is true, why is it upsetting?

CLIENT: It would mean I am a lousy nurse [All-or-nothing thinking]

THERAPIST: Suppose you do always make mistakes and are a lousy nurse. What would that mean?

CLIENT: It would mean that I am a total failure. [Labeling]

THERAPIST: And if you are a total failure, why would that be so bad?

CLIENT: Eventually, everyone would discover that I am no good, that I am worthless. No one would ever respect me. [Mind reading, labeling]

This dialogue reveals several maladaptive assumptions. Bernice believed that she must be perfect to be a good nurse. If she was not successful at all times, she would be a failure. Bernice believed that her worth was determined by her achievement. If she failed at nursing, she would be a worthless individual. Others would not tolerate her imperfection. She could not be respected without being perfect. The therapist discussed this pattern of high standards and all-or-nothing thinking with Bernice and urged her to use a more graduated approach to achieving her goals, and to recognize intermediate steps as accomplishments.

She was also taught to track her negative thoughts using the Daily Thought Record and to dispute these thoughts in therapy using evidence and the generation of reasonable alternatives (see the lower part of Figure 5.1 for an example). Due to Bernice's intelligence and her admittedly negative thoughts about disappointing the therapist if her homework was not fully completed (these automatic thoughts were also discussed in therapy), Bernice began to feel considerably better. By 10th week of treatment, her weekly BDI score had dropped to 14, and she reported that she thought she was no longer depressed, "just sad."

At approximately this point in therapy, an event occurred that tested Bernice's recovery. Her husband filed for a formal legal separation. Bernice's mood slipped as some of her self-critical thoughts became more prominent. Fortunately, she maintained her schedule of activities, including some social events. At one event with a group female students, Bernice divulged her marital situation and received what she found to be an amazing amount of support for herself and criticism of her husband. Her mood rebounded, although she noticed herself feeling more angry than previously. The following interchange reflected some of the process that took place between the therapist and Bernice:

THERAPIST: Mike's decision to divorce really threw you for a loop. [Supportive]

CLIENT: Yes, I found myself reviewing all of my faults—the things I had done wrong that led us to this point.

THERAPIST: It is amazing how strong some of these patterns are when we have to say

Situation	Automatic thought(s)	Emotion(s)	Adaptive response	Outcome
What actual event or stream of thoughts, or daydreams or recollection led to the unpleasant emotion? What (if any) distressing physical sensations did you have?	What thought(s) and/or image(s) went through your mind? How much did you believe each one at the time?	What emotion(s) did you feel at the time? How intense (0-100%) was the emotion?	What cognitive distortion did you make? Response to the automatic thought(s)? How much do you believe each response?	How much do you now believe each automatic thought? What emotion(s) do you feel now? How intense (0-100%) is the emotion? What will you do (or did you do)?
Watching TV in the evening, thinking that I did not exercise today like I was supposed to.	• What a slob. • I'm a mess. • I will never get better if I can't even exercise some. • I can't even get the energy to get off of this couch.	Disgust—85% Depression—50% Hopelessness—20%	• I'm labeling myself. • Although I did not exercise today, I have been doing better in the past. • It was me who assigned the exercise, so I can give myself "permission" not to, as well. • Maybe I deserve a night off. • Energy comes from getting active.	• Disgust—50% • Depression—25% • Hopelessness—10% • I got up and went to the corner store for milk for the morning; pleasure—30%.

FIGURE 5.1. Dysfunctional thought record. From J. Beck (1995). Copyright 1995 by The Guilford Press. Adapted by permission.

certain things to ourselves. It seems like your schema of being unlovable and having to be perfect to get love really rose to the surface. [Describing the cognitive process linked to feeling] And yet, you were able to counteract this tendency. Tell me about that. [Reinforcing change]

CLIENT: Well, I-I just talked about it to some friends—I don't think I would even have done that before therapy! But they were really supportive, pointing out how it was his issue, his fault.

THERAPIST: So their tendency was to criticize him in order to support you? [Clarifying]

CLIENT: Yes. And that helped—mostly knowing that they were supportive. But I guess what helped the most was *my* realization that I don't really have to blame him or me. It's sad to divorce, but I think it is actually the best right now.

THERAPIST: So knowing you are supported is important; and that is why keeping up your social contacts is so critical right now. But it sounds like a really important change in your thinking—knowing that you are okay, and that Mike is okay, even if you both are in this sad situation. [Restating cognitive reframe, and its benefit]

CLIENT: Yeah. It's okay to be sad right now, but I don't have to get depressed—or angry.

At this stage of therapy, the therapist began to probe more of the underlying beliefs and meanings that Bernice gave to different situations. By this time, the therapist had seen several instances in which the theme of inadequacy, and the need to compensate for this inner sense of inadequacy through high standards and self-criticism, had reared its head. The therapist and Bernice reviewed this pattern and agreed that it was likely a major force in her life. The therapist constructed an experiment to test this belief: Bernice went to work and was purposely only "average"; she did not do any of the things she commonly did in the emergency room that other nurses did not do. Although reluctant to try this assignment, she reported that no one had commented to her afterward about not doing her usual job, patients were not endangered, and she had time for her full rests and meal breaks, which was rare.

The therapist and Bernice worked together to frame the way her belief in her own inadequacy had likely emerged through historical reconstruction and influenced her life. An alternative, more adaptive belief—"I'm okay, without having to be excellent"—was generated, and they discussed the short- and long-term advantages and disadvantages of her past and this new belief, and several ways that Bernice could act "as if" she had adopted the new belief, including lowering her demands at work and school, and giving herself permission to have more fun and take better care of herself. Bernice implemented these ideas well; for example, she visited San Francisco on her own, which she reported enjoying considerably. By Session 15, her BDI score was a 6, where it stayed pretty much through the end of therapy (see Figure 5.2).

The other major problem in Bernice's life that posed a continuing threat to her sense of well-being was her marital separation and her continuing sense of being unlovable and alone. As with the previous belief, the historical reasons for the development of this belief and its role in her current life were reviewed. When the therapist sought a healthy alternative, Bernice suggested, "It might be better to be happy and alone, than married and miserable." Although the therapist was not certain that this was a more adaptive belief, as it did not directly address her underlying belief in being unlovable, and it also seemed dichotomous and rigid, it was difficult for Bernice to see other, more adaptive

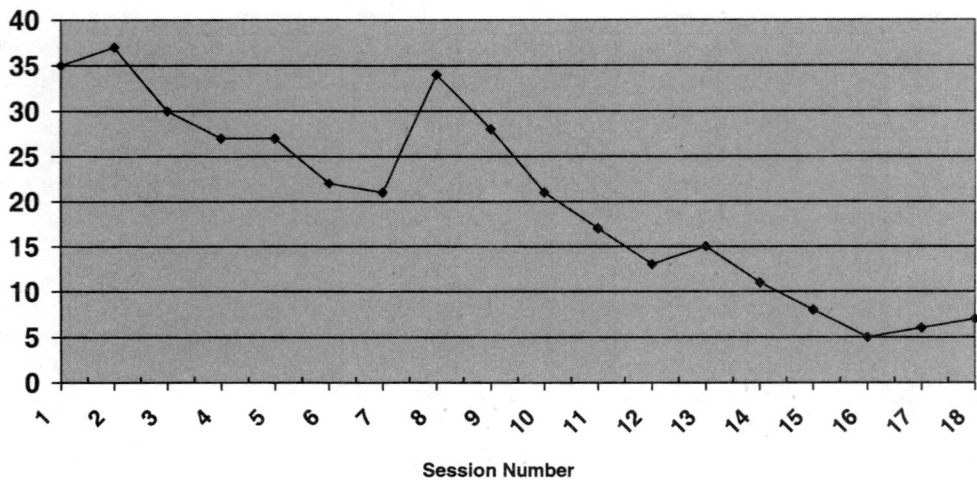

FIGURE 5.2. Bernice's progress in therapy as measured by the Beck Depression Inventory.

middle points. As such, the therapist and Bernice worked together to design applications of this new belief. Although the therapist had expected Bernice to feel some continuing sense of being unlovable by adopting more of a solitary lifestyle, in fact, this did not happen. Bernice pursued relationships with other women and joined a rowing club, in addition to her nursing and MBA program. She set her sights on the completion of her program, now approximately 6 months away, and began to consider a career shift into hospital management. Over time, she became more invested in developing the life of a single career woman.

At Session 24, Bernice reported to the therapist that she felt she had learned a lot through the course of therapy, and had made some excellent personal choices that would help her as she continued on her own. The therapist and Bernice spent two sessions reviewing the methods that had been used in her case, the original beliefs associated with her depression, her current beliefs, and future threats that could precipitate another depression. The therapist predicted that Bernice might still be vulnerable to depression in the area of intimate relationships, and it was agreed that she could return for future sessions if she perceived the need, or if she felt herself becoming depressed. About 1 year later, though, the therapist received a postcard from San Diego. Bernice had taken a nursing management position at a hospital there and was, by her own report, happy. She indicated that she was making some female friends through a sailing club, which would also help prevent future depression.

CONCLUSIONS

This chapter presents the clinical theory and major techniques associated with the treatment of clinical depression. Although this treatment is most often applied in an outpatient setting, such as a private practice office or mental health clinic, it can also be adapted to more serious inpatient cases. The case of "Bernice" is a fairly typical example, though, of how the treatment methods can be integrated into a meaningful outpatient treatment package to address life problems that people face. Although the case was not a complete success, in that her belief about being "unlovable" was not fully challenged or changed, Bernice was able to regain her sense of self-esteem and accomplish important life goals.

In our experience, one of the most challenging aspects of cognitive therapy is not only to have patients realize the effect of their core beliefs on their past and current functioning, but also to be willing and motivated to change these beliefs. As has been noted elsewhere (Young, 1994), core beliefs form a kind of protective layer around the individual and are resistant to change. In many instances, if a natural crisis does convince patients of the need to make significant changes in their basic values or beliefs, it is necessary for the therapist to try to coengineer a critical test to help them to realize that such a change is adaptive. This work is not easy; it requires courage and often a large leap of faith on the part of the patient to achieve change. The therapist is privileged not only to help restore patients to nondepressive functioning but also to help them make more fundamental changes in the way they construct meaning in their lives.

This chapter has not dealt with the research on cognitive therapy for depression in any great depth. Several excellent sources do so (e.g., Clark, Beck, & Alford, 1999; DeRubeis, Tang, & Beck, 2001; Ingram et al., 1998), and the interested reader is referred there for further information. One important point that derives from this current chapter is that cognitive therapy is a complex, multicomponent treatment that requires training and skill to apply well. As has been discussed elsewhere (Dobson, Backs-Dermott, & Dozois, 2000) the essential aspects of cognitive therapy are not yet understood. No doubt, continuing research on this treatment will continue, and we will know more in years to come about the core elements associated with the effectiveness of this successful treatment (Dobson & Khatri, 2000).

REFERENCES

Abraham, I. L., Neudorfer, M. M., & Currie, L. J. (1992). Effects of group interventions on cognition and depression in nursing home residents. *Nursing Research, 41,* 196–202.

Barlow, D. H. (1994). Psychological interventions in the era of managed competition. *Clinical Psychology, Science and Practice, 26,* 574–585.

Beck, A. T. (1963). Thinking and depression: I. Idiosyncratic content and cognitive distortions. *Archives of General Psychiatry, 9,* 324–333.

Beck, A. T. (1964). Thinking and depression: II. Theory and therapy. *Archives of General Psychiatry, 10,* 561–571.

Beck, A. T. (1967). *Depression: Clinical, experimental, and theoretical aspects.* New York: Harper & Row.

Beck, A. T. (1976). *Cognitive therapy and the emotional disorders.* New York: International Universities Press.

Beck, A. T. (1987). Cognitive models of depression. *Journal of Cognitive Psychotherapy, 1,* 5–37.

Beck, A. T., Rush, A. J., Shaw, B. F., & Emery, G. (1979). *Cognitive therapy of depression.* New York: Guilford Press.

Beck, A. T., Steer, R. A., & Garbin, G. K. (1996). *Beck Depression Inventory manual* (2nd. ed.). San Antonio, TX: Psychological Corporation.

Beck, A. T., Ward, C. H., Mendelson, M., Mock, J., & Erbaugh, J. (1961). An inventory for measuring depression. *Archives of General Psychiatry, 4,* 561–571.

Beck, J. S. (1995). *Cognitive therapy: Basics and beyond.* New York: Guilford Press.

Beckham, E. E., & Leber, W. R. (Eds.). (1995). *Handbook of depression* (2nd ed.). New York: Guilford Press.

Chambless, D. L., Sanderson, W. C., Shoham, V., Bennett Johnson, S., Pope, K. S., Crits-Christoph, P., Baker, M., Johnson, B., Woody, S. R., Sue, S., Beutler, L., Williams, D. A., & McCurry, S. (1996). *An update on empirically validated therapies.* Unpublished manuscript, University of North Carolina, Chapel Hill.

Clark, D. A., Beck, A. T., & Alford, B. A. (1999). *Scientific foundations of cognitive theory and therapy of depression.* New York: Wiley.

Comas-Diaz, L. (1981). Effects of cognitive and behavioral group treatment on the depressive symptomatology of Puerto Rican women. *Journal of Consulting and Clinical Psychology, 49,* 627–632.

DeRubeis, R. J., & Feeley, M. (1990). Determinants of change in cognitive therapy for depression. *Cognitive Therapy and Research, 14,* 469–482.

DeRubeis, R. J., Gelfand, L. A., Tang, T. Z., & Simons, A. D. (1999). Medications versus cognitive behavior therapy for severely depressed outpatients: Mega-analysis of four randomized comparisons. *American Journal of Psychiatry, 156,* 1007–1013.

DeRubeis, R. J., Tang, T. Z., & Beck, A. T. (2001). Cognitive therapy. In K. S. Dobson (Ed.), *Handbook of cognitive-behavioral therapies* (2nd ed., pp. 349–392). New York: Guilford Press.

Dobson, K. S. (1989). A meta-analysis of the efficacy of cognitive therapy for depression. *Journal of Consulting and Clinical Psychology, 57,* 414–419.

Dobson, K. S., Backs-Dermott, B., & Dozois, D. J. A. (2000). Cognitive and cognitive-behavioral therapies. In C. R. Snyder & R. E. Ingram (Eds.), *Handbook of psychological change: Psychotherapy process and practices for the 21st century* (pp. 409–428). New York: Wiley.

Dobson, K. S., & Khatri, N. (2000). Cognitive therapy: Looking backward, looking forward. *Journal of Clinical Psychology, 56,* 907–923.

Doyle, A. B. (1998). Are empirically validated treatments valid for culturally diverse populations? In K. S. Dobson & K. D. Craig (Eds.), *Empirically supported therapies: Best practice in professional psychology* (pp. 93–103). Thousand Oaks, CA: Sage.

Elkin, I., Shea, M. T., Watkins, J. T., Imber, S. D., Sotsky, S. M., Collins, J. F., Glass, D. R., Pilkonis, P. A., Leber, W. R., Docherty, J. P., Fiester, S. J., & Parloff, M. B. (1989). National Institute of Mental Health Treatment of Depression Collaborative Research Program. *Archives of General Psychiatry, 46,* 971–982.

Garvey, M. J., Hollon, S. D., & DeRubeis, R. J. (1994). Do depressed clients with higher pretreatment stress levels respond better to cognitive therapy than imipramine? *Journal of Affective Disorders, 32,* 45–50.

Gloaguen, V., Cottraux, J., Cucherat, M., & Blackburn, I. M. (1998). A meta-analysis of the effects of cognitive therapy in depressed clients. *Journal of Affective Disorders, 49,* 59–72.

Gotlib, I. H., & Hammen, C. L. (1992). *Psychological aspects of depression: Toward a cognitive-interpersonal integration.* Chichester, UK: Wiley.

Hollon, S. D. (1996). The efficacy and effectiveness of psychotherapy relative to medications. *American Psychologist, 51,* 1025–1030.

Ingram, R. E., Miranda, J., & Segal, Z. V. (1998). *Cognitive vulnerability to depression.* New York: Guilford Press.

Jacobson, N. S., & Hollon, S. D. (1996). Prospects for future comparisons between drugs and psychotherapy: Lessons from the CBT-versus-pharmacotherapy exchange. *Journal of Consulting and Clinical Psychology, 64,* 74–80.

Jarrett, R. B., Eaves, G. G., Brannemann, B. D., & Rush, A. J. (1991). Clinical, cognitive, and demographic predictors of response to cognitive therapy for depression: A preliminary report. *Psychiatry Research, 37,* 245–260.

Paykel, E. S. (1992). *Handbook of affective disorders* (2nd ed.). New York: Guilford Press.

Persons, J. B., Burns, D. D., & Perloff, J. M. (1988). Predictors of dropout and outcome in cognitive therapy for depression in a private practice setting. *Cognitive Therapy and Research, 12,* 557–575.

Sacco, W. P., & Beck, A. T. (1995). Cognitive theory and therapy. In E. E. Beckham & W. R. Leber (Eds.), *Handbook of depression* (2nd ed., pp. 329–351). New York: Guilford Press.

Segal, Z. V., & Ingram, R. E. (1994). Mood priming and construct activation in tests of cognitive vulnerability to unipolar depression. *Clinical Psychology Review, 14,* 663–695.

Shapiro, D. A., Barkham, M., Rees, A., Hardy, G. E., Reynolds, S., & Startup, M. (1994). Effects of treatment duration and severity of depression on the effectiveness of cognitive-behavioral and psychodynamic–interpersonal psychotherapy. *Journal of Consulting and Clinical Psychology, 62,* 522–534.

Speier, P. L., Sherak, D. L., Hirsch, S., & Cantwell, D. P. (1995). Depression in children and adolescents. In E. E. Beckham & W. R. Leber (Eds.), *Handbook of depression* (2nd ed., pp. 467–493). New York: Guilford Press.

Thase, M. E., Reynolds, C. F., Frank, E., Simons, A. D., Garamoni, G. D., McGeary, J., Harden, T., Fasiczka, A. L., & Cahalane, J. F. (1994). Response to cognitive-behavioral therapy in chronic depression. *Journal of Psychotherapy Practice and Research, 3,* 204–214.

Thase, M. E., Simons, A., McGeary, J., Cahalane, J. F., Hughes, C., Harden, T., & Friedman, E. (1992). Relapse after cognitive behavior therapy of depression: Potential implications for longer courses of treatment. *American Journal of Psychiatry, 149,* 1046–1052.

Weissman, A. N. (1979). The Dysfunctional Attitudes Scale: A validation study (Doctoral dissertation, University of Pennsylvania). *Dissertation Abstracts International, 40,* 1389B–1390B.

Young, J. E. (1994). *Cognitive therapy for personality disorders: A schema-focused approach* (Rev. ed.). Sarasota, FL: Professional Resource Press.

6

Cognitive-Behavioral Therapy for the Management of Bipolar Disorder

MICHAEL W. OTTO
NOREEN REILLY-HARRINGTON

Bipolar disorder is severe and chronic, affecting approximately 1% of the population (Kessler, Rubinow, Holmes, Abelson, & Zhao, 1997), with higher estimates for bipolar spectrum disorders (Akiskal et al., 2000). The most common clinical course is a pattern of repeated episodes of depression and mania/hypomania that are disabling in their own right but may be compounded by the financial, family, and social disruptions that may occur during or following severe episodes (Miklowitz & Goldstein, 1997). In addition, coping with bipolar disorder may be further compromised by high rates of psychiatric comorbidity. For example, in a sample of 288 outpatients with bipolar disorder, 42% met criteria for a comorbid anxiety disorder, 42% for comorbid substance use disorder, and 5% for an eating disorder (McElroy et al., 2000). Bipolar disorder also appears to be a particularly lethal disorder in terms of suicidal risk. In a recently published study, Brown, Beck, Steer, and Grisham (2000) described the 20-year outcome for nearly 7,000 psychiatric outpatients in Pennsylvania, and found that, among the diagnostic categories, patients with bipolar disorder had the strongest risk for completed suicide, followed by major depression and personality disorders. Specifically, bipolar patients were found to have a nearly fourfold increase in suicide risk compared to other psychiatric patients, whereas major depression accounted for a threefold increase in risk (Brown et al., 2000).

Somatic treatments have been particularly emphasized in the management of bipolar disorder, but even with the broad array of mood stabilizing, antipsychotic, antidepressant, and antianxiety medications available, the most common course of bipolar disorder continues to be one of regular relapses to either depression or mania/hypomania. For example, longitudinal data suggest relapse rates as high as 40% in 1 year, and 60% in 2 years despite the use of mood stabilizers (Gitlin, Swendsen, Heller, & Hammen, 1995; see also O'Connell, Mayo, Flatlow, Cuthbertson, & O'Brien, 1991). Ongoing medication adherence brings its own challenges. Lifelong medication use is frequently recommended for bipolar patients. However, poor medication compliance is evident in one-half to two-thirds of patients within the first 12 months of treatment (Keck et al., 1996, 1998), with some data indicating a modal length of compliance with a mood stabilizer of only 2 months (Johnson & McFarland, 1996). These findings encourage the further development of psychosocial strategies to aid the management of bipolar disorder.

Descriptions of adjunctive cognitive-behavioral programs to help manage bipolar disorder received renewed attention in the mid-1990s (e.g., Basco & Rush, 1996; Scott, 1996), and have been complemented by more recent treatment approaches and protocols (e.g., Newman, Leahy, Beck, Reilly-Harrington, & Gyulai, 2001; Otto, Reilly-Harrington, Kogan, Henin, & Knauz, 1999). Also, early work by Cochran (1984) set the stage for a spate of recent, controlled studies of cognitive-behavioral therapy (CBT) for bipolar disorder. Cochran examined the effects of a six-session protocol of CBT focusing on the improvement of medication adherence in bipolar patients. The treatment was associated with significantly better adherence and fewer hospitalizations over a 6-month follow-up period compared to a treatment-as-usual comparison condition.

In a more recent study, Lam and colleagues (2000) examined the outcome of CBT in a sample of 25 bipolar outpatients randomized either to routine care or to routine care combined with a flexible schedule (12–20 sessions) of CBT delivered over the next 6 months. These patients had a mean history of seven manic episodes and nine depressive episodes, but were taking mood stabilizers and were not in an acute episode at the time of the pretreatment evaluation. The CBT emphasized education about bipolar disorder and its management, as well as cognitive restructuring, problem-solving, and routine- and sleep-management interventions. Ratings by an independent assessor at 6 and 12 months revealed that treatment with CBT was associated with significantly fewer manic, hypomanic, and depressed episodes than the comparison condition. In terms of categorical outcomes, 10 of 12 patients treated with CBT had no mood episodes during follow-up compared to only 2 of 11 patients in the comparison condition.

Scott, Garland, and Moorhead (2001) examined outcome for CBT compared to a waiting-list (treatment-as-usual) comparison condition in a sample of 42 patients with bipolar disorder. Treatment consisted of information, regulation of activities and sleep, stress management, cognitive restructuring, interventions for medication adherence, and relapse prevention efforts. Patients in this trial primarily (81%) had bipolar I disorder and rich comorbidity, including a 60% rate of Axis II disorders as assessed by the Personality Diagnostic Questionnaire—Revised (PDQ-R). At 6-month follow-up, patients who received CBT had significantly greater improvements in global functioning and, particularly, depression symptoms. Furthermore, long-term follow-up of 29 patients who eventually received CBT indicated that relapse rates in the 18 months after starting CBT were 60% below the values for the 18 months prior to the initiation of CBT.

Finally, interim results from an ongoing study (Hirshfeld et al., 1998) support the efficacy of CBT offered in a group setting. These researchers examined the effects of an adjunctive, 11-session group program designed to reduce symptoms and help protect against relapse. Elements of treatment included psychoeducation, cognitive restructuring, assertiveness and problem-solving training, activity management, and medication adherence. In analyses to date, this treatment was successful in significantly reducing the number of new episodes and increasing euthymic periods relative to a medication-alone comparison condition.

Together, these four, small, controlled trials (Cochran, 1984; Hirshfeld et al., 1998; Lam et al., 2000; and Scott et al., 2001) provide a consistent picture of the potential efficacy of CBT for reducing relapse among patients with bipolar disorder. There is also tentative evidence for the role of CBT in treating bipolar depression as well. Given the well-documented efficacy for treating unipolar depression (for a review, see Deckersbach, Gershuny, & Otto, 2000; Dobson, 1989), including treatment-resistant and endogenous samples (Fava, Savron, Grandi, & Rafanelli, 1997; Simons & Thase, 1992; Thase, Bowler, & Harden, 1991; Thase, Simons, Cahalane, & McGeary, 1991), there has been hope that these treatment effects would extend to bipolar depression as well. Tentative support for this hypothesis was provided in an uncontrolled study by Zaretsky, Segal, and Gemar (1999). These researchers found that in a case series of unipolar and bipolar patients, both samples of patients demonstrated equal response to CBT.

This evidence for CBT joins other evidence for the efficacy of psychosocial treatments in improving the course of bipolar disorder. In a randomized trial of 79 bipolar patients, Miklowitz and colleagues (2000) found that 21 sessions of family-focused therapy (FFT; Miklowitz & Goldstein, 1997; see also Miklowitz, Chapter 8, this volume) reduced both depressive and manic symptoms, and offered better protection against the recurrence of depression compared to a condition that offered pharmacological treatment and case management alone. Interpersonal and social rhythm therapy (IPSRT; Frank et al., 1994; see also Swartz, Markowitz, & Frank, Chapter 7, this volume) also holds promise for the management of bipolar disorder. Although initial study did not demonstrate efficacy (Frank et al., 1997, 1999), additional investigation has revealed that IPSRT may promote periods of euthymia (Frank & Hlastala, 2000).

It is noteworthy that both FFT and IPSRT share a common focus on psychoeducation and medication adherence, social or family problem solving, and communication training. These elements of treatment are also part of CBT protocols for bipolar disorder (see, e.g., Otto et al., 1999). Thus, although these treatments differ significantly in terms of theoretical assumptions and practical strategies, they do share some of the same targets and elements of treatment. Each of these treatments—CBT, FFT, and IPSRT—are under study in the large, multicenter National Institutes of Health–funded Systematic Treatment Enhancement Program (STEP) for bipolar disorder, which seeks to randomize up to 500 patients in a controlled investigation of these treatments.

The CBT under study in the STEP protocol is a manualized treatment (Otto et al., 1999; see also Henin, Otto, & Reilly-Harrington, 2001) organized into two pathways. One pathway is for patients presenting with bipolar depression (30 sessions), and the other targets patients who are recovering from a manic/hypomanic episode and are in the need of relapse prevention (21 sessions, with patients entering treatment at Session 10 of the 30-session format). In the 30-session protocol, treatment proceeds in four formal stages: a depression-focus phase (9 sessions), a treatment-contract phase (3 sessions), a problem-list phase (14 sessions), and a well-being phase (4 sessions). In each phase, similar cognitive-behavioral procedures are utilized, but the targets and style of therapy shift according to the treatment phase.

TREATMENT PHASE 1: TARGETING BIPOLAR DEPRESSION

The first phase of treatment consists of nine sessions devoted to the treatment of depressive symptoms and utilizes the psychoeducational, cognitive restructuring, and activity assignment interventions commonly applied to unipolar depression (e.g., J. Beck, 1995; Beck, Rush, Shaw, & Emery, 1979). Treatment is initiated with a discussion of a model of the disorder and a rationale for CBT, combined with instruction on the interplay between thoughts, feelings, and behavior. This didactic information is complemented by self-monitoring assignments in which patients are to observe their own experiences, test the model, and identify for themselves the role of thoughts in influencing mood.

Especially at the outset of treatment, attention is placed on the use of vivid metaphors and stories to crystallize important information on the nature of the disorder, the process of change, or a specific assignment or skill. Therapeutic stories and metaphors are suggested to help patients draw on their own knowledge and experiences to sum up treatment principles for use in relevant moments of their life. For example, patients may be provided with a vivid image of the role of negative thoughts in depression, so that the image helps them with the process of self-monitoring and restructuring of these thoughts (see Otto, 2000).

Early sessions are also devoted to helping patients adopt a "therapeutic perspective" toward their own care, emphasizing self-empathy in response to distress and the search for useful problem-solving alternatives ("What would help me now?"). This perspective is seen as a general skill that will aid the acquisition and utilization of skills taught later in treatment. The therapeutic perspective also provides a natural segue to monitoring one's thoughts and correcting the distorted and dysfunctional evaluations that characterize depression.

To complete cognitive restructuring exercises, patients are asked to be aware of their emotions in the moment, and upon detecting an emotional change, to examine both the external situation ("What is going on?") and their internal environment ("What have I been saying to myself?"). This process, by its nature, demands a degree of emotional acceptance; patients are asked to perceive and tolerate an emotion while treating it as a signal for problem solving. This skill is modeled by the therapist virtually every session. In particular, the therapist's comfort with the patient's emotion, and the delivery of appropriate empathy in conjunction with a problem-solving approach, provides a model for the skills to be acquired by the patient. This modeling is considered an essential feature of this program of CBT. In addition, more formal cognitive restructuring interventions (J. Beck, 1995) are complemented by activity assignments that are designed to help return the patient to adaptive behavior and potentially pleasant events that can sustain improvements in mood.

Cognitive interventions in Phase 1 are also concerned with the identification of cognitive themes (core beliefs) that play themselves out over and over again in daily dysfunctional thoughts. Early identification of these themes can help speed application of cognitive interventions for the wide range of topics to be encountered in subsequent phases of treatment.

Case Example: Core Belief Identification

Molly, a 55-year-old woman with a diagnosis of bipolar I disorder, has been married for 30 years and has two adult children. Molly's story begins quite tragically. She was born the youngest of three children in a very poor family. Her parents were immigrants who both suffered from alcoholism and mood disorders. Molly reports that she was told by her parents again and again that she was a "mistake" that deprived the family of money to buy food and other goods, and was repeatedly threatened with being sent to an orphanage because she was "bad." In contrast, her older brother was favored and protected from this verbal abuse. Molly's father committed suicide when she was 13 years old. Her mother often blamed the children for his suicide, saying that he had been under too much stress caring for their family. However, Molly was a tough kid and excelled in school.

Despite being labeled "bad" by her family, she never got into trouble at school and successfully graduated from high school. She began working in business and eventually opened her own office. Molly was savvy, personable, and able to entertain customers with her colorful style, particularly when she was hypomanic. She suffered two severe postpartum depressive episodes after the births of her children and still reports tremendous guilt about not being able to care for them adequately during this time period. During one of her manic episodes, she was swindled in a deal with a business partner and wound up $400,000 in debt. She lost her business and was forced to file bankruptcy. Following this loss, her depressive episodes became more frequent and resistant to pharmacotherapy. It was at this point that her psychiatrist then referred her for adjunctive CBT.

The cognitive portion of her treatment focused on modification of her core beliefs from childhood and the associated, daily dysfunctional thoughts. The Cognitive Conceptualization Diagram developed by J. Beck (1995) is useful in illustrating the connections between the meaning of Molly's negative automatic thoughts, her childhood experiences, and her underlying core beliefs of badness and helplessness (Figure 6.1).

The three situations at the bottom of the diagram illustrate three typical situations Molly discussed in treatment. The underlying meanings of Molly's automatic thoughts in these situations relate directly to her core beliefs. The Cognitive Conceptualization Diagram also guides the examination of patients' underlying assumptions, or rules about the world, and the strategies that they have developed to compensate for core beliefs.

TREATMENT PHASE 2: TREATMENT CONTRACTING AND GOAL SETTING

In the second phase of treatment, three sessions are devoted to discussion and completion of a treatment contract and delineation of targets for the next phase of treatment (for patients entering treatment at the relapse prevention stage, this phase represents the start of treatment). The treatment contract serves as a means of planning for future mood episodes and enables the patient to communicate a plan for treatment with a personally selected cohort of support people (the extended treatment team). The contract is in part designed as an educational tool; the patient describes his or her affective, cognitive, and behavioral symptoms of mania and depression to better target early warning signs of a mood episode. Emphasis is then placed on the problem-solving responses to be taken by the patient and by the treatment team upon signs of a relapse. Of particular importance is the identification of the initial signs of hypomania, to allow early detection and protective action against a potential manic episode. Next, patients develop a set of directives, stating ways in which they and their support systems can be helpful in preventing and managing acute episodes. Strategies of this kind (early detection and intervention) have been found to reduce significantly the rate of occurrence and number of manic episodes (Perry, Tarrier, Morriss, McCarthy, & Limb, 1999).

When the contract is formulated, members of the extended treatment team are asked to review, ask questions, modify in conjunction with the patient, and then sign the contract. If the contract is correctly formulated, the therapist and others who apply the contract become agents of the patient's planning rather than people imposing their own restrictions on the patient. An example contract is available at the Web site *manicdepressive.org*; this contract is an outgrowth of previous work geared toward actively engaging patients in written plans for managing bipolar illness (Bauer & McBride, 1996; Hirshfeld et al., 1998).

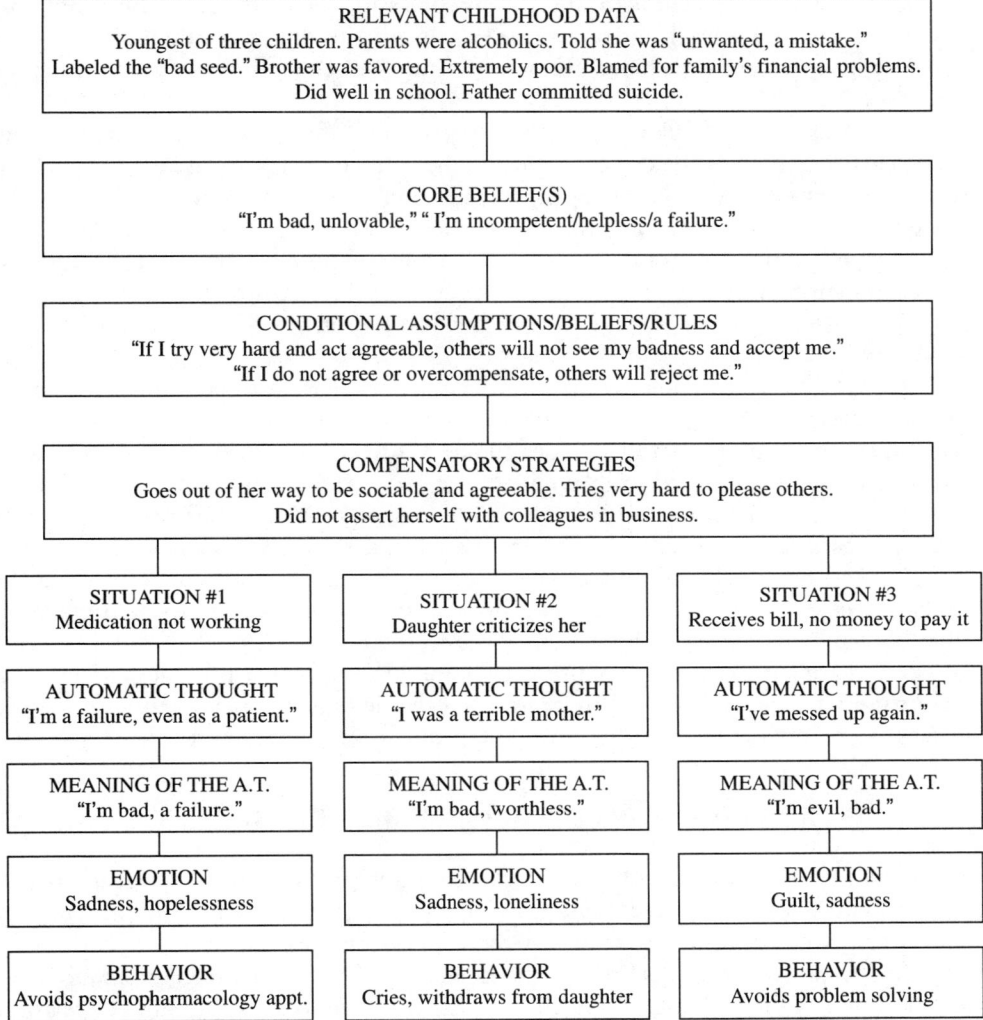

FIGURE 6.1. Cognitive Conceptualization Diagram for Molly's core beliefs. From J. S. Beck (1995). Copyright 1995 by The Guilford Press. Adapted by permission.

Discussions associated with the treatment contract are also designed to define areas where the patient is most at risk for relapse. Untreated disorders are, of course, one prime area of risk, and this phase of treatment serves as a time when problem areas are defined for more intensive treatment in the next phase.

TREATMENT PHASE 3: THE PROBLEM LIST PHASE

The third phase a treatment utilizes a modular design to target problem areas of most concern to the patient and therapist. The goal of this phase is to ensure that treatment can be flexibly applied while maintaining a manualized treatment format that can be replicated across studies (Henin et al., 2001). The case conceptualization worksheets direct the therapist to relevant instrumental outcomes for each patient. Instrumental outcomes, as defined by Rosen and Proctor (1981), are the outcomes therapists wish to manipulate in treatment to achieve ultimate outcomes, such as the resolution of depression or prevention of relapse.

Although use of a modular approach will result in differences in the content among patients, each session is to be conducted using the same problem-focused format: (1) review of the previous week's learning; (2) formulation and completion of the agenda for the session, with attention to in-session rehearsal of concepts; (3) review of the session content; (4) assignment of homework; and (5) troubleshooting homework completion. This format maintains a consistent focus on the step-by-step, goal-oriented, skills acquisition approach that is central to cognitive-behavioral treatments for depression (see, e.g., J. Beck, 1995).

Tables 6.1 and 6.2 provide examples of the case formulation choice points used in the Otto and colleagues (1999) treatment manual. In the manual, the worksheets are constructed in an "if–then" format that guides clinicians toward specific interventions or treatment modules for the specified problem area. The purpose of the first case conceptualization worksheet is to help therapists evaluate the degree to which patients have learned some of the core skills utilized in treatment. As treatment progresses, the patient will be required repeatedly to call upon these skills as they are applied to new instrumental goals.

The purpose of the second case conceptualization worksheet is to help clinicians troubleshoot potential reasons for nonresponse to interventions for depression or select targets for treatment as part of relapse prevention efforts, which provide patients with an opportunity to hone cognitive-behavioral skills while reducing risk factors for relapse. This list is to be reviewed monthly during the problem list phase of treatment.

TREATMENT PHASE 4: WELL-BEING THERAPY

The final phase of treatment adopts a *well-being* perspective and is designed to help patients extend and solidify treatment gains by applying cognitive-behavioral strategies for improving well-being rather than just reducing symptoms (Fava, 1999; Fava et al., 1998). This treatment is well suited to the heterogeneity of needs (e.g., residual symptoms, additional skills building, or return to or enhancement of work, leisure, or relationship activities) that may be present at the end of a successful treatment episode. Typically, the introduction of the well-being focus occurs at Session 27 of 30. However, if the patient is doing well, the principles of well-being therapy can be introduced as early as Session 23 to complement the focus on improving the enjoyment of life that is part of the problem list phase.

REDUCING THE RISK OF RELAPSE: TARGETS FOR TREATMENT

A variety of evidence suggests that psychosocial variables play a crucial role in influencing the course of bipolar disorder. For example, negative life events appear to alter significantly the course of recovery from episodes in patients with bipolar disorder. Johnson and Miller (1997) found that negative life events were associated with a threefold increase in time to recovery in a sample of 67 patients with bipolar disorder hospitalized for mania or depression. Negative life events also appear to affect relapse, with Ellicott, Hammen, Gitlin, Brown, and Jamison (1990) finding a 4.5 higher relapse rate over 2 years among patients with high negative-life-event scores.

TABLE 6.1. Assessment Portion of the Case Conceptualization Worksheet 1

In the treatment manual, therapists are directed to therapeutic interventions associated with failure to achieve checklist items.

1. Therapeutic Attitude

Has the patient learned an empathetic attitude toward herself or himself with an orientation toward stepwise problem solving? Elements of this skill include:

_____ Able to recognize when one is hurt by symptoms or problems and to be oriented toward self-care rather than criticism.
_____ Able to inhibit self-criticism and examine useful responses to negative affect.
_____ Oriented toward learning new skills, and aware of the potential benefits of new skills.
_____ Aware of depression as a syndrome, including thought biases and the source of somatic symptoms, disruptions of activity levels and energy, etc.
_____ Aware of bipolar disorder as a disorder, including the need for the acquisition of specific skills to reduce the risk of relapse.
_____ Able to apply skills learned in session to problem areas.

2. Cognitive Restructuring

Some of the more common targets of cognitive restructuring include the patient's conceptualization of events (particularly social or performance events), the patient's evaluation of his or her own performance, and ongoing evaluation and modification of core beliefs. In these domains, the therapist should be particularly sensitive to themes of presumed rejection by others, and failure-focused attention (noticing what is not proceeding well) combined with perfectionistic or overly rigid self-standards. In addition to this sensitivity, therapists need to ensure that component parts of self-monitoring and cognitive restructuring are being applied. The following checklist should be used to assess the adequacy with which patients have adopted basic cognitive restructuring skills. Problem solving is included as a cognitive skill that patients should by applying in daily life.

_____ Able to identify affect.
_____ Able to identify automatic thoughts (after the fact).
_____ Able to identify automatic thoughts as they occur.
_____ Able to generate alternative thoughts.
_____ Able to feel a shift in affect from cognitive restructuring.
_____ Able to recognize habitual negative thoughts.
_____ Able to apply problem-solving techniques out of the session.

3. Activity Assignments

Activity assignments provide a format for the "doing" component of CBT. The goal of activity assignments is to structure life events and activities that best provide a buffer from negative mood states and that directly contribute to a stable, positive affect

_____ Sufficient buffering events during the week to allow breaks from ongoing stressors (including breaks from boredom).
_____ Regular pleasurable events occur.
_____ Regular mastery/achievement events occur.
_____ Moments of pleasure occur in response to positive events.
_____ Patient attends to positive events once completed.
_____ Activity schedule is manageable given the constraints of bipolar disorder.
_____ Aversive events occur at a low frequency.
_____ Patient is able to enjoy unstructured time.

Note. From Otto, Reilly-Harrington, Kogan, Henin, and Knauz (1999). Reprinted by permission of the authors.

TABLE 6.2. Assessment Portion of Case Conceptualization Worksheet 2

In the treatment manual, therapists are directed to therapeutic interventions associated with each checklist item.

- _____ Patient is noncompliant with medication regimen.
- _____ Patient reports irregular sleep or sleep disruption.
- _____ Substance use is of concern.
- _____ Anxiety interferes with activity goals or pleasant events.
- _____ Avoidance interferes with activity goals or pleasant events.
- _____ Interpersonal relationships are not satisfying.
- _____ Aversive interpersonal events contribute to symptoms.
- _____ Repeated emotional crises interfere with application of skills.
- _____ Patient's goals are not adequately achieved.

Note. From Otto, Reilly-Harrington, Kogan, Henin, and Knauz (1999). Reprinted by permission of the authors.

Cognitive style also appears to play an important role in modulating the impact of life events on symptoms. In combination with negative life stressors, bipolar individuals with dysfunctional attitudes or depressogenic attributional styles are more likely to develop affective symptoms (Alloy, Reilly-Harrington, Fresco, Whitehouse, & Zechmeister, 1999; Reilly-Harrington, Alloy, Fresco, & Whitehouse, 1999). Moreover, dysfunctional and overemotional family communication patterns also appear to exert a significant influence on relapse rates. Miklowitz, Goldstein, Neuchterlein, Snyder, and Mintz (1988) examined the outcome of 23 bipolar patients discharged to families characterized as either high or low in expressed emotion (a critical and hostile communication style coupled with emotional overinvolvement). High expressed emotion families had over five times the relapse rate as families low in expressed emotion.

Finally, several studies suggest that disruptions in sleep–wake cycles may place bipolar patients at risk for new episodes. In particular, negative life events that trigger sleep disruption may be more likely to lead to mania than those that do not (Malkoff-Schwartz et al., 1998). Management of sleep cycles is likewise assumed to aid the control of episodes in bipolar disorder, with support for this proposition provided by case studies (Wehr, 1991; Wehr et al., 1998; Wirz-Justice, 1999).

These risk factors for relapse—negative events, cognitive style, family communication patterns, and sleep patterns—are targeted during Phases 1–3 of treatment with a combination of cognitive restructuring, assertiveness, problem-solving, and activity level interventions. For sleep management, we recommend a two-stage process (Otto, Reilly-Harrington, & Sachs, in press). In the first, the clinician educates the patient about the role of disruptions in the sleep–wake cycle in evoking new episodes and discusses with the patient what level of activity and sleep the patient recommends for him- or herself. Once the desired hours of sleep have been identified, the therapist helps the patient calculate a regular bedtime relative to daily demands and waking times. To aid compliance, the clinician should also identify cues (e.g., television programs) to prompt preparation to sleep.

MEDICATION ADHERENCE

Pharmacological management of bipolar disorders faces some of the classic challenges of any preventive program utilizing medication; at the time the medication is taken, there may be no disorder-related symptoms and, accordingly, no symptom relief to either cue or reward pill taking. Furthermore, emergent side effects may further reduce motivation for pill taking. Whereas a variety of preventive programs may face similar difficulties, bipolar disorder brings with it the additional challenge that past hypomanic episodes may be remembered fondly and may be desired, and patients may also be unconvinced of the need for preventive treatment (see Jamison & Akiskal, 1983; Keck et al., 1996). Under these conditions, it is no surprise that adherence to mood stabilizers is so poor (see, e.g., Keck et al., 1998).

Accordingly, we recommend use of a motivational interviewing approach (Otto et al., in press), an empirically supported strategy for enhancing engagement in treatment (Rollnick & Miller, 1995; Yahne & Miller, 1999). Specifically, we encourage adoption of a life history approach to first eliciting relevant patient information on the impact of bipolar episodes on personal and family goals. This evidence can then be used to help the patient decide whether alternative treatments, or greater adherence to current treatments, is a reasonable strategy to adopt. When successful, patients may adopt a balanced perspective that incorporates more consistent medication use: "You know I really miss my hypomanic episodes, but when I take my medication, my life works better; I am not in trouble all the time."

Enhancing motivation for medication use is only a part of the adherence interventions. Regular self-monitoring and cueing of medication use, as have been adopted for other disorders (see, e.g., Safren, Otto, & Worth, 2000), to help establish and maintain a habit of regular self-care are also recommended for bipolar disorder.

EARLY INTERVENTION STRATEGIES

A variety of CBT protocols (Basco & Rush, 1996; Newman et al., 2001; Otto et al., 1999), emphasize early intervention strategies to reduce the impact of hypomanic or manic episodes should they occur. These interventions are designed to help prevent full manic episodes and the poor financial, social, or sexual decisions that accompany them. Many of the preventive strategies are outlined in the treatment contract, and range from specification of when members of the treatment team should be contacted and act, to rules for risky actions such as using credit cards or making investment decisions. A variety of procedures have been developed (see Newman et al., 2001) to help reduce poor decisions upon the escalation of manic symptoms. Table 6.3 provides a summary of some of these strategies.

For example, Newman and colleagues (2000) describe a "two-person feedback rule," where patients are taught to test out any new plan or idea with at least two trusted advisors. Attention is placed on helping patients identify the difference between the hypomanic symptom of ideas "feeling" correct even though they may not "be" correct. With the two-person feedback rule, patients are taught that if an idea is actually useful, then two other people should be able to find it reasonable.

TREATMENT OF COMORBIDITY

Treatment of comorbid conditions is an additional role for CBT. Recent research has shown that anxiety comorbidity in bipolar disorder is associated with longer times to remission (Feske et al., 2000), a finding that underscores the importance of treating anxiety as part of efforts to speed recovery. CBT and pharmacotherapy (particularly, treat-

TABLE 6.3. Early-Intervention Strategies for Hypomania

- Explore medication solutions (e.g., dosage or medication changes).
- Establish rules to counteract impulsivity, with the help of others (e.g., giving credit cards to someone to hold, avoiding alcohol use).
- Avoid confrontative situations.
- Avoid irreversible decisions ("No big decisions" rule).
- Use the two-person feedback rule (check out any new plan or idea with two trusted friends or family members before acting on them).
- Use the 48-hour rule (allow at least 2 full days with 2 nights' sleep before acting on risky decisions).
- Challenge overpositive cognitions (as recorded in thought records).
- Review the wish to stay manic or nostalgia about previous episodes.
- Maintain adequate sleep and reduce activity levels.
- Increase time sitting and listening.
- Use relaxation techniques.

Note. From Newman, Leahy, Beck, Reilly-Harrington, and Gyulai (2001).

ment with antidepressants) represent the treatment modalities with the best empirical support for efficacy with anxiety disorders, with CBT offering comparable, short-term outcome and the advantage of longer term maintenance of treatment gains, without the need for ongoing treatment (e.g., Christensen, Hadzi-Pavlovic, Andrews, & Mattick, 1987; Gould, Buckminster, Pollack, Otto, & Yap, 1997; Gould, Otto, & Pollack, 1995; Gould, Otto, Pollack, & Yap, 1997; Otto, Penava, Pollock, & Smoller, 1996). Furthermore, CBT has the additional advantage of being free of the manic-inducing effects sometimes associated with antidepressant use in patients with bipolar disorder. Other comorbid conditions also occur at high rates in bipolar disorder. Substance use disorders have been identified in 40–60% of bipolar patients (see, e.g., Chengappa, Levine, Gershon, & Kupfer, 2000; McElroy et al., 2000), and are linked with a poorer course of the disorder (Salloum & Thase, 2000). These findings further motivate the application of a range of psychosocial interventions (e.g., Weiss et al., 2000) for the treatment of these comorbid conditions as part of the overall management of bipolar disorders.

SUICIDE PREVENTION STRATEGIES

As we noted at the outset of this chapter, patients with bipolar disorder are at particular risk of suicide, relative to other diagnostic groups. Accordingly, suicide prevention strategies should be considered as a matter of course with these patients.

In a recent review of the psychosocial literature, Gray and Otto (2001) identified 17 studies that provide controlled outcome data on suicide rates associated with these interventions. Many of these studies were conducted with inadequate power; consequently, effect sizes were used to examine the magnitude of treatment benefits relative to control conditions. Three separate types of interventions were supported by the effect-size analysis: (1) facilitating of a patient's ability to elicit emergency care using simple interventions (printed cards) that can be applied at times of distress, (2) training in problem-solving strategies (particularly social problem solving), and (3) utilizing more comprehensive interventions that combine a problem-solving emphasis with intensive rehearsal of cognitive, social, emotional labeling, and distress-tolerance skills.

Based on this empirical review, Gray and Otto (2001) recommended the following strategies as standard elements of a suicide prevention program for patients with bipolar disorder: (1) vigorously treating the bipolar disorder; (2) overrehearsing help options for times of distress, including the facilitation of help from support networks; (3) training in problem-solving skills; (4) cognitive restructuring for hopelessness-based cognitions; (5) enhancing "reasons for living"; and (6) training in emotional tolerance/regulation skills. As can be noted from this list, many of these elements are already encompassed within the contract-driven and comprehensive CBT programs discussed earlier, but additional attention to each of these strategies is encouraged when working with higher risk patients with bipolar disorder.

CONCLUDING COMMENTS

In recent years, a number of clinical and research programs have adapted cognitive-behavioral interventions to the management of bipolar disorder. Regardless of whether these interventions have focused primarily on increasing adherence to medications or more directly seeking to alter the symptoms of bipolar disorder, multiple small studies have provided evidence of efficacy and encourage the further application of these strategies. With this success, CBT joins two other forms of psychotherapy—family-focused therapy (Miklowitz & Goldstein, 1997) and interpersonal psychotherapy with a social rhythm component (Frank et al., 1994)—in providing empirically based psychosocial treatment for the adjunctive management of bipolar disorder. More data on the overall and relative efficacy of these treatments will be forthcoming as part of the very large Systematic Treatment Enhancement Program (STEP) for bipolar disorder.

REFERENCES

Akiskal, H. S., Bourgeois, M. L., Angst, J., Post, R., Moller, H., & Hirschfeld, R. (2000). Reevaluating the prevalence of and diagnostic composition within the broad clinical spectrum of bipolar disorders. *Journal of Affective Disorders, 59*(Suppl. 1), 5–30.

Alloy, L. B., Reilly-Harrington, N. A., Fresco, D. M., Whitehouse, W. G., & Zechmeister, J. S. (1999). Cognitive styles and life events in subsyndromal unipolar and bipolar disorders: Stability and prospective prediction of depressive and hypomanic mood swings. *Journal of Cognitive Psychotherapy: An International Quarterly, 13*, 21–40.

Basco, M. R., & Rush, A. J. (1996). *Cognitive-behavioral therapy for bipolar disorder.* New York: Guilford Press.

Bauer, M., & McBride, L. (1996). *Structured group psychotherapy for bipolar disorder: The life goals program.* New York: Springer.

Beck, A. T., Rush, A. J., Shaw, B. F., & Emery, G. (1979). *Cognitive therapy of depression.* New York: Guilford Press.

Beck, J. S. (1995). *Cognitive therapy: Basics and beyond.* New York: Guilford Press.

Brown, G. K., Beck, A. T., Steer, R. A., & Grisham, J. R. (2000). Risk factors for suicide in psychiatric outpatients: A 20-year prospective study. *Journal of Consulting and Clinical Psychology, 68*, 371–377.

Chengappa, K. N., Levine, J., Gershon, S., Kupfer, D. J. (2000). Lifetime prevalence of substance or alcohol abuse and dependence among subjects with bipolar I and II disorders in a voluntary registry. *Bipolar Disorder, 2*, 191–195.

Christensen, H., Hadzi-Pavlovic, D., Andrews, G., & Mattick, R. (1987). Behavior therapy and tricyclic medication in the treatment of obsessive–compulsive disorder: A quantitative review. *Journal of Consulting and Clinical Psychology, 55*, 701–711.

Cochran, S. (1984). Preventing medical noncompliance in the outpatient treatment of bipolar affective disorders. *Journal of Consulting and Clinical Psychology, 52,* 873–878.

Deckersbach, T., Gershuny, B. S., & Otto, M. W. (2000). Cognitive-behavioral therapy for depression: Applications and outcome. *Psychiatric Clinics of North America, 23,* 795–809.

Dobson, K. S. (1989). A meta-analysis of the efficacy of cognitive therapy for depression. *Journal of Consulting and Clinical Psychology, 57,* 414–419.

Ellicott, A., Hammen, C., Gitlin, M., Brown, G., & Jamison, K. (1990). Life events and the course of bipolar disorder. *American Journal of Psychiatry, 147,* 1194–1198.

Fava, G. A., Savron, G., Grandi, S., & Rafanelli, C. (1997). Cognitive behavioral treatment of drug resistant major depression disorder. *Journal of Clinical Psychiatry, 58,* 278–282.

Feske, U., Frank, E., Mallinger, A. G., Houck, P. R., Fagiolini, A., Shear, M. K., Grochocinski, V. J., & Kupfer, D. J. (2000). Anxiety as a correlate of response to the acute treatment of bipolar I disorder. *American Journal of Psychiatry, 157,* 956–962.

Frank E., & Hlastala, S. (2000, November 16–19). *Interpersonal and social rhythm therapy for bipolar disorder.* Paper presented at the meeting of the Association for Advancement of Behavior Therapy, New Orleans, LA.

Frank E., Hlastala, S., Ritenour, A., Houck, P., Tu, X. M., Mark, T. H., Mallinger, A. G., & Kupfer, D. J. (1997). Inducing lifestyle regularity in recovering bipolar disorder patients. *Biological Psychiatry, 41,* 1165–1173.

Frank, E., Kupfer, D. J., Ehlers, C. L., Monk, T. H., Cornes, C., Carter, S., & Frankel, D. (1994). Interpersonal and social rhythm therapy for bipolar disorder: Integrating interpersonal and behavioral approaches. *Behavior Therapist, 17,* 143–149.

Frank, E., Swartz, H. A., Mallinger, A. G., Thase, M. E., Weaver, E. V., & Kupfer, D. J. (1999). Adjunctive psychotherapy for bipolar disorder: Effects of changing treatment modality. *Journal of Abnormal Psychology, 108,* 579–587.

Gitlin, M. J., Swendsen, J., Heller, T. L., & Hammen, C. (1995). Relapse and impairment in bipolar disorder. *American Journal of Psychiatry, 152,* 1635–1640.

Gould, R. A., Buckminster, S., Pollack, M. H., Otto, M. W., & Yap, L. (1997). Cognitive-behavioral and pharmacological treatment for social phobia: A meta-analysis. *Clinical Psychology: Science and Practice, 4,* 291–306.

Gould, R. A., Otto, M. W., & Pollack, M. H. (1995). A meta-analysis of treatment outcome for panic disorder. *Clinical Psychology Review, 15,* 819–844.

Gould, R. A., Otto, M. W., Pollack, M. P., & Yap, L. (1997). Cognitive-behavioral and pharmacological treatment of generalized anxiety disorder: A preliminary meta-analysis. *Behavior Therapy, 28,* 285–305.

Gray, S. M., & Otto, M. W. (2001). Psychosocial approaches to suicide prevention: Applications to patients with bipolar disorder. *Journal of Clinical Psychiatry, 62*(Suppl. 25), 56–64.

Henin, A., Otto, M. W., & Reilly-Harrington, N. A. (2001). Introducing flexibility in manualized treatment: Application of recommended strategies to the cognitive-behavioral treatment of bipolar disorder. *Cognitive and Behavioral Practice, 8,* 317–328.

Hirshfeld, D. R., Gould, R. A., Reilly-Harrington, N. A., Morabito, C., Guille, C., Fredman, S. J., & Sachs, G. (1998, November). *Cognitive-behavioral group therapy for bipolar disorder: A controlled trial.* Paper presented at the 32nd Annual Meeting of the Association for Advancement of Behavior Therapy, Washington, DC.

Jamison, K. R., & Akiskal, H. S. (1983). Medication compliance in patients with bipolar disorders. *Psychiatric Clinics of North America, 6,* 175–192.

Johnson, R. E., & McFarland, B. H. (1996). Lithium use and discontinuation in a health maintenance organization. *American Journal of Psychiatry, 153,* 993–1000.

Johnson, S. L., & Miller, I. (1997). Negative life events and time to recovery from episodes of bipolar disorder. *Journal of Abnormal Psychology, 106,* 449–457.

Keck, P. E., McElroy, S. L., Strakowski, S. M., Stanton, S. P., Kizer, D. L., Balistreri, T. M., Bennett, J. A., Tugrul, K. C., & West, S. A. (1996). Factors associated with pharmacologic noncompliance in patients with mania. *Journal of Clinical Psychiatry, 57,* 292–297.

Keck, P. E., McElroy, S. L., Strakowski, S. M., West, S. A., Sax, K. W., Hawkins, J. M., Bourne, M. L., & Haggard, P. (1998). 12-Month outcome of patients with bipolar disorder following hospitalization for a manic or mixed episode. *American Journal of Psychiatry, 155,* 646–652.

Kessler, R. C., Rubinow, D. R., Holmes, C., Abelson, J. M., & Zhao, S. (1997). The epidemiology of DSM-III-R bipolar I disorder in a general population survey. *Psychological Medicine, 27,* 1079–1089.

Lam, D. H., Bright, J., Jones, S., Hayward, P., Schuck, N., Chisholm, D., & Sham, P. (2000). Cognitive therapy for bipolar disorder: A pilot study of relapse prevention. *Cognitive Therapy and Research, 24,* 503–520.

Malkoff-Schwartz, S. F., Frank, E., Anderson, B., Sherrill, J. T., Siegel, L., Patterson, D., & Kupfer, D. J. (1998). Stressful life events and social rhythm disruption in the onset of manic and depressive bipolar episodes: A preliminary investigation. *Archives of General Psychiatry, 55,* 702–707.

McElroy, S. L., Atshuler, L. L., Suppes, T., Keck, P. E., Frye, M. A., Denicoff, K. D., Nolen, W. A., Kupka, R. W., Leverich, G. S., Rochussen, J. R., Rush, A. J., & Post, R. M. (2000). Axis I psychiatric comorbidity and its relationship to historical illness variables in 288 patients with bipolar disorder. *American Journal of Psychiatry, 159,* 420–426.

Miklowitz, D. R., & Goldstein, M. J. (1997). *Bipolar disorder: A family-focused treatment approach.* New York: Guilford Press.

Miklowitz, D. R., Goldstein, M. J., Nuechterlein, K. H., Snyder, K. S., & Mintz, J. (1988). Family factors and the course of bipolar affective disorder. *Archives of General Psychiatry, 45,* 225–231.

Miklowitz, D. J., Simoneau, T. L., George, E. L., Richards, J. A., Kalbag, A., Sachs-Ericsson, N., & Suddath, R. (2000). Family-focused treatment of bipolar disorder: One-year effects of a psychoeducational program in conjunction with pharmacotherapy. *Biological Psychiatry, 48,* 582–592.

Newman, C. F., Leahy, R. L., Beck, A. T., Reilly-Harrington, N. A., & Gyulai, L. (2001). *Bipolar disorder: A cognitive therapy approach.* Washington, DC: American Psychological Association.

O'Connell, R. A., Mayo, J. A., Flatlow, L., Cuthbertson, B., & O'Brien, B. E. (1991). Outcome of bipolar disorder on long-term treatment with lithium. *British Journal of Psychiatry, 159,* 123–129.

Otto, M. W. (2000). Stories and metaphors in cognitive-behavior therapy. *Cognitive and Behavioral Practice, 7,* 166–172.

Otto, M. W., Penava, S. J., Pollock, R. A., & Smoller, J. W. (1996). Cognitive-behavioral and pharmacologic perspectives on the treatment of posttraumatic stress disorder. In M. H. Pollack, M. W. Otto, & J. F. Rosenbaum (Eds.), *Challenges in clinical practice: Pharmacologic and psychosocial strategies* (pp. 219–260). New York: Guilford Press.

Otto, M. W., Reilly-Harrington, N., Kogan, J. N., Henin, A., & Knauz, R. O. (1999). *Cognitive-behavior therapy for bipolar disorder: Treatment manual.* Unpublished manual, Massachusetts General Hospital, Boston.

Otto, M. W., Reilly-Harrington, N., & Sachs, G. (in press). Psychoeducational and cognitive-behavioral strategies in the management of bipolar disorder. *Journal of Affective Disorders.*

Perry, A., Tarrier, N., Morriss, R., McCarthy, E., & Limb, K. (1999). Randomised controlled trial of efficacy of teaching patients with bipolar disorder to identify early warning signs or relapse and obtain treatment. *British Medical Journal, 318,* 149–153.

Reilly-Harrington, N. A., Alloy, L. B., Fresco, D. M., & Whitehouse, W. G. (1999). Cognitive styles and life events interact to predict bipolar and unipolar symptomatology. *Journal of Abnormal Psychology, 108,* 567–578.

Rollnick, S., & Miller, W. R. (1995). What is motivational interviewing? *Behavioural and Cognitive Psychotherapy, 23,* 325–334.

Rosen, A., & Proctor, E. K. (1981). Distinctions between treatment outcomes and their implications for treatment evaluations. *Journal of Consulting and Clinical Psychology, 49,* 418–425.

Safren, S. A., Otto, M. W., & Worth, J. (2000). Life-Steps: Applying cognitive-behavioral therapy to patient adherence to HIV medication treatment. *Cognitive and Behavioral Practice, 6*, 332–341.

Salloum, I. M., & Thase, M. E. (2000). Impact of substance abuse on the course and treatment of bipolar disorder. *Bipolar Disorder, 2*, 260–280.

Scott, J. (1996). Cognitive therapy for clients with bipolar disorder. *Cognitive and Behavioral Practice, 3*, 19–51.

Scott, J., Garland, A., & Moorhead, S. (2001). A pilot study of cognitive therapy in bipolar disorders. *Psychological Medicine, 31*, 459–467.

Simons, A. D., & Thase, M. E. (1992). Biological markers, treatment outcome, and 1-year follow-up in endogenous depression: Electroencephalographic sleep studies and response to cognitive therapy. *Journal of Consulting and Clinical Psychology, 60*, 392–401.

Thase, M.E., Bowler, K., & Harden, T. (1991). Cognitive behavior therapy of endogenous depression: Part 2. Preliminary findings in 16 unmedicated inpatients. *Behavior Therapy, 22*, 469–477.

Thase, M. E., Simons, A. D., Cahalane, J. F., & McGeary, J. (1991). Cognitive behavior therapy of endogenous depression: Part 1: An outpatient clinical replication series. *Behavior Therapy, 22*, 457–467.

Wehr, T. A. (1991). Sleep-loss as a possible mediator of diverse causes of mania. *British Journal of Psychiatry, 159*, 576–578.

Wehr, T. A., Turner, E. H., Shimada, J. M., Lowe, C. H., Barker, C., & Leibenluft, E. (1998). Treatment of a rapidly cycling bipolar patient by using extended bed rest and darkness to stabilize the timing and duration of sleep. *Biological Psychiatry, 43*, 822–828.

Weiss, R. D., Griffin, M. L., Greenfield, S. F., Najavits, L. M., Wyner, D., Soto, J. A., & Hennen, J. A. (2000). Group therapy for patients with bipolar disorder and substance dependence: Results of a pilot study. *Journal of Clinical Psychiatry, 61*, 361–367.

Wirz-Justice, A. (1999). A rapid-cycling bipolar patient treated with long nights, bedrest, and light. *Biological Psychiatry, 45*, 1075–1077.

Yahne, C. E., & Miller, W. R. (1999). Enhancing motivation for treatment and change. In B. S. McCrady & E. E. Epstein (Eds.), *Addictions: A sourcebook for professionals* (pp. 235–249). New York: Oxford University Press.

Zaretsky, A. E., Segal, Z. Z. V., & Gemar, M. (1999). Cognitive therapy for bipolar depression: A pilot study. *Canadian Journal of Psychiatry, 44*, 491–494.

7

Interpersonal Psychotherapy for Unipolar and Bipolar Disorders

HOLLY A. SWARTZ
JOHN C. MARKOWITZ
ELLEN FRANK

Interpersonal psychotherapy (IPT) is a time-limited, focused psychotherapy developed by Klerman, Weissman, and colleagues for the acute treatment of unipolar depression (Klerman, Weissman, Rounsaville, & Chevron, 1984; Weissman, Markowitz, & Klerman, 2000). Like some psychotherapies discussed in this volume (cf. cognitive-behavioral therapy for depression), IPT was designed to treat a specific disorder and has been subjected to systematic evaluation in randomized, controlled research trials. Since its inception, IPT has been modified to treat a range of mood disorders in diverse populations. Most notably, Frank and colleagues at the University of Pittsburgh have reconceptualized IPT as a long-term prevention strategy for patients with recurrent unipolar and bipolar disorders. The first part of this chapter describes IPT in its original form. The second part discusses modified IPT, in combination with medication, as a maintenance treatment for bipolar disorder. We conclude with summaries of the empirical evidence supporting the efficacy of IPT as a treatment for unipolar depression and bipolar disorder, and a discussion of predictors of response to IPT.

HISTORICAL AND THEORETICAL BACKGROUND

IPT rests in part on the theories of Adolf Meyer and Harry Stack Sullivan, founders of the interpersonal school of psychology. Departing from the intrapsychic models of psychopathology popularized by psychoanalysis, Meyer and Sullivan emphasized the interpersonal and psychosocial antecedents of mental disorders (Meyer, 1957; Sullivan, 1953). In their interpersonal approach, assessment and intervention focused on the patient and his or her primary social group rather than on internal mental processes. In developing IPT, Klerman, Weissman and colleagues integrated the conceptual work of the interpersonal theorists with empirical research on psychosocial aspects of depression. Brown and Harris (1978), for example, provided evidence that confiding interpersonal relationships were protective against depression, while Walker, MacBride, and Vachon (1977) found that social support diminished stress among recently bereaved individuals. The epidemiological research of Weissman, Klerman, Paykel, Prusoff, and Hanson (1974) and Henderson, Byrne, Duncan-Jones, Scott, and Adcock (1980), respectively, demonstrating higher rates of marital discord among depressed women and more impaired social relationships among a population at risk for developing neuroses, provided substantiating data for an "interpersonal stressor" model of depression. In addition, data from Coyne (1976) and others underscored the importance of the erosive effects of depression in an interpersonal context as impairments in mood, communication, and activity rupture the social bond. These studies led Weissman and Klerman to articulate a treatment paradigm that targets the reciprocal interactions between mood and life events.

In the early 1970s, psychotherapy was a largely untested, heterogeneous procedure that was administered in an inconsistent manner for the treatment of poorly specified disorders. Klerman and Weissman planned from the outset to test IPT systematically in order to establish its efficacy. Intended for use in clinical trials, IPT is described in a manual (Klerman et al., 1984) and can be delivered in a standardized manner across therapists (Rounsaville, Chevron, Weissman, Prusoff, & Frank, 1986). The earliest test of IPT compared it to antidepressant medication (amitriptyline) in a relatively homogeneous sample of women suffering from major depression (Klerman, DiMascio, Weissman, Prusoff, & Paykel, 1974). Rather than focusing on the psychotherapeutic process (as did many psychodynamic treatments of the day), the major outcomes of interest were symptom reduction and social adjustment.

WHAT IS INTERPERSONAL PSYCHOTHERAPY?

IPT is a practical, focused, time-limited (12–16 weeks) psychotherapy that attends to the reciprocal interactions between mood and current life events. It is also a therapy of life change, encouraging patients to make substantial alterations in problematic roles and relationships in order to resolve depressive symptoms. The treatment first described in the manual by Klerman and colleagues (1984) was recently updated by Weissman and colleagues (2000). The reader is referred to these texts for a more comprehensive description of IPT. In this section, we review the core principles of IPT, summarize basic IPT strategies, and briefly describe the techniques employed in IPT sessions.

Core Principles

Link between Mood and Life Events

Life events themselves do not produce depression. Indeed, most of us experience numerous life events without developing symptoms. However, as discussed earlier, social psychologists have demonstrated links between depression and problematic interpersonal relationships in individuals who are biologically vulnerable to mood disorders. Research suggests that this relationship is bidirectional: that is, negative life events can lead to depression in predisposed individuals, and depressed individuals, in turn, have more difficulty managing interpersonal problems. IPT therapists help patients understand and identify the link between their mood disorder and a specific interpersonal problem. For example, a woman who became depressed in the context of marital difficulties learned in the course of IPT to communicate more productively with her husband and to assert herself more effectively in their relationship. She also discovered that problems with her social role (as a wife) and relationship (with her husband) directly affected her mood. Actively working to optimize her marital relationship improved both her marriage and her depressive symptoms. Although IPT does not impute causality, patients generally accept the idea that their depression has "something to do with" a life event or a relationship. The inherent plausibility of the model enhances its acceptability in clinical settings.

Focused Treatment

Unlike psychotherapies that attempt to address chronic issues such as character pathology, early childhood conflict, or multiple psychiatric disorders, IPT remains steadfastly focused on current depressive symptoms and a carefully selected interpersonal problem area (see the section on strategies). In its acute form, the duration of IPT is specified from the outset. The patient and the therapist explicitly agree to focus on a circumscribed problem area (i.e., complicated bereavement, a marital dispute, etc.) for the duration of treatment. Despite this apparently narrow focus, many patients gain social skills and find themselves better equipped to manage a variety of stressors, even if not explicitly addressed in the treatment, after IPT concludes. Even seeming character pathology may "resolve" as the depression abates, reinforcing the axiom that Axis II and trait diagnoses should not be made in the setting of an active Axis I disorder (Hirschfeld et al., 1983).

Time-Limited Treatment

In its acute form, IPT is administered as a 12- to 16-week treatment. Some therapists elect to specify the treatment duration very precisely from outset (e.g., "We will meet 12 times, and the last appointment is scheduled for June 2 at 10:00 A.M."). Other therapists identify the time frame in more general terms (e.g., "We will meet weekly over the next 3 to 4 months") and specify the exact termination date later in treatment. In either case, the therapist notifies the patient from the outset that treatment duration is limited. This time limit helps both the patient and therapist to concentrate their efforts, work efficiently, and maintain a tight focus. The therapist can use the time limit as leverage, encouraging the patient to take risks in the interest of meeting treatment goals within the designated time period.

A "Here-and-Now" Treatment

At the beginning of the 21st century, prevailing cultural beliefs about psychotherapy remain strongly influenced by the psychodynamic theories of Freud and his successors. Some patients may enter psychotherapy expecting to explore childhood conflicts and early memories. IPT, however, demands that the therapist focus on the events of recent months or year(s), gently discouraging patients' digressions into their distant past. Thus, we conceptualize IPT as a "here-and-now" treatment that focuses primarily on current symptoms, recent relationships, and proximal life events. A history of past relationships may be used to understand recurrent patterns that affect contemporary relationships, but the sessions focus on the events of the week rather than decade-old memories. It should be noted that "here-and-now" does *not* refer to the relationship between the patient and therapist (i.e., transference). Instead, the patient is encouraged to talk about recent conversations, interactions, and dilemmas with people in his or her "real" life.

Medical Model of Depression

The therapist conceptualizes the patient's "problem" as a medical illness characterized by specific symptoms linked to biological processes. IPT equates depression with medical illnesses such as diabetes or heart disease. The therapist educates the patient, making direct statements about diagnosis, heritability of the disorder, and treatment options. Adjunctive use of antidepressant medication, although not always necessary, is fully compatible with the IPT medical model. The IPT therapist diagnoses a major depressive episode using standardized criteria such as DSM-IV (American Psychiatric Association, 1994). This approach, in addition to ensuring an accurate diagnosis, relieves the patient of the guilt associated with this syndrome. The patient learns that his or her lack of energy, poor sleep, feelings of helplessness, and so on, are symptoms of a mood disorder, thereby emphasizing the medical (rather than the moral) etiology of depression. Moreover, the disorder is *treatable*, its symptom of hopelessness notwithstanding. During the initial phase of treatment, the therapist gives the patient the *sick role* (Parsons, 1951), which encourages the patient to participate actively in treatment, helps him or her to accept that symptoms are a manifestations of a medical condition, and relieves the patient of unmanageable social obligations. The therapist conceptualizes the sick role as a temporary status for the patient, who is expected to work in treatment toward resuming the healthy role. Over the course of IPT, the therapist serially administers a standardized measure of depressive symptoms such as the Hamilton Rating Scale for Depression (HRSD; Hamilton, 1960), helping the patient to see (presumably) diminishing scores as treatment progresses.

Active Therapist

The IPT therapist is very active in treatment sessions, working intensively to maintain the treatment focus and intervening when necessary with practical suggestions, role play, and psychoeducation. The therapist adopts a warm, encouraging stance that counters the depressed patient's pessimism with an equal and opposite optimistic realism. In psychodynamic terms, the IPT therapist cultivates a positive transference. Tardiness and lack of participation are understood as sequelae of depression rather than as evidence of an underlying conflictual relationship with the therapist in particular or authority figures in general. The therapist might intervene by saying, "It's hard to feel enthusiastic about therapy when your depression makes it hard to enjoy anything." The therapist blames the depression rather than the patient and uses the time limit to encourage compliance.

Practical Treatment

Well grounded in theory and strongly supported by extant data, IPT is also a very pragmatic treatment. Many of the techniques used in IPT (see later discussion) were adapted from approaches employed by skilled practitioners at the time IPT was developed. Therapists who are new to IPT often comment that although the unifying strategies of IPT are innovative, many of the skills used in IPT are not. Good therapists will say, "It's sort of what I've been doing all along." The relatively intuitive nature of IPT makes it an easy treatment for many clinicians to add to their repertoire.

Nonspecific Factors

Frank identified six therapeutic factors common to all forms of psychotherapy:

> 1) An intense, emotionally charged, confiding relationship with a helping person . . . , 2) A rationale, or myth, which includes an explanation of the cause of the patient's distress and a method for relieving it . . . , 3) Provision of new information concerning the nature and sources of the patient's problems and possible alternative ways of dealing with them . . . , 4) Strengthening the patient's expectations of help through the personal qualities of the therapist, enhanced by his status in society . . . , 5) Provision of success experiences which . . . enhance his sense of mastery . . . , [and] 6) [F]acilitation of emotional arousal. (1971, pp. 355–357)

IPT, like all therapies, offers relief to patients, in some measure, because of these nonspecific factors. Unlike many other psychotherapies, however, IPT has been demonstrated to be more efficacious than a control psychotherapy (Markowitz, Kocsis, et al., 1998), indicating that, in some populations, its activity is greater than its nonspecific effects.

Interpersonal Psychotherapy Strategies

Initial Phase

The initial phase (the first one to three sessions) begins as an enriched psychiatric evaluation. The clinician conducts a psychiatric interview, assesses symptoms, makes a diagnosis of major depression according to the criteria set forth by DSM-IV (American Psychiatric Association, 1994), and offers the patient the *sick role* (Parsons, 1951). As early as the first session, the clinician begins to educate the patient about his or her medical illness (depression) and its treatment options. If the patient is considered a likely candidate for IPT, the therapist will initiate the *interpersonal inventory*, an interpersonally focused anamnesis, which reviews all important past and present relationships as they relate to the current episode of depression. In addition to outlining the "cast of characters" in the patient's life, the interpersonal inventory probes the quality of those relationships, asking the patient to describe unmet expectations of others, satisfying and unsatisfying aspects of relationships, and aspects of relationships that the patient would like to change.

The information collected in the psychiatric interview and the interpersonal inventory allows the therapist to select one of four possible *interpersonal problem areas* (grief, role disputes, interpersonal role transitions, or interpersonal deficits) as the patient's treatment focus. The chosen interpersonal problem area should have both affective valence for the patient and a temporal link to the onset or maintenance of the current episode of depression. The initial phase of treatment concludes with an *interpersonal case formulation*, a summary statement that reiterates the patient's diagnosis and links it to one (or at most two) interpersonal problem areas. For example, the therapist might offer the following interpersonal case formulation to a patient:

> "You have had a difficult year. You first lost your father to cancer last February and then developed back problems in May. But it seems that your depression began in September, just after your youngest son left home to enter the military. I know that you are proud of your son and believe that military training will be good for him. But it is also clear to me that you have felt empty and sad without him at home. Of all the problems you've faced this year, it seems that watching your last son leave home has been the most troublesome for you. You have devoted the last 23 years to caring for

and raising three sons, so it makes sense that this would be a hard time for you. We call this a role transition. I believe that the difficult transition from full-time Mom to retired Mom contributes to your depression. I suggest that we spend the next 2 to 3 months working on this problem. We'll spend time understanding how it feels to be the mother of grown children and thinking about new things for you to do with your time, now that the children are out of the house. As you find ways to adjust to this role transition, your mood should also improve. Does that make sense to you?"

As in this example, the therapist concludes by eliciting the patient's explicit agreement with the treatment focus. The therapist can later invoke this verbal contract if the patient strays too far from the agreed-upon focus. If the patient disagrees with the formulation, the therapist attempts to understand the source(s) of disagreement, working with the patient to reformulate the case until it makes sense to both patient and therapist. If necessary, the therapist can choose two different treatment foci, although, in order to prevent the treatment from becoming too diffuse, a single focus is preferable. The case formulation is also a therapeutic statement that provides reassurance and hope, helps the patient understand the genesis of the episode, and sets the agenda for the remainder of the treatment (Markowitz & Swartz, 1997).

Middle Phase

The second phase of IPT, comprising most of the 12–16 sessions of a typical treatment for depression, focuses on the interpersonal problem area selected in the initial phase and described in the case formulation. Below is a description of each of the four problem areas and a summary of the strategies used to resolve them.

Grief. Grief or complicated bereavement becomes the focus of treatment when the onset of depression is connected to the death of an important person in the patient's life. Treatment strategies include facilitating the mourning process by reviewing in detail the relationship with the deceased person, encouraging the expression of previously suppressed affect in order to facilitate catharsis, and helping the patient recognize distorted (either overly positive or overly negative) memories of the relationship with the deceased. The therapist may suggest that the patient visit the grave, bring in old photographs, speak with mutual friends, and so on, in order to reawaken feelings about the deceased and enable the patient to assess the negative and positive aspects of the relationship realistically. As the mourning process unfolds, the therapist encourages the patient to make role changes that will help him or her reengage in activities and relationships, with the goal of finding satisfactory substitutes for the person lost. A case example follows.

Mr. A, a 79-year-old retired lawyer, sought treatment for depression 1 year after his wife of 52 years died of metastatic breast cancer. Mr. A admitted that although he missed his wife terribly, he had tried to "put her out of my mind" because he found the feelings of loss so overwhelming. Since his wife's death, Mr. A had begun to avoid everything that reminded him of her. He refused invitations to go to the movies because he and his wife had frequently enjoyed movies together; he stopped eating breakfast, so as not to be reminded of mornings spent reading newspapers together over bowls of cereal; he even limited his contact with their children, because he found them too painful a reminder of his wife. In spite of initial resistance, Mr. A's therapist gently encouraged him to talk about his wife, especially her final, difficult year in a hospice.

With the therapist's support, Mr. A discussed both positive memories of their marriage and previously unexpressed angry feelings about her "deserting" him ("I always thought I would be the first one to go"). The therapist encouraged Mr. A to focus on both memories of their life together and the impact of her absence on his current life. By encouraging both catharsis and an active reengagement in previously pleasurable activities, the therapist was able to help Mr. A move through the grieving process. By the end of treatment, Mr. A no longer avoided activities that evoked his wife's memory and was contemplating taking a trip abroad with a senior citizen group. As Mr. A resumed his previously active lifestyle, his HRSD scores dropped from 22 (moderately depressed) to 7 (not depressed).

Interpersonal Role Dispute. A "role dispute" is defined as a relationship in which the individuals have nonreciprocal or conflicting expectations of each other. For instance, an individual may develop depressive symptoms in the context of repeated disagreements with a spouse about the distribution of household responsibilities or the management of shared finances. The goals of treatment are to identify the dispute (which may be covert), develop a plan for change, and modify both communication patterns and role expectations. Likened to unilateral couple therapy (Markowitz, 1998), strategies for treating a role dispute include communication analysis, role play, and an exploration of realistic options. Satisfactory outcomes, depending on the circumstances, include either successful resolution of the dispute or dissolution of the relationship, if resolution of conflict is deemed impossible or undesirable. An example of a role dispute follows:

Ms. B, a 41-year-old computer programmer, experienced a major depression in the context of a role dispute with her partner of 8 years, Amy. Ms. B and Amy disagreed about whether or not to have children. In deference to her partner's wishes to not have any children, Ms. B rarely discussed her yearnings to become a parent. As her depression intensified, she stopped doing her work and, instead, spent hours surfing the Internet in search of agencies that facilitated international adoptions for gay couples. When she entered treatment, her HRSD score was 19.

The therapist helped Ms. B identify and articulate her feelings about having children: She wanted to have a child, and did not want to raise a child by herself, but feared that Amy would leave her if she brought up the issue. Using role play and communication analysis, the therapist helped Ms. B confront Amy with her feelings and wishes. Although this strategy initially created increased friction in relationship, the couple began a very productive dialogue about their respective needs and wishes. Honest communication was very reassuring to Ms. B, and her symptoms improved as she felt she could be emotionally open with her partner. As IPT came to an end, Amy and Ms. B planned to join a group for potential adoptive parents in order to learn more about parenting and adoption. Although they had not yet decided whether to adopt, Ms. B felt relieved that the issue was again "on the table," and that they were now working as a couple to make an informed decision. Her HRSD score after 16 IPT sessions was 4.

Role Transition. Role transitions include any major life change, such as getting a new job, moving to a new city, being diagnosed with a medical illness, or retiring. The patient becomes depressed in the context of difficulties meeting the demands of the new role or inability to let go of the old role. Treatment focuses on helping the patient to appraise realistically both the old and new roles, establish a more balanced view of each role, mourn the loss of the positive aspects of the old role, and develop the skills necessary to manage the new role more successfully.

Because the category of role transitions affords a relatively broad focus, it can be invoked when the patient presents with several potential foci. Subsuming several possible foci under a single problem area prevents the treatment from becoming too diffuse. The following vignette illustrates a case that could have been conceptualized as a series of role disputes (with the boyfriend and the son) but was instead managed successfully as a role transition (to single parenthood).

> Ms. C, a 34-year-old divorced mother of three, became depressed several months after Michael, her boyfriend of 5 years, was incarcerated for robbery. Although he was not the father of her children, Michael had become the primary disciplinarian in the household and seemed to be the only person who could "talk sense into" Ms. C's oppositional 16-year-old son (the biological father did not have contact with the family). Treatment focused on helping Ms. C successfully make the transition to the status of single parent. Early sessions focused on the pros and cons of life with Michael. Ms. C felt that he helped her manage her children and provided companionship. With probing from the therapist, Ms. C also acknowledged that Michael had been verbally abusive at times and drank too much. She admitted that she was relieved to get away from Michael's angry outbursts but was worried about her ability to manage her children without him.
> With help from her therapist, Ms. C developed strategies to set clearer limits with her children, building on her previous experience as a single mother before she met Michael. When the 16-year-old's behavior worsened in the face of these limits, her therapist helped Ms. C decide to seek professional treatment for her son. She reestablished ties with friends to provide companionship and support in Michael's absence. As Ms. C became more comfortable with her newfound independence, her depressive symptoms diminished (HRSD scores moved from 29 to 9). Although still planning to reunite with Michael upon his release from prison, at the end of treatment Ms. C was proud of her ability to function without him.

Interpersonal Deficits. Interpersonal deficits is a default category: The patient has experienced neither complicated bereavement nor a role dispute or role transition. The category is reserved for patients who have a long history of impoverished or unsuccessful interpersonal relationships, and there is no evidence of an acute precipitant of the depressive episode. These patients may have underlying character pathology that interferes with attachments or, more likely, long-standing low-grade depression (dysthymic disorder) that interferes with the formation of lasting relationships (Weissman et al., 2000). Not surprisingly, these patients are more difficult to treat with any psychotherapy, and perhaps more so with IPT, because of their deficits in the area where IPT works (Sotsky et al., 1991). Treatment focuses on helping the patient to expand his or her social skills and to understand the link between mood symptoms and social impairment. The therapist can use role play, hypothetical social situations, and—unusual for IPT—the relationship with the therapist to enhance the patient's repertoire. Markowitz (1998) has developed a modified form of IPT designed to treat patients suffering from dysthymic disorder. This model introduces the concept of an iatrogenic role transition; that is, the therapist moves the patient from chronic depression to euthymia in IPT, concurrently helping the patient develop a new set of skills to manage interpersonal relationships. Chronic depression, which inhibits social functioning, may explain the presentation of patients without recent life events; it may be easier to treat the problem as dysthymic disorder *rather than* using the interpersonal deficits model to treat acute depression. This has not, however, been studied to date.

Mr. D, a 20-year-old college student, describes himself as "computer nerd" who maintains a 4.0 grade point average in a difficult engineering major. Mr. D sought treatment after taking an on-line depression screening test that suggested he obtain professional advice. He met DSM-IV criteria for major depression, with a baseline HRSD score of 17, but had difficulty specifying the onset of his symptoms. Conducting an interpersonal inventory clarified for the therapist that Mr. D was very isolated. Aside from lectures, regular chats with on-line "cyber buddies," and weekly phone calls to his parents in another state, Mr. D had virtually no social contacts. Treatment focused on helping Mr. D to build social skills, first with on-line friends, and then with other students in his class. The therapist made ample use of role play to help Mr. D achieve some comfort initiating social interactions. At first, he was even reluctant to speak with his therapist. Thus, the therapist used Mr. D's growing experience with self-disclosure in therapy as another vehicle to expand his limited repertoire of social skills. Treatment gains were slow, and Mr. D continued to experience a moderate degree of symptoms as treatment ended (HRSD score was 12). The therapist deemed the treatment partially effective and referred Mr. D for medication and a trial of cognitive-behavioral psychotherapy after IPT concluded.

Termination

By the final phase of IPT (the last three sessions of treatment), the patient has usually improved. The therapist announces the approaching end to therapy and begins to review with the patient his or her progress in treatment—which is often considerable. It is helpful to reexamine the curve of improvement in HRSD scores (or their equivalent) and once again link changes in mood to resolution of the interpersonal problem area. These maneuvers help to shore up the patient's sense of self-sufficiency and facilitate his or her growing independence from the therapist. The therapist acknowledges that it is sad to break up a good team and encourages the patient to voice his or her thoughts about the end of treatment. Patients often express mixed feelings about "graduating" from psychotherapy, though most are pleased to feel better without an interminable course of treatment. This process affords the therapist an opportunity to help the patient distinguish between sadness (a normal response to separation) and depressed affect. The therapist reviews the symptoms of depression, the potential for recurrence, and the interpersonal issues that might be likely to trigger a relapse for the patient in the immediate future.

Because the goals of treatment are both specified and specific, the therapist and patient can discuss explicitly the degree to which depressive symptoms have resolved and interpersonal goals have been met. In the event that a patient remains symptomatic, the therapist blames the treatment rather than the patient (who is often predisposed to self-blame) and helps the patient find new therapeutic options. Sometimes, although no longer depressed, a patient who still struggles with unresolved concerns (e.g., uncertainty about long-term career goals) will request a referral for another form of help (e.g., career counseling or psychodynamic psychotherapy) to explore issues that were identified but not addressed in IPT.

Interpersonal Psychotherapy Techniques

Opening Question

IPT sessions typically begin with the question "How have you been since we last met?" This deceptively ordinary query serves several important functions. First, it focuses the patient's attention on the here and now ("since we last met") and elicits information about the preceding week. It then prompts either a symptom update (e.g., "I've been less weepy") or an interpersonally focused response detailing a recent life event (e.g., "I had a big fight with my parents on Tuesday"). If the patient begins with a symptom, the therapist, following the patient's lead, reviews the depressive symptoms in greater detail (i.e., inquiring about sleep, appetite, concentration, etc.) and then attempts to link the depressive affect to the week's events. For example, the therapist might say,

> "It sounds like your mood has improved a little. Is there something that happened this week that might have affected your mood?"

If the patient responds with an interpersonal issue, the therapist first obtains additional details about the event and then asks the patient to report on his or her symptoms, now linking life events to mood:

> "So the fight with your parents didn't go the way you would have liked. We can discuss some other options you might have to deal with their displeasure about your decision to withdraw from summer school. But first I'd like to hear about your depressive symptoms this week. How has your mood been? Is there any connection between fluctuations in your mood and the argument with your parents?"

Eclectic Techniques

Each interpersonal problem area is associated with a specific set of IPT strategies designed to address the interpersonal issue and resolve the depressive symptoms. These strategies, described generally here and more fully in the manual (Klerman et al., 1984; Weissman et al., 2000), are unique to IPT. By contrast, in each session, the therapist selects from an array of eclectic techniques, many of which will be familiar to the therapist from other forms of psychotherapy. For example, the therapist uses empathetic listening and open-ended questions to build rapport and elicit information, an approach used in many supportive treatments. IPT encourages expression of affect and exploration of suppressed feelings to facilitate catharsis, an approach also used in psychodynamic psychotherapy (Markowitz, Svartberg, & Swartz, 1998). Although not a cognitive-behavioral treatment, IPT includes some techniques typically associated with cognitive and behavioral therapies, such as role play, communication analysis, decision analysis, and behavioral activation. These techniques are used to build rapport, explore affect, and then move the patient from *feelings* to *action*.

Eliciting Details

In order to better understand a patient's relationships and interpersonal functioning, the therapist elicits considerable detail about the patient's interpersonal experiences. The more vivid the picture in the therapist's mind, the better able the therapist will be to guide the patient to more productive interpersonal relationships. When describing events, the patient should be encouraged to report details of conversations ("He said . . . , and then I said . . . , and he replied . . . "), how the patient felt at each juncture in the interchange, the specific context of the event ("I had just come home from work and she had spent the whole day with the children at our community swimming pool"), and the timing of the interplay between mood and events ("I got a letter from my ex-boyfriend on Wednesday and noticed that my mood got worse"). These specific descriptions enable the therapist to assess more accurately communication patterns, the effect of mood on interpersonal functioning, and the nature of interpersonal conflicts. Elaborating the minutiae of interpersonal exchanges will often intensify the patient's affective memory of the event, in turn facilitating catharsis.

Exploring Options

A technique often used in IPT is helping patients generate and explore a list of options to better address an interpersonal problem. Depressed patients often feel trapped or "stuck," generally the result of negative cognitions associated with the depression rather than an accurate appraisal of the situation. The therapist works with the patient to find options where he or she previously felt there were none. If the patient is profoundly anergic, the therapist initially may need to supply suggestions. However, the goal of treatment is to help the patient generate his or her own list of alternatives and to select a new option that may lead to a better interpersonal outcome for the patient. For example, the therapist might say,

> "You feel your only choice under these circumstances is to put up with your malicious coworker or quit your job. Being depressed makes it feel like you are stuck, without options. But that may not be true. Let's think together about other ways you might respond to your coworker. Maybe you can think of some things that you would like to change, things that would enable you to stay at your job, without feeling so mistreated."

Optimistic Stance

IPT is fundamentally an optimistic, forward-looking treatment. In order to counteract the depressed patient's pessimistic outlook, the therapist adopts an optimistic stance that encourages the patient to "think out of the box," consider hitherto unexplored possibilities, and take interpersonal risks that may help him or her achieve previously unattainable goals. Acting as interpersonal cheerleaders, therapists gently push patients to try out new interpersonal strategies between sessions, even if patients doubt their capacity to succeed. The therapist then offers positive feedback when the patient reports taking interpersonal risks, underscoring the patient's incredible tenacity in the face of a debilitating depression. Patients are commended for their courageous efforts to bring about change, and every sign of improvement (i.e., a drop in HRSD scores, newfound pleasures, diminished conflict) is identified and applauded. On the other hand, if a patient experiences difficulties during treatment, the therapist blames the depression (not the patient) and helps the patient identify smaller, more manageable, interim goals.

Applications of Interpersonal Psychotherapy

IPT has been adapted to treat a wide range of depressive disorders. Originally designed as an acute treatment for major depression (Klerman et al., 1984; Weissman et al., 2000), IPT has subsequently been adapted to treat antepartum depression (Spinelli, 1997), postpartum depression (O'Hara, Stuart, Gorman, & Wenzel, 2000), late-life depression (Reynolds et al., 1999), depressive symptoms in individuals who are HIV-seropositive (Markowitz, Kocsis, et al., 1998), and depressed adolescents (Mufson, Weissman, Moreau, & Garfinkel, 1999). IPT has also been used as a maintenance treatment to prevent new episodes of depression in patients with histories of recurrent major depression (Frank et al., 1990; Reynolds et al., 1999) and as a treatment for patients with dysthymic disorder (Markowitz, 1998). Investigators have reformatted IPT as a couple intervention for depressed patients with marital disputes (Foley, Rounsaville, Weissman, Sholomskas, & Chevron, 1989) and as a group therapy (Wilfley, Mackenzie, Welch, Ayres, & Weissman, 2000). Pilot studies under way at the University of Pittsburgh are testing a brief form of IPT (eight sessions) for depression, and IPT plus a behavioral intervention for patients with depression and comorbid panic-spectrum anxiety symptoms. IPT for bipolar disorder (discussion follows) is perhaps the most radical adaptation of the model yet described.

INTERPERSONAL AND SOCIAL RHYTHM THERAPY FOR BIPOLAR DISORDER

Depression by Any Other Name

Some authors have argued that bipolar depression does not differ fundamentally from unipolar depression (Joffe, Young, & MacQueen, 1999). Indeed, diagnostic criteria for the two syndromes are identical, and major depressive disorder is distinguishable only by history from bipolar I disorder, most recent episode depressed (American Psychiatric Association, 1994). Nevertheless, researchers have identified several features of bipolar depression that may distinguish it from unipolar depression, including longer episode duration, increased probability of psychotic symptoms, and limited efficacy of antidepressant medications (Goldberg & Kocsis, 1999). Bipolar depression is often characterized by the so-called "atypical" symptoms of depression, including hypersomnia, hyperphagia, and psychomotor retardation (Goodwin & Jamison, 1990), and may be more difficult to treat (Hlastala et al., 1997). Unlike correctly diagnosed unipolar disorder, bipolar depression is haunted by the specter of mania (Goodwin & Jamison, 1990).

Treatment approaches to unipolar and bipolar depression also overlap but differ in several important ways. For both forms of depression, antidepressant medications are essential treatment ingredients. For patients with bipolar disorder, however, antidepressant medications pose the dual problems of limited efficacy and the risk of precipitating mania (Altshuler et al., 1995). When prescribed for bipolar disorder, antidepressant medications are administered in conjunction with a mood stabilizer in order to confer protection against antidepressant-induced mania and to promote longitudinal mood stability (Sachs, Printz, Kahn, Carpenter, & Docherty, 2000). Psychotherapy for bipolar depression should also be administered with a mood stabilizer because of the ever-present risk of mania. Thus, psychotherapy designed for the treatment of bipolar depression always addresses the issue of medication adherence, whereas psychotherapy for unipolar depression, which can be administered in lieu of pharmacotherapy, addresses the choice between medication and psychotherapy or the need, or wish, to combine the two.

Psychotherapy for Bipolar Disorder

Although extensive data demonstrate the efficacy of psychosocial treatments for unipolar depression, few psychotherapies have been developed and tested for the treatment of bipolar disorder (Craighead, Miklowitz, Vajk, & Frank, 1998). None is specifically designed for the depressive phase of the disorder. Nevertheless, a review of the literature suggests that psychotherapies used across the phases of bipolar disorder may have selectively positive effects on bipolar depression (Swartz & Frank, 2001). In consensus guidelines summarizing expert opinions on optimal treatment strategies for bipolar disorder, groups from Canada (Kusumakar et al., 1997) and the United States (Bauer et al., 1999; Hirschfeld et al., 1994) recommend adjunctive psychosocial interventions as part of the overall treatment strategy but do not endorse any particular type of psychotherapy. These relatively vague recommendations stem from a paucity of clinical trials documenting the efficacy of psychotherapy for bipolar disorder.

Interpersonal and social rhythm therapy (IPSRT), a modified form of IPT, has been developed as an adjunctive treatment for bipolar disorder (Frank, Swartz, & Kupfer, 2000) and is currently being tested in a randomized, controlled trial at the University of Pittsburgh. Designed for use across the phases of bipolar disorder, it is among a handful of psychotherapies that seems to have a selectively positive effect on bipolar depression (Swartz & Frank, 2001). We describe IPSRT, discuss its relationship to IPT for unipolar depression, and comment on its role as a treatment for bipolar *depression* in particular.

Overview of Interpersonal and Social Rhythm Therapy and Theoretical Background

IPSRT helps patients with bipolar disorder to address interpersonal problems and regulate their social rhythms (Frank, Swartz, et al., 2000). It combines the principles of IPT for unipolar depression with a behavioral strategy designed to regularize daily routines (social rhythm therapy) and psychoeducation to enhance adherence to medication regimens. IPSRT focuses on (1) the identification and management of affective symptoms; (2) the link between mood and life events; (3) the maintenance of regular daily rhythms as elucidated by the Social Rhythm Metric (SRM); (4) the identification and management of potential precipitants of rhythm dysregulation, with special attention to interpersonal triggers; and (5) the facilitation of mourning the lost healthy self.

The social rhythm therapy component of IPSRT evolved from research suggesting that individuals with bipolar disorder have a genetic predisposition to circadian rhythm and sleep–wake cycle abnormalities that may be responsible, in part, for the symptomatic manifestations of the illness (Goodwin & Jamison, 1990). It also evolved from a theory of *social Zeitgebers* (persons, social demands, or tasks that *set* the biological clock) and *Zeitstörers* (physical, chemical, or psychosocial events that *disturb* the biological clock) as the putative bridges between life events and mood symptoms (Ehlers, Frank, & Kupfer, 1988; Ehlers, Kupfer, Frank, & Monk, 1993). Thus, the social rhythm therapy component of IPSRT is based on the assumption that helping patients to maintain more regular rhythms will lead to greater mood stability.

Interpersonal events pose the dual risks of psychological distress and disrupted social rhythms. For example, a new baby may cause not only emotional upheaval but also dramatic changes in sleep patterns, leisure activities, and exercise routines. The death of a spouse may lead to grief as well as shifts in meal times, socializing, and sleep habits. These kinds of life events, therefore, change one's circadian and social rhythms. For an individual with the genetic predisposition to bipolar disorder, dysregulation of these rhythms may perturb his or her vulnerable central nervous system, leading to mood symptoms. Research suggests that, in patients with bipolar disorder, life events that disrupt social rhythms are significantly associated with the onset of manic—but not depressive—episodes (Malkoff-Schwartz et al., 1998). IPSRT modulates the effects of interpersonal problems on mood by the traditional IPT strategies outlined previously, and by minimizing the disrupting effects of interpersonal experiences on daily routines.

Interpersonal Psychotherapy versus Interpersonal and Social Rhythm Therapy

IPSRT is an adaptation of IPT and therefore retains most of the key features of IPT discussed earlier in this chapter. In order to highlight the distinctions between the two therapies, however, we focus on aspects of the treatment that are either unique to IPSRT or represent significant modifications of the IPT approach. We summarize these differences in Table 7.1.

Treatment Duration

IPT was originally developed as an acute treatment for a single episode of depression. Recognizing that many patients suffer from recurrent episodes of major depression, Frank and colleagues extended the model and developed a maintenance form of IPT (IPT-M) that is administered monthly to prevent subsequent recurrences (Frank, 1991). Although half of patients who experience depression will suffer only a single episode, all

TABLE 7.1. Comparing IPT to IPSRT

Domain	IPT	IPSRT
Goals	Resolution of depressive episode	Prevention of mania and depression
Duration of treatment	12–16 weeks	Variable (about 2 years)
Frequency of sessions	Weekly	Weekly for several months, then monthly
Techniques	Link mood to life events	Link mood to life events and search for specific triggers of rhythm disruption
	Encourage change	Help patients adapt to change
	Encourage increased activity to combat depression	Find a healthy balance between spontaneity and stability
	Encourage return to previous level of functioning	Grieve the lost healthy self; optimize functioning given limitations of chronic illness
Adjunctive medication	Optional (unless proscribed by a research study)	Necessary; treatment supports medication adherence
Social rhythm therapy	No	Yes; complete and discuss Social Rhythm Metric weekly
Psychoeducation	Yes	Yes, including discussion of medications and their side effects
Involvement of family member/significant other	Optional (to resolve an interpersonal role dispute)	Recommended (to develop a safety plan)
Efficacy	Well established	Efficacy trial in progress

patients suffering from bipolar disorder are at high risk for recurrence (Keller et al., 1993).

Thus, IPSRT is designed as a maintenance treatment (akin to IPT-M) that is administered over several years in order to prevent the recurrence of affective episodes. Even in its recurrent form, however, the course of unipolar disorder is far more predictable than the hectic, bidirectional course of bipolar disorder (Frank, Swartz, et al., 2000). Thus, the duration and timing of the phases of IPSRT are much more variable than IPT or IPT-M.

IPSRT can begin when a patient is fully symptomatic, subsyndromal, or euthymic. Depending on the severity of the patient's symptoms, the duration of the initial phase of treatment may vary from several weeks to several months. For example, if a patient is manic, it is usually impossible to obtain an accurate interpersonal inventory until symptoms diminish. Treatment will focus on symptom management and containment—rather than the specific content areas of IPSRT—until the patient recovers sufficiently to participate in the more structured treatment activities. In contrast, a moderately depressed or euthymic patient may complete the initial phase of treatment rather quickly and move on to the case formulation and intermediate phase of treatment within the first few weeks. The intermediate phase of IPSRT, equivalent to the middle phase of IPT, focuses on an interpersonal problem area and social rhythms. Again, the duration of the intermediate phase can vary from several months to longer than a year, depending on the patient's symptoms. After symptoms remit, treatment frequency decreases to monthly visits. During this time, the patient consolidates treatment gains, increases confidence in his or her capacity to apply IPSRT techniques outside of sessions, and self-monitors for early warning signs of recurrence. Because many patients experience symptom flare-ups during a period of "remission," extra sessions can be scheduled during the maintenance phase to address these transient subsyndromal episodes. In our study, this phase of treatment lasts for 2 years.

The goal of IPSRT is to smooth the course of a chronic and chaotic disorder. It is administered across the phases of the disorder both to address current symptoms and to prevent future episodes. We have defined the maintenance period of IPSRT as a 2-year interval in our clinical trial. It is unclear, however, whether 2 years represents an optimal treatment duration for this population. On the one hand, several investigators have demonstrated that patients suffering from bipolar disorder continue to experience psychosocial deficits many years after symptom remission (Coryell et al., 1993; Goldberg, Harrow, & Grossman, 1995; Tohen et al., 2000). These findings suggest that targeted psychotherapy should be delivered for at least 2 to 5 years following remission in order to address persistent deficits in functioning. On the other hand, some patients (or their managed care companies) may elect to terminate psychotherapy and continue treatment with a psychiatrist for medication monitoring alone.

Therapist Role

IPSRT assumes that the therapist is familiar with bipolar disorder and its treatments. The therapist must be cognizant of the prodromal symptoms of mania and depression (in order both to intervene and to help the patient to recognize these symptoms), and the medications used to treat bipolar disorder (in order to encourage medication adherence and help the patient recognize side effects). Because patients with bipolar disorder may require monitoring by family members in order to detect early warning signs of recurrence, IPSRT therapists obtain permission to contact significant others and must therefore be comfortable interacting with family members. Thus, IPSRT is best administered by an experienced clinician with versatile therapeutic skills. On the other hand, therapists with prior experience treating bipolar disorder can acquire a working knowledge of IPSRT with 8 hours of training and two supervised cases.

Link between Mood and Life Events

As in IPT, the IPSRT therapist establishes a link between the patient's current episode and interpersonal events. In IPSRT, however, the therapist conducts an even more extensive *search for triggers of rhythm disruption*. The therapist elicits in great detail the events leading up to current and previous manic and depressive episodes, searching for evidence of alterations in the patient's daily routines that preceded the development of symptoms, and combing the patient's history for external sources of social rhythm disruption (i.e., a transcontinental flight, a new work schedule, or an interpersonal conflict). These historical details help the therapist understand the patient's patterns of illness and aid in the identification of potential episode triggers. IPSRT, then, encourages the patient to make life changes in order to protect the integrity of circadian rhythms and the sleep–wake cycle.

Balancing Stability and Spontaneity

At some point in the recovery process, most patients with bipolar disorder question the need for protecting the integrity of their social rhythms. To someone with a long history of fluctuating mood states and erratic social rhythms, a very regular lifestyle can seem "boring" and unappealing. The therapist addresses this crucial issue on several levels. First, the therapist can help the patient find a healthy *balance between stability and spontaneity*. This process requires a spirit of careful experimentation on the parts of both therapist and patient in order to determine how much sleep, stimulation, and regularity are associated with an optimal mood state for each individual. Extreme inactivity, on the one hand, can contribute to isolation and depressive symptoms; excess stimulation, on the other hand, may precipitate mania. It is helpful to pursue this aspect of treatment over many months, since seasonal variation in mood and energy often occurs in bipolar patients. Some patients, for example, may find they benefit from a busier schedule during the winter months, when they would typically tend toward depression, but must learn to curtail these same activities during the summer months, when they are at increased risk for a mania.

IPT encourages depressed patients to take risks and make fairly drastic changes in their lives. The social rhythm component of IPSRT, however, introduces a cautionary note into treatment. The therapist encourages the patient to explore options and improve relationships, but to make changes more gradually. In IPSRT, the impetus to change is tempered by attention to social rhythm integrity and by distinguishing between an impulsive behavior (a symptom of mania) and a goal-directed action (a therapeutic outcome). Indeed, a goal of IPSRT is often to slow the process of change (i.e., defer travel plans, reduce course loads, cut back an overextended work schedule). Thus, in IPSRT, changes are made sparingly and in a graded fashion, with considerable attention paid to the potentially disrupting effects of shifts in activity, stimulation, and relationships. If IPT for unipolar depression is a therapy of change, then IPSRT is a therapy of stabilization.

Social Rhythm Therapy

Social rhythm therapy is a behavioral intervention designed to help patients regulate their daily rhythms. The Social Rhythm Metric (SRM), a self-report instrument that measures social rhythm regularity (Monk, Flaherty, Frank, Hoskinson, & Kupfer, 1990), is used as a therapeutic tool to help patients stabilize their routines. On this 17-item form, patients rate their mood and record daily activities (e.g., time out of bed, first contact with another person, meal times, bedtime), whether each activity occurred alone or with others present, and how stimulating (i.e., quiet versus interactive) these other activities were. Patients fill out SRMs daily at home and then bring them into the office to review with the therapist. The social rhythm therapy component of IPSRT begins with a review of the first 3 or 4 weeks of "free-running" SRMs in order to find those rhythms that seem to be particularly unstable. For example, is the patient having dinner at 5:00 P.M. one day, skipping dinner the next, and going out for dinner at 10:00 P.M. on the third? Is there evidence of regularity during the week but extreme deviation on the weekend? Every effort is made to determine whether the patient's social rhythm instability results from untreated/prodromal bipolar symptoms or from a self-imposed lifestyle choice. In either case, the therapist will encourage the patient to work toward stabilization.

If the rhythm instability is related to symptoms, patients learn that stabilizing rhythms can help diminish these symptoms. If the therapist determines that the rhythm instability is a lifestyle choice, he or she explains that disrupting circadian integrity may prevent a complete recovery. The therapist and patient identify sequential SRM goals, including short-term goals (e.g., going to bed before midnight for seven consecutive days), intermediate goals (e.g., no napping for a month), and long-term objectives (e.g., finding a job with a more regular work schedule). General strategies for regulating rhythms include minimizing overstimulation, monitoring the frequency and intensity of social interactions, and working toward graduated SRM goals. The therapist also uses the SRMs to help patients understand the dynamic interplay among instabilities in daily routines, patterns of social stimulation, sleep–wake times, and mood fluctuations. The following case example illustrates an application of both interpersonal and social rhythm therapy techniques:

> Mr. E, a 50-year-old corporate executive with a long history of bipolar disorder, entered treatment in a depressive episode that began 1 month after his wife of 25 years announced her plans to leave him. Although the patient did not initially volunteer the information, an interview with his wife revealed that she wanted to end the marriage because of Mr. E's recurrent promiscuous behavior. His responsibilities to a multinational company required frequent brief trips across time zones, including regular travel from North America to Europe and the Middle East. Mr. E admitted that while traveling and hypomanic, he had had several brief extramarital liaisons. He later regretted these affairs but felt unable to stop his behavior. Both Mr. E and his wife expressed a desire to resolve their marital problems. The IPSRT problem area was conceptualized as a role dispute with his wife. In addition to deploying the usual IPT strategies for a role dispute, the therapist helped the patient understand the relationships among his travel schedule, rhythm disruptions, mood shifts, and marital conflict. For instance, it became apparent that Mr. E's travel led him to miss doses of medications and lose entire nights of sleep.
>
> He would then arrive at his destination in a hypomanic state that impaired his judgment, increased his sex drive, and led to his promiscuity and the subsequent conflict with his wife.

The therapist and Mr. E carefully evaluated his erratic social rhythms. Their first goal was to assess the importance of each business trip, eliminating all nonessential travel that might contribute to social rhythm disruption. Mr. E discovered that he was able to accomplish a surprising amount of work via conference calls and e-mail, decreasing his travel by almost half. These changes enabled him to develop more stable daily rhythms and contributed to a more even mood. When trips could not be avoided, the therapist worked with Mr. E and his psychiatrist to discuss timing of medication doses and the addition of a sleeping medication on long flights to ensure that he got some sleep (an intermediate goal). They also worked toward eliminating unnecessarily stimulating activities (e.g., late-night social events) and maintaining a schedule that approximated his home sleep–wake schedule while abroad. As Mr. E's mood stabilized and the promiscuity abated, his relationship with his wife improved; they began to discuss the possibility of downsizing their lifestyle in order to allow Mr. E to take a less lucrative but lower pressure job (long-term objective).

Adapting to Changes in Routines

Changes in routine are an inexorable part of life. Some changes are predictable (e.g., graduation, the birth of a child); others are not (e.g., physical illness, winning the lottery). IPSRT helps patients adapt to changes in routine. In the event of a predictable change, the therapist encourages the patient to entrain his or her rhythms gradually to a new schedule, thereby minimizing the disruptive effects of the change. For example, the therapist may suggest that a patient shift her wake time backwards by a half-hour each week over a 3-week period in preparation for a new schedule that will require her to be ready for work earlier than before.

Unanticipated changes, however, may require considerable therapist effort to address both unexpected alterations in schedules and their psychological meaning to the patient. For example, following the unexpected death of a patient's dog, the therapist offered her patient both an opportunity to grieve and practical suggestions to help protect his social rhythms. This patient had always awakened at 8:00 A.M. to walk his dog. Thus, the therapist encouraged the patient to plan to meet friends for breakfast over the next few weeks—both to mitigate against the loss and to ensure that he find a substitute rationale to reinforce his 8:00 A.M. wake-up time.

Use of Interpersonal Psychotherapy Strategies

IPSRT uses the interpersonal strategies of IPT to address both an interpersonal problem area and the rhythm-specific complexities of interpersonal stressors and life events that may be instrumental in precipitating affective episodes. IPRST therefore extends the role of IPT strategies to include both the improvement of interpersonal functioning and the indirect enhancement of more stable social rhythms. For example, a patient with bipolar disorder struggled with her teenage daughter's late-night outings and failure to adhere to household curfews. The patient stayed up late on consecutive nights worrying and wanting to confront her daughter immediately upon her return. The sleep deprivation and late-night arguments contributed to a subsequent hypomanic episode. The problem was labeled a role dispute. In addition to trying to improve communication between the patient and her daughter, IPSRT also focused on ways of addressing the dispute that specifically avoided social rhythm disruptions.

Grieving the Lost Healthy Self

In IPT for unipolar disorder, the problem area of grief is *not* invoked when the patient experiences symbolic losses, such as the loss of a job or loss of function from physical illness; these issues would be handled as role transitions. Patients with bipolar disorder, however, frequently grieve for the person they were before the illness, or the person they might have become if they did not suffer from bipolar disorder. In IPSRT, the process of *grieving for the lost healthy self* utilizes the IPT techniques associated with grief to help the patient mourn this loss. The therapist encourages the patient to express painful feelings about lost hopes, ruined relationships, interrupted careers, and missed opportunities. This technique also provides a forum for the patient to mourn lost "highs," struggle with denial, and balance spontaneity and stability. As the patient mourns the passing of a former self, the therapist encourages him or her to develop new relationships, to establish new, more realistic goals, and to focus on future opportunities.

Addressing Medication Adherence

Adherence to medication regimens is difficult for many patients with bipolar disorder. Most of the medications used to treat the illness (i.e., lithium, sodium divalproex, neuroleptics) have side effects that can be difficult to tolerate, including tremor, weight gain, dry mouth, and hair loss. Furthermore, many individuals are ambivalent about staying on medications that deprive them of seductive hypomanias. Therapists use strategies such as psychoeducation and grieving the lost healthy self to address some of these issues. They also work with the psychopharmacologist (in the instance of a split treatment) to manage side effects aggressively and to help the patient discuss openly any concerns about medications. Finally, reviewing serial serum blood levels of mood stabilizers provided by the psychiatrist can help the therapist both to detect covert nonadherence and to provide an opportunity for positive feedback when there is evidence of improved adherence.

Integrating and Balancing Interpersonal Psychotherapy and Social Rhythm Therapy Components

As for IPT, the IPSRT manual is written as a guideline rather than a "cookbook." In general, the therapist first encourages social rhythm regularity and then explores the interpersonal meaning of an event. The instincts of the individual therapist play an important role in balancing the disparate techniques of IPSRT. For example, in a given session, the therapist might focus on a particularly urgent interpersonal problem and defer a discussion of SRMs. Alternatively, the therapist might opt to work on medication adherence issues for a period of time before addressing either the interpersonal problem area or SRMs. IPSRT should be delivered as a seamless treatment that is administered flexibly to meet the needs of an individual patient.

EMPIRICAL FINDINGS

IPT is one of a few psychotherapies to have demonstrated efficacy for the treatment of a variety of disorders under controlled research conditions. We do not attempt to describe all extant research on IPT, but we do summarize major findings. For a fuller discussion, the reader is referred to Weissman and colleagues (2000).

Acute Treatment for Major Depression

IPT has been subjected to testing in two large, randomized, controlled trials for the treatment of acute depression. The first study was a 16-week trial conducted in Boston and New Haven comparing IPT, amitriptyline alone, amitriptyline plus IPT, and a control condition for the treatment of major depression ($n = 81$) (DiMascio et al., 1979). Patients assigned to the control condition were told to call if they were very distressed, but no treatment sessions were scheduled. Both IPT and amitriptyline performed comparably, yielding a greater reduction in symptoms than the control condition.

The NIMH sponsored the next large study, the Treatment of Depression Collaborative Research Program (TDCRP) (Elkin et al., 1989), in which 250 outpatients meeting DSM-III criteria for major depression were randomly assigned to one of four treatment cells: IPT, cognitive-behavioral therapy (CBT), imipramine plus clinical management (CM), or placebo plus CM. After 16 weeks, all four groups showed improvement in depressive symptoms, with nonstatistically significant differences across cells. However, a secondary analysis of the data suggested that both imipramine and IPT (but not CBT) were significantly more efficacious than the placebo–CM condition for more severely depressed patients (Sotsky et al., 1991).

Maintenance Treatment for Recurrent Major Depression

Frank and colleagues at the University of Pittsburgh adapted IPT for the long-term, prophylactic treatment of patients with histories of highly recurrent depression (Frank et al., 1990; Frank, Kupfer, Wagner, McEachran, & Cornes, 1991). An important innovation in the development of IPT, this approach used the acute strategies of IPT to prevent subsequent depressive episodes. They enrolled 128 acutely ill patients with at least three (and an average of seven) prior episodes of major depression and treated them to remission with acute, weekly IPT plus imipramine. Following 4 months of continuation treatment consisting of *both* imipramine and IPT, patients were randomly assigned to one of five treatment cells: the monthly maintenance form of IPT (IPT-M) alone, IPT-M plus imipramine, IPT-M plus placebo, medication clinic plus placebo, or medication clinic plus imipramine. Imipramine was administered in the same doses used to treat acute symptoms (mean dose 200 mg/day), whereas IPT was tapered from weekly to monthly sessions in the maintenance phase. Both imipramine and IPT-M yielded significantly longer survival times (i.e., fewer relapses) than did placebo. Perhaps not surprisingly, "high-dose" imipramine performed better than "low-dose" monthly IPT, and IPT-M conferred no additional benefit to treatment with imipramine. That even a monthly dosage of IPT-M had significant benefit for these high-risk patients is impressive.

Reynolds and colleagues (1999), also from the University of Pittsburgh, implemented a study of similar design in a population of depressed geriatric patients (> age 60). After 16 weeks of stable depression scores, of the 180 patients with recurrent, nonpsychotic unipolar major depression who were treated acutely with nortriptyline (NTP) and IPT, 107 subjects were randomly assigned to one of four monthly maintenance therapy conditions: medication clinic plus NTP, medication clinic plus placebo, IPT-M plus NTP, or IPT-M plus placebo. Using survival analyses, the investigators demonstrated that subjects assigned to any of the active treatments had a significantly greater chance of remaining depression-free than those assigned to medication clinic plus placebo. The best outcome was observed in patients assigned to the combined treatment condition, with 80% remaining depression-free over a 3-year period.

Adaptations of Interpersonal Psychotherapy for Other Depressive Disorders and Comorbid Conditions

HIV-Positive Patients

Markowitz and colleagues (1995) at Cornell University modified IPT to treat HIV-seropositive patients with depressive symptoms. Adaptations of IPT included a focus on having two medical illness (HIV and depression) and on "living out your fantasies" in order to make the most of however much life remained. Modeled on the TDCRP, investigators randomly assigned 101 HIV-positive subjects with depressive symptoms to treatment with IPT, CBT, supportive psychotherapy (SP), or imipramine plus SP. Although all groups improved, subjects who received IPT alone or imipramine plus SP had significantly greater improvement in depressive symptoms than those receiving CBT or SP alone (Markowitz, Kocsis, et al., 1998).

Dysthymic Disorder

Patients with dysthymic disorder, by definition, have suffered from a mood disorder for at least 2 years, and often for decades. Markowitz (1998) has modified IPT to address the chronic mood symptoms and concomitant social skills deficits of this population. Retaining IPT's original acute format, IPT for dysthymic disorder (IPT-D) conceptualizes the treatment period itself as an iatrogenic role transition that moves the patient from chronic depression to euthymia. During treatment, the patient learns that he or she has been suffering from a chronic mood disorder (an example of IPT's use of the medical model) rather than, as most patients believe, character flaws or a depressive personality. The therapist helps the patient understand that the long-standing depressive symptoms have interfered with social skills acquisition, which in turn has led to compromised interpersonal functioning. Continuing the cycle, unsatisfactory relationships maintain the mood disorder. In IPT-D, patients learn to function in the new—and initially difficult—role of a nondepressed individual. In most instances, 6 months of monthly continuation sessions are administered after acute treatment to consolidate the gains of responders. Investigators at Cornell University are currently conducting a randomized, controlled study comparing IPT-D, antidepressant medication (sertraline), and SP for the treatment of dysthymic disorder (Weissman et al., 2000).

In a separate undertaking, Steiner and colleagues (1998) from McMaster University in Canada treated over 700 patients with dysthymic disorder in community settings. Subjects were randomly assigned to 4 months of treatment with IPT (12 sessions), sertraline, or IPT plus sertraline. Of subjects assigned to IPT, 51% responded to treatment compared to 63% and 62% response rates in subjects assigned to sertraline and combination treatment, respectively. A 2-year follow-up evaluation of health care and social services utilization showed that assignment to IPT (either alone or in combination with sertraline) was associated with lower services utilization and cost. Thus, although treatment that included IPT was more costly than treatment with sertraline alone, psychotherapy was associated with a reduction in overall health care costs. The investigators deemed combination treatment the most *cost-effective* intervention because it was associated with both higher response rates and a reduction in overall costs.

Primary Care Settings

Investigators at the University of Pittsburgh evaluated the effectiveness of IPT delivered in a primary care setting (Schulberg et al., 1996) with 276 primary care patients meeting DSM-III-R criteria for current major depression. Subjects were randomly assigned to 8 months of treatment with NTP, IPT (delivered by a psychiatrist or clinical psychologist), or usual care (delivered by a primary care physician). Subjects assigned to either NTP or IPT experienced a more rapid and complete reduction of depressive symptoms than subjects assigned to usual care. At 8 months, in both intent-to-treat and completer analyses, there were significant differences in symptoms scores between usual care and both IPT and NTP subjects. There were high levels of attrition from both the IPT and NTP conditions.

Pregnant and Postpartum Women

Although the risks of antidepressant medication during pregnancy and lactation are acceptable under some circumstances (Stowe et al., 1997, 2000; Wisner, Gelenberg, Leonard, Zarin, & Frank, 1999), women of childbearing age may prefer treatment with psychotherapy. Thus, psychotherapy may play a central role in the treatment of depressed women during their reproductive years. Spinelli (1997) at Columbia University, has modified IPT to treat women who are depressed and pregnant. In a 16-week, open, pilot trial of IPT for 13 pregnant women who met criteria for major depression, she found that mean depression rating scores decreased significantly over the 16-week study period. A larger, randomized, controlled trial is planned.

O'Hara and Stuart from the University of Iowa have adapted IPT for the treatment of postpartum depression (Stuart & O'Hara, 1995). A large sample ($n = 120$) of postpartum women who met DSM-IV criteria for major depression were randomly assigned to IPT or a waiting-list control condition. Subjects assigned to IPT showed significantly greater improvement in depressive symptoms and psychosocial functioning, and were more likely to achieve syndromal remission than control subjects (O'Hara et al., 2000).

Adolescents

Investigators at Columbia University have adapted IPT to treat depressed adolescents (IPT-A; Mufson, Moreau, Weissman, & Klerman, 1993). Modifications include the addition of a fifth interpersonal problem area, the single-parent family, and parental involvement in the initial phase of treatment. Mufson and colleagues randomly assigned 48 depressed adolescents to 12 weeks of treatment with IPT-A or a clinical monitoring condition. Patients were predominantly Latino and of low socioeconomic status. Of the patients assigned to IPT-A, 75% met remission criteria by the end of treatment compared to less than 50% of the patients assigned to the control condition. Patients assigned to IPT-A also showed significantly greater improvement in overall social functioning (Mufson et al., 1999). Rossello and colleagues randomly assigned 71 depressed Puerto Rican adolescents to treatment with IPT, CBT, or a waiting-list control condition. Subjects assigned to IPT or CBT showed greater improvement in depressive symptoms than control subjects. On measures of functioning and self-esteem, subjects assigned to IPT fared better than those assigned to CBT (Rossello & Bernal, 1999).

Bipolar Disorder

A single, large trial of IPSRT as an adjunctive treatment for bipolar disorder is currently under way at the University of Pittsburgh. Acutely ill bipolar patients are treated with medication and randomly assigned to either IPSRT or intensive clinical management (CM). Once stabilized (defined as 4 weeks of symptom scores averaging ≤ 7 on the HRSD and ≤ 7 on the Bech–Rafaelsen Mania Scale [Bech, Bolwig, Kramp, & Rafaelsen, 1979] while on a stable medication regimen), patients are reassigned to either IPSRT or CM (in conjunction with the medication regimen that led to stabilization) for 2 years of monthly preventive treatment.

Although the study is not yet complete, several preliminary reports have been published. Among the first 42 patients treated acutely with either IPSRT or CM, those treated for mania achieved clinical remission significantly more quickly than those treated for depression (Hlastala et al., 1997). Although there were no statistically significant effects of treatment assignment, among the 22 depressed patients, median time to remission was 21 weeks with IPSRT versus 40 weeks with CM, suggesting that IPSRT may hasten recovery from a depression more effectively than a nonspecific "medication clinic" intervention. Among the first 82 patients to enter the preventive phase of treatment, patients who received the same treatment for both acute and preventive phases (either CM followed by CM, or IPSRT followed by IPSRT) had lower rates of recurrence (< 20% vs. > 40%) and levels of symptomatology over the subsequent 52 weeks than those reassigned to the alternate modality (either IPSRT followed by CM, or CM followed by IPSRT) (Frank et al., 1999). Subsequent analyses, however, have suggested that losing IPSRT (i.e., assignment to IPSRT in the acute phase followed by CM in the preventive phase) put patients at particular risk of depressive (but not manic) recurrence (Frank, Swartz, et al., 2000). Finally, it seems that patients assigned to IPSRT in the preventive phase suffer fewer subsyndromal depressive symptoms than those assigned to CM, but they have the same rate of manic recurrences (Frank, 1999). These reports suggest that IPSRT may exert a selectively favorable effect on the depressive component of the disorder.

Bipolar Patients with Comorbid Borderline Personality Disorder

Frank, Pilkonis, and colleagues at the University of Pittsburgh are conducting an open trial of IPSRT combined with pharmacotherapy for acutely ill patients with comorbid bipolar I disorder and borderline personality disorder. They hypothesize that the interpersonal sensitivity and affective lability of patients with borderline personality disorder will respond to the interpersonal and behavioral strategies of IPSRT. Preliminary analyses of the first 11 patients enrolled in this protocol suggest that these patients are difficult to treat, requiring complex pharmacotherapy regimens and long courses of psychotherapy. Compared to patients with bipolar I disorder only, patients with comorbid borderline personality disorder showed a trend toward requiring a greater number of medications and higher average symptom scores over time (Swartz et al., 2000). Only 3 subjects have met stringent stabilization criteria, with a mean time to stabilization of 76 weeks (vs. 35 weeks to stabilization for subjects with bipolar disorder alone [$n = 122$]). Dropout rates were high (7 out of 11 subjects), but some subjects showed improvements in symptoms and interpersonal functioning over a long treatment period and following numerous medication trials.

PREDICTORS OF RESPONSE TO INTERPERSONAL PSYCHOTHERAPY

A pressing question in psychotherapy research—and, indeed, in much of medicine—is "What works for whom?" (Roth & Fonagy, 1996). We know that IPT is an efficacious treatment for depression, which, in practical terms, means that 50–75% of patients treated with a full course of IPT will experience significant relief from their symptoms. Do we know which patients are most and least likely to benefit from IPT? Yes and no. Researchers have retrospectively identified some predictors of response to IPT, which include biological markers, symptom severity, symptom profile, and characteristics of the patient–therapist dyad. Most IPT studies exclude subjects with active suicidal ideation, psychosis, and severe cognitive dysfunction; therefore, we know very little about how IPT might function in these groups of patients. For any single patient, however, clinical judgment will figure prominently in the decision of whether to initiate treatment with IPT.

Thase and colleagues (1997) demonstrated that depressed subjects with abnormal sleep profiles were less likely than depressed subjects with normal sleep profiles to remit with IPT alone. These same subjects showed a robust response when pharmacotherapy was added to IPT. Investigators from the TDCRP established that patients with low social dysfunction are likely to respond to IPT, whereas patients with low cognitive dysfunction are likely to respond to CBT. They also demonstrated that patients with more severe depressive symptoms had a better response to IPT and imipramine than to CBT or placebo with CM (Sotsky et al., 1991). According to investigators at the University of Pittsburgh, recurrently depressed women with lifetime histories of panic disorder, elevated levels of lifetime panic symptoms, and/or high levels of somatic anxiety are significantly less likely to remit with IPT alone than depressed patients without these panic-spectrum symptoms (Feske, Frank, Kupfer, Shear, & Weaver, 1998; Frank, Shear, et al., 2000). Interestingly, comorbid anxiety symptoms were also shown to predict nonremission for patients treated for bipolar I disorder with medications and either IPSRT or intensive CM (Feske et al., 2000). These analyses suggest that IPT may be a good choice for patients with more severe depressive symptoms, who already possess some social skills, but it may be less desirable as monotherapy for patients with comorbid panic-spectrum symptoms and/or abnormal sleep EEG recordings.

Relatively few data are available to help us predict response to IPT or IPSRT as maintenance strategies. The Pittsburgh group demonstrated that patients with recurrent major depression who received maintenance IPT were less likely to experience a recurrence of depression over a 2-year period if the IPT sessions achieved and maintained a high level of interpersonal focus. The authors attributed the capacity to maintain focus to characteristics of the patient–therapist dyad, which may have included therapy quality, level of patient difficulty, and match between therapist and patient (Frank et al., 1991). Although data are not yet available to support this assertion, clinical experience suggests that IPSRT may be particularly helpful for patients experiencing problematic interpersonal relationships and/or stressful life events in addition to their mood symptoms. Because IPT is a life-event-based treatment, it is probably most helpful for people who have had life events. Patients whose lives are devoid of identifiable events might fare better with intrapsychic or cognitive treatments.

CONCLUSIONS

IPT has grown in scope and popularity since its conceptualization in the 1970s. A treatment that is both intuitive and rigorous, IPT has withstood the test of multiple randomized, controlled clinical trials to emerge as a clearly efficacious treatment for depression. IPSRT, in relatively early stages of testing, seems a promising maintenance strategy for bipolar disorder. Individuals with IPT expertise can now be identified in 18 countries across five continents, and researchers have begun the task of testing IPT with new populations and for new disorders (Weissman et al., 2000). The absence of a formalized system for IPT training and lack of experience with psychotherapy dissemination strategies have limited the rate of its uptake in wider clinical settings. As investigators and clinicians become increasingly cognizant of the gap between efficacy and effectiveness (Wells, 1999), the next challenge facing IPT researchers will be to test IPT in routine practice settings and with more heterogeneous patient populations.

ACKNOWLEDGMENTS

Preparation of this chapter was supported in part by Grant Nos. MH-60473 (to Holly A. Swartz), MH-49635 (to John C. Markowitz), and MH-29618 (to Ellen Frank) from the National Institute of Mental Health.

REFERENCES

Altshuler, L. L., Post, R. M., Leverich, G. S., Mikalauskas, K., Rosoff, A., & Ackerman, L. (1995). Antidepressant-induced mania and cycle acceleration: A controversy revisited. *American Journal of Psychiatry, 152,* 1130–1138.

American Psychiatric Association. (1994). *Diagnostic and statistical manual of mental disorders* (4th ed.). Washington, DC: Author.

Bauer, M. S., Callahan, A. M., Jampala, C., Petty, F., Sajatovic, M., Schaefer, V., Wittlin, B., & Powell, B. J. (1999). Clinical practice guidelines for bipolar disorder from the Department of Veterans Affairs. *Journal of Clinical Psychiatry, 60,* 9–21.

Bech, P., Bolwig, T. G., Kramp, P., & Rafaelsen, O. J. (1979). The Bech–Rafaelsen Mania Scale and the Hamilton Depression Scale: Evaluation of homogeneity and inter-observer reliability. *Acta Psychiatrica Scandinavica, 59,* 420–430.

Brown, G. W., & Harris, T. (1978). *Social origins of depression: A study of psychiatric disorders in women.* New York: Free Press.

Coryell, W., Scheftner, W., Keller, M., Endicott, J., Maser, J., & Klerman, G. L. (1993). The enduring psychosocial consequences of mania and depression. *American Journal of Psychiatry, 150,* 720–727.

Coyne, J. C. (1976). Depression and the response of others. *Journal of Abnormal Psychology, 85,* 186–193.

Craighead, W. E., Miklowitz, D. J., Vajk, F. C., & Frank, E. (1998). Psychosocial treatments for bipolar disorder. In P. E. Nathan & J. M. Gorman (Eds.), *A guide to treatments that work* (pp. 240–248). New York: Oxford University Press.

DiMascio, A., Weissman, M. M., Prusoff, B. A., Neu, C., Zwilling, M., & Klerman, G. L. (1979). Differential symptom reduction by drugs and psychotherapy in acute depression. *Archives of General Psychiatry, 36,* 1450–1456.

Ehlers, C. L., Frank, E., & Kupfer, D. J. (1988). Social *zeitgebers* and biological rhythms. *Archives of General Psychiatry, 45,* 948–952.

Ehlers, C. L., Kupfer, D. J., Frank, E., & Monk, T. H. (1993). Biological rhythms and depression: The role of *zeitgebers* and *zeitstorers*. *Depression, 1,* 285–293.

Elkin, I., Shea, M. T., Watkins, J. T., Imber, S. D., Sotsky, S. M., Collins, J. F., Glass, D. R., Pilkonis, P. A., Leber, W. R., Docherty, J. P., Fiester, S. J., & Parloff, M. B. (1989). National Institute of Mental Health Treatment of Depression Collaborative Research Program: General effectiveness of treatments. *Archives of General Psychiatry, 46,* 971–982.

Feske, U., Frank, E., Kupfer, D. J., Shear, M. K., & Weaver, E. (1998). Anxiety as a predictor of response to interpersonal psychotherapy for recurrent major depression: An exploratory investigation. *Depression and Anxiety, 8,* 135–141.

Feske, U., Frank, E., Mallinger, A. G., Houck, P. R., Fagiolini, A., Shear, M. K., Grochocinski, V. J., & Kupfer, D. J. (2000). Anxiety as a correlate of response to the acute treatment of bipolar I disorder. *American Journal of Psychiatry, 157,* 956–962.

Foley, S. H., Rounsaville, B. J., Weissman, M. M., Sholomskas, D., & Chevron, E. (1989). Individual versus conjoint interpersonal psychotherapy for depressed patients with marital disputes. *International Journal of Family Psychiatry, 10,* 29–42.

Frank, E. (1991). Interpersonal psychotherapy as a maintenance treatment for patients with recurrent depression. *Psychotherapy, 28,* 259–266.

Frank, E. (1999). Interpersonal and social rhythm therapy prevents depressive symptomatology in bipolar 1 patients [Abstract]. *Bipolar Disorders, 1,* 13.

Frank, E., Kupfer, D. J., Perel, J. M., Cornes, C., Jarrett, D. B., Mallinger, A. G., Thase, M. E., McEachran, A. B., & Grochocinski, V. J. (1990). Three-year outcomes for maintenance therapies in recurrent depression. *Archives of General Psychiatry, 47,* 1093–1099.

Frank, E., Kupfer, D. J., Wagner, E. F., McEachran, A. B., & Cornes, C. (1991). Efficacy of interpersonal psychotherapy as a maintenance treatment of recurrent depression: Contributing factors. *Archives of General Psychiatry, 48,* 1053–1059.

Frank, E., Shear, M. K., Rucci, P., Cyranowski, J. M., Endicott, J., Fagiolini, A., Grochocinski, V. J., Houck, P., Kupfer, D. J., Maser, J. D., & Cassano, G. B. (2000). Influence of panic-agorophobic spectrum symptoms on treatment response in patients with recurrent major depression. *American Journal of Psychiatry, 157,* 1101–1107.

Frank, E., Swartz, H. A., & Kupfer, D. J. (2000). Interpersonal and social rhythm therapy: Managing the chaos of bipolar disorder. *Biological Psychiatry, 48,* 593–604.

Frank, E., Swartz, H. A., Mallinger, A. G., Thase, M. E., Weaver, E. V., & Kupfer, D. J. (1999). Adjunctive psychotherapy for bipolar disorder: Effects of changing treatment modality. *Journal of Abnormal Psychology, 108,* 579–587.

Frank, J. (1971). Therapeutic factors in psychotherapy. *American Journal of Psychotherapy, 25,* 350–361.

Goldberg, J. F., Harrow, M., & Grossman, L. S. (1995). Course and outcome in bipolar affective disorder: A longitudinal follow-up study. *American Journal of Psychiatry, 152,* 379–384.

Goldberg, J. F., & Kocsis, J. H. (1999). Depression in the course of bipolar disorder. In J. F. Goldberg (Ed.), *Bipolar disorders: Clinical course and outcome* (pp. 129–147). Washington, DC: American Psychiatric Press.

Goodwin, F., & Jamison, K. (1990). *Manic–depressive illness.* New York: Oxford University Press.

Hamilton, M. (1960). A rating scale for depression. *Journal of Neurology, Neurosurgery, and Psychiatry, 25,* 56–62.

Henderson, S., Byrne, G., Duncan-Jones, P., Scott, R., & Adcock, S. (1980). Social relationships, adversity and neurosis: A study of associations in a general population sample. *British Journal of Psychiatry, 136,* 574–583.

Hirschfeld, R. M., Clayton, P. J., Cohen, I., Fawcett, J., Keck, P., McClellan, J., McElroy, S., Post, R., & Satloff, A. (1994). Practice guideline for the treatment of patients with bipolar disorder. *American Journal of Psychiatry, 151,* 1S–36S.

Hirschfeld, R. M., Klerman, G. L., Clayton, P. J., Keller, M. B., McDonald-Scott, P., & Larkin, B. H. (1983). Assessing personality: Effects of the depressive state on trait measurement. *American Journal of Psychiatry, 140,* 695–699.

Hlastala, S. A., Frank, E., Mallinger, A. G., Thase, M. E., Ritenour, A. M., & Kupfer, D. J. (1997). Bipolar depression: An underestimated treatment challenge. *Depression and Anxiety, 5,* 73–83.

Joffe, R. T., Young, L. T., & MacQueen, G. M. (1999). A two-illness model of bipolar disorder. *Bipolar Disorders, 1,* 25–30.

Keller, M. B., Lavori, P. W., Coryell, W., Endicott, J., & Mueller, T. I. (1993). Bipolar I: A five-year prospective follow-up. *Journal of Nervous and Mental Disease, 181,* 238–245.

Klerman, G. L., DiMascio, A., Weissman, M. M., Prusoff, B. A., & Paykel, E. S. (1974). Treatment of depression by drugs and psychotherapy. *American Journal of Psychiatry, 131*, 186–191.

Klerman, G. L., Weissman, M. M., Rounsaville, B. J., & Chevron, E. S. (1984). *Interpersonal psychotherapy of depression*. New York: Basic Books.

Kusumakar, V., Yatham, L. N., Haslam, D. R. S., Parikh, S. V., Matte, R., Sharma, V., Silverstone, P. H., Kutcher, S. P., & Kennedy, S. (1997). The foundations of effective management of bipolar disorder. *Canadian Journal of Psychiatry, 42*, 69S–73S.

Malkoff-Schwartz, S., Frank, E., Anderson, B., Sherrill, J. T., Siegel, L., Patterson, D., & Kupfer, D. J. (1998). Stressful life events and social rhythm disruption in the onset of manic and depressive bipolar episodes. *Archives of General Psychiatry, 55*, 702–707.

Markowitz, J. C. (1998). *Interpersonal psychotherapy for dysthymic disorder*. Washington, DC: American Psychiatric Press.

Markowitz, J. C., Klerman, G. L., Clougherty, K. F., Spielman, L. A., Jacobsberg, L. B., Fishman, B., Frances, A. J., Kocsis, J. H., & Perry, S. W. (1995). Individual psychotherapies for depressed HIV-positive patients. *American Journal of Psychiatry, 152*, 1504–1509.

Markowitz, J. C., Kocsis, J. H., Fishman, B., Spielman, L. A., Jacobsberg, L. B., Frances, A. J., Klerman, G. L., & Perry, S. W. (1998). Treatment of depressive symptoms in human immunodeficiency virus-positive patients. *Archives of General Psychiatry, 55*, 452–457.

Markowitz, J. C., Svartberg, M., & Swartz, H. A. (1998). Is IPT time-limited psychodynamic psychotherapy? *Journal of Psychotherapy Practice and Research, 7*, 185–195.

Markowitz, J. C., & Swartz, H. A. (1997). Case formulation in interpersonal psychotherapy of depression. In T. D. Eells (Ed.), *Handbook of psychotherapy case formulation* (pp. 192–222). New York: Guilford Press.

Meyer, A. (1957). *Psychobiology: A science of man*. Springfield, IL: Thomas.

Monk, T. K., Flaherty, J. F., Frank, E., Hoskinson, K., & Kupfer, D. J. (1990). The Social Rhythm Metric: An instrument to quantify the daily rhythms of life. *Journal of Nervous and Mental Disease, 178*, 120–126.

Mufson, L., Moreau, D., Weissman, M. M., & Klerman, G. L. (1993). *Interpersonal psychotherapy for depressed adolescents*. New York: Guilford Press.

Mufson, L., Weissman, M. M., Moreau, D., & Garfinkel, R. (1999). Efficacy of interpersonal psychotherapy for depressed adolescents. *Archives of General Psychiatry, 57*, 573–579.

O'Hara, M. W., Stuart, S., Gorman, L. L., & Wenzel, A. (2000). Efficacy of interpersonal psychotherapy for postpartum depression. *Archives of General Psychiatry, 57*, 1039–1045.

Parsons, T. (1951). Illness and the role of the physician: A sociological perspective. *American Journal of Orthopsychiatry, 21*, 452–460.

Reynolds, C. F., III, Frank, E., Perel, J. M., Imber, S. D., Cornes, C., Miller, M. D., Mazumdar, S., Houck, P. R., Dew, M. A., Stack, J. A., Pollock, B. G., & Kupfer, D. J. (1999). Nortriptyline and interpersonal psychotherapy as maintenance therapies for recurrent major depression: A randomized controlled trial in patients older than 59 years. *Journal of the American Medical Association, 281*, 39–45.

Rossello, J., & Bernal, G. (1999). The efficacy of cognitive-behavioral and interpersonal treatments for depression in Puerto Rican adolescents. *Journal of Consulting and Clinical Psychology, 67*, 734–745.

Roth, A., & Fonagy, P. (1996). *What works for whom?: A critical review of psychotherapy research*. New York: Guilford Press.

Rounsaville, B. J., Chevron, E. S., Weissman, M. M., Prusoff, B. A., & Frank, E. (1986). Training therapists to perform interpersonal psychotherapy in clinical trials. *Comprehensive Psychiatry, 27*, 364–371.

Sachs, G. S., Printz, D. J., Kahn, D. A., Carpenter, D., & Docherty, J. P. (2000, April). The expert consensus guideline series: Medication treatment of bipolar disorder 2000. *Postgraduate Medicine Special Report*, pp. 1–104.

Schulberg, H. C., Block, M. R., Madonia, M. J., Scott, C. P., Rodriguez, E., Imber, S., Perel, J.,

Lave, J., Houck, P. R., & Coulehan, J. L. (1996). Treating major depression in primary care practice: Eight-month clinical outcomes. *Archives of General Psychiatry, 53*, 913–919.

Sotsky, S. M., Glass, D. R., Shea, M. T., Pilkonis, P. A., Collins, J. F., Elkin, I., Watkins, J. T., Imber, S. D., Leber, W. R., Moyer, J., & Oliveri, M. E. (1991). Patient predictors of response to psychotherapy and pharmacotherapy: Findings in the NIMH Treatment of Depression Collaborative Research Program. *American Journal of Psychiatry, 148*, 997–1008.

Spinelli, M. G. (1997). Interpersonal psychotherapy for depressed antepartum women: A pilot study. *American Journal of Psychiatry, 154*, 1028–1030.

Steiner, M., Browne, G., J. R., Gafni, A., Byrne, C., Bell, B., & Dunn, E. (1998). *Sertraline and IPT in dysthymia: One year follow-up*. Poster presented at the 38th Annual Meeting of the NIMH New Clinical Drug Evaluation Unit (NCDEU), Boca Raton, FL.

Stowe, Z. N., Cohen, L. S., Hostetter, A., Ritchie, J. C., Owens, M. J., & Nemeroff, C. B. (2000). Paroxetine in human breast milk and nursing infants. *American Journal of Psychiatry, 157*, 185–189.

Stowe, Z. N., Owens, M. J., Landry, J. C., Kilts, C. D., Ely, T., Llewellyn, A., & Nemeroff, C. B. (1997). Sertraline and desmethylsertraline in human breast milk and nursing infants. *American Journal of Psychiatry, 154*, 1255–1260.

Stuart, S., & O'Hara, M. W. (1995). Interpersonal psychotherapy for postpartum depression: A treatment program. *Journal of Psychotherapy Practice and Research, 4*, 18–29.

Sullivan, H. S. (1953). *The interpersonal theory of psychiatry*. New York: Norton.

Swartz, H. A., & Frank, E. (2001). Psychotherapy for bipolar depression: A phase-specific strategy? *Bipolar Disorders, 3*, 11–22.

Swartz, H. A., Pilkonis, P. A., Frank, E., Mallinger, A., Cherry, C. R., & Kupfer, D. J. (2000, January). *Bipolar disorder and comorbid borderline personality disorder: Treatment course and pharmacotherapy*. Poster presented at the Eli Lilly and Society for Biological Psychiatry Symposium on Bipolar Disorders, Phoenix, AZ.

Thase, M. E., Buysse, D. J., Frank, E., Cherry, C. R., Cornes, C. L., Mallinger, A. G., & Kupfer, D. J. (1997). Which depressed patients will respond to interpersonal psychotherapy?: The role of abnormal EEG sleep profiles. *American Journal of Psychiatry, 154*, 502–509.

Tohen, M., Hennen, J., Zarate, C. M., Jr., Baldessarini, R. J., Strakowski, S. M., Stoll, A. L., Faedda, G. L., Suppes, T., Gebre-Medhin, P., & Cohen, B. M. (2000). Two-year syndromal and functional recovery in 219 cases of first-episode major affective disorder with psychotic features. *American Journal of Psychiatry, 157*, 220–228.

Walker, K. N., MacBride, A., & Vachon, M. L. (1977). Social support networks and the crisis of bereavement. *Social Science and Medicine, 11*, 35–41.

Weissman, M. M., Klerman, G. L., Paykel, E. S., Prusoff, B. A., & Hanson, B. (1974). Treatment effects on the social adjustment of depressed patients. *Archives of General Psychiatry, 30*, 771–778.

Weissman, M. M., Markowitz, J. C., & Klerman, G. L. (2000). *Comprehensive guide to interpersonal psychotherapy*. New York: Basic Books.

Wells, K. B. (1999). Treatment research at the crossroads: The scientific interface of clinical trials and effectiveness research. *American Journal of Psychiatry, 156*, 5–10.

Wilfley, D. E., Mackenzie, K. R., Welch, R. R., Ayres, V. E., & Weissman, M. M. (2000). *Interpersonal psychotherapy for group*. New York: Basic Books.

Wisner, K. L., Gelenberg, A. J., Leonard, H., Zarin, D., & Frank, E. (1999). Pharmacologic treatment of depression during pregnancy. *Journal of the American Medical Association, 282*, 1264–1269

8

Family-Focused Treatment for Bipolar Disorder

David J. Miklowitz

Bipolar disorder, formerly known as manic–depressive illness, is a debilitating psychiatric condition affecting between 1.2% and 1.6% of the population (Kessler et al., 1994; Regier et al., 1990). It is usually treated with mood-stabilizing medications during acute periods of illness and long-term maintenance. More recently, various forms of psychosocial treatment have emerged as adjuncts to standard pharmacotherapy.

This chapter offers the rationale, theoretical background, empirical basis for, and clinic methods central to one such approach—*family-focused therapy* (FFT; Miklowitz & Goldstein, 1997). FFT is a 9-month outpatient psychoeducational program for patients living with or in close association with parents, a spouse, or siblings. It is given during the interval following acute mood episodes and consists of three interrelated modules: *psychoeducation* about the nature, course, origins, treatment, and self-management of bipolar disorder; *communication enhancement training* to interrupt negative cycles of family interaction; and *problem-solving skills training* to address illness-related family conflicts. As I indicate here, it has been found to be an efficacious adjunct to medications in improving the longitudinal course of bipolar disorder over periods of up to 2 years.

THE BIPOLAR SYNDROME AND ITS TREATMENT

Bipolar disorder is characterized by extreme shifts in mood, thinking, and behavior from the highest of highs ("manias") to the lowest of lows (depressions). Manic episodes are characterized by elevated or irritable mood, a decreased need for sleep, an increase in energy and goal-directed behavior, rapidity of thinking and speech, impulsiveness, and inflated self-esteem (or, in extreme cases, grandiose delusions). Depressions are usually characterized by sad mood, loss of interests, psychomotor agitation or retardation, insomnia, lethargy or fatigue, loss of concentration, feelings of worthlessness, and suicidal thinking and behavior.

Episodes of bipolar disorder can vary from several days to several months, with depressive periods typically lasting longer than manic periods. Patients with bipolar I disorder show the most dramatic shifts, from severe depressions to severe, debilitating manias. Patients with bipolar II disorder show shifts from severe depressions to milder, shorter, less debilitating periods of activation called "hypomania."

Many bipolar patients show a cycle characterized by manias followed by depressions, with "euthymic" or normal mood periods in between. Others cycle from depression to mania and back again. About 40% of bipolar I patients have "mixed" affective episodes characterized by mania and depressive symptoms simultaneously. About 15% of bipolar I and II patients have periods of "rapid cycling" in which manic, mixed, hypomanic, or depressive episodes appear four or more times in a single year (Calabrese, Fatemi, Kujawa, & Woyshville, 1996). It is common for bipolar patients to have residual symptoms of hypomania, depression, or dysthymia between major episodes (Harrow, Goldberg, Grossman, & Meltzer, 1990).

Bipolar disorder is usually treated with standard mood stabilizers such as lithium carbonate or the anticonvulsants (divalproex sodium [Depakote] or carbamazepine [Tegretol]), either alone or in combination. Newer mood stabilizers in the anticonvulsant class include lamotrigine (Lamictal), topiramate (Topamax), and gabapentin (Neurontin). These latter agents are usually used as adjuncts to standard mood stabilizers, although there is some evidence that bipolar depressions respond well to lamotrigine alone (Calabrese et al., 1999). Antipsychotic agents are often recommended alongside of mood stabilizers, particularly the "novel antipsychotic" agents such as olanzapine, risperidone, clozapine, quetiapine, and ziprasidone. Adjunctive antidepressant agents such as paroxetine, bupropion, or venlafaxine can sometimes help the patient recover more rapidly from severe depressions, but they carry the risk of sudden switches into mania, mixed disorder, or acceleration of cycles (Altshuler et al., 1995).

The manic pole, while quite dramatic and often very debilitating, usually responds at least partially to antimanic and antipsychotic agents (Keck & McElroy, 1996; McElroy & Keck, 2000; Thase & Sachs, 2000). The mood stabilizers control the manic pole of the illness better than the depressive pole: About 50–70% of patients respond to lithium, divalproex sodium, or carbamazepine "monotherapy" during acute episodes of mania (McElroy & Keck, 2000) and between 30% and 50% during acute episodes of depression (Thase & Sachs, 2000). As a result, the challenge facing psychiatrists, psychologists, and other mental health professionals is often treatment of the depressive pole of the disorder.

Once patients stabilize from an acute episode, *relapse prevention* becomes the central objective of treatment. On standard mood-stabilizing medications, about 37% of patients have a recurrence within 1 year, and about 60% within 2 years (Gelenberg et al., 1989; Gitlin, Swendsen, Heller, & Hammen, 1995). Furthermore, bipolar patients have a host of psychosocial impairments that persist even when they take medication (Coryell et al., 1993; Hammen, Gitlin, & Altshuler, 2000; Harrow et al., 1990; Goldberg, Harrow, & Grossman, 1995). The disorder is associated with low occupational functioning, high rates of separation and divorce, family conflict, and problems in the adjustment of offspring. Combining pharmacotherapy and psychosocial intervention has the potential to alleviate the psychosocial impairments not addressed by medication alone.

A pitfall in the drug treatment of bipolar disorder is the reluctance or even outright refusal of many patients to take medications on an ongoing basis. Many do not see the reason to continue on drug regimens when they feel well; others complain bitterly about side effects such as weight gain, mental sluggishness, or abdominal distress. Some patients enjoy their manic periods and resent that the medications take away these feelings of exhilaration, yet do little to repair their depressions. As many as 59% of patients are fully or partially nonadherent with medications in the year after a hospitalized episode (Strakowski et al., 1998), and as many as two-thirds discontinue medications altogether at some point in their lives (Colom et al., 2000). Predictors of medical nonadherence include younger age, male gender, comorbid alcohol or substance use disorders, denial of the illness, side effects, and lack of a supportive family or social network (Colom et al., 2000; Goodwin & Jamison, 1990; Keck et al., 1996; Keck, McElroy, Strakowski, Bourne, & West, 1997). Adjunctive psychosocial intervention has the potential to enhance the patient's consistency with medication, particularly if education is provided about the long-term effects of the disorder's cycling and the underlying influences of biological vulnerability.

STRESS AS A TRIGGER FOR BIPOLAR EPISODES

Why is the cycling of bipolar disorder so variable from patient to patient? Various theories have been proposed, including the notion that the illness takes on an autonomous, self-perpetuating quality over time (Post, 1992), that certain constellations of symptoms (e.g., psychosis, mixed episodes, comorbid substance use) bode poorly for longer term outcome (e.g., Calabrese et al., 1996; Strakowski, DelBello, Fleck, & Arndt, 2000; Tohen, Waternaux, & Tsuang, 1990), that treatment with antidepressants accelerates the cycling of the disorder (Altshuler et al., 1995), or that nonadherence to medications—particularly rapid discontinuation of lithium or other agents—stimulates sudden relapses (Strober, Morrell, Lampert, & Burroughs, 1990; Suppes, Baldessarini, Faedda, Tondo, & Tohen, 1993). Other theories focus on "stress triggers"—life events or family disturbances that may become breeding grounds for increased cycling of the disorder.

It is reasonably well-established that certain kinds of life events precede bipolar episodes. Notably, life events that have the potential to disrupt patients' "social rhythms" (patterns of expectable daily activity and sleep–wake cycles) are potent precipitators of manic episodes. Examples of rhythm-disruptive life events include the birth of a baby, "cramming" late at night for final exams, or taking transatlantic flights (Malkoff-Schwartz et al., 1998). Events that promote "goal attainment" also appear to precede increases in manic symptoms (e.g., winning a contest, getting married, getting promoted; Johnson et al., 2000). Associations have also been found between life events and the onset or recovery from bipolar depressive episodes (see, e.g., Johnson & Miller, 1997; Johnson & Roberts, 1995).

A separate literature concerns the role of family or marital relationships in the course of bipolar disorder. Much of this work has focused on "expressed emotion" (EE), a well-established predictor of relapse in schizophrenia and recurrent major depressive illness (for a review, see Butzlaff & Hooley, 1998). EE refers to the *emotional attitudes* of criticism, hostility, or emotional overinvolvement (overprotectiveness) held by close relatives at the time of a patient's acute illness episode, attitudes that are presumed to persist among relatives as the patient recovers. There are three naturalistic studies indicating that high levels of EE (high criticism, hostility, or overinvolvement) in close relatives are associated with a more pernicious course of bipolar illness over periods of 9 months or more (Miklowitz, Goldstein, Nuechterlein, Snyder, & Mintz, 1988; O'Connell, Mayo, Flatow, Cuthbertson, & O'Brien, 1991; Priebe, Wildgrube, & Muller-Oerlinghausen,

1989). The EE–illness course association has also been observed in two randomized psychosocial treatment studies of bipolar patients (Honig, Hofman, Rozendaal, & Dingemanns, 1997; Miklowitz, Simoneau, et al., 2000).

The mechanisms by which life events or family stress affect the course and outcome of bipolar disorder are unclear. Stressors may interact with biological vulnerabilities believed to be central to the pathophysiology of bipolar disorder, such as the functioning of the hypothalamic–pituitary–adrenal axis or abnormal activity of the protein kinase C signaling cascade. For example, it has been proposed in animal paradigms that long-term stress and overproduction of glucocorticoids damage or destroy cells in the hippocampus. The hippocampus is an important component of the limbic system, which regulates emotional states, sleep, and arousal (Manji, 2001; Sapolsky, 2000).

THE ROLE OF PSYCHOSOCIAL TREATMENT

The interactive roles of stress and biological vulnerability, the ceilings on the efficacy of pharmacotherapy in controlling illness recurrences, and the problem of nonadherence to medication all raise the possibility that combining psychosocial treatment with pharmacotherapy may improve the course of bipolar illness over time. The underlying assumption of psychosocial treatment, in contrast to medication, is that the patient can learn skills for coping with bipolar disorder and the stress agents that elicit its cycling. Thus, psychosocial treatment is considered part of the prophylactic, maintenance treatment of the disorder rather than part of its acute treatment.

The goals of adjunctive therapy include assisting patients in (1) understanding the nature and the precipitants of their illness episodes (typically, using the most recent illness period as an example); (2) planning to prevent future episodes; (3) accepting the realities of the disorder, the need for maintenance medications, and the social and occupational limitations the disorder imposes; (4) distinguishing the disorder from personality traits or everyday ups and downs; (5) identifying and coping with triggers for mood cycling; and (6) improving function within the family, social, and occupational milieu.

Various forms of psychotherapy have been proposed and, in some cases, empirically tested as adjuncts to pharmacotherapy for bipolar disorder. These models include but are not limited to interpersonal and social rhythm therapy (see Swartz, Markowitz, & Frank, Chapter 7, this volume), cognitive-behavioral therapy (see Otto & Reilly-Harrington, Chapter 6, this volume), and FFT. The remainder of this chapter is devoted to the FFT model and its associated empirical base. For more general reviews of psychotherapy outcome studies in bipolar disorder, see Craighead and Miklowitz (2000), Huxley, Parikh, and Baldessarini (2000), or Miklowitz and Craighead (2001).

FAMILY-FOCUSED THERAPY: THEORETICAL BACKGROUND AND EMPIRICAL BASIS

FFT has its theoretical roots in the behavioral family management model for treating patients with schizophrenia and their family members (see Falloon, Chapter 1, this volume). This outpatient treatment is based on the assumption that families of schizophrenic patients are not "dysfunctional" or directly causal in the pathway from biological vulnerability to episodes of schizophrenia. Rather, families are seen as needing knowledge about the disorder and the skills for communicating and solving problems relevant to it.

In the absence of these skills, families will rely on coercion, overprotectiveness, or various aversive control tactics to manage the stress related to the illness.

Families of bipolar patients also need education and skills building to deal with the disorder, but three important differences stand out. First, bipolar patients are often higher functioning than schizophrenic patients and usually play a more active role in their own illness management. As a result, family members' expectations can often be set higher. Second, bipolar patients are more likely to be married or partnered, whereas schizophrenic patients more frequently rely on parent caregivers. Thus, educational strategies need to be adjusted to the needs of marital units, often those involving young children. Third, families of bipolar patients seem to enjoy fast-paced, lively interchanges, and do not like feeling bridled by overly structured, directed forms of communication. As a result, skills training has to allow for greater flexibility in communication styles (Miklowitz & Goldstein, 1997).

Data from one open trial and two randomized trials support the efficacy of FFT in the outpatient treatment of bipolar disorder. In the first (Miklowitz & Goldstein, 1990), 9 patients with recent episodes of bipolar, manic disorder were given 21 sessions over 9 months (12 weekly sessions, followed by 6 biweekly and 3 monthly sessions). In the first phase, psychoeducation (7 sessions), patients and relatives were given information about how to recognize signs of bipolar disorder and cope with its cycling. This included didactic material on symptoms, etiology (with a focus on vulnerability–stress interactions), medical and psychosocial treatments, and self-management. It also included a relapse prevention drill, in which patients and relatives were taught to identify early warning signs (prodromal symptoms) and develop steps for averting major relapses (e.g., having family members call to arrange an emergency medical appointment). Later modules of FFT included communication enhancement training (7–10 sessions), in which patients and relatives were taught, via a behavioral rehearsal format, skills such as active listening, or delivering positive or negative feedback to other family members. In the final module, problem solving (4–5 sessions), patients and relatives learned to identify circumscribed problems and go through the steps of solving and implementing solutions to these problems, particularly those that arose during the postepisode phase.

The 9 patients were given standard pharmacotherapy for bipolar disorder (lithium, carbamazepine, and adjunctive antipsychotic, antidepressant, or anxiolytic agents). The comparison group was 23 historical control patients from an earlier follow-up study, who received similar, aggressive delivery of pharmacotherapy but no family treatment (Miklowitz et al., 1988). Over 9 months, only 1 of 9 (11%) FFT-treated patients relapsed; in contrast, 14 of the 23 historical controls (61%) relapsed during a 9-month follow-up.

The first randomized trial, conducted at the University of Colorado (Miklowitz, Simoneau, et al., 2000), assigned 101 bipolar I patients in a 1:2 randomization strategy to the 9-month FFT program (the protocol used in the previous study) plus standard medication ($n = 31$) or a comparison condition called crisis management (CM) plus standard medication ($n = 70$). Patients in CM were given two sessions of family education covering some of the same material as the more intensive FFT model, but in abridged form. They also received follow-up crisis intervention sessions or phone consultations as needed over 9 months. All family education or communication/problem-solving sessions in both conditions were administered in the patients' home setting.

All patients began in an acute manic, depressed, or mixed episode. Of the 101 patients, 79 completed 9 months of treatment and an additional 3 months of research follow-up; 35 of these 79 had relapses of mania or depression. FFT was associated with a lower relapse rate (29%) among treatment completers than was CM (53%)—a significant difference. A survival analysis model, which included data on the 22 treatment dropouts, indicated that FFT was superior to CM in prolonging survival intervals (time without relapsing) in the community. FFT was associated with differential reductions in depressive but not manic relapses.

Analysis of specific symptom clusters confirmed that FFT led to greater reductions in the severity of depressive symptoms than CM over the year of treatment and follow-up. The effects were strongest among patients in high EE families, who showed the most dramatic shifts in depressive symptoms from baseline to 1 year. Preliminary results from a 2-year follow-up of patients in this study suggest that the differential effects of FFT on depression severity scores are maintained well beyond the active treatment period (Miklowitz, Richards, George, Suddath, & Wendel, 2000).

An analysis of a subset of families from the Colorado study (Simoneau, Miklowitz, Richards, Saleem, & George, 1999) identified at least one mechanism by which FFT has its clinical effects. Among 22 families who took part in interaction task assessments at baseline and again after the 9-month FFT protocol, levels of positive affective communication (notably, nonverbal acknowledgment) increased robustly. Positive communication dropped slightly over the same interval in 22 families from the CM group. Moreover, increases in levels of positive nonverbal behavior among patients were correlated with their degree of symptomatic improvement over the year of treatment and follow-up. No differential treatment effects were found on EE or negative interactional behavior, however. Thus, FFT may exert its effects in part through increasing the buffering, protective effects of the family or marital environment rather than decreasing its risk properties.

The second randomized trial, conducted at the University of California, Los Angeles (UCLA; Goldstein, Rea, & Miklowitz, 1996; Rea et al., 2001), examined 53 patients, 28 of whom were assigned to FFT plus medication, and 25 to a comparison condition called individually focused patient treatment (IFPT) plus medication. In the latter treatment, patients met with a clinician for 30-minute individual therapy sessions administered with the same frequency as FFT sessions (21 sessions over 9 months). The treatment was problem-focused, supportive, and educational, and included a focus on symptom management, medication adherence, and coping with life stressors. The UCLA study also examined the generalizability of FFT beyond the home setting by providing all treatment within a University outpatient clinic. Finally, the UCLA sample was more ethnically diverse (40% were African American, Hispanic American, or Asian American) than the Colorado sample (16%).

A proportional hazards survival analysis by the Anderson–Gill method, which took into account "multiple failure events" (multiple relapses over time in the same patient), indicated that patients in FFT had fewer relapses during the full 2-year study interval than those in IFPT. In fact, patients in FFT were less likely to relapse in the posttreatment interval than those in IFPT, although both groups were equally likely to relapse during the active 9-month treatment. Likewise, patients who participated in FFT were less likely to be hospitalized over the 2-year treatment and follow-up interval than those in IFPT, although group differences were again limited to the posttreatment period. Finally, patients in family treatment were significantly less likely to be hospitalized when they did relapse than those in IFPT. Thus, FFT may have helped patients and relatives to avoid hospitalizations, perhaps through teaching them to recognize relapses early and obtain emergency medical treatment.

FFT appears to be an efficacious adjunct to pharmacotherapy for patients with bipolar disorder who begin in an acute period of illness. Data from the Colorado and UCLA studies, however, suggest that the effects of FFT are often delayed. In the Colorado study, the FFT and CM groups did not differ in the severity of depressive symptoms until the 9-month follow-up interview. Likewise, in the UCLA study, patients in FFT only showed an advantage during the posttreatment period. Possibly, the education and skills training central to the FFT approach must be "absorbed" before their effects relative to comparison interventions can be observed.

The remainder of this chapter outlines the clinical methods of FFT. The reader who wishes for more detailed descriptions of the modules and additional clinical case studies is referred to the published FFT manual (Miklowitz & Goldstein, 1997).

TECHNIQUES OF FAMILY-FOCUSED TREATMENT

Clinical Setting

FFT is generally administered within an outpatient clinic setting. Patients attend up to 21 sessions with their parents, spouse, or siblings, and are in concurrent pharmacotherapy with a psychiatrist or primary care provider who regularly communicates with the family clinician.

FFT clinicians are usually master's degree level or above. No particular theoretical orientation is required, although an awareness of the nature of family systems is usually essential (i.e., the mutual influence of one family member on another; that symptomatic behaviors can affect as well as be affected by the family or marital context). Clinicians must also be open to—and knowledgeable about—the psychobiological bases of the disorder.

Pretreatment Assessment of the Patient and Family

FFT begins with a thorough diagnostic assessment of the patient. Documenting the bipolar diagnosis is central to the decision to offer or not offer FFT, the content of which would be off the mark for a patient who is not truly bipolar. Diagnostic interviews often lead to surprising findings: Patients who have long believed they have bipolar disorder may not meet the DSM-IV criteria, or may have comorbid "border" conditions as well as bipolar disorder (e.g., borderline personality disorder, attention-deficit/hyperactivity disorder, eating disorders, or substance abuse/dependence disorders). The most popular standardized diagnostic interview is probably the Structured Clinical Interview for DSM-IV Axis I Disorders (First, Spitzer, Gibbon, & Williams, 1995). Often, family members offer critical information to aid the diagnostic evaluation.

Once the diagnosis is established, the clinician conducts a series of family assessments. Within the research setting, these assessments are usually formalized, and consist of the Camberwell Family Interview for assessing expressed emotion (Vaughn & Leff, 1976) and direct family interaction tasks designed to assess family affect and communication (Goldstein, Judd, Rodnick, Alkire, & Gould, 1968). Clinicians administering FFT in community settings can conduct assessments in a less formalized manner, through observation of communication processes within treatment sessions: Do family members allow each other to finish sentences? How often do they speak for each other or cut each other off? Do they acknowledge each others' viewpoints? Is communication clear and succinct? Do problems get adequately defined? Are potential solutions generated and evaluated? Do members engage in "negative escalation cycles" of criticism followed by countercriticism?

More generally, the clinician tries to determine whether the family is in crisis. Many couples or families are upset by the occurrence of a manic or depressive episode in one member, but some are able to resolve this crisis and go on living their lives once the patient has achieved a degree of clinical stability. For others, the manic or depressive episode is a highly disruptive event that can ultimately lead to the disintegration of the family. The Global Assessment of Relational Functioning, a 1–100 scale of family adjustment, can help place a given family on a continuum of health relevant to its organization, problem solving, and emotional climate (American Psychiatric Association, 1994; Dausch, Miklowitz, & Richards, 1996). The duration and intensity of FFT treatment can be adjusted to the level of impairment or distress of the family.

Psychoeducation

Once a baseline assessment is accomplished, clinicians begin seven or more weekly sessions of education about bipolar disorder. Psychoeducation enables the family or couple to develop a shared understanding of the illness. The topical outline of the psychoeducation module is presented in Table 8.1.

The module begins when the clinician asks the patient, after reviewing a symptom list, to describe his or her most recent manic or depressive episode. The clinician also asks family members to describe what they observed as the illness was developing; these observations may or may not match the patient's experiences. For example, the clinician says:

> One of the ways we want to help you is to look at the symptoms of bipolar disorder and show you how a diagnosis is made. We want to identify which of these symptoms you had so we can know what you went through during your episode, as well as when you were becoming ill. Some people find it easy to talk about their symptoms, and others find it hard—they feel embarrassed or ashamed, or sometimes they just can't remember. But let's give it a try. (Miklowitz & Goldstein, 1997, p. 101)

Note that the clinician attends to two issues here: the patient's and family members' intellectual understanding of the patient's illness and symptoms, and their affective reactions to it. Much of FFT combines information giving with exploration of the affect associated with receiving this information.

Clarifying the symptoms during the recent acute episode (as well as the more muted symptoms accompanying the recovery period) often brings to the surface the family's disagreements over the disorder. In some couples or families, relatives "overidentify" the patient with the disorder (attribute all or most of his or her behavior during the postepisode period to the illness), whereas others "underidentify" the patient with the disorder (claim that the patient's symptoms of manic illness are really due to his or her irritable or grandiose personality style, or that his or her depression is really just laziness or entitlement). Likewise, some patients overidentify themselves with the disorder ("I'm unable to ever work again") or underidentify with it ("What others are calling mania is really just who I am").

Consider the following interchange between Dwayne, age 35, and his wife Lynn, 33. Dwayne's recent manic episode had led to significant conflicts between himself and his two boys.

DWAYNE: Yeah, I get irritable with you and the kids, but that's the bipolar talking. I don't really have those feelings about you or Ben. No matter who got in my way, I would just run right over them.

TABLE 8.1. Issues in Psychoeducation

The symptoms and course of the disorder
- The signs and symptoms of bipolar disorder
- The development of the most recent episode
- The recent life events survey
- Discussing the hospitalization experience
- Variations in prognosis: The course of the disorder

The etiology of bipolar disorder
- The vulnerability–stress model
- The roles of stress and life events
- Genetic and biological predispositions
- Risk and protective factors

Intervening within the vulnerability–stress model
- Types of medication and what they do
- Psychosocial treatments
- How the family can help
- The self-management of the disorder
- The relapse drill

Note. From Miklowitz and Goldstein (1997). Copyright 1997 by The Guilford Press. Reprinted by permission.

LYNN: Well, knowing it's part of your illness doesn't necessarily make it any easier. You launch into those loud verbal tirades. . . . It's kind of like getting hit by a driver who you later find out had a vision problem or something. He shouldn't have been on the road in the first place. Why can't you try harder to keep it under control?

In this example, Dwayne identifies his irritability as a symptom of his disorder. Lynn, in contrast, sees purposefulness in his behavior and believes he could change it if he tried harder. Often, the tendency to see controllability in symptomatic behaviors underlies the expression of high-EE attitudes (Hooley, 1987). Nonetheless, Lynn may be correct that Dwayne could make a greater effort to control his affective reactions to their young son. Psychoeducation may help Lynn and Dwayne to determine which aspects of Dwayne's irritability are truly disorder-driven and which are reactions attributable to stress triggers within the family.

Discussing the Disorder's Etiology and Treatment

As the psychoeducation module progresses, participants are exposed to a vulnerability–stress model for understanding bipolar episodes. They are encouraged to recognize the interactive roles of socioenvironmental factors (recent life events, sudden family arguments, life transitions), genetic predisposition (as reflected in a family history of major affective disorder), risk factors (e.g., sudden changes in sleep–wake cycles, abrupt discontinuation of medications, family conflicts, alcohol and drug abuse) and protective factors (e.g., maintaining regular blood levels of mood-stabilizing medications, keeping the family environment low-key during the recovery period, engaging in regular psychosocial treatment sessions, keeping track of one's sleep and mood on a daily chart).

The importance of adherence to medication regimens is constantly emphasized. For some families, it is useful to review the specific biological vulnerabilities believed to be associated with the disorder. Patients and family members may see a greater justification for long-term maintenance medication if they understand that there are neurophysiological or neuroanatomical abnormalities that remain dormant but can become activated under conditions of stress.

The material on etiology comes alive for participants when they begin to discuss how each environmental risk or protective factor applies to them, and when they consider their family pedigree. The family history discussion takes the patient off of the hot seat, in that he or she is no longer relegated to the role of being the only "patient" in the family. Drew, a 25-year-old, was quite surprised to learn that his father, who presented as a very well-adjusted, somewhat emotionally restricted man, had had a psychotic depressive episode in college. Although describing this experience was difficult for his father, it helped Drew to feel less stigmatized.

The Relapse Prevention Drill

The discussion of symptoms and etiological mechanisms leads into the relapse prevention drill. Patients and relatives generate a list of prodromal symptoms that herald the development of new manic or depressive episodes (using the most recent episode as an example). They also list the environmental circumstances in which these symptoms are most likely to occur (e.g., in the context of significant family or work stress; during certain seasons of the year). Then, using a problem-solving format, participants generate ideas for how to intervene should one or more of these signs and its associated environmental context appear. For example, Robert, who had had several manic episodes, said that his prodromal symptoms included mild irritability, distrustfulness of others, and a subjective feeling of mental clarity. His girlfriend Jessie observed that he stood too close to people and talked too loud. They both agreed that these symptoms usually appeared when he had more stress at work. Their prevention plan included (1) Robert agreeing to call his physician when one or more prodromal symptoms appeared, or Jessie doing so if he would not; (2) as a couple, trying to reinstitute regular sleep–wake rhythms if their routines had been disrupted by his escalating symptoms; (3) Jessie encouraging Robert to get away from his immediate work stress; and (4) Jessie accompanying Robert to the hospital emergency room, if necessary. The relapse prevention drill is often best done as a verbal or even a written contract that families troubleshoot and revise from time to time.

Communication Enhancement Training

Once patients and relatives have a general understanding of the syndrome of bipolar disorder, they can move on to tasks that are more mutual in nature, notably, tasks that involve restructuring patterns of communication. Most families and especially couples coping with bipolar disorder are acutely aware of difficulties in communicating during the postepisode period. Communication training is perhaps the most direct method used in FFT to modify the EE attitudes of criticism and hostility, which are often reflected among relatives and patients in negative, back-and-forth verbal interchanges (Simoneau, Miklowitz, & Saleem, 1998).

Communication training generally occupies 7–10 sessions in months 3, 4, and 5 of the FFT contract. Clinicians begin with a rationale for this module:

A person can be at risk for another relapse of bipolar disorder if the home environment is tense and there is much conflict. In contrast, good communication and problem-solving ... can be among those "protective factors" against stress that we talked about before. ... We want to help you communicate in the most clear and the least stressful way possible, so that everyone's voice is heard and problems get solved. (Miklowitz & Goldstein, 1997, p. 191)

The participants are then acquainted with four skills: expressing positive feelings (acknowledging other members of the family even for seemingly minor positive behaviors), active listening (keeping eye contact, reflective paraphrasing, and asking clarifying questions), making positive requests for change in other family members' behaviors, and expressing negative feelings (Falloon, Boyd, & McGill, 1984; Liberman, Wallace, Falloon, & Vaughn, 1981). The format by which the clinician teaches these skills is through in-session role playing, the steps of which are outlined in Table 8.2.

Learning a communication skill is an iterative process, in which patients or relatives practice with each other and are coached by the family clinician until they have grasped it. Families sometimes resist this approach because it can feel phony, staged, or unnatural. As mentioned earlier, patients with bipolar disorder and their relatives are often accustomed to high voltage, unpredictable, affectively charged interchanges (Miklowitz & Goldstein, 1997). Yet the structure provided by role-playing exercises does much to decrease conflict within the family or couple and increase participants' sense of collaboration. The awkwardness in learning the skills is acknowledged by the clinician. He or she encourages the participants to practice the skills between sessions, until the skills feel more natural and begin to generalize to the home setting.

Problem-Solving Skills Training

The problem-solving module occupies the final four to five sessions of FFT. During this interval, sessions have been tapered to biweekly and, in the last 12 weeks, monthly. Participants are first familiarized with the problem-solving method (Falloon et al., 1984; Liberman et al., 1981), which involves defining specific problems, brainstorming solutions, evaluating the advantages and disadvantages of each potential solution, choosing solutions, and finally, developing an implementation plan.

Problem solving focuses on the specific areas of conflict that often arise during the postepisode phases of bipolar (notably, manic) illness, including medication nonadherence (or family disagreements about the use of medication), resumption of prior work and social roles, "life trashing" (repairing the damage done to friendships, finances, or

---

TABLE 8.2. Steps for Role Playing of Communication Skills

- Model the skill for the participants.
- Ask participants to turn their chairs toward one another.
- Ask the participants to role-play an interchange involving use of a skill.
- Elicit feedback from all family members.
- Model alternative ways of using the skill.
- Conduct new rehearsal of the skill with coaching.
- Offer praise for the participants' efforts.
- Give a homework assignment.

Note. Adapted from Miklowitz and Goldstein (1997). Copyright 1997 by The Guilford Press. Adapted by permission.

work opportunities during the acute episode), and relationship or living situation conflicts. Clinicians encourage the family to choose and try to solve specific problems within these larger topical areas, first within sessions and later, between sessions.

An example from a family of a bipolar adolescent illustrates this technique.

Nathan, an 18-year-old, was in a depressed phase following his hospitalization for a manic episode. The episode had interfered with his plan to graduate from high school and go to college in France. His mother, with whom he and his two younger brothers lived, became increasingly irritated that he seemed to be using his illness to justify inactivity, lack of direction, and laziness. She insisted that he find a job and move out. He argued that she was not recognizing the limitations imposed by his disorder and that he wasn't yet capable of being independent, although he also argued that he should be able to go out "partying" with his friends until late at night. These disagreements over the controllability of his symptoms led to considerable conflict in the household, to the point that his mother considered "shipping him back East to see if his father can handle it."

In problem solving, this mother–son pair was able to break down these larger conflicts over independence into a series of specific problems, which included the irregular hours Nathan kept, his lack of effort in seeking a job, their differing views on his disorder, and their troublesome communication. The result was two agreements: Nathan agreed to get himself up at a specific time (notably, on weekends) if his mother agreed not to enter his room before 10:00 A.M., and he agreed to obtain 10 hours of after-school paid work at a school-operated food court. Negotiating these agreements required considerable use of active listening by the two members of this family: Both had to validate each other's point of view before any specific agreements could be reached.

Families of bipolar patients often resist the problem-solving approach, arguing that it does not address the underlying issues of which the specific problems are reflections. At times, the clinician simply forges ahead with the belief that one or more successful attempts at solving circumscribed problems will give the family a sense of confidence in its ability to negotiate larger conflicts. At other times, he or she may agree that exploration of larger themes is appropriate. In the case of this family, exploring Nathan's anxiety over independence and the possibility of his illness getting worse led Nathan to acknowledge that he often solicited his mother's caregiving, while simultaneously reacting negatively to it. This discussion helped him realize that he needed to take more responsibility for his illness and its management, and to focus on short-term goals that would eventually take him toward greater independence. His mother also agreed that she needed to give him more room to make mistakes (a dilemma parents face even with the healthiest of teenagers).

Termination of FFT

The final phases of FFT involve reviewing the patient's and family's progress with reference to the previously listed goals of psychotherapy (e.g., Has the functioning of the family improved? Do the patient and family members recognize his or her vulnerability to future episodes? The need for maintenance medication?). Typically, the relapse prevention drill is reviewed and modified as appropriate. Referrals are made as necessary for ongoing psychosocial treatment, including individual therapy for the patient, additional couple or family therapy, or mutual support and informational groups, such as the National Alliance for the Mentally Ill (*www.nami.org*), the National Depressive and Manic–

Depressive Association (*www.ndmda.org*), or the Child and Adolescent Bipolar Foundation (*www.bpkids.org*).

FUTURE DIRECTIONS

Family-focused treatment has been shown to be effective for recently episodic bipolar patients in one open trial and two randomized trials conducted within laboratory settings. Future research should examine the applicability of this approach within community settings that treat ethnically and socioeconomically diverse patients, patients with comorbid alcohol/drug abuse or dependence disorders, or patients with medical problems. Studies should also examine the effectiveness of FFT as delivered by the clinicians that work within community settings, and within their usual time constraints. The Systematic Treatment Enhancement Program for Bipolar Disorder (Gray, Frankle, & Sachs, 2001; Sachs, 1998) examines the effectiveness of FFT and pharmacotherapy in a large, unselected sample of patients treated at numerous clinical centers around the country, as compared with various forms of individual psychotherapy and pharmacotherapy.

The applicability of FFT to early-onset and geriatric bipolar populations deserves examination. Adolescent bipolar patients, who are at especially high risk for a pernicious course of illness, psychosocial impairment, suicidality, and medical nonadherence, may be especially well-suited to this approach (Geller & Luby, 1997). A treatment development study of FFT for early-onset bipolar patients (NIMH Grant No. MH62555, David J. Miklowitz, principal investigator) is currently underway in a collaboration between the University of Colorado and the University of Pittsburgh School of Medicine. Finally, no psychosocial treatment studies have been undertaken with older bipolar patients, who are often difficult to diagnose, treatment refractory, at high suicide risk, and who require complex combinations of anticonvulsants, atypical antipsychotics, and other drugs (McDonald, 2000). Developing adjunctive psychosocial interventions for these frequently neglected patients is an important direction for future research.

ACKNOWLEDGMENTS

Preparation of this chapter was supported in part by National Institute of Mental Health Grant Nos. MH43931, MH55101, and MH62555, and by a Distinguished Investigator Award to David J. Miklowitz from the National Alliance for Research on Schizophrenia and Depression.

REFERENCES

Altshuler, L. L., Post, R. M., Leverich, G. S., Mikalauskas, K., Rosoff, A., & Ackerman, L. (1995). Antidepressant-induced mania and cycle acceleration: A controversy revisited. *American Journal of Psychiatry, 152,* 1130–1138.

American Psychiatric Association. (1994). *Diagnostic and statistical manual of mental disorders* (4th ed.). Washington, DC: Author.

Butzlaff, R. L., & Hooley, J. M. (1998). Expressed emotion and psychiatric relapse: A meta-analysis. *Archives of General Psychiatry, 55,* 547–552.

Calabrese, J. R., Bowden, C. L., & Sachs, G. S., Ascher, J. A., Monoaghan, E., & Rudd, G. D. (1999). A double-blind placebo-controlled study of lamotrigine monotherapy in outpatients with bipolar I depression: Lamictal 602 Study Group. *Journal of Clinical Psychiatry, 60,* 79–88.

Calabrese, J. R., Fatemi, S. H., Kujawa, M., & Woyshville, M. J. (1996). Predictors of response to mood stabilizers. *Journal of Clinical Psychopharmacology, 16*(Suppl. 1), 24–31.

Colom, F., Vieta, E., Martinez-Aran, A., Reinares, M., Benabarre, A., & Gasto, C. (2000). Clinical factors associated with treatment noncompliance in euthymic bipolar patients. *Journal of Clinical Psychiatry, 61,* 549–555.

Coryell, W., Scheftner, W., Keller, M., Endicott, J., Maser, J., & Klerman, G. L. (1993). The enduring psychosocial consequences of mania and depression. *American Journal of Psychiatry, 150,* 720–727.

Craighead, W. E., & Miklowitz, D. J. (2000). Psychosocial interventions for bipolar disorder. *Journal of Clinical Psychiatry, 61*(Suppl. 13), 58–64.

Dausch, B. M., Miklowitz, D. J., & Richards, J. A. (1996). A Scale for the Global Assessment of Relational Functioning, II: Reliability and validity in a sample of families of bipolar patients. *Family Process, 35,* 175–189.

Falloon, I. R. H., Boyd, J. L., & McGill, C. W. (1984). *Family care of schizophrenia: A problem-solving approach to the treatment of mental illness.* New York: Guilford Press.

First, M. B., Spitzer, R. L., Gibbon, M., & Williams, J. B. W. (1995). *Structured clinical interview for DSM-IV Axis I disorders.* New York: Biometrics Research Department, New York State Psychiatric Institute.

Gelenberg, A. J., Kane, J. N., Keller, M. B., Lavori, P., Rosenbaum, J. F., Cole, K., & Lavelle, J. (1989). Comparison of standard and low serum levels of lithium for maintenance treatment of bipolar disorders. *New England Journal of Medicine, 321,* 1489–1493.

Geller, B., & Luby, J. (1997). Child and adolescent bipolar disorder: A review of the past 10 years. *Journal of the American Academy of Child and Adolescent Psychiatry, 36,* 1168–1176.

Gitlin, M. J., Swendsen, J., Heller, T. L., & Hammen, C. (1995). Relapse and impairment in bipolar disorder. *American Journal of Psychiatry, 152*(11), 1635–1640.

Goldberg, J. F., Harrow, M., & Grossman, L. S. (1995). Course and outcome in bipolar affective disorder: A longitudinal follow-up study. *American Journal of Psychiatry, 152,* 379–385.

Goldstein, M. J., Judd, L. L., Rodnick, E. H., Alkire, A., & Gould, E. (1968). A method for studying social influence and coping patterns within families of disturbed adolescents. *Journal of Nervous and Mental Disease, 147,* 233–251.

Goldstein, M. J., Rea, M. M., & Miklowitz, D. J. (1996). Family factors related to the course and outcome of bipolar disorder. In C. Mundt, M. J. Goldstein, K. Hahlweg, & P. Fiedler (Eds.), *Interpersonal factors in the origin and course of affective disorders* (pp. 193–203). London: Gaskell.

Goodwin, F. K., & Jamison, K. R. (1990). *Manic–depressive illness.* New York: Oxford University Press.

Gray, S. M., Frankle, W. G., & Sachs, G. S. (2001). STEP-BD: A design for evaluating effectiveness of treatment for bipolar disorder. *Economics of Neuroscience, 3,* 65–68.

Hammen, C., Gitlin, M., & Altshuler, L. (2000). Predictors of work adjustment in bipolar I patients: A naturalistic longitudinal follow-up. *Journal of Consulting and Clinical Psychology, 68,* 220–225.

Harrow, M., Goldberg, J. F., Grossman, L. S., & Meltzer, H. Y. (1990). Outcome in manic disorders: A naturalistic follow-up study. *Archives of General Psychiatry, 47,* 665–671.

Honig, A., Hofman, A., Rozendaal, N., & Dingemanns, P. (1997). Psychoeducation in bipolar disorder: Effect on expressed emotion. *Psychiatry Research, 72,* 17–22.

Hooley, J. M. (1987). The nature and origins of expressed emotion. In K. Hahlweg & M. J. Goldstein (Eds.), *Understanding major mental disorder: The contribution of family interaction research* (pp. 176–194). New York: Family Process Press.

Huxley, N. A., Parikh, S. V., & Baldessarini, R. J. (2000). Effectiveness of psychosocial treatments in bipolar disorder: State of the evidence. *Harvard Review of Psychiatry, 8,* 126–140.

Johnson, S., & Miller, I. (1997). Negative life events and recovery from episodes of bipolar disorder. *Journal of Abnormal Psychology, 106,* 449–457.

Johnson, S. L., & Roberts, J. E. (1995). Life events and bipolar disorder: Implications from biological theories. *Psychological Bulletin*, 117, 434–449.

Johnson, S. L., Sandrow, D., Meyer, B., Winters, R., Miller, I., Solomon, D., & Keitner, G. (2000). Increases in manic symptoms following life events involving goal-attainment. *Journal of Abnormal Psychology*, 109, 721–727.

Keck, P. E., Jr., & McElroy, S. L. (1996). Outcome in the pharmacological treatment of bipolar disorder. *Journal of Clinical Psychopharmacology*, 16(Suppl. 1), 15–23.

Keck, P. E., Jr., McElroy, S. L., Strakowski, S. M., Bourne, M. L., & West, S. A. (1997). Compliance with maintenance treatment in bipolar disorder. *Psychopharmacology Bulletin*, 33, 87–91.

Keck, P. E., Jr., McElroy, S. L., Strakowski, S. M., Stanton, S. P., Kizer, D. L., Balistreri, T. M., Bennett, J. A., Tugrul, K. C., & West, S. A. (1996). Factors associated with pharmacologic noncompliance in patients with mania. *Journal of Clinical Psychiatry*, 57, 292–297.

Kessler, R. C., McGonagle, K. A., Zhao, S., Nelson, C. B., Hughes, M., & Eshleman, S., Wittchen, H. U., & Kendler, K. S. (1994). Lifetime and 12-month prevalence of DSM-III-R psychiatric disorders in the United States: Results from the National Comorbidity Survey. *Archives of General Psychiatry*, 51, 8–19.

Liberman, R. P., Wallace, C. J., Falloon, I. R. H., & Vaughn, C. E. (1981). Interpersonal problem-solving therapy for schizophrenics and their families. *Comprehensive Psychiatry*, 22, 627–629.

Malkoff-Schwartz, S., Frank, E., Anderson, B., Sherrill, J. T., Siegel, L., Patterson, D., & Kupfer, D. J. (1998). Stressful life events and social rhythm disruption in the onset of manic and depressive bipolar episodes: A preliminary investigation. *Archives of General Psychiatry*, 55, 702–707.

Manji, H. K. (2001). The neurobiology of bipolar disorder. *Economics of Neuroscience*, 3, 37–44.

McDonald, W. M. (2000). Epidemiology, etiology, and treatment of geriatric mania. *Journal of Clinical Psychiatry*, 61(Suppl. 13), 3–11.

McElroy, S. L., & Keck, P. E. (2000). Pharmacologic agents for the treatment of acute bipolar mania. *Biological Psychiatry*, 48, 539–557.

Miklowitz, D. J., & Craighead, W. E. (2001). Bipolar affective disorder: Does psychosocial treatment add to the efficacy of drug therapy? *Economics of Neuroscience*, 3, 58–64.

Miklowitz, D. J., & Goldstein, M. J. (1990). Behavioral family treatment for patients with bipolar affective disorder. *Behavior Modification*, 14, 457–489.

Miklowitz, D. J., & Goldstein, M. J. (1997). *Bipolar disorder: A family-focused treatment approach*. New York: Guilford Press.

Miklowitz, D. J., Goldstein, M. J., Nuechterlein, K. H., Snyder, K. S., & Mintz, J. (1988). Family factors and the course of bipolar affective disorder. *Archives of General Psychiatry*, 45, 225–231.

Miklowitz, D. J., Richards, J. A., George, E. L., Suddath, R., & Wendel, J. S. (2000). *Family-focused psychoeducation for bipolar disorder*. Paper presented at the 34th meeting of the Association for the Advancement of Behavior Therapy, New Orleans, LA.

Miklowitz, D. J., Simoneau, T. L., George, E. L., Richards, J. A., Kalbag, A., Sachs-Ericsson, N., & Suddath, R. (2000). Family-focused treatment of bipolar disorder: One-year effects of a psychoeducational program in conjunction with pharmacotherapy. *Biological Psychiatry*, 48, 582–592.

O'Connell, R. A., Mayo, J. A., Flatow, L., Cuthbertson, B., & O'Brien, B. E. (1991). Outcome of bipolar disorder on long-term treatment with lithium. *British Journal of Psychiatry*, 159, 132–129.

Post, R. M. (1992). Transduction of psychosocial stress into the neurobiology of recurrent affective disorder. *American Journal of Psychiatry*, 149, 999–1010.

Priebe, S., Wildgrube, C., & Muller-Oerlinghausen, B. (1989). Lithium prophylaxis and expressed emotion. *British Journal of Psychiatry*, 154, 396–399.

Rea, M. M., Tompson, M., Miklowitz, D. J., Goldstein, M. J., Hwang, S., & Mintz, J. (2001). *Family-focused treatment vs. individual treatment for bipolar disorder: Results of a randomized clinical trial*. Manuscript submitted for publication.

Regier, D. A., Farmer, M. E., Rae, D. S., Locke, B. Z., Keith, S. J., Judd, L. L., & Goodwin, F. K. (1990). Comorbidity of mental disorders with alcohol and other drug abuse: Results from the Epidemiologic Catchment Area (ECA) Study. *Journal of the American Medical Association, 264*, 2511–2518.

Sachs, G. (1998). *Treatments for bipolar disorder*. Unpublished grant proposal (NIMH Contract No. N01MH80001).

Sapolsky, R. M. (2000). The possibility of neurotoxicity in the hippocampus in major depression: A primer on neuron death. *Biological Psychiatry, 48*, 755–765.

Simoneau, T. L., Miklowitz, D. J., Richards, J. A., Saleem, R., & George, E. L. (1999). Bipolar disorder and family communication: Effects of a psychoeducational treatment program. *Journal of Abnormal Psychology, 108*, 588–597.

Simoneau, T. L., Miklowitz, D. J., & Saleem, R. (1998). Expressed emotion and interactional patterns in the families of bipolar patients. *Journal of Abnormal Psychology, 107*, 497–507.

Strakowski, S. M., DelBello, M. P., Fleck, D. E., & Arndt, S. (2000). The impact of substance abuse on the course of bipolar disorder. *Biological Psychiatry, 48*, 477–485.

Strakowski, S. M., Keck, P. E., McElroy, S. L., West, S. A., Sax, K. W., Hawkins, J. M., Kmetz, G. F., Upadhyaya, V. H., Turgul, K. C., & Bourne, M. L. (1998). Twelve-month outcome after a first hospitalization for affective psychosis. *Archives of General Psychiatry, 55*, 49–55.

Strober, M., Morrell, W., Lampert, C., & Burroughs, J. (1990). Relapse following discontinuation of lithium maintenance therapy in adolescents with bipolar I illness: A naturalistic study. *American Journal of Psychiatry, 147*, 457–461.

Suppes, T., Baldessarini, R. J., Faedda, G. L., Tondo, L., & Tohen, M. (1993, September–October). Discontinuation of maintenance treatment in bipolar disorder: Risks and implications. *Harvard Review of Psychiatry, 1*, 131–144.

Thase, M. E., & Sachs, G. S. (2000). Bipolar depression: Pharmacotherapy and related therapeutic strategies. *Biological Psychiatry, 48*, 558–572.

Tohen, M., Waternaux, C. M., & Tsuang, M. T. (1990). Outcome in mania: A 4-year prospective follow-up of 75 patients utilizing survival analysis. *Archives of General Psychiatry, 47*, 1106–1111.

Vaughn, C. E., & Leff, J. P. (1976). The influence of family and social factors on the course of psychiatric illness: A comparison of schizophrenia and depressed neurotic patients. *British Journal of Psychiatry, 129*, 125–137.

9

Treatment of Marital Discord and Coexisting Depression

K. DANIEL O'LEARY

In the 1970s and 1980s, marriage was considered to be a risk factor for depression, especially in women (Bernard, 1972; Hafner, 1986). In fact, Bernard argued that men are bullish on marriage because it serves them well, but that it has a negative impact on women. However, recent studies have contradictory findings: Married men and women actually have a lower risk for the incidence and recurrence of major depression compared to divorced, single, or separated men and women (e.g., Amenson & Lewinson, 1981; Anthony & Petronis, 1991; Aseltine & Kessler, 1993; Coryell, Endicott, & Keller, 1991). Studies of subclinical depression have demonstrated that married men and women also report lower levels of depressive symptoms as measured by interviews and questionnaires than do separated or divorced men and women (Amenson & Lewinsohn, 1981; Anthony & Petronis, 1991). Taken together, these findings have prompted researchers to investigate the link between marriage and depression more thoroughly, since it does not seem that marriage, in and of itself, is a predictor of depression. Beach, Sandeen, and O'Leary (1990) suggested that poor marital quality, and not simply marriage itself, seems to be the key risk factor in increased depressive symptomatology.

Our model of treating marital discord and coexisting depression is based on the assumption that marital discord can cause clinical depression (Beach et al., 1990). The model is based on the further assumption that alleviating marital discord reduces depression. We do not believe that the marital discord–depression link is unidirectional. In fact, we have published data showing that, under some circumstances, namely, the presence of chronic dysphoria, marital discord may develop (Beach & O'Leary, 1993). However, we believe that in many circumstances, marital discord leads to clinical depression, and I present data in this chapter to support this belief. Moreover, if a client believes that his or her depression is caused by marital discord, then treating the depression itself, without addressing the marital discord, will not be clinically effective in the long run (O'Leary, Riso, & Beach, 1990); that is, the client's attributions about the cause of his or her depression should be taken into account when deciding on a treatment plan.

It is possible that a certain type of marital discord leads to clinical depression, whereas other types do not. For example, I have seen enough cases to lead me to believe that discovery of an affair, learning that one's spouse is leaving, and severe and/or unexpected physical aggression often lead to clinical depression in women. For men, a wife's physical aggression appears to be much less devastating than discovery of an affair or learning that she is leaving. These types of marital problems, which usually have a sudden onset, may have a much greater impact on depressive symptoms than long-standing general marital strife emanating from communication problems, lack of affection and caring, and differences over child rearing. Whatever specific stressors cause or significantly contribute to marital problems, I review the literature on the marital discord–depression link to provide the reader with a sense of the magnitude of this problem.

In reviewing the association between marital discord and depression, studies are separated according to the type of design used. Specifically, in discussing the association of marital discord and depressive *symptoms*, studies are divided into four types: (1) Correlational, (2) retrospective, (3) longitudinal, and (4) immediate impact. In discussing the association of marital discord and a diagnosis of *major depression*, a clinical entity, studies are divided into two types: (1) relative risk studies and (2) immediate impact studies. For a more detailed discussion on the association of marital discord and depression, see O'Leary and Cano (2001). Because this chapter is about treatment of depression and coexisting marital discord, I selectively review studies on marital discord and depression simply to provide a rationale for our treatment strategy.

MARITAL DISCORD AND DEPRESSIVE SYMPTOMS

Correlational Studies

Three community-based studies have shown that marital discord is positively correlated with depressive symptomatology. Renne's (1970) data from a study of 5,163 individuals in the Berkely Longitudinal Research Project provided us (O'Leary, Christian, & Mendell, 1994) with data to calculate the correlation of marital discord and depressive symptomatology. Weiss and Aved (1978) and Beach, Arias, and O'Leary (1987) used smaller samples of married couples (Beach et al., $n = 131$; Weiss & Aved, $n = 104$). In these three studies, the correlations of marital discord and depressive symptomatology ranged from .35 to .40 for wives and from .32 to .47 for husbands.

Whiffen and Gotlib (1989) used a questionnaire to assess a sample of husbands and wives attending a prenatal medical clinic. The couples comprised four categories: (1) both partners reporting marital distress, (2) the wife reporting marital distress, (3) the husband reporting marital distress, and (4) neither spouse reporting marital distress. Whiffen and Gotlib found that men and women reporting marital distress experienced significantly more depressive symptoms than those who did not report marital distress. Additionally, men's martial discord predicted women's depressive symptoms (i.e., men's marital discord was associated with both their own and their wives' depressive symptoms). However, wives' marital discord was associated only with their own depressive symptomatology.

O'Leary and colleagues (1994), in a community sample of 328 married couples, found that men *and* women in discordant marriages were approximately 10 times more likely to report depressive symptomatology than were men and women in satisfactory marriages. These results were not simply a result of spousal depression: The odds of an individual in a discordant marriage experiencing depressive symptomatology were significant even when the researchers held constant both the level of the spouse's depressive symptomatology and marital discord.

The relationship between marital discord and depression has also been assessed in clinical samples. In a sample of 139 couples seeking marital therapy, Christian, O'Leary, and Vivian (1994) assessed the link between depressive symptoms and marital discord. In this group, mean Beck Depression Inventory (BDI) scores were 14.40 for women and 9.64 for men. Christian and colleagues found that 39% of the wives and 24% of the husbands scored above the cutoff of 14 (designed to separate individuals with no significant level of depression from those with a significant level of depression). When examining moderate depression, as indicated by a BDI score above the cutoff of 19, 22% of wives and 9% of husbands scored in the moderately depressed range (Beck, Steer, & Garbin, 1988). Women reported significantly more depressive symptoms than men, as evidenced by the BDI scores of each group. Additionally, women reported more marital discord than men. Despite these significant gender differences in both level of depressive symptomatology and reported marital discord, the two variables were positively correlated for both genders. Christian and colleagues' (1994) results provide further support for the assertion that depression and marital discord are associated in both males and females.

Longitudinal Studies

Using a community sample of 241 couples assessed at 6 and 18 months after marriage, Beach and O'Leary (1993) addressed the role of marital discord both cross-sectionally and prospectively. As predicted, there was a significant increase in the concurrent correspondence between marital discord and depressive symptomatology from premarriage to 18 months for both men and women. The correlation increased from approximately .35 to approximately .50 for both genders. In addition, the investigators found that marital discord was predictive of later depressive symptomatology for both men and women.

Fincham, Beach, Harold, and Osborne (1997), examining the longitudinal link between depressive symptoms and marital satisfaction, assessed 116 couples from the community on two occasions, 18 months apart. Depressive symptoms and marital satisfaction were significantly related when examined both cross-sectionally and longitudinally. Fincham and colleagues also evaluated causal models of the relationship and found opposite relationships for men and women; that is, as expected, based on past research, marital discord was a predictor of depressive symptoms in women but not men. However, depressive symptoms were a predictor of marital discord for men. This was one of the first longitudinal studies to investigate gender differences in the association between marital discord and depression. In an interpretation of their results, Fincham and colleagues suggest that, as a result of depression, men may act in ways destructive to their marital relationships more than women. With the longitudinal methodology, the unidirectional and bidirectional influences of marital discord and depression were explicated. Further research of this type should continue to examine the reason for gender differences in the marital discord–depression link. Such research is necessary; replication of the Fincham results would point to a need for different types of marital interventions for depressed men and women.

Some studies have found that depressive symptoms may lead to marital stress and discord. Davila and colleagues (Davila, Bradbury, Cohan, & Tochluk, 1997; Davila, Hammen, Burge, Paley, & Daley, 1995) conducted two longitudinal studies and found that depressive symptoms generated relationship stress in both dating and married women.

Beach and O'Leary (1993), in another longitudinal study of 264 young married women, found that women diagnosed with dysthymia were more likely to have discordant marriages than women without such a diagnosis. Wives with dysthymia experienced a 23-point average decline in their scores on a measure of marital satisfaction during the first 18 months of marriage, whereas wives without dysthymia experienced a decline of only 4 points.

Some studies, however, question the association between depressive symptoms and marital discord. Burns, Sayers, and Moras (1994), using structural equation modeling to examine the causal link between these two variables, assessed 115 patients undergoing cognitive-behavioral treatment for various types of mood disorders, including major depressive disorder, dysthymic disorder, adjustment disorder with depressed mood, and depressed with comorbid anxiety disorders. Patients in the study were either married or in a relationship with a significant other. Through structural equation modeling, Burns and colleagues attempted to account for reciprocal associations between marital discord and depression, which they suggested may have inflated previous estimates of the association. In this study, patients completed questionnaires assessing depressive symptoms and relationship discord at a pretreatment screening. Burns and colleagues found a weak causal association when depressive symptoms and relationship discord were assessed at the 12-week follow-up. However, depressive symptoms were not found to cause relationship discord. Based on these results, they concluded that the link between relationship discord and depression had been overestimated in previous studies due to methodological variance; that is, studies not using methods such as structural equation modeling may fail to account for the reciprocal link between relationship discord and depression, and thus overestimate their association. The research of Burns and colleagues is an important addition to the literature due to its critical examination of the association between marital discord and depression with different statistical techniques and populations. However, one very important difference exists between this study and other previous studies: Burns and colleagues used a population of individuals who had mood disorders, whereas other studies have been conducted with community-based samples or samples seeking marital therapy. Research regarding the association of marital problems and depressive symptomatology in a sample of patients with mood disorders would be quite useful.

In summary, many studies show a significant association between depressive symptoms and marital discord. Studies from the 1970s conducted without standardized measures of marital discord or depression showed a significant relationship between the two variables (for a review of these early correlational studies, see O'Leary et al., 1994). A significant, albeit moderate, correlation ($r = .35$) between depressive symptoms and marital discord consistently demonstrated in those early studies. In addition, this relationship existed for both genders. Relatively few studies have examined the relationship between chronic, milder forms of depression, such as dysthymia, and marital discord. However, results of these studies indicate that dysthymia is associated with marital discord both cross-sectionally and longitudinally.

Whisman (2001) conducted a meta-analysis of the association between depressive symptoms and marital dissatisfaction. Data were analyzed separately for both genders in order to facilitate the evaluation of gender differences in the marital discord–depression link. The results of this meta-analysis further confirmed the relationship between marital discord and depression discussed earlier; that is, depressive symptoms and marital quality were inversely related. Across the 26 studies included in the meta-analysis, the correlation between depressive symptoms and marital satisfaction was $-.42$ for women and $-.37$ for men. Correlations were significant for both genders. Furthermore, the difference in the magnitude of the correlations between women and men was significant, with the association between depressive symptoms and marital dissatisfaction being greater for women.

Retrospective Studies

Finlay-Jones and Brown (1981) investigated the role of "loss events" on the development of depression and found that a depressive episode was significantly associated with a severe loss, such as death of a loved one, unemployment, and separation from a loved one 3 months prior to the depressive episode. Sixty-five percent of women diagnosed with depression experienced at least one severe loss prior to the onset of depression.

Expanding the research on the context of negative events in marriage and close relationships, Brown, Harris, and Hepworth (1995) identified "humiliation" and "entrapment" events. A humiliation event devalues the individual in relation to the self or others (e.g., discovery of an affair, verbal or physical attacks by anyone; separation or divorce initiated by the partner). Entrapment refers to ongoing difficult events that have existed for at least 6 months and make leaving a relationship difficult (e.g., a child with lifelong illness, a paralyzed husband). Both humiliation and entrapment events, as opposed to danger and loss, were most associated with depression in women. Unfortunately, there is little research in the United States regarding the distinction between types of marital events that are and are not associated with the development of depressive symptomatology and clinical depression. Furthermore, there is almost no research regarding the personality types or coping styles of women who do and do not become depressed in the face of negative events in marriage (Christian, 1993).

MARITAL DISCORD AND MAJOR DEPRESSION

Relative Risk Studies

In a now classic study, Weissman (1987) showed that marital problems increase risk of being depressed approximately 25-fold. Despite the fact that this study did not use a standard measure of either marital satisfaction or discord, the findings represented an important acknowledgment of the risk for clinical depression given some level of marital problems. Women who reported that they "did not get along" with their spouse had a 6-month prevalence rate of 45.5%; those who reported that they "did get along" with their spouse, however, had only a 2.9% prevalence of major depression at 6 months. In men reporting that they did not get along with their spouse, the 6-month prevalence rate of major depression was 14.9%; in men who did get along with their spouse, the rate was only 0.6%. Despite the gender differences in overall prevalence rates, the odds ratios (ORs) for men and women were quite similar (women: OR = 28.1; men: OR = 25.8).

Whisman and Bruce (1999) used similar methodology to assess marital problems and the incidence of a major depressive episode (MDE) across a 1-year period. They utilized a sample of 904 individuals from the New Haven Epidemiologic Catchment Area Program, who did not meet criteria for an MDE at baseline. In accordance with their predictions, Whisman and Bruce found that participants reporting marital problems at the initial assessment were more likely to have experienced an MDE at 1-year follow-up than were participants not initially reporting marital problems. Incidence rates of MDE were 5.3% for the former group and only 2.1% for the latter group. Data on depressed individuals could not be analyzed separately by gender due to the small number in the sample who became depressed ($n = 26$), so ORs could not be compared with the findings of Weissman (1987). In their sample, Whisman and Bruce (1999) did not exclude individuals who had previously experienced MDEs. Therefore, there is the possibility that marital distress at the initial assessment may have been a consequence of the history of major depression. To assess this possibility, Whisman and Bruce controlled for history of major depression and found that participants reporting marital distress were still more likely to develop MDEs than participants who reported no marital distress.

Immediate Impact Studies (Depression Shortly after Negative Marital Events)

Christian-Herman, O'Leary, and Avery-Leaf (2001) examined women reporting a major negative marital event within the past month, such as an affair, a threat of separation or divorce, or an incident of physical abuse. Only women who had never been depressed were included in the sample. Following the occurrence of the major marital stressor, 38% of the women became clinically depressed. Moreover, the results of the path analysis demonstrated a significant association between marital discord and later depressive symptomatology. In contrast, the path analyses did not demonstrate an association of depressive symptoms with later marital discord.

In a related study, Cano and O'Leary (2000) assessed women who had recently experienced a highly negative martial event (as in the Christian-Herman et al. study described earlier). They compared these women to a control group of women who had not experienced a negative event in their marriage. Unlike the study just described, Cano and O'Leary did not exclude women previously diagnosed with depression. They found that 72% of the women who had experienced a highly negative marital stressor became clinically depressed within 1 month after the event, whereas only 12% of the controls became depressed.

In short, the two related studies assessing women shortly after experiencing a major marital stressor show convincingly that highly negative events in marriage can lead directly to clinical depression. Both studies were with women; we do not know about the impact of such stressors on men. On the one hand, I have seen enough cases in which the wife is seeking a divorce to know that many men experience clinical depression when their wives leave them. On the other hand, I am not aware of enough studies of men's responses to significant marital stressors to have any clear sense of the strength of the impact that such marital stressors have on men.

TREATMENT OF COEXISTING MARITAL DISCORD AND MAJOR DEPRESSIVE DISORDER

Recent research advances have been instrumental in solidifying the conceptual foundation for martial therapy as an intervention for depression. More specifically, widespread recognition of the robust relationship between marital discord and depression, acknowledgment of the bidirectional nature of the relationship, and the realization that marital discord may interact with personal vulnerabilities and result in both increased depressive symptomatology and exacerbation of interpersonal difficulties have all been crucial in solidifying this foundation (Beach, 2001).

In our own work with couples for over 20 years, my associates and I have screened out the couples we believed would not profit from dyadic therapy. Our criteria included

(1) drug and/or alcohol abuse and (2) the presence of an ongoing affair. In both cases, such factors would likely interfere with the progress of marital therapy.

More recently, we have also begun screening out couples with significant psychological and physical aggression. In some facilities, all couples are screened out if there has been any physical aggression by the male partner against the female partner in the last year. This selection criterion seems far too exclusive to me, since there is considerable evidence that physical aggression exists in approximately 30–40% of young community couples (O'Leary, 1999a). In addition, about half of couples presenting for marital problems report some level of physical aggression in their relationship (O'Leary, in press). The key issue for which we have almost no data at present is the extent to which physical and/or psychological aggression interferes with marital therapy specifically focused on reducing such aggression. My own clinical experience leads me to believe that high levels of psychological aggression by either partner are much more detrimental to improvement in marital therapy than low levels of physical aggression (e.g., pushing or slapping by one or both partners). Consequently, in individual sessions with each partner, I assess the potential for such psychological aggression by asking how often arguments occur and how heated they become. If I believe that one or both partners will not be able to contain their anger in a conjoint session, I suggest that they receive individual therapy to address such issues before beginning marital therapy.

The frequency and intensity of physical aggression must also be addressed. Our practice has been to exclude not only couples whose aggression has led to physical injury requiring medical attention but also couples in which the wife does not feel that she will be able to speak openly and freely in a conjoint session. It should be noted, however, that we have a highly specific dyadic therapy designed to reduce psychological and physical aggression (O'Leary, Heyman, & Neidig, 1999). While I believe that exclusion of all couples with any physical aggression is too restrictive, I believe that we should exclude couples (1) if there have been more than three instances of physical aggression in the past year, (2) if the psychological aggression appears intense, (3) if there have been any injuries requiring medical attention resulting from acts of physical aggression, and (4) if the wife indicates that she feel uncomfortable talking about her problems in a conjoint context.

When a couple presents with both depression and marital discord, Beach has (2001) argued that the clinician must first assess how likely the depressed individual is to benefit from this type of intervention. He highlighted three issues to be addressed before beginning marital therapy for depression: (1) the salience of the marital problems; (2) the perceived etiology of the marital problems, and (3) suicidal ideation.

Beach argued that when considering the salience of the marital problems, one first needs to ascertain their relative salience compared to other problems in the depressed individual's life. If the marital problems are significant and a cause of distress to the individual, then marital therapy for depression should certainly be considered. If marital problems exist but other issues appear to be leading to the depression, such as job loss or coping with illness of a relative, then marital therapy would probably be ill-advised.

Second, it is beneficial to assess the depressed individual's understanding of his or her difficulties in life and to ascertain how he or she sees the marital problems relative to these other difficulties. More specifically, it is important to assess whether the client sees his or her marital problems as causes of the depression. In a study regarding prediction of response to treatment, O'Leary and colleagues (1990) asked patients which problem came first, depression or marital discord. They found that women who reported that marital problems preceded their depression had worse marital outcomes in a cognitive therapy intervention condition than did women reporting the same sequence of problems who were assigned to marital therapy. More specifically, the marital problems did not improve in cognitive therapy. In contrast, women in marital therapy improved their marital satisfaction. Accordingly, we suggested that marital therapy should be a high priority for depressed individuals who indicate that their marital problems preceded their current level of depressive symptomatology.

Third, if the depressed individual is suicidal, marital therapy may not be appropriate. Many clinically depressed individuals have some level of suicidal ideation; thus, it is important that the therapist assess for the frequency of current suicidal ideation, whether there is a plan for the suicidal ideation, and whether it appears likely that the individual would act on the ideation. If there is persistent and active suicidal ideation, individual therapy is advised (O'Leary, Sandeen, & Beach, 1987), since conduct of therapy is difficult when the client is experiencing significant suicidal ideation.

A fourth issue when one addresses an issue of depression and marital discord is the degree of commitment to the marriage. If commitment to the marriage is low (i.e., 50% or less on a scale from 1 to 100), we have found that one partner may have already decided to leave the marriage and/or has a "significant other." When the commitment is as low as 50%, it is wise to consider carefully the amount of verbalized caring and love in the relationship. If caring and love are quite low, we are cautious in proceeding to marital therapy.

TREATMENT STRATEGIES TO ENHANCE THERAPEUTIC EFFECTIVENESS

Several issues should be addressed when tailoring marital therapy for a couple in which one or both partners are depressed, including assessment of anger and psychological abuse, the impact of the depression on marital interactions, hope/hopelessness, the need for support from the nondepressed partner, and the need for positive marital interactions. It has been recommended that the therapist meet with each partner individually for at least one session to assess these areas thoroughly relative to each partner. Then the therapist can meet with the couple together (and individually, as needed).

Let us now consider each of these issues and how they can be addressed in the therapy itself. To minimize the adverse impact of anger and psychological abuse in therapy, ground rules are useful. More specifically, the therapist can alert clients that if the anger and psychological abuse erupts frequently and intensely, he or she may cease providing marital therapy and suggest individual therapy as an alternative. In addition, I have found it useful to tell the clients that if they feel they are likely to explode at their partners at home, they should call me anytime of the day for a phone session. This admonition is designed to indicate how important it is that therapy progress not be set back by highly angry outbursts.

In considering the role of depression in marital functioning, it seems appropriate to discuss how a major depressive episode can affect the marriage; that is, it is wise to tell the nondepressed partner about the effects of depression on marital interactions. In general, one can describe the symptoms of a major depressive episode and note how those symptoms can impact on a relationship. For example, I discuss the fact that sexual desire in depressed individuals is often low. I note that some of the negativity in the relationship may be due to depression itself, and that concentration is often low when one is depressed. I discuss these symptoms and their likely impact on the relationship so that the nondepressed individual can attribute some of the difficulties in the relationship to the depression itself—instead of simply thinking that the partner lacks sexual interest and is hostile.

Generating hope for improvement is important in any kind of therapy, but generation of such hope is of even greater importance when treating a depressed client in a troubled marriage. The therapist can describe the kinds of clinically significant gains one generally obtains in marital satisfaction (average increases in 1 standard deviation in marital satisfaction) and the reductions that one can expect in depressive symptomatology (average decreases of 15–18 points in depressive symptomatology [BDI]). Both types of changes are of sufficient magnitude to allow a therapist to realistically convey hope about the kinds of changes one can expect in marital therapy when one of the partners is depressed. The generation of hope fits particularly well with the data seen on changes in depressive symptomatology that occur in the first five to six sessions of treatment for depression, whether that change is observed in marital or cognitive therapy for depression. The role of a therapist in providing hope for the client has been discussed in the therapy literature for decades (e.g., Franks, 1973), and the need to provide such hope is not any less today. Hopelessness may generate stress and prompt a negative perception of the hopeless individual. In turn, the negative perception may produce critical communications from others to the hopeless individual (Joiner, 2001). Finally, such critical communications can predict depression and its reoccurrence (Hooley & Teasdale, 1989).

PHASES OF THERAPY FOR MARITAL PROBLEMS AND COEXISTING DEPRESSION

Behavioral marital therapy for depression tends to be of relatively short duration and quite problem-focused. In our own work, we have a series of three intervention phases. The first phase of therapy involves an intense focus on stressors in the relationship and a concomitant effort to reestablish positive activities in the relationship. The second phase of therapy is a bit broader in focus, examining the spouses' communication, problem-solving abilities, and quality of day-to-day interactions. In the third and final phase of therapy, the therapist helps the couple prepare for termination and helps to identify situations that are likely to trigger relapse of depression or an increase in marital discord (Beach et al., 1990). It is not my purpose in this chapter to provide a session-by-session guide or therapeutic cookbook. The interested reader can consult Beach and colleagues (1990) for such a session-by-session guide for 15 sessions of martial therapy with couples that have a depressed partner.

Several interventions are herein noted to provide a flavor for the ways in which a therapist may help clients bring about change in the initial phases of therapy to accomplish the following goals: (1) increase marital cohesion, (2) increase self-esteem support, and (3) reduce or eliminate severe, recurrent marital stressors. The strategies used to increase marital cohesion were drawn from the pool of support–understanding strategies described by Weiss (1978) over two decades ago. Those strategies include increasing companionship activities, caring gestures, caring days, sexual interactions, and individual activities. The therapist must use his or her best judgment, since the amount of caring and/or hostility between the partners often dictates whether he or she suggests these activities. If the level of hostility is high due to a past affair, a degrading insult of the partner, or past physical abuse, the therapist can help the clients find their own level of interactions with which they feel most comfortable. As I have stated, especially when first getting to know a couple, the therapist should make no assumptions about their abilities to carry out "simple" assignments (Beach et al., 1990). In this regard, when encouraging companionship activities, it is wise for the therapist to assign responsibilities for various aspects of a task to one or the other partner, since "joint responsibility" frequently translates into "no one's responsibility."

Relatedly, sexual interactions may not be desired by one or both parties early in a therapy. Such activities may have to follow days or weeks of positive interactions, as exemplified by helping the partner with household activities and other caring gestures. The purpose of suggestions that reflect caring is to initiate a warmer emotional climate, to increase the likelihood of both parties desiring sexual interactions.

Strategies used to increase self-esteem support include encouraging verbalizations that communicate appreciation or acknowledgment of the other person's good qualities. Such positive communication has long been a hallmark of behavioral marital therapy (Jacobson & Margolin, 1979). Because this kind of positive communication should not be dependent upon the other person's behavior, it is less likely to fail than more complicated interactions, such as problem solving. To obtain a sense of the ease with which the clients can implement positive communication, it is useful to ask each partner to compliment or verbalize appreciation to the other in the session. If they have difficulty doing so, they can be asked to compliment each other for the kinds of things they used to appreciate in one another. In turn, the therapist can use this appreciation diagnostically to learn what each partner may be able to do now to enable the other to feel positive about him or her.

The elimination of major stressors in the relationship is a crucial step in the initial phase of therapy. Before healing of the relationship can proceed, it is necessary to help the clients cease highly destructive patterns of interaction. Indeed, negative behavior has been shown to be more highly associated with marital satisfaction than positive behavior (see, e.g., Broderick & O'Leary, 1986), and more recent studies regarding psychological aggression also show the direct effect of such negativity on marital satisfaction and physical aggression (O'Leary, 1999b). In this vein, we ask that the partners reduce explicitly denigrating spousal references, severe criticisms, and blame. We also tell the couple that in a longitudinal study, blame of partner has been shown to predict a decrease in marital satisfaction (Fincham & Bradbury, 1993), and emphasize that partner blame in or out of the session can be very detrimental.

We ask partners not to threaten divorce, especially in anger. Instead, we ask that they hold their feelings about separation and divorce in abeyance until they have given marital therapy a reasonable try. Usually, we request that they agree to participate in marital therapy for 4 months, although clients and therapists often may be able to get a sense about whether any progress is likely within the 6 weeks.

TREATMENT MANUALS AND THERAPY PLANNERS

Beach and colleagues (1990) provide a treatment manual with guides for 15 sessions of marital therapy. Like any manual, this is basically a guide for the therapist treating a couple with a depressed partner. I later present evidence to document the effectiveness of this therapeutic approach, and a case illustration at the end of this chapter to provide a more clinical sense of how I have proceeded in treating cases of coexisting marital discord and depression.

The interested reader can also consult O'Leary, Heyman, and Jongsma's *The Cou-*

ples Psychotherapy Treatment Planner (1998), which provides behavioral definitions of the presenting problems, long- and short-term goals, and therapeutic interventions tied to long- and short-term objectives. Furthermore, there are diagnostic suggestions regarding Axis I and II disorders and an electronic add-on upgrade module to *Therascribe 3.0 for Windows: The Computerized Assistant to Treatment Planning*. Most relevant to this chapter on treatment of coexisting marital discord and depression is the chapter, "Depression Due to Relationship Problems." (There is also a chapter called "Depression Independent of Relationship Problems"). In the former are 39 therapeutic interventions described in concrete ways. For example, "Have each partner describe whether and why he/she believes the depression was caused by problems in the relationship" or "Have each partner complete an assessment of love/caring for the other partner" (p. 75).

A third approach is contained in *Brief Therapy for Couples* by Halford (2001), where the essential strategy is to help partners help themselves. There is also a strong emphasis on brief therapy. Whereas depression is not a focus of this book at all, an interested reader can obtain an important sense of how some therapists have been able to get the clients themselves to take responsibility for changing many things. In this self-regulation approach, a dyadic formulation is still often the rubric for therapy, but it is followed by each partner, self-selecting behavior changes for him- or herself. For a depressed individual in a discordant relationship, such an emphasis could be useful, just as in individual cognitive-behavioral therapy for depression (O'Leary & Beach, 1990). As Halford stresses, "I believe that commitment to self-change is necessary to achieve relationship improvement in distressed couples" (p. 48). I happen to share this belief.

In my opinion, many clients can get along quite well with others outside the marriage; they do not need communication "training." Overall, what may be most crucial is that the therapist help to motivate individuals to want to improve themselves and, in turn, their relationship. Halford uses an approach that emphasizes individual change, albeit in a dyadic context. A useful research endeavor would be to assess different strategies early in the therapy process for motivating clients to want to change. Marital therapy, like many other therapies, is most likely to be effective if change is made early in treatment. Comparing emphases on (1) self-change, (2) relationship/dyadic change, and (3) insight into relationship etiology would be quite informative and such research could potentially have quite practical results.

OUTCOME STUDIES

In order to evaluate the efficacy of different treatment modalities for depression, O'Leary and Beach (1990) compared behavioral marital therapy (BMT) to cognitive therapy (CT) (Beck, Rush, Shaw, & Emery, 1979). Participants in the study included couples randomly assigned to individual CT, individual CT with conjoint BMT, or a wait-list condition. Both BMT and CT effectively reduced depressive symptomatology, as evidenced by significantly lower BDI (Beck et al., 1988) scores in the two treatment groups than in the wait-list group. The two treatment conditions did not differ significantly in reduction of depressive symptomatology.

When marital satisfaction was compared across the three groups, as predicted, the BMT group was found to have higher marital satisfaction scores than the other two groups at the end of therapy. The CT and wait-list groups did not differ significantly on marital satisfaction. These couples were reassessed 1 year after the end of treatment. The BMT group continued to have significantly higher marital satisfaction scores than the

CT group at 1-year follow-up. However, BDI scores of the BMT and CT groups continued not to differ significantly at follow-up. Of interest to the clinician facing a decision about whether marital therapy can be effective regardless of the level of depressive symptomatology, there was not a significant association of initial and posttreatment BDI scores.

In a similar study, Jacobson, Dobson, Fruzzetti, Schmaling, and Salusky (1991) randomly assigned 60 married couples to BMT, CT, or a combined treatment condition. All wives in the study were diagnosed with major depression, but couples were both maritally distressed and maritally nondistressed. Where there was no marital distress, individual CT was superior to BMT in treating depression. However, in maritally distressed couples, CT and BMT were equally effective in treating depression. The combined treatment was not more effective than either CT or BMT, regardless of the initial level of marital distress. Overall, this study, and a related study by Beach and O'Leary (1992), showed that BMT alleviates depression by enhancing the marital environment, whereas CT for depression works through a cognitive change process.

ANTIDEPRESSANT MEDICATION AS A CONCURRENT TREATMENT

When a couple presents for marital therapy and one of the partners is clinically depressed, the question naturally arises about concurrent medication use for depression, anxiety, and/or mood regulation. If the depression has been severe and recurrent, antidepressant medication is well-advised (Thase et al., 1997). Relatedly, if the depressed partner is suicidal, antidepressant medication is also in order (O'Leary et al., 1987). Leff and colleagues (2000) compared antidepressant medication to couple therapy in 77 depressed individuals. The primary antidepressant medication consisted of desipramine, with trazadone and fluvoxamine used as backup medications. Couple therapy consisted of 12–20 sessions as needed to "help the patient and partner gain new perspectives on the presenting problems, to attach different meanings to the depressive types of behavior and to experiment with new ways of relating to each other" (Leff et al., 2000, p. 96). The medication group had a dropout rate three times higher than the couple therapy group. Both groups improved significantly in depressive symptomatology, but the couple therapy group made significantly greater gains than the medication group. At a 2-year follow-up, the advantage of the couple treatment over medication remained significant in terms of reduction in depressive symptomatology. Unfortunately, information was not presented on the changes in relationship distress.

As noted earlier, a case is presented to describe concretely how one can proceed with a couple and to illustrate certain kinds of problems one encounters in treating couples in which one partner is depressed.

CASE EXAMPLE OF TREATING A DEPRESSED WOMAN WITH COEXISTING MARITAL DISCORD

Pamela, a 52-year-old woman, is a nurse. Her husband Larry is a teacher. Pamela has been depressed periodically for the 3 years since she discovered that her husband had a close relationship with another woman named Lisa. While the relationship did not involve sexual intercourse, it did involve some physical intimacy, though Pamela did not know the specific extent of the intimacy. Marital therapy initially involved a detailed assessment of the marital history with the husband and wife separately and included an agreement on the husband's part not to see his female friend at all.

This marriage was quite positive in many ways. The couple had two children, one in high school and one in college. Both were doing well academically, and both were athletes in high school. The husband, however, felt that his wife was quite controlling; Larry said that he sensed the control from the day they got engaged. In fact, he felt pressured to get engaged. Pamela, on the other hand, said that Larry basically did what he wanted to do all his life. A popular teacher who was asked to chaperone school events, he coached football each fall (which meant that he did not get home for dinner until after Pamela and the children had eaten). In terms of the family of origin, Pamela was raised by her mother; her father left her mother for another woman when Pamela was 6 years old. Larry was raised by his mother and father, but he rarely saw his father except on Sundays.

Intervention

Initially, the focus of the intervention was on describing the role of depression and anxiety in this relationship, and its impact on the marital relationship. Pamela's depression clearly resulted from her discovery of Larry's relationship with Lisa, and both Pamela and Larry agreed on the etiology of Pamela's depression and periodic bouts of anxiety. Thus, there was a need to consult with each of them separately to address issues discussed in this chapter: assessment of anger and psychological abuse, hope/hopelessness, the need for support from the nondepressed partner, and the need for positive marital interactions. I discussed the likelihood of Pamela's periodic angry outbursts in detail with Larry, as well as his need to predict their occurrence and to be patient when confronted with Pamela's anger. Hope was generated by having Pamela and Larry focus on the positive qualities of the relationship, especially the good relationship they each had with the children, and their mutual enjoyment of them. The mutual friends they shared and did not wish to lose also generated hope. Finally, the commitment that they each had to the other was a factor that gave them both hope. In some individual sessions, I prompted Larry to do positive things for Pamela that she would like, such as buying her a CD or book, commenting about her physical attractiveness to him, or saying how he respected her opinion on many issues. In turn, as Pamela became comfortable with joint activities such as going to dinner and the movies, I encouraged them to engage in such activities.

Problems Along the Way

Pamela's anger outbursts and jealousy made progress difficult. As much as Larry tried to assure her that the relationship with his female friend was over, Pamela had thoughts of Larry calling, sending e-mails, and meeting his female friend in public places such as shopping malls. Relatedly, thoughts of Pamela's father leaving her mother intruded. In fact, Pamela's jealousy pushed Larry away from her, and he himself had bouts of anger toward her. He threatened to leave the marriage. Larry's patience, and an antidepressant medication, seemed to facilitate change. In addition, Pamela's determination to control her own feelings, as well as some specific steps to occupy her attention with nonproblem, issues were important factors in facilitating change. Such steps included brisk walks, taking a speciality course in pediatric nursing, having lunch twice a month with a friend, and decorating the house.

ACKNOWLEDGMENTS

Support during the writing of this chapter came from NIMH Grant No. MH5798502.

REFERENCES

Amenson, C. S., & Lewinsohn, P. M. (1981). An investigation into the observed sex difference in prevalence of unipolar depression. *Journal of Abnormal Psychology, 90,* 1–13.

Anthony, J., & Petronis, K. R. (1991). Suspected risk factors for depression among adults 18–44 years old. *Epidemiology, 2,* 123–132.

Aseltine, R. H., & Kessler, R. C. (1993). Marital disruption and depression in a community sample. *Journal of Health and Social Behavior, 34,* 237–251.

Beach, S. R. H. (2001). Marital therapy for co-occurring marital discord and depression. In S. R. H. Beach (Ed.), *Marital and family processes in depression: A scientific foundation for clinical practice* (pp. 205–224). Washington, DC: American Psychological Association.

Beach, S. R. H., & O'Leary, K. D. (1992). Treating depression in the context of marital discord: Outcome and predictors of response for marital therapy vs. cognitive therapy. *Behavior Therapy, 23,* 507–528.

Beach, S. R. H., & O'Leary, K. D. (1993). Marital discord and dysphoria: For whom does the marital relationship predict depressive symptomatology? *Journal of Social and Personal Relationships, 10,* 405–420.

Beach, S. R. H., Arias, I., & O'Leary, K. D. (1987). The relationship of marital satisfaction and social support to depressive symptomatology. *Journal of Psychopathology and Behavioral Assessment, 8,* 305–316.

Beach, S. R. H., Sandeen, E. E., & O'Leary, K. D. (1990). *Depression in marriage: A model for etiology and treatment.* New York: Guilford Press.

Beck, A. T., Rush, A. J., Shaw, B. F., & Emery, G. (1979). *Cognitive therapy of depression.* New York: Guilford Press.

Beck, A. T., Steer, R. A., & Garbin, M. G. (1988). Psychometric properties of the Beck Depression Inventory: Twenty-five years of evaluation. *Clinical Psychology Review, 8,* 77–100.

Bernard, J. (1972). *The future of marriage.* New York: World.

Broderick, J. E., & O'Leary, K. D. (1986). Contributions of affect, attitudes, and behavior to marital satisfaction. *Journal of Consulting and Clinical Psychology, 54,* 514–517.

Burns, D. D., Sayers, S. L., & Moras, K. (1994). Intimate relationships and depression: Is there a causal connection? *Journal of Consulting and Clinical Psychology, 62,* 1033–1043.

Cano, A., & O'Leary, K. D. (2000). Infidelity and separations precipitate major depressive episodes and symptoms of nonspecific depression and anxiety. *Journal of Consulting and Clinical Psychology, 68,* 774–781.

Christian, J. L. (1993). *The impact of negative events in marriage on depression.* Unpublished doctoral dissertation, State University of New York at Stony Brook, Stony Brook, NY.

Christian, J. L., O'Leary, K. D., & Vivian, D. (1994). Depressive symptomatology in maritally discordant women and men: The role of individual and relationship variables. *Journal of Family Psychology, 8,* 32–42.

Christian-Herman, J. L., O'Leary, K. D., & Avery-Leaf, S. (2001). The impact of negative events in marriage on depression. *Journal of Social and Clinical Psychology, 20,* 25–41.

Coryell, W., Endicott, J., & Keller, M. (1991). Major depression in a nonclinical sample: Demographic and clinical risk factors for first onset. *Archives of General Psychiatry, 49,* 117–125.

Davila, J., Bradbury, T. N., Cohan, C. L., & Tochluk, S. (1997). Marital functioning and depressive symptoms: Evidence for a stress generation model. *Journal of Personality and Social Psychology, 73,* 849–861.

Davila, J., Hammen, C., Burge, D., Paley, B., & Daley, S. E. (1995). Poor interpersonal-problem solving as a mechanism of stress generation in depression among adolescent women. *Journal of Abnormal Psychology, 104,* 592–600.

Fincham, F. D., Beach, S. R. H., Harold, G. T., & Osborne, L. N. (1997). Marital satisfaction and depression: Different causal relationships for men and women? *Psychological Science, 8,* 351–357.

Fincham, F. D., & Bradbury, T. N. (1993). Marital satisfaction, depression, and attributions: A longitudinal analysis. *Journal of Personality and Social Psychology, 64,* 442–452.

Finlay-Jones, R., & Brown, G. W. (1981). Types of stressful life events and the onset of anxiety and depressive disorders. *Psychological Medicine, 11,* 803–815.

Franks, J. (1973). *Persuasion and healing: A comparative study of psychotherapy* (Rev. ed.). Baltimore: Johns Hopkins University Press.

Hafner, R. J. (1986). *Marriage and mental illness: A sex-roles perspective.* New York: Guilford Press.

Halford, W. K. (2001). *Brief therapy for couples: Helping partners help themselves.* New York: Guilford Press.

Hooley, J., & Teasdale, J. D. (1989). Predictors of relapse in unipolar depressives: Expressed emotion, marital distress, and perceived criticism. *Journal of Abnormal Psychology, 98,* 229–235.

Jacobson, N. S., Dobson, K., Fruzzetti, A. E., Schmaling, D. B., & Salusky, S. (1991). Marital therapy as a treatment for depression. *Journal of Consulting and Clinical Psychology, 59,* 547–557.

Jacobson, N. S., & Margolin, G. (1979). *Marital therapy: Strategies based on social learning and behavior exchange principles.* New York: Brunner/Mazel.

Joiner, T. E. (2001). Nodes of consilience between interpersonal–psychological theories of depression. In S. R. H. Beach (Ed.), *Marital and family processes in depression* (pp. 129–138). Washington, DC: American Psychological Association.

Leff, J., Vearnals, S., Brewin, C. R., Wolff, G., Alexander, B., Asen, E., Dayson, D., Jones, E., Chisholm, D., & Everitt, B. (2000). The London Depression Intervention Trial: Randomized controlled trial of antidepressants v couple therapy in the treatment and maintenance of people with depression living with a partner: Clinical outcome and costs. *British Journal of Psychiatry, 177,* 95–100.

O'Leary, K. D. (1999a). Developmental and affective issues in assessing and treating partner aggression. *Clinical Psychology: Science and Practice, 6,* 400–414.

O'Leary, K. D. (1999b). Psychological abuse: A variable deserving critical attention in domestic violence. *Violence and Victims, 14,* 3–23.

O'Leary, K. D. (in press). Conjoint therapy for partners who engage in physically abusive behavior. *Journal of Aggression, Maltreatment, and Trauma.*

O'Leary, K. D., & Beach, S. R. H. (1990). Marital therapy: A viable treatment for depression and marital discord. *American Journal of Psychiatry, 147,* 183–186.

O'Leary, K. D., & Cano, A. (2001). Marital discord and partner abuse: Correlates and causes of depression. In S. R. H. Beach (Ed.), *Marital and family processes in depression* (pp. 163–182). Washington, DC: American Psychological Association.

O'Leary, K. D., Christian, J. L., & Mendell, N. R. (1994). A closer look at the link between marital discord and depressive symptomatology. *Journal of Social and Clinical Psychology, 13,* 33–41.

O'Leary, K. D., Heyman, R. E., & Neidig, P. H. (1999). Treatment of wife abuse: A comparison of gender specific and conjoint approaches. *Behavior Therapy, 30,* 475–505.

O'Leary, K. D., Heyman, R. E., & Jongsma, A. E., Jr. (1998). *The couples psychotherapy treatment planner.* New York: Wiley.

O'Leary, K. D., Riso, L. P., & Beach, S. R. H. (1990). Attributions about the marital discord/depression link and therapy outcome. *Behavior Therapy, 21,* 413–422.

O'Leary, K. D., Sandeen, E. E., & Beach, S. R. H. (1987, November). *Treatment of suicidal, maritally discordant clients by marital therapy or cognitive therapy.* Paper presented at the 21st Annual Meeting of the Association for the Advancement of Behavior Therapy, Boston, MA.

Renne, K. S. (1970). Correlates of dissatisfaction in marriage. *Journal of Marriage and the Family, 32,* 54–67.

Thase, M. E., Greenhouse, J. B., Frank, E., Reynolds, C. F., Pilkonis, P., Hurley, K., Grochonoski, V., & Kupfer, D. J. (1997). Treatment of major depression with psychotherapy or psychotherapy–pharmacotherapy combinations. *Archives of General Psychiatry, 54,* 1009–1015.

Weiss, R. L. (1978). The conceptualization of marriage from a behavioral perspective. In T. Paolino, Jr. & B. McCrady (Eds.), *Marriage and marital therapy: Psychoanalytic, behavioral, and systems theory perspectives* (pp. 165–297). New York: Brunner/Mazel.

Weiss, R. L., & Aved, B. M. (1978). Marital satisfaction and depression as predictors of physical health status. *Journal of Consulting and Clinical Psychology, 46,* 1379–1384.

Weissman, M. M. (1987). Advances in psychiatric epidemiology: Rates and risk for major depression. *American Journal of Public Health, 77,* 445–451.

Whiffen, V. E., & Gotlib, I. H. (1989). Stress and coping in maritally distressed and nondistressed couples. *Journal of Social and Personal Relationships, 6,* 327–344.

Whisman, M. A. (2001). The association between depression and marital dissatisfaction. In S. R. H. Beach (Ed.), *Marital and family processes in depression: A scientific foundation for clinical practice* (pp. 3–24). Washington, DC: American Psychological Association.

Whisman, M. A., & Bruce, M. L. (1999). Marital distress and incidence of major depressive episode in a community sample. *Journal of Abnormal Psychology, 108,* 674–678.

10

Treatment of Suicidality

A Family Intervention for Adolescent Suicide Attempters

MARY JANE ROTHERAM-BORUS
ALISON M. GOLDSTEIN
AMY S. ELKAVICH

Adolescent suicide and attempted suicide are significant public health problems, with almost 2 million adolescents attempting to kill themselves annually and 700,000 requiring medical treatment (Centers for Disease Control, 1998; U.S. Bureau of the Census, 1996). These rates reflect a tripling in the rate of completed suicide in the last 50 years, making adolescent suicide attempters the most common psychiatric emergency in their age group (Holinger, 1990). About half who once attempt suicide repeat their attempt (Shaffer & Piacentini, 1994), 10% within 3 months (Spirito et al., 1992). Attempted suicide is then a significant risk factor for completed suicide (Andrews & Lewinsohn, 1992; Groholt, Ekeberg, Wichstrom, & Haldorsen, 1997; Martunen, Hillevi, Henriksson, & Lonnqvist, 1992). In addition to dying prematurely, adolescent attempters are at increased risk of substance abuse, delinquency, school dropout, and mental health disorders (Spirito, Jelalian, Rasile, Rohrbeck, & Vinnick, 2000). For example, 40–50% of suicidal youth are clinically depressed (Andrews & Lewinsohn, 1992; Kovacs, Goldston, & Gastonis, 1993; Piacentini, Rotheram-Borus, Gillis, et al., 1995); suicidal youth are also likely to have disruptive behavior disorders and to abuse alcohol and drugs more frequently than nonsuicidal youth (Andrews & Lewinsohn, 1992). Adolescents who attempt suicide tend to retain their psychiatric problems, with both occupational and social ramifications into adulthood (Berman & Jobes, 1994). Considering the high level of problem behaviors and related risk associated with adolescent suicidality, it is vital that these young suicide attempters receive intervention immediately following their suicide attempt.

Many youth do not receive any mental health intervention, and few adhere to the recommendations of their physicians to attend outpatient treatment (Spirito et al., 2000).

Among those youth who do attend treatment, the recommended interventions are typically aimed at reducing depression and improving mood, presuming that suicide emerges from a depressive disorder (Pfeffer et al., 1994). There is a high correlation between depression and suicidal behavior in adults (Klimes-Dougan, 1998; Merikangas, Wicki, & Angst, 1994). However, a number of studies of adolescent suicide attempters suggest that only about half of the attempters are currently depressed (DeMaso, Ross, & Beardslee, 1994; Metha, Chen, Mulvenon, & Dode, 1998; Piacentini, Rotheram-Borus, & Cantwell, 1995; Summerville, Kaslow, Abbate, & Cronan, 1994; Trautman, Rotheram-Borus, Dopkins, & Lewin, 1991). Treatments focusing on an affective disorder may only work for a subgroup of suicidal adolescents. In addition, those most in need of services are least likely to respond to treatment (Bickman, 1996; Pfeffer et al., 1994). For example, youth with the most serious psychiatric problems may receive intensive mental health services delivered consistently over many years, yet their mental health symptoms may not remit (Bickman, 1996). Therefore, treating suicide attempters is a major challenge. Treatments are needed that specifically focus on suicidality and are planned to improve treatment adherence as a first step in the interventions.

Successful Negotiation/Acting Positively (SNAP) therapy is a brief and highly structured, short-term family treatment program for suicidal adolescents delivered in outpatient settings (Rotheram-Borus et al., 1996, 1999). A six-session outpatient intervention designed on the basis of cognitive-behavioral theory, it focuses on adolescents and their parents regarding the anticipation, identification, and coping strategies for family members of youth with suicidal feelings. SNAP therapy allows maximization of the family's involvement in and adherence to treatment (Rotheram-Borus et al., 1999). Concentrating on troublesome situations rather than focusing on difficult individuals within the family system meets this goal, creating a more positive atmosphere for the family, both in therapy and at home. Some of the tools used to achieve an effective model for family problem solving and increasing coping skills within the family are behavioral contracting, cognitive restructuring, therapist modeling, structured role playing, and reframing. Structured activities are used not only to create unique cognitive and social competencies but also to break down barriers to change within the family fueled by misconceptions, negative attitudes, and misinformation.

The goal of this chapter is to review SNAP, a treatment program for suicidal youth. However, prior to implementing the SNAP program, we review the emergency room (ER) treatment of youth, issues that must be addressed with youth's families, and how to identify youth in imminent danger of suicide (in contrast to a general risk factor that may be carried throughout a lifespan). Unless these issues are addressed, it is unlikely that youth will attend any treatment sessions that allow for intervention. Once the setting for treatment has been addressed, the theoretical foundations and format of each of the six sessions of SNAP treatment are described.

EMERGENCY ROOM TREATMENT OF SUICIDE ATTEMPTERS

When interviewed in the ER following a suicide attempt, both the family and the adolescent often report that it was a "big mistake," and that the adolescent had no intention of suicide; the youth was simply upset and it will not reoccur (Piacentini, Rotheram-Borus, & Cantwell, 1995). Adolescent suicide attempts are typically not medically serious or life threatening, leading many internists and psychiatrists to agree with the family's perceptions that the attempt was not a serious health threat. Less than 50% of adolescent suicide attempters in the ER are referred for follow-up treatment, and of those, only half who do receive referrals attend even one session (Piacentini, Rotheram-Borus, Gillis, et al., 1995; Spirito, Brown, Overholser, & Fritz, 1989). Research also shows that those who do attend are rarely compliant with the treatment procedure (up to 77%; Piacentini, Rotheram-Borus, & Cantwell, 1995; Taylor & Stansfield, 1984; Trautman, Stewart, & Morishima, 1993). After a suicide attempt, even one therapeutic contact can prove helpful in reducing the risk for future attempts, as well as positively affect the mental state of the adolescent attempter (Shaffer & Piacentini, 1994). Though these treatment adherence rates may be similar to those of other pediatric disorders (La Greca, 1990; Litt & Cuskey, 1980), attempters, their families, and clinicians treating these families need to recognize the importance of referral and adherence to outpatient therapy.

The ER experience has a direct impact on the follow-up treatment of the attempter (Rotheram-Borus et al., 1999; Shaffer, Garland, Gould, Fisher, & Trautman, 1988). Oftentimes, the ER requires tedious paperwork, long waiting periods, and family members being repeatedly asked for the same information by staff in different roles within the ER (receptionists, internists, psychiatrists, nurses, residents, trainees). Families develop or are reinforced for negative attitudes toward the ER, the hospital, and the entire follow-up treatment process (Haynes, 1979; Hazzard, Hutchinson, & Krawiecki, 1990). Although not all aspects of ER care can be improved (e.g., waiting periods), the way the provider interacts with attempters and their families can be more effective.

Implementing brief interventions with staff can improve treatment adherence (Rotheram-Borus, Piacentini, et al., 1996; Rotheram-Borus, Walker, & Ferns, 1996). A specialized ER program was designed to support the suicide attempter, the attempter's relatives, and staff throughout the intervention process (Rotheram-Borus et al., 1999). The follow-up treatment adherence of the adolescent suicide attempter is influenced by a number of things: (1) the family's expectations of both treatment and the referral process, (2) the establishment of a positive rapport with the attempter, (3) the expectations of therapy for the family as well as the attempter, (4) perceptions of the medical setting, and (5) the provision of a timely and specific referral. To address each of these issues, the recommended ER outpatient program in conjunction with SNAP focuses on three major components: staff training, providing a videotape orientation on treatment, and conducting a family therapy session in the ER.

Staff Training

The ER provides an opportunity for providers both to establish the family's expectations about outpatient treatment and to define the suicide attempt in a way that does not induce guilt and blame. Families often expect quick and drastic improvements through treatment (Hirschfeld et al., 1997), whereas providers anticipate improvement occurring over an extensive period of time (Trautman et al., 1993). Furthermore, patients may develop a negative outlook of the treatment programs recommended to suicide attempters and their families if the ER experience is inefficient and unpleasant (Shaffer et al., 1988). Therefore, the first component of the specialized ER program is staff training.

At least six professional groups are typically involved in ER care of adolescent suicide attempters: receptionists, physicians, security guards, residents, child psychiatry fellows, and nurses. Each professional has a different role in relation to the suicide attempter and his or her family and receives training commensurate to that role. However, it is important to note that all specialized training must be brief or it will not be implemented. Staff changes are common in the ER, and it is typical to expect that training will have to be provided twice annually for each of three shifts (i.e., nighttime, daytime, swing shift). A training manual is available for a 2-hour training program for each staff subgroup (Miller, Rotheram-Borus, Piacentini, & Graae, 1992). The content for each of the professional groups is as follows:

1. *ER physicians* are trained to acknowledge cultural differences and identify language barriers to increase the rate of return for follow-up treatment (i.e., encouraging family therapy). Some physicians wanted to induce fear and make the ER experience aversive in order to increase fear among the family. However, the physician is encouraged to alleviate confusion, anxiety, and fears of the parents who may blame themselves for their child's attempt.

2. *Residents* inform the family of ER suicide procedure, dispel any confusion or disorientation, and clarify any misconceptions concerning the ER (i.e., the ER is concerned with the long-term health of your child, not just the immediate medical situation). Reinforcing positive behavior in the family members, as well as the suicidal youth, improves self-esteem while easing the anxiety of discussing personal family matters with strangers (i.e., thanking the family members for sharing how they feel, clearly defining the importance of involving the entire family in the follow-up process).

3. *ER child psychiatric fellows* discuss the possible reasons for the suicide attempt with family members and concentrate on identifying negative thought processes (i.e., "This is all my fault and I just want to die") and how to change them into positive influences in the future (i.e., "Things are tough right now, but I'll get through it with help and want to live my life"). Negative thought processes may occur in the entire family. Both the suicidal adolescent and the family members are taught to reevaluate their modes of thinking in the six-session intervention.

4. *Nursing staff* must also stress treatment adherence while dealing with the attempter in less than desirable circumstances (i.e., induce vomiting by having the youth drink charcoal to deter future attempts). Nurses function daily in the hectic environment of the ER and are able to use that training to create a sense of privacy and safety for both the attempter and his or her family by clearly describing the steps involved in the treatment and care of a suicide attempter to alleviate any fears or distrust in the ER procedure.

5. *Security personnel* are trained to keep the ER environment free of trash and debris, and are also made aware of potential interaction of a questionable nature with the attempter. Since youth suicide attempters are three to nine times more likely to be female, guards must be prepared to deal with confrontations of a potentially sexual nature (i.e., flirting) while remaining on guard and protecting the attempter's well-being.

6. *Receptionists* set the tone of interaction with the family (i.e., is the ER a caring environment or a large bureaucracy?). Because all ER care is typically long, boring, and repetitive, we developed "care packages" consisting of a comb, a magazine, and a candy bar to assist the family to alleviate boredom.

The specialized ER program helps staff members to identify their own fears in relating to suicidal youth and their families. The ER intervention manual acknowledges the stressful work environment and then guides staff members through the tasks they must accomplish to treat the suicidal patient successfully. "Self-talk" examples are outlined in the manual to aid the staff when the suicidal youth becomes aggressive or emotional (i.e., Nurse: "I won't let him or her provoke me; stay cool, stay focused"). ER staff adherence to the specialized procedures is essential in creating effective lines of communication with the suicidal youth and their families, as well as easing any fears the family may have regarding treatment and hospitals in general (Deykin, Hsieh, Joshi, & McNamara, 1986; Rogawski & Edmundson, 1971; Rotheram-Borus et al., 2000; Welu, 1977). In addition to staff training, the ER program includes two other components: showing (1) a soap opera videotape to the attempter and his or her family to set expectations regarding therapy and the consequences of suicide attempts, and (2) a therapy session.

Setting Expectations: A Soap Opera Videotape

Families frequently ignore didactic instructions by clinicians: Information that many attempters reattempt suicide and that death could occur often induces guilt and leads to avoidance. A rational argument alone does not have the same potency as information presented to motivate clients toward action (Fisher et al., 1993). After piloting a variety of strategies to deliver information about what occurs in therapy and the consequences of adolescent suicidal acts, a soap opera video format was developed. Soap operas are the most popular television programs for many ethnic groups, particularly Latinos (Schilling, Duan, & Rotheram-Borus, 2001). The video was filmed in an ER and presents a vignette of two adolescent attempters: a young man who has made a second suicide attempt and dies as a result of it, and a young woman who has made her first attempt. The video follows the treatment of the young woman as her family interacts with the internist and the psychiatrist, indicating the parameters of treatment within the context of the attempter's ER experience: the number of sessions, the length of each session, who should attend, the types of intervention activities, and the outcomes of therapy. In every ER interaction, each professional is encouraged to support the family and to identify the strengths of the family's coping abilities. In the context of a caring and supportive environment, the problems in the family are more likely to emerge.

Family Session in the ER

Most adolescents are dependent on their parents for both financial and emotional support. Therefore, the treatment process for a suicidal youth is likely to be more effective if the attempter's family is involved in the treatment. How the family copes as a unit has proven to be the main factor in distinguishing adolescent suicide attempters from non-attempters (Asarnow, 1992: Asarnow, Carlson, & Guthrie, 1987; Shaffer, 1974). For example, a depressed mother is at greater risk for having a suicidal child; therefore, treating the mother's depression may ultimately reduce the child's risk (Klimes-Dougan, 1998). Additionally, if the mother has a positive attitude toward therapy, she is much more likely to insist that her child adhere to and attend therapy sessions; the parent's participation in treatment with a suicidal adolescent has increased the success of the treatment (Piacentini, 1994). Finally, family conflict is a common precipitant of adolescents' suicidal behavior; therefore, the family's involvement in the treatment of the suicidal youth and their dedication to decrease conflict within the family will greatly influence the success or failure of the treatment (Rotheram-Borus & Trautman, 1988). In addition, to ensure that there is supervision for the youth, most adolescents will not be released from the ER until the parent or guardian arrives. Because parents are required to come to the ER, there is an opportunity for intervention. The opportunity may be lost at an outpatient therapy session; parents are not required to attend the session.

Given the potential influence of parents, our specialized program includes a family therapy session delivered in the ER, which is based on principles of building a family's motivation to attend therapy and providing a framework to understand their child's suicidality. The therapist has four assigned tasks to accomplish in the session: (1) Identify positive feelings among family members; (2) teach family members a tool for labeling and assessing their affective states; (3) distinguish imminent danger of suicide from risk for suicidal acts; and (4) make a family plan about how to cope if the youth feels suicidal again.

Positive Family Feelings

While in the ER, families must cope with conflicting feelings: confusion regarding ER procedures, guilt over the suicide attempt, anger at the attempter, and frustration with the ER experience (Rotheram-Borus, Piacentini, et al., 1996). Concurrently, suicidal youth often report feeling "numb" and are unable to identify their affective states. In order to enhance motivation for the family to participate in therapy, the therapist attempts to remind family members of their strong caring for each other. He or she begins the session not by asking the family about the problems it is experiencing, but about the last time that the youth felt love for the parents. The youth and parents are each asked to identify the last time that they shared a positive experience together. Remembering positive feelings and good times works in sharp contrast to the feeling of wanting to kill oneself. By focusing on the caring, both youth and parents are motivated to change the situation that led to the suicide attempt. Neither parents nor youth are blamed for the attempt; not having the skills to cope with suicidal feelings and events is framed as the precipitant of the event.

The Feeling Thermometer

Adolescent attempters and their family members are often unable to recognize and, consequently, to regulate, intense emotional states such as anger, depression, and hopelessness. Many adolescent attempters have trouble recognizing the correlation between the event that triggered their suicidal attempt, their feelings and thoughts regarding the event, and their ultimate decision to attempt suicide. Youth commonly describe a feeling of numbness, followed by an overwhelming sense of panic directly before they attempt suicide. The ability to report their affective states is a key skill that the SNAP therapy program attempts to improve. The "Feeling Thermometer" is a tool used by the therapist to help the family members establish a vocabulary to convey their feelings to each other and to the therapist. A vocabulary for feelings is most important for monitoring the status of the suicide attempter's suicidal feelings.

The Feeling Thermometer is a self-rating scale ranging from 0 to 100. One hundred represents the most uncomfortable (i.e., frustrated, anxious, scared, and sad) feeling state possible, and 0 represents the most positive, comfortable state possible. The Feeling Thermometer is utilized so that attempters and their families are able to discern different levels of emotionality specifically surrounding suicide. A sample Feeling Thermometer is presented in Figure 10.1.

Once youth are able to identify elevations in their level of emotional arousal, they can take the needed steps to cope with these changes and, we hope, distinguish signs of the possible onset of a suicidal crisis. By using the Feeling Thermometer, family members are able to express their feelings to each other before these emotions interfere with effective problem solving or lead to negative and potentially painful situations. After the

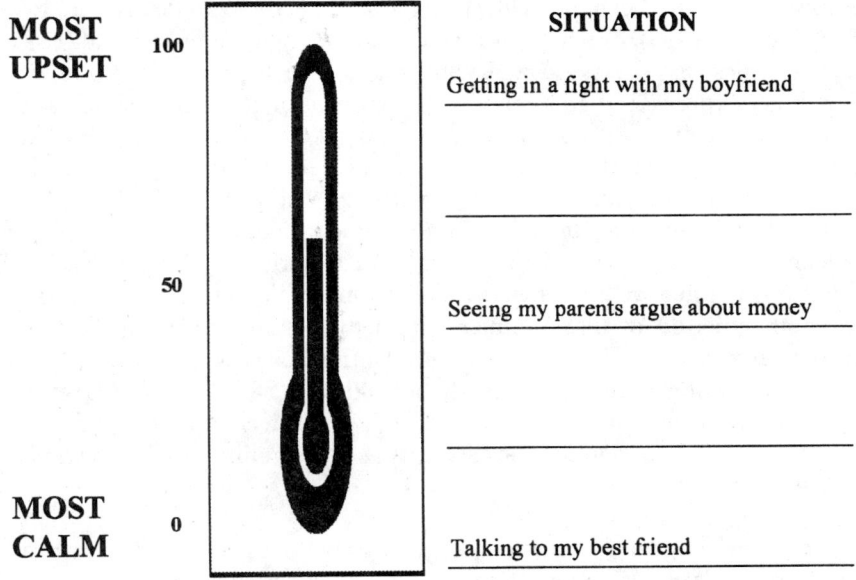

FIGURE 10.1. Sample Feeling Thermometer. From Miller, Rotherman-Borus, Piacentini, Graae, and Castro-Blanco (1992).

Feeling Thermometer is presented to the family, the therapist then reinforces the connection between interpersonal problem situations and high levels of emotional arousal, using the thermometer as a tool to help family members recognize when their own level of discomfort has been reduced, and to implement behavioral strategies for regaining self-control. In the SNAP therapy, family members link difficult family situations to each level of the feeling thermometer, similar to the way a behavioral therapist would use a problems hierarchy to rank-order difficult situations for systematic desensitization or relaxation therapy (Lazarus, 1992; Wolpe, 1950).

Distinguishing Imminent Danger of Suicide from Risk for Suicidal Acts

It is key to distinguish between general risk for suicide and the factors that lead a youth to be in imminent danger for suicide (Rotheram-Borus, 1987). Many individual, relationship, and environmental factors have been linked to risk for suicide. For example, as noted earlier, being depressed places youth at increased risk for suicide (Pfeffer et al., 1994). Youth who perceive negative events as their fault and pervasive in every area of their lives have an attributional style that is associated with depression. Concurrently, youth with this perceptual style typically assume that positive events are happenstance, atypical occurrences, isolated within a unique moment (Rotheram-Borus, 1987; Schwartz, Kaslow, Seeley, & Lewinsohn, 2000). Youth who are poor problem solvers are at increased risk for suicide attempts (Rotheram-Borus, Walker, et al., 1996), as are substance/alcohol abusers (Kotila, 1989). Impulsivity is associated with increased risk for suicide (Asarnow et al., 1987; Kashden, Fremouw, Callahan, & Franzen, 1993; Levenson, 1974; Orbach, Rosenheim, & Hary, 1987; Rotheram-Borus, Trautman, Dopkins, & Shrout, 1990). Most suicide attempters have experienced conflict within their families; their parents are more likely to be depressed (Brent & Perper, 1995; Piacentini, Rotheram-Borus, & Cantwell, 1995). While each of these factors may be linked with risk for suicide, these statistics may be associated with risk over a lifespan. When, how, or why does this risk get expressed in an adolescent's suicide attempt on a specific day?

Imminent danger for suicide is a concept that takes into account the youth's emotional state, an environment that may elicit suicidal ideation, and modalities and personal resources available to the youth for coping with every day stressors (Bradley & Rotheram-Borus, 1989; Rotheram-Borus, 1987). Once identified, certain events that provoke suicidal feelings may be anticipated based on prior experience. For example, if the first attempt was precipitated by a conflict within the family, a second attempt may be triggered by another period of high conflict within the familial unit. One way to assess imminent danger for suicide is to evaluate the youth's behavior and decide if his or her behavior is incompatible with suicide. Rotheram-Borus (1987) identified a set of actions and coping styles that may indicate incompatibility with feeling and acting suicidal. To identify the current style of coping, the therapist assesses abilities of youth to perform in each of the following five areas:

1. Identify three positive events or positive personal attributes (demonstrating that they are not viewing the world as a negative experience that is unchanging and pervades all areas of their life).
2. Identify their current emotional state and situations that may trigger suicidal feelings (countering a general numbness or disassociation between affect and behavior).
3. Plan three ways to cope with a situation that elicits suicidal acts (their problem-solving ability remains intact).
4. Make a written commitment for no suicidal behavior, and contact and promise to speak personally to the therapist prior to taking any action, if and when suicidal feelings emerge.
5. Identify persons who could and would provide social support if suicidal feelings emerge.

Whereas establishing the validity of this risk assessment is very difficult, there are indications that if youth are able to meet all five criteria, they are at low risk of imminent danger of suicide (Piacentini, Rotheram-Borus, & Cantwell, 1995). If they cannot meet these criteria, then they should be evaluated as serious risks in imminent danger for suicide and be referred for a full psychiatric evaluation. This model that identifies when youth are highly suicidal assists therapists, families, and youth to monitor the status of an adolescent's imminent danger for suicide. In addition to being used in the ER, this brief assessment becomes the foundation for the SNAP treatment program for youth who have attempted suicide, or who have suicidal ideation. During the family therapy session in the ER, the imminent danger assessment is administered.

Planning with a Family to Cope Effectively in the Future

The imminent danger assessment begins to provide parents with a framework to understand behavioral markers that indicate when their children are coping in an ineffective manner. It also helps the family make a plan to anticipate situations that may elicit attempts in the future, and to identify the steps they will make to avert suicidal actions. In order to conceptualize a family plan, family members must be invested in the treatment process as well as the recovery of the suicidal adolescent. In SNAP treatment, families are taught coping skills and methods of problem solving that will aid them successfully resolving future suicide-provoking situations.

There are subgroups of suicidal youth who suffer from major psychiatric disorders, such as bipolar disorder, conduct disorder, and affective disorders, with a history of past attempts (D'Angelo & Walsh, 1967; Reisinger, 1976; Shaffer, 1974). Clearly, these youth need adjunctive treatment for their major psychiatric disorders. However, the SNAP model still proves helpful in coping with suicidality among these youth.

SUCCESSFUL NEGOTIATION/ ACTING POSITIVELY THERAPY

The reduction of future adolescent suicide attempts is the ultimate and primary goal of the SNAP therapy (Miller, Rotheram-Borus, Piacentini, Graae, & Castro-Blanco, 1992). To accomplish this goal, SNAP therapy is based on four assumptions regarding attempters and their families:

1. Under duress, little change occurs; only when individuals feel good about themselves and have positive feelings about other family members are they motivated to change.
2. Each family has a road map or current conceptualization of the problem that typically involves a set of behaviors, rules, social roles, and social identities for each family member; reframing the current road map in each of these areas allows flexibility in the family's future actions.
3. Most suicide attempts involve a failure to resolve conflict; increasing conflict resolution skills assists in reducing motivation for future attempts.
4. Suicidal acts are behaviors that can be extinguished via a behavioral paradigm using the tasks in the imminent danger assessment: A goal is set to reduce suicidal actions, triggers are identified, a hierarchy of triggers is established (i.e., a problem hierarchy), the emotional states associated with each trigger are identified, and methods of intervening with each trigger are planned and rehearsed.

Family members work with the therapist to identify and integrate the cognitive, emotional, and social skills needed in order to achieve each of the four tasks successfully. Working collaboratively to accomplish these four tasks within six sessions of therapy instills feelings of self-efficacy and competence among family members and challenges their previous negative attitudes and misinformation. Using tasks that are both interactive and structured, involving repetition and feedback, each session is structured to encourage positive family interactions, to support family problem solving while extinguishing suicidality, and to reinforce the therapist's credibility and value to the family.

SNAP therapy is to be administered in six 1-hour weekly sessions, with additional meetings recommended on a case-by-case basis (Miller, Rotheram-Borus, Piacentini, Graae, & Castro-Blanco, 1992). SNAP therapy should be conducted with the entire family for best results; this may include family members outside the nuclear family who play a significant role in the life of the attempter. If younger members of the family are thought to be disruptive, distracting, or unable to benefit from the discussions, they need not be in attendance. Parents and adolescents are critical members of the family constellation. If there is no immediate family, explore other support systems with the adolescent suicide attempter and attempt to bring those individuals into therapy.

As treatment aims to decrease suicidality, the attempter is screened for current suicidal feelings and actions at each of the six sessions. As outlined earlier, the therapist must assess whether the youth is behaving in a manner that is inconsistent with the suicidal acts (Bradley & Rotheram-Borus, 1989; Rotheram-Borus, 1987). Specifically, the therapist must be able to discern whether the adolescent (1) can enter a contract that specifies he or she will not engage in suicidal behavior for a specified period of time, (2) can express positive statements about him- or herself and family members who are present, (3) can assess his or her own feelings and identify suicide-provoking situations, (4) can produce coping strategies to deal with suicide-provoking situations, and (5) can identify social support persons to contact in the event of a crisis. In accomplishing these tasks, the therapist attempts to elicit a positive connection using support and encouragement. Being unable to connect sufficiently in a relationship with the therapist to accomplish these tasks is likely evidence of serious, debilitating depression. The adolescent who is unable to complete each of these tasks should be considered at imminent risk for suicide, and alternatives to outpatient weekly treatment may need to be recommended.

SNAP therapy also aims to increase family members' conflict resolution skills, particularly for situations that may provoke adolescents' suicidal acts or feelings. Within the SNAP therapy context, suicidal behavior is presented as an ineffective method of problem resolution. More effective problem-solving strategies must be learned by the family in order to avoid further suicidal behavior. A step-by-step social problem-solving model is the first step in educating family members about the central components of SNAP therapy. This model includes (1) defining the problem, (2) creating and identifying alternative solutions, (3) choosing and implementing a solution, and (4) assessing the efficacy of the chosen solution. A secondary set of skills is presented to augment families' problem-solving abilities, including (1) ascertaining and modifying prior expectations and assumptions concerning other family members; (2) recognizing and changing or eliminating obstacles to problem solving, such as those found in overly rigid family rules, roles, and beliefs; (3) determining the benefits of keeping the current style of conflict resolution; (4) developing coping repertoires; and (5) improving positive negotiation skills.

Oftentimes, the families of adolescent suicide attempters have chronic problem situations, with an intensity that varies over time but never completely resolves (Kagan & Schlosberg, 1989). These problems may affect an individual in the family (e.g., anxiety, bipolar disorder), the entire family unit (e.g., marital or parent–child conflict, single-parent family), and stem from external influences (e.g., financial problems, unstable or inadequate living situation), or a combination of the three. Due to the time constraints of the SNAP therapy intervention, families are advised that it is unrealistic to expect that they will be able to stay within the confines of SNAP therapy. Instead, the therapist encourages family members to learn and practice problem-solving techniques in therapy and use these techniques to deal with family problems and crises when they arise. The primary focus of problem solving within SNAP therapy is to improve coping with situations that elicit suicidal thoughts, feelings, and actions from a family member (Miller, Rotheram-Borus, Piacentini, Graae, & Castro-Blanco, 1992). Families are encouraged to contact the therapist when a situation in other areas of their life becomes overwhelming or beyond their control. In order to begin creating a stable environment for the family to access in the future, if necessary, but not only must the clinical setting be perceived as a safe place to go for future assistance, but the therapist must also establish credibility in order to effect maximum treatment adherence.

Strategies for Shaping Behavior in New Ways

There are two techniques used to create a positive atmosphere within the treatment setting: (1) tokens—a way of validating individual and family strengths, and encouraging positively balanced communications; and (2) reframing—redefining the suicidal episode and ongoing family problems in a more neutral context.

Tokens

Tokens are typically poker chips, bingo markers, or small 1" × 1" pieces of construction paper that are distributed to each family member (10 tokens each) at the beginning of each session. These are to be given to each other and to the therapist whenever positive verbal statements are made to another member. The therapist also generously distributes tokens to assist in shaping positive interactions among family members. Tokens are not exchanged for tangible rewards but acquire reinforcing power throughout the session as positive behaviors are identified. Adolescents who, at the beginning of Session 1, proclaim, "These are useless," have proudly asserted, "I got eight tokens. How many did you get?" at the end of a session.

Reframing

A positive family atmosphere is established by modeling how to reframe problems or conflict situations (Watzlawick, 1978). Reframing is used to reduce the level of perceived blame among family members by attributing negative consequences (e.g., overprotectiveness) to situational causes (e.g., dangerous neighborhoods). The therapist's goal is to emphasize situations that elicit negative interactions within the family rather than focusing on a specific negative behavior. In order to achieve this goal, the actual intent, as opposed to the perceived intent, of negative interactions must be emphasized (Gottman, Notarius, Gonso, & Markman, 1976). For example, rules concerning curfew or dating must be redefined as an expression of parental concern instead of a reflection of the parent's lack of trust. On the other hand, the therapist may also need to help reframe the adolescent's desire to spend more time away from home in the context of normal adolescent social development rather than as a sign of disrespect or decreased love for the family. Reframing family problems so that they are perceived as a group effort to solve, counteract, or defeat "external" circumstances serves to promote cohesion within the family. Reframing is encouraged throughout therapy, whenever it is necessary. This technique of reframing is employed to alleviate blame and negative feelings, and to facilitate successful family problem solving and negotiation throughout treatment.

Description of Individual Sessions

SNAP therapy is based on a series of highly interactive, structured tasks involving repeated practice and feedback, always in a way that encourages a positive family atmosphere, as outlined in Table 10.1. The SNAP manual is available at *http://chipts.ucla.edu*, and a description of the sessions is summarized here.

Session 1

The first session aims to establish a positive family atmosphere and to promote problem solving within the family. The therapist must provide a clear and simple understanding

TABLE 10.1. Outline of the Session Content for Each SNAP Therapy Session

Session	Primary goals
1	Establish positive family environment; create therapist's credibility.
2	Create family problem hierarchy; select midrange problem to work on.
3	Analyze family obstacles (i.e., rules, roles, assumptions) that might interfere with successful problem resolution.
4	Review coping strategies and negotiation techniques; brainstorm solutions to selected problems.
5	Evaluate solutions; select best solution; negotiate implementation of solution.
6	Repeat process with important family problem; review course of treatment and address any termination issues.

of both his or her role and the underlying beliefs and structure of SNAP therapy. In order to validate his or her credibility during the first session, the therapist uses a handout titled "What Happens If . . . Therapy" to ensure that family members understand the goals of SNAP therapy and the steps taken to achieve these goals. After this, the therapist draws up a written contract with the family for the six-session protocol. The contract promises no suicidal acts without contacting the therapist personally and to attend the next session of treatment. The contract also indicates that the therapy is for six sessions' duration.

In the first session, family members are asked to generate a list of things they like about themselves and other family members. They then generate a list of strengths for the whole family. Individuals making these communications are rewarded with tokens in an effort to draw attention to positive communication. All family members are involved in identifying the family's strengths, as is the therapist, who distributes tokens. The therapist then instructs family members to give a token to another person when he or she makes a positive, affirmative, or constructive statement to or about that person. Family members are also encouraged to promote constructive communication by rewarding the positive exchanges directed at others. For example, the therapist might give the father a token for honestly expressing his feelings about his child. The therapist must be comfortable in using the tokens in order for the family to accept the use of them as well. It is important that the therapist encourage the use of tokens in each session to facilitate positive expression and encouragement.

At the end of the first session, the therapist works with each family member to think of some behavior that he or she would like to change in the upcoming week:

"I want Mom to kiss me good-bye when she leaves for work."
"I want Mary to ask me for permission to go out with her boyfriend instead of just doing it."
"I want Dad to let me stay out a little later with friends on the weekend."

Successfully completing this exercise serves as a preview of the family's problem-solving and negotiating skills that will be covered in the following five sessions, as well as reinforcement of the therapist's credibility and effectiveness. The exercise also identifies individual needs within the family and increases the chances that they will return for Session 2. In order to continue to encourage the supportive family tone, the family members are assigned the task of giving tokens to each other at least once before the next session.

Session 2

The process of learning effective problem solving begins in Session 2. The goals of this session are (1) to present the family with a step-by-step model to aid in solving interfamilial problems and (2) to develop a systematic family problem hierarchy that will serve as the foundation for all following sessions. In each session, the therapist's first task is to review the events of the past week, emphasizing positive interactions, activities, and feelings. Tokens are again given as reinforcement for behaviors that led to successes in reaching goals (e.g., no suicidal feelings) over the last week. The main points of Session 1 and the homework assignment are also reviewed. The therapist then must assess any suicidal ideation or behaviors the attempter might have experienced since the last session. If any suicidal ideation or behavior did occur, the assessment of imminent danger (discussed earlier) is employed to ascertain present risk status. If no suicidal behavior is reported, the therapist commends both the attempter and family members for their success in avoiding any suicide-inducing situations over the past week or dissipating those situations that did take place. The plan of coping with suicidal situations from Session 1 is then reviewed and revised as needed.

The family and therapist discuss the role of conflict as a precursor to suicidal ideation and actions. The therapist sets the framework: Conflict is normative (i.e., all families argue). The treatment aims to help families develop a new set of rules that allow them to "fight fairly" and manage conflict situations. The family is given a handout outlining the rules, including (1) talking and discussing to replace physical or verbal assault and suicidal behavior; (2) telling others how one feels (e.g., stating emotions such as anger or sadness) instead of acting; (3) listening to others and respecting their opinions (demonstrated in eye contact, nonverbal behavior); and (4) attempting to resolve issues as they occur rather than saving a list of grievances.

> THERAPIST: Don't just yell about [the problem] or walk away or bury it. . . . Try to figure out a way to work the problem out. You need to listen hard so that you can tell them what you heard. . . . If an emergency comes up, do you agree to contact your therapist or clinic immediately? Are the rules clear? Do you agree to these rules and can you live with them? (Miller, Rotheram-Borus, Piacentini, Graae, & Castro-Blanco, 1992, p. 113).

Once the family reviews the rules, the therapist has everyone agree to follow the guidelines in future problem situations.

An outline of the family problem-solving model is introduced to the family and explained in detail. The five-step process for resolving familial difficulties handed to all family members is the foundation for all discussion and resolution exercises:

1. State the goal in one sentence: What do you want to increase?
2. Brainstorm potential solutions—the quality of alternatives is not as important as the quantity.
3. List the costs and benefits of each potential solution and what it will take to implement them.
4. Choose a solution to the problem and implement it.
5. Reevaluate the success of the solution and restate the goal.

Once positive family traits from the last session have been reviewed, the family creates a *family problem hierarchy*. Each member of the family makes a personal list of family problem situations. The family then reviews each list as a group. Using a round-robin-style inquiry for each person's list limits conflict and disagreement during the review of each family member's problem hierarchy. The therapist also assists individual family members by clarifying generalized complaints (e.g., "He hates me") into specific behavioral goals ("I want him to say he loves me three times a week").

THERAPIST: What is it that bothers you about your mom?

MARY: She's always nagging me.

THERAPIST: How does she do that?

MARY: Nothing I do is good enough for her. My room is never clean enough, my clothes are always dirty, and she doesn't like the people I hang out with.

THERAPIST: How would you like her to treat you?

MARY: I don't want her yelling at me so much.

THERAPIST: What would you like her to do instead?

MARY: Well, she could ask me to clean my room, and when I do it, she could thank me.

THERAPIST: (*to the mother*) Do you think that's something you could try to do next time you'd like Mary to clean her room?

MOTHER: I'll try.

Next, each family member consults his or her Feeling Thermometer for each situation in the hierarchy. The therapist then ranks these scores within the confines of the family problem hierarchy, taking an active role as mediator in this exercise by reinforcing positive interaction. The family problem hierarchy is utilized over the course of treatment in order to develop various problem situations, so that family members are able to practice improving their coping skills without high levels of conflict. At first, the family selects a low- to moderate-level problem for skills practice; less important problems are easier to resolve than significant problems. Over time, the family becomes more adept at problem solving and chooses more difficult situations to address.

The homework for Session 2 consists of having family members (1) rate three problem situations using the Feeling Thermometer over the next week, and (2) provide "caring days" for each other, whereby each individual receives one day of special attention during the week (e.g., favorite meal, extra help with household tasks, flowers or other small trinkets, etc.; Stuart, 1980). The therapist chooses the family member who is least engaged in the intervention process to be the recipient of a caring day.

Session 3

The third session's goal is to select a problem on the family hierarchy and analyze it from both a cognitive-behavioral and a family systems perspective. The exercises in which the family engages during this session are generated to (1) create concise working definitions of the behaviors they have designated to be changed; (2) facilitate family members' skills at identifying differences between actual and perceived intent of an action; (3) examine the role that each family member plays in generating family conflict; and (4) articulate the ways in which family beliefs, rules, and roles can restrict problem resolution. The therapist uses tools such as structured role playing, naming each person's role in the family (e.g., the bad guy, the baby, or the protected person in the family), and scripted vignettes, which provide the family with a framework to understand their interactions.

THERAPIST: What is it you want from your daughter?
FATHER: She doesn't respect me.
THERAPIST: What do you mean by that?
FATHER: You can just tell. She doesn't show me any respect.
THERAPIST: What would she do or say if she showed you respect?
FATHER: She would act respectful.
THERAPIST: Give me a concrete example of what she would say or do.
FATHER: Okay. When I tell her to be home by 8 o'clock, I want her home.
THERAPIST: So you want your daughter to be at home by 8 at night unless you tell her she can stay out later.
FATHER: That's right. That's showing respect. (Miller, Rotheram-Borus, Piacentini, Graae, & Castro-Blanco, 1992, p. 41)

The framework does not have to be definitive, nor a 100% accurate description of the family routine. Verbally providing a definition of what occurs within the family supplies a vocabulary to understand the interactions (similar to the function of the Feeling Thermometer); future conflicts can be analyzed using this framework. When some family members are uncomfortable in the roles that appear to be operating, the family can use the framework to change the existing system.

The therapist aids family members in recognizing their assumptions surrounding the family's problem situations and outlines how these expectations can result in family conflict. Additionally, the therapist helps family members understand the gap between the intentions and outcomes of their behaviors. By making their intentions clear and understood, family members are able to see that an action may have been perceived as negative but the intention was positive:

INEZ: I am so miserable.
MOTHER: What's the matter?
INEZ: I just know that Antonio is going to break up with me.
MOTHER: What makes you think this will happen?
INEZ: I always knew it would happen. I'm so ugly, and I have such terrible luck with boys.
MOTHER: You're not ugly!! I am struck every day by how beautiful you are.
INEZ: I can't do anything right. I might as well be dead.
MOTHER: I know it hurts a lot when you break up, but it hasn't even happened yet. Besides, there are plenty of other boys who like you.
INEZ: Nobody else is like Antonio. I'm so depressed. (Miller, Rotheram-Borus, Piacentini, Graae, & Castro-Blanco, 1992, pp. 44–45)

Family members are asked to write down their own and others' roles in a conflict situation during the next week as homework.

Session 4

The goals for this session are (1) to improve coping skills and negotiation strategies, and (2) to formulate alternative solutions to a family problem. After reviewing the homework for the past week and checking for any emerging suicidal feelings or actions, a number of different coping strategies are introduced (e.g., take an action, control your feelings, seek social support, escape the scene, change the meaning of the situation, solve the problem; Folkman & Lazarus, 1980). The therapist demonstrates how these coping skills are alternative methods of coping with conflict situations and gives examples of coping styles that have typically been used by different family members. The family problem hierarchy is repeatedly used to demonstrate previous coping styles and conflict resolution strategies used by each family member. Using a conflict from the previous week, the therapist analyzes each person's style of coping. For example, there was a fight about whether the family would go to church; the fight ended with the mother getting angry and leaving alone; the daughter went into her room and was depressed and suicidal; the father watched a football game. The coping strategy of each person is identified and alternative styles are considered. The more repetition, analysis, and rehearsal of successful resolution of family problem situations, the greater the odds of the intervention having a positive impact.

Families discuss the components of a successful negotiation with the therapist, using a set of guidelines:

1. Be specific and brief when stating what you want.
2. Use positive statements—identify what you want to have increased.
3. State what you think others want.
4. State your goals without placing blame.
5. Listen without interrupting.
6. Take time-outs when you need to cool down before proceeding.

Both scripted and semistructured role-play situations enable the family to practice negotiation skills. Family members are asked to create a list of potential solutions to a problem they have been working on over the last two sessions. Tokens affirm the efforts of the family while permitting the familial unit to function as independently as possible. As homework, the family is asked to try and negotiate any very small problem that arises before the next session.

Session 5

The family reviews resolutions of family problem situations during the previous week, and the therapist checks for current suicidal ideation or actions. The family studies possible solutions from the list generated during the previous week and discusses potential problem solutions and its success in evaluating the situation. The therapist and the family review the list of solutions created in the previous session, revising plans as needed. One principle is reasserted each session: Each time a plan is made, it will need to be revised; the first attempts at problem solving are not likely to be optimal but will improve over time as they are modified. The family uses a handout of sample problems and solutions to identify strategies for successful problem evaluation and generation of solutions. Family members assign their own solutions and then evaluate the costs and benefits of each. Whereas Session 4 focused on the generation of solutions, Session 5 emphasizes evaluation of the appropriateness of each potential solution. The discussion of the consequences of each solution is a test of the family's negotiation skills. As in Session 4, the therapist allows the family to interact as independently as possible, rewarding positive and constructive behaviors and assisting only when needed to resolve and guide the interaction. The final homework assignment is to identify the areas in which conflict might emerge in the future.

Session 6

In the last session, the family endeavors to solve a most difficult and prominent problem situation within the family hierarchy of stressful issues. In many cases, the problem has diminished throughout the course of the SNAP intervention. The therapist, serving as both consultant and observer, assists if the family requests help and, if needed, subtly redirects the quality of the family interactions in order to continue in a positive working environment. Once the family has finished the problem-solving task, each family member is asked to discuss what he or she liked most about his or her performance, and also to identify another strategy that could have been utilized. In order to increase family members' ability to cultivate positive problem-solving skills, the therapist reinforces positive performance with tokens and social praise, then gives feedback to each person.

The contract that initiated treatment outlines the termination point at the end of the sixth session. Termination focuses on the accomplishments made during SNAP and long-term memories of positive feelings that have been exchanged among family members. Persistent problems that may demand future attention are identified. The therapist stresses that the aim of SNAP therapy was not to resolve all of the family's issues over the short series of sessions, but to educate the family in basic methods to resolve possible situations in the future, especially those likely to provoke suicidal feelings in a family member. The family receives encouragement from the therapist to persist in practicing and employing the problem-solving and negotiating techniques learned throughout the sessions. Through repetition, the family will be able to support a more positive family environment and diminish the tendency and frequency of those conflict situations that often lead to suicidal behavior. Finally, the therapist asserts that there is still a potential for certain problems to feel overwhelming and encourages the family to contact him or her, or the clinic, if the learned negotiation skills do not assist the family unit in resolving a difficult issue.

CASE EXAMPLE

In order to demonstrate the implementation of the program, we provide the case example of Camilia, a 15-year-old Puerto Rican adolescent who took 15 tylenol following the arrival of her father for a visit from Puerto Rico. Her mother had gone to dinner with her father the night before the attempt. Camilia was depressed and had no formal history of a past attempt. Her 32-year-old mother had another child, a boy, 9 years old. The family included a grandmother, who was living in the household. The mother had a boyfriend that she had been dating for about 8 months, and was well-liked by the grandmother. In the ER, the family asserted that the suicide attempt was a mistake, that Camilia did not really intend to kill herself, and no further attempts would reoccur. The bilingual therapist met with family in the ER; Camilia and her mother (Antonia), brother (Carlos), and grandmother (Mrs. Fuentes) were in the ER. Camilia said she had been suicidal repeatedly, typically triggered by her father's visits to Chicago. Her greatest fear was to be alone with her father in the family apartment. There had not been a history of sexual abuse in the family; however, Camilia did perceive her father as potentially abusive. The father had battered the mother when the children were young.

During the first session, the family demonstrated a high level of cohesion and easily identified strengths and shared positive events. The daughter and the mother were perceived as closely bonded; Camilia performed several roles as the "mother" to her mother. She cautioned her mother about dating "dangerous" men and how to protect herself. Camilia was worried about her mother attending the church's social club dance each Sunday night. In contrast, Antonia hoped that Camilia would go with her and meet young men on Sunday night. In the first session, a $3'' \times 5''$ file card was used to generate alternative solutions for Camilia about what she would do if her father arrived at the family apartment while she was home alone. Camilia felt comfortable that she could cope with the situation after the family discussed the trigger of her suicidal event.

Throughout the sessions, the family built a "family hierarchy" for conflict situations and situations likely to elicit suicidal feelings. Carlos, Camilia's younger brother, attended each session. After the list of situations was built, the family began problem-solving how to cope, starting with easy situations. Over the sessions, the family identified the roles adopted by Camilia, Carlos, Antonia and Mrs. Fuetentes. Camilia was identified as often operating in the role of "mother." Antonia (the mother) was identified as the family's adolescent. Carlos was the family clown and baby. Whenever tension emerged among the women in the family, Carlos made jokes and distracted the family from the conflict. This strategy resulted in many family fights remaining unresolved. The problem-solving strategies would become derailed. Similarly, Mrs. Fuetentes, the grandmother, also helped distract the family from resolving problems. She would get sick or needy whenever a high level of family conflict emerged. The family roles were oriented toward keeping potential conflict between Antonia and Camilia from becoming critical and resolving conflicts effectively. The family reviewed the current "rules" for conflict resolution that emerged during the sessions when the problem hierarchies were reviewed. Similarly, the roles within the family became a repeated topic of discussion. When dysfunctional patterns emerged during the session (e.g., Carlos making jokes to distract the family, or Mrs. Fuentes becoming ill or needy), the therapist would label the patterns and implement a new problem-solving strategy. The jokes and neediness of family members were addressed as soon as the conflict situation was resolved to the satisfaction of all family members. The man the mother was dating was evaluated as "a good man" by all family members. Encouraging and providing status and power to Antonia and decreasing Camilia's inappropriate power was a constant theme within the family. The therapist encouraged Camilia to be the "daughter" and emphasized the wide range of situations in which she was not the person to make decisions. Her "job" as daughter was to go to school, date, play with her friends and Carlos. Antonia's job was defined as "mother" (i.e., taking responsibility, making decisions, and providing financially for the family). The impact of her decisions regarding men with whom she was involved in romantic relationships was discussed as a "family" issue and was not the pervue of Antonia alone. At each session, suicidal feelings that emerged during the previous week were resolved. Because the trigger situations were very specific (when the father returned), there was little reemergence of imminent danger of suicide. In particular, early in therapy, Antonia committed not to reunite with her ex-husband. Fear of the parents reuniting had been a major fear of both children.

No further suicide attempts occurred over the next 3 years. Camilia did marry at age 16.5 years and became pregnant about 6 months later. Antonia remarried about a year later. The two families lived in the same building. The family remained close and reported many strong, positive relationships over time.

SUMMARY

SNAP therapy is a short, intensive, structured, outpatient family treatment program for adolescent suicide attempters. Similar approaches are utilized with adults when suicidal ideation and actions occur. Based on the principles of cognitive-behavioral and family therapy, the goal of SNAP therapy is to create a family environment that focuses on positive interpersonal relationships and feelings, defining family members' roles and rules for negotiating conflict in an effective manner. The situations likely to elicit suicidal feelings are identified; individuals and families learn practical ways to solve the problems that could potentially lead to suicidal situations. Perceptual styles of seeing one's life and family as perpetually and pervasively negative are challenged and countered by a focus on the strengths and loving feelings of the suicidal individual and the family. Vocabularies for describing feelings, roles, and rules for conflict are articulated to help family members describe future conflict situations. SNAP therapy also works to address both the role of family conflict in triggering suicidal behavior and the high rates of nonadherence that are typical for this population. The SNAP treatment is only one component of establishing a comprehensive and coordinated system of care for attempters. The ER procedures, interventions, and the definition of suicidal events, as well as the therapeutic contact must be engineered. The utility of the intervention continues to be evaluated, although initial evaluations have been positive (Rotheram-Borus et al., 2000; Rotheram-Borus, Piacentini, et al., 1996).

REFERENCES

Andrews, J., & Lewinsohn, P. M. (1992). Suicidal attempts among older adolescents: Prevalence and co-occurrence with psychiatric disorders. *Journal of the American Academy of Child and Adolescent Psychiatry, 31,* 655–662.

Asarnow, J. (1992). Suicidal ideation and attempts during middle childhood: Associations with perceived family stress and depression among child psychiatric inpatients. *Journal of Clinical Child Psychology, 21,* 35–40.

Asarnow, J., Carlson, G., & Guthrie, D. (1987). Coping strategies, self-perceptions, hopelessness, and perceived family environments in depressed and suicidal children. *Journal of Consulting and Clinical Psychology, 55,* 361–366.

Berman, A. L., & Jobes, D. A. (1994). Treatment of the suicidal adolescent. *Death Studies, 18*(4), 375–389.

Bickman, L. (1996). A continuum of care: More is not always better. *American Psychologist, 51,* 689–701.

Bradley, J., & Rotheram-Borus, M. J. (1989). *Imminent danger assessment and suicide risk among adolescents: A training manual for runaway shelter staff.* Tulsa: University of Oklahoma Press.

Brent, D. A., & Perper, J. A. (1995). Research in adolescent suicide: Implications for training, service delivery, and public policy. *Suicide and Life-Threatening Behavior, 25*(2), 222–230.

Centers for Disease Control and Prevention. (1998). Youth risk behavioral surveillance in the United States, 1997. *Morbidity and Mortality Weekly Report, 47*(SS-3), 1–89.

D'Angelo, R., & Walsh, J. (1967). An evaluation of various therapy approaches with lower socioeconomic group children. *Journal of Psychology, 76,* 59–64.

DeMaso, D., Ross, L., & Beardslee, W. (1994). Depressive disorders and suicidal intent in adolescent suicide attempters. *Developmental and Behavioral Pediatrics, 15,* 74–77.

Deykin, E., Hsieh, C., Joshi, N., & McNamara, J. (1986). Adolescent suicidal and self-destructive behavior: Results of an intervention study. *Journal of Adolescent Health Care, 7,* 88–95.

Fisher, P. W., Shaffer, D., Piacentini, J., Lapkin, J., Kafantaris, V., Leonard, H., & Herzog, D. B. (1993). Sensitivity of the diagnostic interview schedule for children, 2nd ed. (DISC-2.1) for specific diagnoses of children and adolescents. *Journal of the American Academy of Child and Adolescent Psychiatry, 32,* 666–673.

Folkman, S., & Lazarus, R. S. (1980). An analysis of coping in a middle-aged community sample. *Journal of Health and Social Behavior, 21,* 219–239.

Gottman, J. M., Notarius, C., Gonso, J., & Markman, H. (1976). *A couple's guide to communication.* Champaign, IL: Research Press.

Groholt, B., Ekeberg, O., Wichstrom, L., & Haldorsen, T. (1997). Youth suicide in Norway, 1990–1992: A comparison between children and adolescents completing suicide and age- and gender-matched controls. *Suicide and Life-Threatening Behavior, 27*, 250–263.

Haynes, R. B. (1979). Introduction. In R. B. Haynes, D. W. Taylor, & D. Sackett (Eds.), *Compliance and health care* (pp. 1–13). Baltimore: Johns Hopkins University Press.

Hazzard, A., Hutchinson, S. J., & Krawiecki, N. (1990). Factors related to adherence to medication regimens in pediatric seizure patients. *Journal of Pediatric Psychology, 15*, 543–555.

Hirschfeld, R. M., Keller, M. B., Panico, S., Arons, B. S., Barlow, D., Davidoff, F., Endicott, J., Froom, J., Goldstein, M., Gorman, J. M., Marek, R. G., Maurer, T. A., Meyer, R., Phillips, K., Ross, J, Schwenk, T. L., Sharfstein, S. S., Thase, M. E., & Wyatt, R. J. (1997). The National Depressive and Manic–Depressive Association consensus statement on the undertreatment of depression [see comments]. *Journal of the American Medical Association, 277*(4), 333–40.

Holinger, P. (1990). The causes, impact, and preventability of childhood injuries in the United States. *American Journal of Diseases of Childhood, 144*, 670–676.

Kagan, R., & Schlosberg, S. (1989). *Families in perpetual crisis.* New York: Norton.

Kashden, J., Fremouw, W., Callahan, T., & Franzen, M. (1993). Impulsivity in suicidal and nonsuicidal adolescents. *Journal of Abnormal Child Psychology, 21*, 339–353.

Klimes-Dougan, B. (1998). Screening for suicidal ideation in children and adolescents: Methodological considerations. *Journal of Adolescence, 21*(4), 435–444.

Kotila, L. (1989). Age-specific characteristics of attempted suicide in adolescence. *Acta Psychiatrica Scandinavica, 79*(5), 436–443.

Kovacs, M., Goldston, D., & Gastonis, C. (1993). Suicidal behaviors and childhood-onset depressive disorders: A longitudinal investigation. *Journal of the American Academy of Child and Adolescent Psychiatry, 32*, 8–20.

La Greca, A. (1990). Treatment of suicide ideators: A problem-solving approach. *Behavioral Therapy, 21*, 403–411.

Lazarus, A. A. (1992). The multimodal approach to the treatment of minor depression. *American Journal of Psychotherapy, 46*(1), 50–57.

Levenson, M. (1974). Cognitive correlates of suicidal risk. In C. Neuringer (Ed.), *Psychological assessment of suicidal risk* (pp. 150–163). Springfield, IL: Thomas.

Litt, I., & Cuskey, W. (1980). Compliance with medical regimens during adolescence. *Pediatric Clinics of North America, 27*, 3–15.

Martunen, M. J., Hillevi, M. A., Henriksson, M. M., & Lonnqvist, J. K. (1992). Adolescent suicide: Endpoint of long-term difficulties. *Journal of the American Academy of Child an Adolescent Psychiatry, 31*, 649–654.

Merikangas, K. R., Wicki, W., & Angst, J. (1994). Heterogeneity of depression: Classification of depressive subtypes by longitudinal course. *British Journal of Psychiatry, 164*(3), 342–8.

Metha, A., Chen, E., Mulvenon, S., & Dode, I. (1998). A theoretical model of adolescent suicide risk. *Archives of Suicide Research, 4*, 115–133.

Miller, S., Rotheram-Borus, M. J., Piacentini, J., & Graae, F. (1992). *Emergency room staff training manual for adolescent suicide attempters.* Los Angeles: Department of Psychiatry, University of California.

Miller, S., Rotheram-Borus, M. J., Piacentini, J., Graae, F., & Castro-Blanco, D. (1992). *Successful Negotiation Acting Positively (SNAP): A brief cognitive-behavioral family therapy manual for adolescent suicide attempters and their families.* New York: Department of Child Psychiatry, Columbia University.

Orbach, I., Rosenheim, E., & Hary, E. (1987). Some aspects of cognitive functioning in suicidal children. *Journal of the American Academy of Child Psychiatry, 26*, 181–185.

Pfeffer, C., Hurt, S., Kakuma, T., Peskin, J., Siefker, C. A., & Nagabhairava, S. (1994). Suicidal children grow up: Suicidal episodes and effects of treatment during follow-up. *Journal of the American Academy of Child and Adolescent Psychiatry, 33*, 225–230.

Piacentini, J. (1994, October). *Family-based interventions to improve treatment adherence and outcome among adolescent suicide attempters.* Paper presented at the annual meeting of the American Academy of Child and Adolescent Psychiatry Meeting, New York, NY.

Piacentini, J., Rotheram-Borus, M. J., & Cantwell, C. (1995). Brief cognitive-behavioral family therapy for suicidal adolescents. In L. Vandecreek, S. Knapp, & T. L. Jackson (Eds.), *Innovations in clinical practice: A source book* (pp. 151–168). Sarasota, FL: Professional Resource Press.

Piacentini, J., Rotheram-Borus, M. J., Gillis, R., Graae, F., Trautman, P. D., Garcia-Leeds, C., Cantwell, C., & Shaffer, D. (1995). Demographic predictors of treatment attendance in adolescent suicide attempters. *Journal of Consulting and Clinical Psychology, 63,* 469–473.

Reisinger, J. (1976). Parents as change agents for their children: A review. *Journal of Community Psychology, 4,* 103–123.

Rogawski, A. B., & Edmundson, B. (1971). Factors affecting the outcome of psychiatric interagency referral. *American Journal of Psychiatry, 127,* 925–934.

Rotheram-Borus, M. J. (1987). Evaluation of imminent danger of suicide in children. *American Journal of Orthopsychiatry, 47,* 59–67.

Rotheram-Borus, M. J., Piacentini, J., Cantwell, C., Belin, T., & Song, J. (2000). The 18-month impact of an emergency room intervention for adolescent female suicide attempters. *Journal of Clinical and Consulting Psychology, 68,* 1081–1083.

Rotheram-Borus, M. J., Piacentini, J., Van Rossem, R., Graae, F., Cantwell, C., Castro-Blanco, D., & Feldman, J. (1996). Enhancing treatment adherence with a specialized emergency room program for adolescent suicide attempters. *Journal of the American Academy of Child and Adolescent Psychiatry, 35,* 654–663.

Rotheram-Borus, M. J., Piacentini, J., Van Rossem, R., Graae, F., Cantwell, C., Castro-Blanco, D., & Feldman, J. (1999). Treatment adherence among Latina female adolescent suicide attempters. *Suicide and Life-Threatening Behavior, 29*(4), 319–331.

Rotheram-Borus, M. J., & Trautman, P. D. (1988). Hopelessness depression, and suicidal intent among adolescent suicide attempters. *Journal of the American Academy of Child and Adolescent Psychiatry, 27,* 700–704.

Rotheram-Borus, M. J., Trautman, P. D., Dopkins, S. C., & Shrout, P. (1990). Cognitive style and pleasant activities among female adolescent suicide attempters. *Journal of Consulting and Clinical Psychology, 58,* 554–561.

Rotheram-Borus, M. J., Walker, J. U., & Ferns, W. (1996). Suicidal behavior among middle-class adolescents who seek crisis services. *Journal of Clinical Psychology, 52*(2), 137–43.

Schilling, R., Duan, N., & Rotheram-Borus, M. J. (2001). *Video adaptation of efficacious HIV prevention groups.* Grant proposal.

Schwartz, J. A., Kaslow, N. J., Seeley, J., & Lewinsohn, P. (2000). Psychological, cognitive, and interpersonal correlates of attributional change in adolescents. *Journal of Clinical Child Psychology, 29,* 188–98.

Shaffer, D. (1974). Suicide in childhood and early adolescence. *Journal of Child Psychology and Psychiatry, 15,* 275–291.

Shaffer, D., Garland, A., Gould, M., Fisher, P., & Trautman, P. D. (1988). Preventing teenage suicide: A critical review. *Journal of the American Academy of Child and Adolescent Psychiatry, 27,* 675–687.

Shaffer, D., & Piacentini, J. (1994). Suicide and attempted suicide. In M. Rutter & E. Taylor (Eds.), *Child psychiatry—modern approaches* (3rd ed., pp. 407–424). London: Blackwell Scientific Publications.

Spirito, A., Brown, L., Overholser, J., & Fritz, G. (1989). Attempted suicide in adolescence: A review and critique of the literature. *Clinical Psychology Review, 9,* 335–363.

Spirito, A., Jelalian, E., Rasile, D., Rohrbeck, C., & Vinnick, L. (2000). Adolescent risk taking and self-reported injuries associated with substance use. *American Journal of Drug and Alcohol Abuse, 26*(1), 113–123.

Spirito, A., Plummer, B., Gispert, M., Levy, S., Kurkjian, J., Lewander, W., Hagberg, S., & DeVost, L. (1992). Adolescent suicide attempts: Outcomes at follow-up. *American Journal of Orthopsychiatry, 62,* 464–468.

Stuart, R. B. (1980). *Helping couples change: A social learning approach to marital therapy.* New York: Guilford Press.

Summerville, M., Kaslow, N., Abbate, M., & Cronan, S. (1994). Psychopathology, family functioning, and cognitive style in urban adolescents with suicide attempts. *Journal of Abnormal Child Psychology, 22,* 221-236.

Taylor, E., & Stansfield, S. (1984). Children who poison themselves: A clinical comparison with psychiatric controls. *British Journal of Psychiatry, 145,* 127-132.

Trautman, P. D., Rotheram-Borus, M., Dopkins, S., & Lewin, N. (1991). Psychiatric diagnoses in minority female adolescent suicide attempters. *Journal of the American Academy of Child and Adolescent Psychiatry, 30,* 617-622.

Trautman, P. D., Stewart, N., & Morishima, A. (1993). Are adolescent suicide attempters non compliant with outpatient care? *Journal of the American Academy of Child and Adolescent Psychiatry, 32,* 89-94.

U.S. Bureau of the Census. (1996). *National and state population estimates* [Online]. Available: *http://www.census.gov.* [January 19, 2001]

Watzlawick, P. (1978). *The language of change: Elements of therapeutic communication.* New York: Basic Books.

Welu, T. (1977). A follow-up program for suicide attempters. *Suicide and Life-Threatening Behavior, 7,* 17-30.

Wolpe, J. (1950). Need-reduction, drive-reduction, and reinforcement: A neurophysiological view. *Psychological Review, 57,* 19-26

III

Psychological Treatments for Substance Use and Abuse Disorders

Substance use disorders, and particularly alcohol dependence and abuse, are among the most prevalent mental disorders in the general population. Addictive behaviors not only cause significant distress and interference with the patient's life, but they also impose significant direct and indirect costs to the nation in medical resources used for care, treatment, rehabilitation, and reduced or lost productivity. Addiction is a complex phenomenon. Biological, genetic, psychological, and social factors all contribute to the development and maintenance of the problem. Once the addictive behavior has developed, it is difficult to change. Prior research has shown that various conditions need to be met for individuals to quit the harmful habits and initiate the process of change.

Prochaska and colleagues postulate six distinct stages of this change process: Precontemplation, contemplation, preparation, action, maintenance, and termination (e.g., Prochaska & DiClemente, 1982; Prochaska & Velicer, 1997). Various personal, interpersonal, and contextual variables contribute to this process of change. Psychological intervention (when delivered at the right time) can greatly facilitate this process. It can influence the decisional balance for discontinuing the habit, raise the patient's sense of self-efficacy, and provide coping strategies to deal with temptations. In addition, basic behavioral principles and social support can greatly motivate patients to initiate change and maintain progress. The following chapters outline a number of specific treatment techniques from different theoretical orientations to facilitate this change process.

Due to the prevalence of alcohol dependence and abuse, most of the chapters in this section discuss specific interventions to treat problem drinking. However, the same principles can also be applied to other addictive behaviors. The first chapter by Nancy Handmaker and Scott Walters (Chapter 11) describes motivational interviewing, a powerful therapeutic method developed by William Miller, which is the direct application of Prochaska's model of behavior change. Chapter 12 by Tracy O'Leary and Peter Monti describes cognitive-behavioral therapy for alcohol addiction. Both types of treatments are delivered in individual treatment sessions. Chapter 13 by Joseph Nowinski outlines the well-known twelve-step group treatment program for problem drinking, a supportive group intervention. Michael Rohrbaugh and Varda Shoham (Chapter 14) provide a description of systemic family consultation, a couple treatment for alcohol abuse. The last chapter in this section (Chapter 15) by Stephen Higgins, Stacey Sigmon, and Alan Budney outlines community reinforcement plus voucher training for the treatment of cocaine dependence. However, similar techniques can also be used for treating other forms of addictive behaviors. We believe that this collection of intervention methods for addictive behaviors represents the most effective and state of the art psychological techniques to treat these debilitating conditions.

REFERENCES

Prochaska, J. O., & DiClemente, C. C. (1982). Transtheoretical therapy: Toward a more integrative model of change. *Psychotherapy: Theory, Research, and Practice, 20,* 161–173.

Prochaska, J. O., & Velicer, W. F. (1997). The transtheoretical model of health behavior change. *American Journal of Health Promotion, 12,* 38–48.

11

Motivational Interviewing for Initiating Change in Problem Drinking and Drug Use

NANCY S. HANDMAKER
SCOTT T. WALTERS

Client acceptance of an "alcoholic" or "addict" label has often been used as a measure of readiness to change in the addictions field. The phrase "in denial" has been applied to ambivalent problem drinkers and drug users who are unwilling to adopt an identity of an "alcoholic" or "addict." Interestingly, this emphasis on labeling as proof of treatment readiness is uncommon in other areas of treatment. For example, it would be unthinkable for a therapist to ask that a client embrace a fixed identity of "depressive." Imagine a first session like the following: "You are a narcissist. You need to acknowledge that before we can begin our work together." What would proceed is predictable: The therapist and client would very likely engage in a dispute. The client might respond: "You think *I'm* a narcissist? What about you? You just me met and you think you know enough to give me a diagnosis?" Similarly, saying "You are an addict. You've got to admit that to change," often sets up the unhealthy situation in which the therapist argues for change while the client argues against it.

AMBIVALENCE AS A NATURAL PART OF CHANGE

An alternative approach is to expect clients to be ambivalent about behavior change, especially at the initial stages of treatment. Prochaska, DiClemente, and Norcross (1992) have developed a transtheoretical model to describe how people change problem behaviors, with and without treatment. People who are not considering change are described as being in the *precontemplation* stage. For clients in this stage, it is most helpful to raise the level of awareness of the risks and problems associated with their current behaviors.

Once people become aware that their behaviors are causing problems or putting them at risk, they may enter the *contemplation* stage and consider whether they should change. Here, individuals begin to weigh the pros and cons of changing versus not changing behaviors. It is characteristic of clients at this stage to be ambivalent, because of the conflict between the reasons for changing versus continuing to drink or use drugs. For example, comments such as "I know drinking this much is not good for me but I can't sleep unless I'm drunk" suggest that the client has good reason both to change and not to change. The task for the counselor thus becomes tipping the balance in favor of changing. As the internal conflict subsides in this stage, ambivalence also declines. Clients tend to make comments such as "What can I do?" or "I've got to do something about this, but what?" This *preparation* stage is a "window of opportunity." At this point, the task for a counselor is to help the client determine the best course of action to take. Individuals in the *action* stage of change are pursuing their goals. Finally, in the *maintenance* stage, clients have already developed new habits and are in the process of maintaining them. Many individuals relapse into old patterns of behavior several times before changing for good. Because these slips are a natural part of the recovery process, a therapist would want to help clients revisit the processes of contemplation, determination, and action, without becoming stuck or demoralized. Several revolutions in the change cycle are common before new patterns of behavior are reliably maintained.

RATIONALE FOR MOTIVATIONAL INTERVIEWING

Motivational interviewing addresses where clients are in the cycle of change and assists them in moving toward change. It is especially designed to address ambivalence in the early stages of change. The "Drinker's Check-Up" (DCU), a single-session method for moving clients from contemplation to action, was the first test of motivational interviewing. The conceptualization underlying the DCU is that personal feedback on alcohol-related impairment delivered by an empathic therapist increases the discrepancy between the client's perceived benefits of drinking or drug use and the consequences. Using a decisional balance as a metaphor, the goal is to tip the balance toward change using personalized feedback about alcohol-related consequences. In an early test of this method, Miller, Sovereign, and Krege (1988) recruited drinkers via a newspaper advertisement offering confidential feedback about their drinking. Participants were randomized to a DCU or a 6-week waiting-list control. At a 6-week follow-up, subjects who received the DCU significantly reduced their drinking whereas waiting-list control subjects showed no change. After receiving the DCU, the waiting-list group showed comparable decreases in their drinking. Both groups maintained their improvement when contacted 12 months later. These findings were replicated in a second study of the DCU (Miller, Benefield, & Tonigan, 1993).

In the largest clinical trial of motivational interviewing, four sessions of motivational enhancement therapy were compared to up to 12 sessions of either cognitive-behavioral therapy or twelve-step facilitation (Project MATCH Research Group, 1997, 1998). The first two motivational enhancement therapy sessions consisted of a DCU and an individualized change plan delivered in a motivational interviewing style. The third and fourth sessions were visits to review client progress, reexamine reasons for change, and adjust the change plan, if necessary. At the 3-year follow-ups, participants in all three conditions showed significant and roughly equivalent reductions in all drinking measures. Thus, motivational enhancement therapy, in four sessions, produced outcomes comparable to the other treatments involving up to three times as many sessions.

MOTIVATIONAL INTERVIEWING AS A COUNSELING STYLE

Motivational interviewing is a "directive, client-centered counseling style for eliciting behavior change by helping clients to explore and resolve ambivalence" (Rollnick & Miller, 1995, p. 325) about change. Rooted in humanistic and existential psychology, the assumptions inherent in the motivational interviewing style are that the client brings to the therapy session a basic capacity for the actualization of a positive self and is responsible for changing. The therapist's role is thus to create those conditions shown to enhance the likelihood that a client will engage in behavior change efforts. Miller and Rollnick (1991) have summarized the elements underlying motivational interviewing in four basic principles: (1) express empathy; (2) develop discrepancy; (3) roll with resistance; and (4) support self-efficacy.

Express Empathy

The therapist's expression of empathy communicates acceptance toward building a working alliance and supporting the client's exploration of his or her ambivalence about change. Thus, fundamental to motivational interviewing is the skill of expressing accurate empathy through reflective listening. The methods for practicing reflective listening have been described extensively (Truax & Carkhuff, 1967) but essentially involve an "active" style of listening. The therapist tracks the verbal and nonverbal responses made by the client and reflects back what he or she believes the client is communicating. This process of reflecting clarifies and enhances the client's thinking. A key strategy of motivational interviewing, described later, involves the selective reflection of a client's statements about change to reinforce them.

Develop Discrepancy

A second basic principle underlying motivational interviewing is that when people perceive a discrepancy between where they are and where they want to be, motivation for change is increased. The motivational interviewer seeks to highlight the inconsistency between the client's behavior and his or her stated values and goals. Offering personalized (or normative) feedback such as the DCU and contrasting values with addictive behaviors and related lifestyles are two widely used techniques that are described later.

Roll with Resistance

The amount of defensiveness or resistance that a client evidences during a session is often the best predictor of whether he or she will change a problem behavior. Furthermore, studies have shown that therapist counseling style is often directly related to the level of client resistance. For example, in an analysis of audiotaped feedback from the DCU an empathic therapist style was found to be predictive of decreased client resistance (Miller et al., 1993). The opposite was also true, in that when the therapist was more overtly confrontational, the client reacted defensively. Moreover, client defensiveness elicited during these single 1-hour sessions was strongly predictive of increased drinking at the 12-month follow-up. Signs of client resistance include arguing, interrupting, bringing up irrelevant matters, and simply failing to participate. When confronted with such actions, it can be tempting to present an intellectual argument for why a client should change the addictive behavior, particularly when there is evidence of a serious health risk. But despite this tendency, efforts to convince clients with direct confrontation have been shown to be less effective at producing long-term behavior change. Rather than arguing with clients, or telling them what they "must" do, client resistance is a signal to respond differently. The drinker is seen as the primary source for finding answers and solutions and is thus the one who should voice the need for change. The most helpful technique for disarming argumentative or resistant speech is to reflect back what has been said. After all, who can argue with his or her own words? For instance, *simple* reflections include restating or paraphrasing what the client has said:

- "You're having a hard time seeing a need to quit."
- "You're surprised that you are at the 99th percentile of drinkers."
- "So your wife has been worrying that your marijuana use is getting out of hand."
- "One thing you've noticed is that you seem to be drinking more than you used to."

The *double-sided* reflection is useful when the client has expressed reasons for change as well as reasons against it. It helps to clarify the dilemma of ambivalence or uncertainty with regard to change, and allows clients to explore further the direction to be taken in a supportive atmosphere.

- "You want to quit, but you're afraid it might be difficult for you."
- "This must be scary for you. On the one hand, you seem to be using drugs quite a bit, but on the other hand, you have trouble seeing yourself as an addict."

Some statements offered by the clients can be reframed and reflected back with a twist. Rather than confronting clients with the inappropriateness or irrationality of their behavior, the therapist uses a sort of "verbal judo," refusing to be baited and adding subtle twists that build momentum toward change. For example, *amplified* reflections are extreme statements under the guise of reflection with which the client will be unlikely to agree:

- "Maybe it's none of your wife's business whether you use drugs or not."
- "So it seems to you that your drinking is perfectly normal."
- "You seem to be saying that if you quit, your friends would reject you."

Though this type of reflection should be used carefully (the therapist must be reasonably sure that the client will not agree with this position, or perceive the comment as mocking), such a technique helps to move the client from an extreme position (i.e., where there are no reasons for anyone to be concerned), to a more moderate one (i.e., there may be some reasons for making a change). Because the therapist occupies the extreme position, the client cannot, and he or she will tend to choose a more moderate one, where movement toward change becomes easier.

Support Self-Efficacy

In the long run, the client, not the therapist, will be responsible for choosing and implementing change. Belief in one's own efficacy has often been seen to be an important predictor of outcome success, and if clients talk about how they would go about changing, and what it might look like, they are more likely to view it as a realistic option. Thus, the therapist listens for and reinforces talk about the client's belief in making a change. For instance, examples of reflective statements that support self-efficacy might include the following:

- "Your success in quitting injecting methamphetamine in the past gives you confidence that you can stop using cocaine."
- "You certainly have a number of friends who would be able to help."
- "Those are some really good ideas about how to cut down on your drinking!"

The client might be asked to make a list of friends and relatives who would support him or her in this decision. We have also found that there are a number of clients, high on desire, who cannot begin to consider a change because they do not think they have the ability. Thus, we might ask clients to outline a plan, providing they have sufficient desire: "It sounds like you might not be ready to make a change, but how would you go about changing *if you wanted to*?" A client who feels trapped may also be encouraged by the past successes of others. The therapist can mention specific stories of past clients who have been successful in changing their behavior. Finally, the counselor's own belief in the person's ability to change can become a self-fulfilling prophecy (Leake & King, 1977).

PHASE 1: BUILDING MOTIVATION

Miller and Rollnick (1991) have conceptualized motivational interviewing in two phases that can take place over one or more sessions, depending on the client's readiness. Phase 1 focuses on building motivation for change. If a client is in the action stage of readiness by the first session, Phase 1 may proceed quite rapidly. For example, it is optional whether the motivational interview includes feedback in a "check-up" format. The goal during Phase 1 is to elicit self-motivational statements, which often include the recognition of problems, the expression of concerns about drinking or drug use, the expression of intention or desire to change, and optimism about change. During Phase 1, the counselor keeps the process going by (1) asking open-ended questions (i.e., questions that do not elicit a simple "yes" or "no" response), (2) reflecting, and (3) making summary statements. This phase of the motivational interview may be conceptualized as "tipping the scale" toward the side of change. When a client shows readiness to change, the emphasis is placed on strengthening commitment and developing a plan during Phase 2.

Beginning the Open-Ended Motivational Session

After the introductions and procedures required by the treatment setting have been completed, the motivational interview might begin as an affirmation and an open-ended question followed by reflection. Examples of these might be "Tell me what led to your coming today? What brought you in for alcohol and drug treatment? What are some of the recent events in your life that led to your seeking treatment?" It is important to be respectful of what the client wants to talk about initially. He or she will respond in a number of ways. The session may proceed with the client providing a story that is indirectly related to his or her alcohol and drug use. Eventually, the therapist directs the discussion to alcohol and drugs. Here is an example of how this might proceed with the fictional case of a 34-year-old man who was brought into treatment by his older sister.

THERAPIST: I appreciate your making this effort to come in to meet with me. Now that we've taken care of some of the necessary paperwork, I'd like to spend the remainder of our time today hearing from you about what led to your coming in. Before we end our meeting, we can talk about where you might want to go from here. Okay?

CLIENT: Yeah.

THERAPIST: What led to your coming in today?

CLIENT: I really didn't want to come here. My sister brought me in because I have been missing work and might lose my job.

THERAPIST: So, it wasn't your idea to come in today. Sounds like your sister is worried about you. Tell me what's been happening at work.

CLIENT: My boss is asking me to work too much overtime.

THERAPIST: You're being asked to work more hours than you want to.

CLIENT: No. It's not that. It's just hard for me to get up on Saturdays. I don't like coming in on the weekends anyway.

THERAPIST: It's difficult to work on the weekends.

CLIENT: Yeah.

THERAPIST: What makes it hard to work on the weekends?

CLIENT: Well, I usually am up late on Friday and Saturday nights.

THERAPIST: You're up late on Friday and Saturday nights, and that makes it difficult to work the next 2 days. How is this connected to your sister's worries?

CLIENT: Well I'm hungover, and my boss has complained because I'm not coming in. He told me no more excuses.

THERAPIST: Your boss has given you an ultimatum.

CLIENT: Yeah. He'll fire me.

THERAPIST: What would that mean for you?

CLIENT: I could lose my apartment and have no place to live. My sister knows that I've lived on the streets before, and she's afraid that will happen again.

THERAPIST: So if you lose your job, you could lose a lot more.

CLIENT: Yeah.

Introducing the Topic of Addictions

A step toward enhancing motivation for change is to relate the client's concerns directly to his use of alcohol or drugs. For example, the client has indicated that it is important to keep his home. The session might proceed with the therapist exploring a connection between the client's keeping his home and his alcohol or drug use.

THERAPIST: Now, you said that the difficulties at work have to do with your finding it hard to get up for work on the weekends.

CLIENT: Yeah.

THERAPIST: What happens on Friday and Saturday nights that makes it hard to get up in the mornings?

CLIENT: Well, we party.

THERAPIST: What do you mean?

CLIENT: I mean my friends and I go out to play pool at a bar and drink until it closes. Then, we usually get together and drink afterwards.

THERAPIST: Your drinking and staying out late make it difficult to work the next day, and that's causing problems between you and your boss. If you lose your job, you could lose your apartment too.

Strategies for Developing Discrepancy

Eliciting Self-Motivational Statements

Throughout Phase 1, the therapist seeks to elicit concerns, problems, and statements about change from the client toward building on the side of change. The therapist may ask questions that directly evoke the client's concerns, problems, intentions, and optimism about change. Examples are "What about your drinking troubles you? What problems does your drinking cause? What are you thinking you'd like to do about your drinking? What is different now that you think that you can be successful in changing?" This process is kept going by using reflective listening and summarizing. Miller and Rollnick (1991) suggest specific questions that elicit further change talk on a specific problem or concern that the client has raised, for example, (1) asking for an elaboration (e.g., "What else?"), (2) asking about extremes (e.g., "What is the worst thing that could happen if you don't stop drinking?"), (3) looking forward (e.g., "How would your life improve if you weren't drinking as much?"), and (4) looking backward (e.g., "What was it like before you began smoking marijuana?"). The following is an example of these approaches with our case illustration:

THERAPIST: So you're saying that being out late and drinking is making it hard to get up for work.

CLIENT: Yeah. I'm pretty hungover the next day.

THERAPIST: What is that like? [Asking for an elaboration]

CLIENT: My head is pounding. I am tired and lately I've been spitting up blood in the morning.

THERAPIST: You feel physically sick after a night of drinking and now you've noticed you're spitting up blood. What do you think this means? [Asking for an elaboration]

CLIENT: I think that I'm doing some damage to my body this time.

THERAPIST: Like what kind of damage? [Asking for an elaboration]

CLIENT: I have a friend who has, like, a hole in his stomach because of his drinking. He spits up blood, too. That doesn't stop him from drinking.

THERAPIST: What is worst that could happen to your friend? [Asking for extremes]

CLIENT: I think he's going to die, if he doesn't stop drinking.

THERAPIST: What do you think will happen to you, if you continue to drink like you are? [Looking forward]

CLIENT: I'm scared sometimes, but it doesn't seem to stop me either.

THERAPIST: You're fearful about what the blood could mean. What was your life like when you didn't have these fears? [Looking backward]

CLIENT: I felt better before all the drinking and drugs.

Exploring the Pros and Cons

The crux of motivational interviewing is resolving ambivalence about change. Exploring the reasons for changing versus staying the same leads to increased understanding about the client's ambivalence. The therapist may want to use a Decisional Balance Sheet like the one illustrated in Table 11.1 to guide this process. The worksheet is helpful in keeping track of the client's statements. It helps guide the process of eliciting self-motivational statements, making selective reflections, and summarizing throughout the interview. This process can build the discrepancy between the reasons for changing versus staying the same. By this point in the session, the therapist would have begun entering information from the client in the column for "Reasons for Changing" in the Decisional Balance Sheet. The therapist may continue this process of exploring items on the side of change by asking open-ended questions about problems in the past or present related to drinking or drug use, demonstrated in the following example:

THERAPIST: What are some of the other difficulties that drinking is causing you, or has caused you in the past?

CLIENT: I've lost everything at one time or another.

THERAPIST: Your drinking has led to some serious losses.

CLIENT: I was living with my girlfriend before I became homeless. She threw me out.

TABLE 11.1. Decisional Balance Sheet

Reasons for not changing	Reasons for changing
(Benefits of addiction)	(Costs of addiction)
Being with friends	Having hangovers
Having a place to play pool	Having threats of job loss
	Possible loss of housing
	Causing harm to health
	Lost relationships in the past
(Costs of changing)	(Benefits of changing)
Losing friends	Being able to work weekends
Feeling lonely and depressed	Keeping job
Staying away from the bar	Keeping apartment
Not playing pool at the bar	

THERAPIST: That is losing a lot. How was the breakup of that relationship connected to your drinking?

After exploring the consequences of drinking and drug use, the therapist may begin to elicit reasons for continuing to drink or use drugs. This may begin with a summary statement and open-ended question:

THERAPIST: You have told me a lot about the losses you've experienced as a result of your drinking in the past, as well as what could happen in the near future if you don't change or cut back on your drinking. You have been so clear about what drinking has cost you and what you are risking now due to your drinking. Help me understand some of the good things about drinking that motivate you to continue to drink in spite of the losses or threats to your future.

CLIENT: I ask myself the same question sometimes. It's more of a habit than anything else. I get off work and get together with my friends, Tito and Josh, and that's what we do. We drink.

THERAPIST: So you've wondered yourself what the attraction is to drinking. You think it's a way of life for you and your friends.

CLIENT: I wouldn't say a way of life, but yeah, it's how we spend our time together.

THERAPIST: What would happen if you didn't drink when you got together with Tito and Josh?

CLIENT: I don't know. I haven't tried it, but I don't think it would be much fun.

THERAPIST: It's hard to imagine not drinking when you're with your friends. In fact, it might even be boring without the alcohol.

CLIENT: It's boring now, sometimes. I tell Tito and Josh I'm going home after the bar closes, but then I end up drinking some more.

THERAPIST: You find yourself drinking with Josh and Tito, and staying out late even when you aren't having fun. What would happen if you didn't go out with them one weekend?

CLIENT: My sister tells me, "Stay home." I've done that and it's worse.

THERAPIST: Staying home is not the solution for you.

CLIENT: I'm lonely and I get depressed. So I usually end up looking for my friends at the bar.

THERAPIST: It's hard for you to be alone.

CLIENT: Yeah. That's been true since I was a kid. I get depressed.

THERAPIST: And maybe drinking helps you deal with the depression.

CLIENT: Yeah. Drinking and playing pool.

After adequately exploring the pros and cons of alcohol and drug use, this open-ended portion of the motivational interview ends with a summary. At this time, the information contained in the Decisional Balance Sheet is offered back to the client:

THERAPIST: So, let me see if I am following you here. On the one hand, you have a hard time staying away from the bars and your drinking friends. Loneliness and depression motivate you to seek them out even when you're trying not to go out. On the other hand, your partying on the weekends involves drinking to the extent that you are suffering from headaches and tiredness, and this is causing some difficulties at your job. While you like to play pool and drink with your friends, it is important for you to keep your job and your apartment, and if you lose your housing, you risk being on the streets, where you have been before. Now you are noticing a change in your health.

Providing "Check-Up" Feedback

Several studies suggest that personalized feedback is often effective at reducing levels of alcohol consumption (Baer et al., 1992; Miller et al., 1988, 1993), even when such feedback is merely mailed to the drinker and no face-to-face meeting occurs (Agostinelli, Brown, & Miller, 1995; Walters, Bennett, & Miller, 2000). Most feedback mechanisms for alcohol, such as the DCU (Miller et al., 1988), include quantity/frequency information, peak blood alcohol levels, tolerance and other risk factors, and norm comparisons. Other feedback forms (e.g., Walters, 2000) have included information shown to be particularly motivational for a specific population, such as percentage of income spent on alcohol and hours spent intoxicated versus hours spent studying (for college students). The therapist may choose to use the DCU developed for motivational enhancement therapy procedures or develop a unique "check-up" based on the agency's pretreatment alcohol and drug assessment. In any case, it is a good idea to provide the feedback session in close time proximity to the initial motivational interview. The following are examples of questions about the feedback that elicit self-motivational statements (Miller & Rollnick, 1991): "What do you make of this? Do the numbers surprise you? Do you notice anything else that concerns you? What part of this concerns you the most? Does this make sense to you?"

Begin the feedback session with an affirmation and check in with the client. Checking in with the client gives the therapist an opportunity to know whether something more immediate needs to be addressed, such as worsening depression, need for medical referral, and so on. If the client detours into another topic that could be addressed in a later session, this should be summarized and noted as something to follow-up on later.

THERAPIST: I'm happy to see you again. You clearly are concerned about the events happening in your life. I am impressed that you have the courage to come in and talk about them. I have what is called a Personal Feedback Form that has information about you based on what you told us during the intake interview and on questionnaires. Before I go over the feedback from your intake, I'd like to hear about how you have been doing since the last time I saw you.

Following a summary of this part of the session, feedback is presented in a written format for the client to view as you are reviewing it. An example of feedback on alcohol use is illustrated in Table 11.2.

THERAPIST: Now let's switch gears. Here is a copy of your Personal Feedback Form. I'd like to begin with information on your drinking. Because alcohol beverages vary in strength, we have converted your drinking pattern into standard drinks. One drink contains about one-half ounce of pure ethyl alcohol. According to what you told us about your typical weekly drinking, you are consuming 67 standard drinks a week, which places you in the 98th percentile of male drinkers. This means that if there

TABLE 11.2. Personal Feedback on Drinking and Norms

Your drinking and drug use	
Standard "drinks" (SDs) per week:	67 SDs
Your drinking compared to U.S. adults (same sex):	98th percentile
Heaviest drinking episode:	36 SDs
Cocaine use:	3 days
Your drug use compared to U.S. adults (same sex):	99th percentile

were 100 men in this room, 98 would be drinking less than you. You and one other would be drinking more than the rest.

CLIENT: Oh yeah? Huh.

THERAPIST: You're not sure what to make of this.

CLIENT: Well, not really. Tito and Josh and I can drink a lot.

THERAPIST: The three of you drink quite heavily sometimes.

CLIENT: Yeah, a lot.

THERAPIST: Maybe more than you planned to sometimes.

CLIENT: Everytime. I say I'll only drink this much, and then I don't stick to what I said I was going to do.

THERAPIST: When you're with Tito and Josh, it's hard to stick to a plan of not drinking as much as they are.

CLIENT: Yeah.

THERAPIST: Let's look at how much you drank during one of your heaviest drinking episodes. Based on what you told us, you drank 24 beers in one day. That was, like, twice what you normally drink.

CLIENT: Yeah, and I drove, too.

THERAPIST: You were also driving that day. What do you think about that?

CLIENT: I could have ended up in jail.

Exploring Values and Goals

Another technique for building discrepancy is to explore how substance use is inconsistent with a client's personal values or goals.

THERAPIST: You mentioned in your intake that you've been arrested for driving while intoxicated and have spent time in jail. What was that like?

CLIENT: That was awful. I hated it.

THERAPIST: You hated it. What was the worst part?

CLIENT: You have nothing to do. It smells bad. People are hitting on you for something. I hate being locked up and not being able to do what I want.

THERAPIST: Sounds pretty bad. One thing that seems very important to you is to have freedom to do what you want.

CLIENT: Yeah.

THERAPIST: It looks like you took a risk of going back to jail just a few weeks ago.

CLIENT: Yeah. I had a bad headache and missed work the next day. It wasn't worth it.

THERAPIST: It wasn't worth the risk of being arrested or what it cost you the next day.

CLIENT: Right.

THERAPIST: Getting back to your feedback form, let's take a look at what you told us about your recent use of substances besides alcohol. In the past month, you told us that you smoked crack cocaine three times.

CLIENT: Yeah.

THERAPIST: Based on what we know, most men (99%) don't smoke crack, so any use puts you into a very small group. What do you think about that?

CLIENT: Not much.

THERAPIST: So nothing comes to mind when you compare your drug use to that of other men.

CLIENT: I know most people don't smoke crack.

THERAPIST: You know that it's an uncommon practice.

CLIENT: I usually only do it when I'm seriously drunk. It's something to do to get high.

THERAPIST: You're likely to smoke crack at times when you are most intoxicated.

CLIENT: I was smoking that night I was driving drunk.

THERAPIST: You take more risks when you smoke crack.

CLIENT: I don't think I would have been driving if I hadn't smoked crack.

As already mentioned, asking the question "What else?" is a strategy to elicit more about a specific area of concern, or information about other areas not yet brought up by the client.

THERAPIST: What else about your crack use worries you?

CLIENT: The times I spit up blood. That happens when I'm smoking crack.

THERAPIST: So one of the most worrisome physical effects that you're experiencing is connected to the crack.

CLIENT: I think I'm drinking too much when I smoke crack. I must be bleeding from somewhere, like my stomach. I could be sick.

THERAPIST: You're worried about what your crack use is doing to your health. Tell me more about your concerns.

CLIENT: When I had hepatitis, I had to stay home all the time.

THERAPIST: You've already experienced what it would be like to be that sick and it really limited what you could do.

CLIENT: Yeah.

THERAPIST: Again, you've brought up how you value your freedom to do things on your own, and being sick limits that.

CLIENT: Yeah.

THERAPIST: By drinking and smoking crack, you're risking your health and the freedom that comes with it to be on your own.

CLIENT: Yeah. I hadn't looked at it that way, but probably what makes me feel the best is being on my own right now.

THERAPIST: Being on your own?

CLIENT: My apartment and now answering to anybody at home.

THERAPIST: So while you get lonely sometimes, you like having your own place and the freedom to do what you like. What happens if you don't change the drinking and drug use?

CLIENT: I'll lose it all.

THERAPIST: You'll lose what is most important to you.

Moving from Phase 1 to Phase 2: Recognizing Readiness for Change

Phase 1 strategies are aimed at tipping the client's decisional balance in favor of change. It is useful to close Phase 1 with a summary that pulls together the client's self-motivational statements from the open motivational interview and the feedback sessions. As clients become more motivated, they tend to stop offering objections, to appear more resolved, and to talk about what it would be like to change. For many clients, there may not be a clear point of decision or determination for change. They may shift back to contemplating change by the next session or waffle about their plans. Clients may also be ambivalent about changing one substance while they are abstaining or cutting back on another. They may be ambivalent about change while attempting to change. A client may get discouraged or frustrated and question his or her choice to change (e.g., "Life isn't so great now that I'm sober. At least when I was drunk, I could get away from all these problems"). Phase 1 strategies can be employed toward resolving ambivalence at any point (e.g., "You feel discouraged. Maybe we should go back over what led to your decision to change. What was going to happen if you didn't stop your drinking?").

Miller and Rollnick have begun incorporating "Readiness Rulers" as brief strategies for assessing motivation for change. Clients are asked to rate how ready they are for change on a scale of 0 to 10: 0, "not at all," and 10, "extremely ready." When a client responds at a low level, the therapist may ask what it would take to get to a higher number of the scale, as a strategy for exploring ambivalence or obstacles to change (or conversely, why the client is not at an even lower number).

CLIENT: I'm at about a 5.

THERAPIST: Although you are interested in changing, you aren't feeling strongly about it.

CLIENT: Right. I know that when I get depressed, I'll want to go out and drink.

THERAPIST: So, maybe if you had other ways of dealing with your feelings, you'd be more ready to cut back the drinking?

CLIENT: Yeah.

When a client indicates that he or she is ready to consider moving forward by cutting back or abstaining from drinking and drug use, it is time to move to Phase 2. This is then followed with a key question, such as "Where would you like to go from here? Now that you've shared these concerns, what would you like to do about them? So what do you think you'd like to do about your drinking?" For example, to the question "What would you like to do about the drinking and crack cocaine?" our client responded:

CLIENT: I'm ready to stop smoking crack, but I'm not ready to quit drinking.

In some cases, such as persons with dual diagnoses, clients will be ready to take action on another problem area that may or may not be related to their drinking and drug use (e.g., depression). It is consistent with a motivational interviewing style to accept what is important to the client. Respond with empathic reflection and develop the change plan with the client's agenda for change.

PHASE 2: STRENGTHENING COMMITMENT TO CHANGE

Following a clear statement of intent to change, you may strengthen the commitment to change by asking open-ended questions about the benefits:

THERAPIST: What are some of the good things about quitting crack?

CLIENT: My health. I am scared about spitting up blood.

THERAPIST: That frightens you. It worries me, too. What about the alcohol? What would be good about cutting back on your drinking?

CLIENT: My boss would back off. My sister wouldn't worry so much.

THERAPIST: You would feel more secure at work, and you would be helping your sister to feel better about you. You care about her.

CLIENT: Well, I care about her, but I care more about being left alone!

THERAPIST: You don't want people to be bugging you about what you're doing.

CLIENT: Got that right.

THERAPIST: Well, it gets back to being independent and being on your own. It's important not to make explanations or feel bad about what you are doing. What does it take not to be constantly monitored by other people?

CLIENT: Not using drugs, for one thing.

THERAPIST: Your independence is important to you. Maybe we could work on a plan to help you keep your apartment and job, and the freedom that comes with them, as well as getting others to back off from keeping track of what you're doing.

CLIENT: I'd like that, but I know what you're going to say is that I have to stop drinking.

THERAPIST: What do you think you should do about your drinking?

CLIENT: I shouldn't drink so much.

THERAPIST: You think it's a good idea to cut back on your drinking.

Developing a Change Plan

Toward the development of a change plan, it can be helpful to conduct a functional analysis. Derived from social learning theory, a functional analysis is a breakdown of the sequence of events that lead up to a drinking or drug-using situation. This procedure, often referred to as a SORC analysis, determines the external Situations; internal Organismic states, including cognitions; Responses or operant behaviors; and Consequences of a drinking or drug-using episode. The Situations and Organismic states are called "triggers" to drinking or drug using. The Consequences are the effects associated with drinking and drug abuse that reinforce the use. The New Roads Brainstorm List, illustrated in Table 11.3, is one exercise that follows a functional-analytic strategy to help clients see that risky drinking behavior has both antecedents and consequences (Miller & Pechacek, 1987). For example, when a client drinks alcohol to move from a negativity to a more desirable state, alcohol functions as a path. For this exercise, the client is asked first to list situations in which he or she is likely to feel like using alcohol. The therapist records the answers in a column under the Triggers heading:

THERAPIST: What I'd like to do now is find out a little about how you see your drinking. When do you most feel like using alcohol? In what situations is it hardest not to use alcohol? What feelings do you have before you drink?

To the right of the Triggers column, is a second column, Effects. Now the client is asked to describe the positive or desirable effects of alcohol:

THERAPIST: What do you like about your drinking? What are the positives? What does it do for you that you like? What are some of the good things about drinking?

In the third step, the therapist draws lines from items in the Triggers column to items in the Effects column that link particular antecedents with their related consequences. For example, "shyness" in the Triggers column might be connected with "feel more comfortable" in the Effects column. In connecting antecedents and consequences, the therapist may find that some items have no corresponding partner in the opposite column. In this case, something is missing from the other list, and the corresponding trigger or effect must be found. At the end, every item on one list should be connected to one (or more) item(s) on the other list. The therapist, who finally can discuss a list of alternatives to drinking, asks the client, "If you chose not to drink, how else might you get from these triggers to these effects?" This begins the search for alternative coping strategies. For

TABLE 11.3. New Roads Brainstorm List

Triggers	Effects
Insomnia	Relieve craving
Fear	Courage
Depression	Accepted by others
Anger	Get to sleep
At bar	Forget, escape
Thirsty	Feel good
Peer pressure	Quench thirst

Note. Data from Miller and Pechacek (1987).

example, possible alternatives for feeling good would be both to increase pleasurable activities and practice methods that challenge negative cognitions. Figure 11.1 illustrates a portion of a Change Plan Worksheet that might result from the New Roads process of identifying alternative paths and the related goals that would address drinking and drug-use goals.

ADAPTING MOTIVATIONAL INTERVIEWING FOR SPECIAL POPULATIONS

Over the past two decades, motivational interviewing and motivational enhancement therapy have yielded beneficial effects in decreasing alcohol consumption and substance use in more than two-dozen clinical trials with diverse populations, including adolescents (Aubrey, 1998), pregnant problem drinkers (Handmaker, Miller, & Manicke, 1999), persons with severe mental illness and comorbid substance use disorders (Daley, Salloum, Zuckoff, Kirisci, & Thase, 1998; Swanson, Pantalon, & Cohen, 1999), binge-drinking college students (Borsari & Carey, 2000), and patients specifically hospitalized for alcohol-related accidents (Gentilello et al., 1999). Motivational interviewing has been used to address marijuana (Stephens, Roffman, Cleaveland, Curtin, & Wertz, 1994), nicotine (Butler et al., 1999), and opiate (Saunders, Wilkinson, & Phillips, 1995) use in a variety of settings and shows an efficacy comparable to other treatments (Burke, Arkowitz, & Dunn, 2002; Miller, Zweben, DiClemente, & Rychtarik, 1995). Most studies have used

---

The changes I want to make are:

    Drink no more than 3 drinks per occasion three times per week.

    Abstain from cocaine and other drugs.

    Learn new skills to:

        Cope with negative moods.

        Manage anger.

        Deal with cravings and urges.

        Refuse alcohol and drugs.

    Increase pleasurable activities other than drinking and using drugs.

    Play pool at nondrinking locations.

FIGURE 11.1. Sample Change Plan Worksheet.

motivational interviewing as a stand-alone intervention rather than as an addition to more extensive clinical treatment. The specific format of motivational interviewing has varied in length from a single counseling session (e.g., Butler et al., 1999) to a two-session assessment and feedback approach (e.g., Miller et al., 1988), to the four-session motivational enhancement therapy (Miller, Zweben, et al., 1995).

There are a few points to keep in mind when adapting motivational interviewing or feedback interventions for a specific population. The first point is the nature of the population and what constitutes problematic alcohol or drug use. The personalized feedback, of course, would be adapted for that specific population. For example, there is no safe level of alcohol consumption during pregnancy. Consequently, the use of population normative data in a feedback "check-up" would not be appropriate. A second point to consider is the goal of the motivational interviewing session. Is referral to treatment the goal? Or to increase treatment adherence? Is the motivational interview a stand-alone treatment option or a prelude to another intensive change effort? The goal of the intervention will determine the focus of the session and the nature of the feedback. For example, Daley and Zuckoff (1998) provided a motivational session for persons with mental illness while they were in a psychiatric hospital, with the goal of increasing the likelihood that they would attend an initial outpatient aftercare session within the dual-diagnosis program. The focus of the intervention was resolving ambivalence about engaging in outpatient care. Alternately, Brown and Miller (1993) tailored their motivational "check-up" session as a prelude to an inpatient chemical dependence program. A third point to consider when adapting motivational interviewing has to do with the available resources. Feedback that was mailed out reached more college-age binge drinkers than alternatives and was more effective at decreasing drinking (Walters, 2000). In primary health care settings, health care practitioners are limited to brief consultations about health behaviors. Consequently, motivational interventions aimed at substance use reduction will need to adapt to the limited time and lack of training among health care practitioners in counseling methods.

SUMMARY AND CONCLUSIONS

Motivational interviewing has been shown to yield consistent, beneficial treatment effects. Even in the relative brevity of a single session, marked and sometimes profound effects have been found (Handmaker et al., 1999), and the largest demonstrated effects from clinical trials of motivational interviewing have been with those persons most seriously addicted (Bien, Miller, & Boroughs, 1993; Brown & Miller, 1993; Handmaker et al., 1999). Furthermore, the outcomes from motivational interviewing seem relatively enduring.

The overwhelming impact of this approach has led researchers to ask what accounts for its success (Miller, 2000). The answer may lie in the empathic counseling approach used in motivational interviewing. Miller believes it is the interpersonal context created by the therapist attributes and skills that inspires change. Said more resolutely, William Miller suggests that agape, a selfless, accepting, sacred form of loving, explains the profound effects of motivational interviewing. He describes this love in the context of the critical conditions of change outlined years ago by Carl Rogers (1957): unconditional regard, acceptance, and profound respect. Miller adds selflessness, patience, and hope to the interpersonal style of an effective therapist. Whether it is the transforming power of love or other, rival hypotheses that account for the effects of motivational interviewing are explorations for the future. Finding the source of transforming therapeutic effects is likened by Miller to the "rediscovery of fire."

REFERENCES

Agostinelli, G., Brown, J. M., & Miller, W. R. (1995). Effects of normative feedback on consumption among heavy drinking college students. *Journal of Drug Education, 25*, 31–40.

Aubrey, L. L. (1998). *Motivational interviewing with adolescents presenting for outpatient substance abuse treatment.* Unpublished doctoral dissertation, University of New Mexico, Albuquerque.

Baer, J. S., Marlatt, G. A., Kivlahan, D. R., Fromme, K., Larimer, M. E., & Williams, E. (1992). An experimental test of three methods of alcohol reduction with young adults. *Journal of Consulting and Clinical Psychology, 60*(6), 974–979.

Bein, T. H., Miller, W. R., & Boroughs, J. M. (1993). Motivational interviewing with alcohol outpatients. *Behavioural and Cognitive Psychotherapy, 21*, 347–356.

Borsari, B., & Carey, K. B. (2000). Effects of a brief motivational intervention with college student drinkers. *Journal of Consulting and Clinical Psychology, 68*(4), 728–733.

Brown, J. M., & Miller, W. R. (1993). Impact of motivational interviewing on participation and outcome in residential alcoholism treatment. *Psychology of Addictive Behaviors, 7*, 211–218.

Burke, B. L., Arkowitz, H., & Dunn, C. (2002). The efficacy of motivational interviewing and its adaptations: What we know so far. In W. R. Miller & S. Rollnick (Eds.), *Motivational interviewing: Preparing people for change* (2nd ed., pp. 217–250) New York: Guilford Press.

Butler, C. C., Rollnick, S., Cohen, D., Russel, I., Bachmann, M., & Stott, N. (1999). Motivational consulting versus brief advice for smokers in general practice: A randomised trial. *British Journal of General Practice, 49*, 611–616.

Daley, D. C., Salloum, I. M., Zuckoff, A., Kirisci, L., & Thase, M. E. (1998). Increasing treatment adherence among outpatients with depression and cocaine dependence: Results of a pilot study. *American Journal of Psychiatry, 155*, 1611–1613.

Daley, D. C., & Zuckoff, A. (1998). Improving compliance with the initial outpatient session among discharged inpatient dual diagnosis clients. *Social Work, 43*, 470–473.

Gentilello, L. M., Rivara, F. P., Donovan, D. M., Jurkovich, G. J., Daranciang, E., Dunn, C. W., Villaveces, A., Copass, M., & Ries, R. (1999). Alcohol interventions in a trauma center as a means of reducing the risk of injury recurrence. *Annals of Surgery, 230*(4), 473–483.

Handmaker, N. S., Miller, W. R., & Manicke, M. (1999). Findings of a pilot study of motivational interviewing with pregnant drinkers. *Journal of Studies on Alcohol, 60*, 285–287.

Leake, G. J., & King, A. S. (1977). Effect of counselor expectations on alcoholic recovery. *Alcohol Health and Research World, 11*(3), 16–22.

Miller, W. R. (2000). Rediscovering fire: Small interventions, large effects. *Psychology of Addictive Behaviors, 14*(1), 6–18.

Miller, W. R., Benefield, R. G., & Tonigan, J. S. (1993). Enhancing motivation for change in problem drinking: A controlled comparison of two therapist styles. *Journal of Consulting and Clinical Psychology, 61*, 455–461.

Miller, W. R., Brown, J. M., Simpson, T. L., Handmaker, N. S., Bien, T. H., Luckie, L. F., Montgomery, H. A., Hester, R. K., & Tonigan, J. S. (1995). What works? A methodological analysis of the alcohol treatment outcome literature. In R. K. Hester & W. R. Miller (Eds.), *Handbook of alcoholism treatment approaches: Effective alternatives* (2nd ed., pp. 12–44). Needham Heights, MA: Allyn & Bacon.

Miller, W. R., & Pechacek, T. F. (1987). New roads: Assessing and treating psychological dependence. *Journal of Substance Abuse Treatment, 4*, 73–77.

Miller, W. R., & Rollnick, S. (1991). *Motivational interviewing: Preparing people to change addictive behavior.* New York: Guilford Press.

Miller, W. R., Sovereign, R. G., & Krege, B. (1988). Motivational interviewing with problem drinkers: II. The Drinker's Check-Up as a preventive intervention. *Behavioural Psychotherapy, 16,* 251–268.

Miller, W. R., Zweben, A., DiClemente, C. C., & Rychtarik, R. G. (1995). *Motivational enhancement therapy manual* (Project MATCH Monograph Series, Vol. 2). Rockville, MD: National Institute on Alcohol Abuse and Alcoholism.

Prochaska, J. O., DiClemente, C. C., & Norcross, J. C. (1992). In search of how people change: Applications to the addictive behaviors. *American Psychologist, 47,* 1102–1114.

Project MATCH Research Group. (1997). Matching alcoholism treatments to client heterogeneity: Project MATCH posttreatment drinking outcomes. *Journal of Studies on Alcohol, 58,* 7–29.

Project MATCH Research Group. (1998). Matching alcoholism treatments to client heterogeneity: Project MATCH three-year drinking outcomes. *Alcoholism: Clinical and Experimental Research, 23*(60), 1300–1311.

Rogers, C. R. (1957). The necessary and sufficient conditions for therapeutic personality change. *Journal of Consulting Psychology, 21,* 95–103.

Rollnick, S., & Miller, W. R. (1995). What is motivational interviewing? *Behavioural and Cognitive Psychotherapy, 23,* 325–334.

Saunders, B., Wilkinson, C., & Phillips, M. (1995). The impact of a brief motivational intervention with opiate users attending a methadone program. *Addiction, 90,* 415–424.

Stephens, R. S., Roffman, R. A., Cleaveland, B. L., Curtin, L., & Wert, J. (1994, November). *Extended versus minimal intervention with marijuana dependent adults.* Paper presented at the annual meeting of the Association for Advancement of Behavior Therapy, San Diego, CA.

Swanson, A., Pantalon, M. V., & Cohen, K. R. (1999). Motivational interviewing and treatment adherence among dually-diagnosed patients. *Journal of Nervous and Mental Disease, 187*(10), 630–636.

Truax, C. B., & Carkhuff, R. R. (1967). *Toward effective counseling and psychotherapy.* Chicago: Aldine.

Walters, S. T. (2000). In praise of feedback: An effective intervention for college students who are heavy drinkers. *Journal of American College Health, 48,* 235–238.

Walters, S. T., Bennett, M. E., & Miller, J. E. (2000). Reducing alcohol use in college students: A controlled trial of two brief interventions. *Journal of Drug Education, 30*(3), 361–372.

12

Cognitive-Behavioral Therapy for Alcohol Addiction

TRACY A. O'LEARY
PETER M. MONTI

The core elements of cognitive-behavioral therapy for alcohol problems are coping and social skills training (CSST). For nearly 30 years, CSST has predominated the research literature as one of the most effective treatments for alcohol abuse and dependence. CSST is firmly grounded in a social learning theoretical foundation (Monti, Abrams, Kadden, & Cooney, 1989). In social learning theory (Abrams & Niaura, 1987; Bandura, 1977), the phenomenon of alcohol abuse is explained by the immediate cognitive and environmental determinants of drinking behavior, referred to as proximal determinants (Abrams & Niaura, 1987), which include the environmental setting, expectations and beliefs, general and drinking-specific coping skills, and the person's emotional, physiological, and cognitive state during the drinking episode (Abrams, 1983). Decisions about drinking are governed by both self-efficacy and outcome expectations. If one's outcome expectations are heavily weighted toward short-term reinforcing effects of alcohol and other positive outcome expectancies from drinking, and these are not countered by awareness of the long-term negative consequences of alcohol misuse, excessive alcohol use may result. Social learning theory is also grounded in cognitive and behavioral factors that moderate and influence person–environment interactions.

Today CSST includes a variety of tailored protocols and programs for prevention and treatment across the spectrum of addictive behaviors, including alcohol, cocaine, and tobacco abuse (Abrams et al., 1991, 1992; Monti & Rohsenow, 1999; Monti, Rohsenow, Colby, & Abrams, 1995b; Monti, Rohsenow, Michalec, Martin, & Abrams, 1997; Rohsenow, Monti, Martin, Michalec, & Abrams, 2000). CSST has been applied in a broad range of settings and interventions, such as early intervention/prevention work in schools (Botvin, Baker, Dusenbury, Tortu, & Botvin, 1990), brief interventions such as the Drinker's Check-Up (Miller & Sovereign, 1989), and motivational enhancement approaches (e.g. Monti, Colby, et al., 1999), behavioral couple therapy (O'Farrell, 1994), relapse prevention (Marlatt & Gordon, 1985), community reinforcement (Higgins, Sigmon, & Budney, Chapter 15, this volume), and cue exposure (Monti et al., 1993b).

The major aim of most CSST approaches for alcohol problems is to enhance one's repertoire of adaptive coping skills for managing real-life situations and events that are "high risk" for relapsing back to problematic alcohol use. A major assumption of CSST is that individuals with alcohol problems lack adequate coping skills due to deficits in affect regulation and in handling interpersonal situations. Coping skills deficits can be the result of person–environment interactions. For example, an individual with a biological predisposition toward alcohol abuse who experiences precipitating stressful environmental demands, such as chronic life stress (e.g., disability, unemployment) and/or the buildup of daily hassles (e.g., relationship problems) may be at heightened risk for using alcohol to cope with problems (Monti et al., 1989). In support of this, Brown, Vik, Patterson, Grant, and Schuckit (1995) found that among individuals with alcohol problems who experienced severe psychosocial stressors, those with improvements in coping skills and social networks had better outcomes after treatment than those who did not.

Using adaptive coping skills in an environment marked by peer pressure to drink and drinking cues can be especially difficult. While in treatment, clients are encouraged to avoid high-risk situations for alcohol use. However, complete avoidance of all alcohol-related cues and situations is neither pragmatic nor realistic. Seeing television advertisements for alcoholic beverages, going to holiday parties, and being asked if one would care for a cocktail before the meal when dining out at a restaurant are commonplace examples of the pervasiveness of alcohol in our culture. Because of this, helping clients to cope with exposure to alcohol cues can be an effective answer to this dilemma. Thus, controlled exposure to alcohol cues plus response prevention has been recently incorporated in several CSST interventions (Monti et al., 1993b, 2001), and our cue exposure treatment (CET) is a standard part of our CSST package (see Rohsenow, Niaura, Childress, Abrams, & Monti, 1990, for a complete discussion of the clinical implications of cue reactivity).

There are four primary content areas in CSST: (1) interpersonal skills for enhancing relationships; (2) cognitive-emotional coping skills for affect regulation; (3) coping skills for managing daily life events, stressful events, and high-risk situations for drinking; and (4) coping with alcohol use cues. Cognitive coping skills include strategies both to cope with psychophysiological or cognitive reactions associated with urges or cravings to drink and to increase self-efficacy in remaining abstinent from alcohol in high-risk situations. Interpersonal skills include techniques to increase positive social interactions and self-confidence, and to minimize negative social interactions and avoidance of others.

In this chapter, we present our model of CSST for alcohol dependence. We also review the assessment and treatment interventions for the model and present empirical evidence of the effectiveness of CSST.

CLIENT CHARACTERISTICS AND SPECIAL CONSIDERATIONS

Cognitive Impairments Due to Intoxication/Withdrawal

When our CSST package was initially developed and tested, treatment for substance abuse was commonly in the form of a 28-day rehabilitation program. Today, the bulk of substance abuse treatment services are delivered in short-term outpatient sessions, with more severely dependent patients and those with co-occurring psychopathology receiving inpatient or partial hospitalization care, along with briefer lengths of stay in the hospital. Because of these factors, we generally begin CSST with clients as soon after admission as possible—3–4 days after substance use ceases and/or detoxification begins. A byproduct of this relatively rapid introduction of CSST is that we treat more clients with mild to moderate cognitive impairment secondary to their substance use or detoxification. Some researchers have raised the concern that because of possible cognitive impairment, clients may not fully benefit from cognitive-behavioral coping skills early in treatment (e.g., Allen, Goldstein, & Seaton, 1997; Schafer et al., 1991; Smith & McCrady, 1991). However, CSST in its original form was expressly designed and developed for individuals with severe psychiatric impairment (Monti, Corriveau, & Curran, 1982; Monti & Kolko, 1985) and was based on a solid foundation of behavioral components. For these reasons, CSST may be more appropriate in early treatment of substance abuse than other forms of therapy. An important feature of our CSST package is the deliberate introduction of more cognitively complex material later in the treatment, so as to allow for better integration of cognitive skills that result from improvements in cognitive functioning following abstinence (see Mann, Gunther, Stetter, & Ackermann, 1999). In addition, we have found that clients from a wide range of educational levels benefit from CSST, further bolstering the argument that CSST is appropriate for individuals regardless of their educational attainments (Rohsenow, Monti, Binkoff, & Liepman, 1991). The content and structure of CSST are in large part responsible for its broad applicability. Using concrete examples, using the client's own preferred beverage in CET, teaching one specific skill in separate session modules, role-playing skills in subsequent sessions, assigning intersession homework, and providing immediate feedback to clients—all of these aspects of CSST contribute to more rapid, effective, and efficient learning and retention.

Cue Reactivity and Cue Exposure Issues

On occasion, we have had clients adamantly tell us prior to the first session of CET that they do not have urges and therefore cannot see how the treatment will benefit them. We have also had clients tell us after completing CET that they initially thought it would be easy for them to pick up their preferred beverage and sniff it. Still others express concerns that they are wasting our time being in CET because they are 100% committed to abstinence and have no desire to drink again. The reality for most of our clients is that they are typically quite taken aback by the strong physical and emotional impact they experience during CET. The experience of going through CET is invaluable to many clients in terms of understanding firsthand the concept of automaticity of urges to drink and learning to apply coping skills during actual urges to drink.

Clients vary in their degree of cue reactivity during CET, which in turn has implications for their outcomes. Studies from our lab have demonstrated that cue reactors—those who report increased urge to drink and have increased salivation in response to the sight and smell of alcohol—appear more responsive to alcohol cues (Monti et al., 1993a, 1993b; Rohsenow et al., 1992). Conceptually, therefore, it could be argued that cue reactors would derive more benefit from CET than nonreactors. However, in another study from our lab, increased salivation during cue reactivity was associated with increased drinking after treatment (Rohsenow et al., 1994). These findings underscore the importance of helping clients to become more adept at identifying their own physiological, interoceptive sensations during alcohol exposure. Such sensations may include increased heart rate, mouth watering, swallowing, and stomach grumbling. By increasing awareness of one's own physical reactions to the presence of alcohol cues, the individual can learn to apply coping skills in the presence of those reactions irrespective of urge levels.

Setting

Currently, no data support the superiority of group versus individual formats for CSST; both approaches can be effective. Traditionally, we have conducted our CSST clinical trials in group-based substance abuse programs within inpatient and partial hospital formats. There are several advantages to group CSST, including efficiency and economy of treating individuals within a group, the ease of doing behavioral rehearsal role plays and giving/receiving feedback from group members, and the support and encouragement that the group members provide for each other in their mutual and public commitment to sobriety. Most significantly, the behavioral rehearsal role plays, which are considered the seminal elements of CSST, are usually much more realistic and impactful when clients' peers are involved. Indeed, there is some evidence that group skills training is better than individual skills training in terms of more rapid gains in social skills (Oei & Jackson, 1980), although reductions in drinking rates tend to be similar across both group and individual formats (e.g., Graham, Annis, Brett, & Venesoen, 1996; Oei & Jackson, 1980).

Extending Coping and Social Skills Training to Significant Others/Family

A more recent line of clinical research has focused on the benefits of including a spouse or partner in cognitive-behavioral treatments for alcohol abuse (cf. Epstein & McCrady, 1998). For example, studies have found that individuals with alcohol problems and their partners who receive couple-based relapse prevention programs with behavioral couple therapy for alcohol abuse report better relationship as well as drinking outcome results compared to those receiving behavioral marital therapy alone (O'Farrell, Choquette, & Cutter, 1998; O'Farrell, Choquette, Cutter, Brown, & McCourt, 1993). In addition, studies show that including a behavioral couple component in alcohol treatment results in more significantly improved drinking and marital outcomes than when focusing on individual alcohol treatment alone (e.g., McCrady, Stout, Noel, Abrams, & Nelson, 1991). Monti and colleagues (1990) compared a communication skills training group (CST), a communication skills training group with family participation (CSTF), and a cognitive-behavioral mood management training group (CBMMT), and found that individuals receiving CST or CSTF drank significantly less alcohol per drinking day during 6-month follow-up than those in CBMMT, with no differences between individuals receiving CST versus CSFT. Clearly, there appear to be benefits of including family or significant others in alcohol treatment, but the findings from Monti and colleagues suggest that there are no additive effects of including a family member or spouse above and beyond the overall effectiveness of CSST.

Individual versus Group Format

For some therapists, it may not be possible to conduct CSST in a group setting due to the nature of their professional setting (e.g., exclusively individual outpatient services, consultations, etc.). Doing CSST with clients individually can be just as effective and has the advantage of being tailored exclusively to that particular client's needs, issues, and high-risk situations. It is important for therapists to assign a sufficient amount of intersession homework to clients in individual-format CSST in order for generalization to occur. In the case of CET homework, clients would, of course, not be encouraged to expose themselves to the sight and smell of alcohol outside of the safety of treatment. Rather, the therapist should promote homework assignments that center on urge-coping skills to deal with naturally occurring urges between sessions.

ALCOHOL COPING SKILLS TRAINING: ASSESSMENT

Coping Skills Assessment

In lieu of observing individuals in their natural environment, the best means for assessing coping skills are via role-play assessments. Three role-play assessment instruments measuring reactions to simulated high-risk situations have shown predictive validity: the Situational Competency Test (Chaney, O'Leary, & Marlatt, 1978), the Adaptive Skills Battery (Jones & Lanyon, 1981), and the Alcohol-Specific Role Play Test (ASRPT; Abrams et al., 1991; Monti, Rohsenow, et al., 1993). We focus our review on the ASRPT and its most recent iteration, the Coping with Alcohol-Relevant Situations Test (CARS; Colby, Monti, & Rohsenow, 1997).

The ASRPT consists of 10 audiotaped situations (five interpersonal and five intrapersonal) that describe a high risk of relapse to alcohol use. At the end of the description, a prompt asks the client what he or she would do in the situation to keep from drinking. Trained raters evaluate the audiotaped response for coping skills (i.e., the probability of solving the problem or managing affect) and anxiety level. After presentation of each audiotaped situation, the client provides self-reports of urge to drink on a 0–10 scale (0 = "not at all," 10 = "as strong as it gets"), level of perceived difficulty in dealing with the situation if it were to occur in real life, and level of anxiety. Latency to first response is also timed, based on the premise that more rapid and skillful responses are associated with improved outcomes. The ASRPT has demonstrated good interrater reliability and internal consistency (Abrams et al., 1991; Monti, Rohsenow, et al., 1993). In one study, individuals who showed more skillful responses, reported lower urges to drink, and had shorter latencies to respond during the ASRPT, drank significantly less after treatment (Monti et al., 1990).

In developing the ASRPT into the CARS, the major aim was to increase the efficiency and ease of measuring coping skills in clinical settings. Like the ASRPT, the CARS utilizes an audiotaped format and demonstrates good reliability and validity (Colby et al., 1997). Similar to findings on the ASRPT, behavioral measures on the CARS have been shown to predict drinking following alcohol treatment. In support of these findings, one study reported that individuals in alcohol treatment who have more difficulty in role plays do better in coping skills training than in interactional therapy (Kadden, Litt, Cooney, & Busher, 1992). This suggests that deficits in skills, as evidenced during the assessment phase, can later be targeted effectively in coping skills training programs.

Cue Reactivity Assessment

Before beginning CET, the therapist should assess the individual's level of cue reactivity to his or her preferred alcoholic beverage. Our Cue Reactivity Assessment (Monti et al., 1987, 1993a) measures urge to drink and salivation in response to the sight and smell of one's preferred alcoholic beverage, compared to one's reactions in response to a neutral beverage. Information from the assessment can greatly assist the therapist in guiding the client to focus on certain aspects of CET. For example, increased salivation during Cue Reactivity Assessment is related to higher risk of relapse after treatment (Rohsenow et al., 1994). A client who reports no urge to drink but experiences increased salivation may have a false sense of security that he or she is not at risk, based on the lack of urges. In this case, the therapist can coach the client to identify and pay closer attention to physical sensations during CET as a means of practicing coping skills in response to physiological reactions.

In the Cue Reactivity Assessment, alcohol and neutral beverage (e.g., water) cues are presented, followed by self-report measures (urge to drink, anxiety level, amount of attention paid to the stimulus) and physiological measures (salivation, blood pressure, heart rate, prepulse inhibition of the startle reflex). The client is assessed after eating lunch, in order to control for the effects of appetite on urges. The client brushes his or her teeth and then sits at a table in an interview room with a one-way mirror. The assessor, sitting behind the mirror, explains the procedure and forms, and tells the client that he or she will first practice the procedure. The client proceeds to practice holding and sniffing a glass in response to audible tone prompts and inserting cotton rolls in his or her mouth to measure salivation. In front of the client is a glass of water and a commercially labeled bottle of water under one inverted opaque container, and a glass of his or her customary alcoholic beverage and its commercial container under another opaque container. A vial containing the cotton rolls is placed directly in front of each beverage container. The client is reminded that no drinking of any beverage is permitted during the assessment. To the surprise of some, we have never had a client drink during the Cue Reactivity Assessment.

At the beginning of the actual assessment, the client relaxes for 3 minutes and then is prompted by audiotape to insert the cotton rolls in his or her mouth, then uncover the first container (water), hold the glass of water, sniff the water for 3 minutes, wait for the signal to place the water back beneath the opaque container, and remove the cotton rolls from his or her mouth and place them in the vial. The client next completes a self-report rating form (urge level, anxiety level, and amount of attention paid to the cues) and relaxes for 3 minutes. Then, he or she is signaled to insert new cotton rolls and repeat the same procedure with the other container (the alcohol). Before and after the assessment, the cotton rolls are weighed to measure amount of salivation, as it is the psychophysiological response with the most predictive validity (Niaura et al., 1988; Rohsenow et al., 1994). Following the Cue Reactivity Assessment, we review the session with the client and address any untoward reactions that he or she may have had during the assessment. For example, if a client reported continued urges to drink alcohol after the assessment is complete, the therapist would discuss how this is a normal reaction, explain that the urges should abate in a matter of time, and wait with the client until his or her reported urge levels were low before allowing him or her to go home.

Drinking Triggers Interview

Imaginal exposure to several high-risk drinking situations is an essential ingredient in CET. Prior to conducting CET, we use the Drinking Triggers Interview to ask the client about the situations that pose the highest risk of relapse for him or her personally (Monti et al., 1993a). During this interview, we ask the client to describe all personally relevant events or situations frequently associated with heavy drinking, strong urges to drink, and/or difficulty resisting urges in the recent past. For clients who have difficulty in coming up with situations, useful prompts include asking about certain places commonly associated with drinking (bars, home, a friend's house), emotions (e.g., depressed, angry, anxious, stressed), interpersonal conflicts (fight with spouse, disagreement with boss), "drinking buddies," or physical states (e.g., hunger, fatigue, feeling hungover).

After writing down the trigger situations described by the client, the assessor asks the client to rank-order them on the following variables: (1) frequency of occurrence, (2) self-efficacy in refraining from drinking in the situation ("If you were in this situation today and not here in treatment, how confident are you that you would not drink?"), and (3) urge to drink in the situation ("If you were in this situation today and not in treatment, how much would you want to have a drink?"). The client reports his or her rankings on the 0–10 scale. From this information, the assessor develops a hierarchy based on the client's urge to drink ratings, assigning higher rankings for trigger situations with greater urge and frequency ratings. Ideally, the hierarchy should have four to six trigger situations with urge ratings ≥ 4 on the 0–10 scale.

TREATMENT

The elements of CSST fall into two broadly defined skills domains: interpersonal/social skills and intrapersonal skills, which focus on urges and emotions related to an increased likelihood of drinking. CSST focuses primarily on teaching interpersonal skills, while cue exposure with urge-coping skills (CET) teaches intrapersonal skills for managing negative emotions and urges to drink. In the descriptions that follow, we describe CSST and its elements in the context of a group format, as we have conducted the majority of our CSST programs in group settings.

Communication and Social Skills Training (CSST)

Overview

At the start of communication skills training, the therapist reviews the rationale and goals for the skills training. For example, the therapist might begin with the following introduction and rationale:

> "There are many high-risk situations for drinking. Often, these situations involve other people in your life—getting into an argument with your spouse, feeling stressed out about a meeting with your boss, and interacting socially with friends and family are just a few examples. Sometimes people drink to cope with these situations and with negative feelings they might be having, such as feeling angry, frustrated, sad, or lonely. For some people, positive feelings can also be a trigger—wanting to have a good time or to celebrate the end of the work week can be associated with increased urges to drink. Others might have avoided these situations altogether when they were drinking and as a result feel lonely, isolated, and unsure of their ability to cope. The goal of this skills training program is to help you identify some of your own high-risk situations, to practice using skills to cope effectively with them, and to increase your self-confidence in handling these situations and not drinking. Practicing these skills here in treatment will help you to feel more comfortable when you're in similar situations in the future, now that you're in sobriety. This program will help you to improve and enhance your

current relationships, decrease negative interactions with people in your life, and reduce the risk of relapsing back to drinking."

At the beginning of each session, the therapist also discusses the rationale and goals for the specific module being covered, and writes out an outline of the skills session on a large board as a visual aid and prompt, so clients can refer back to the skills guidelines during role plays and thereby strengthen their skills building. It is important to present the skills guidelines as suggestions rather than rules that must be followed exactly. The former approach lets clients know that flexibility is important in skills training and that some skills guidelines may be more or less pertinent to their own high-risk situations. Perhaps most significantly, presenting skills guidelines as suggestions sets the stage for a more collaborative rapport with clients. Obviously, clients who feel that they can freely ask questions, request clarification, and share their perceptions about the skills guidelines tend to engage more in role plays and are more willing to try out the skills both within and outside the session.

After reviewing skills guidelines, the therapist models both ineffective and effective responses to a sample high-risk situation. First, the therapist states the goals of the situation, then models an ineffective response with a cotherapist or group member helping out. The therapist then asks the group for specific feedback and suggestions on how to improve the response (e.g., "Don't raise your voice—keep it low," "Look at the person in the eye when you're talking to them," "Stick to one topic at a time and be brief when you're stating what's bothering you," etc.). After generating a short discussion, the therapist repeats the role play using a more effective response based on the skills guidelines. Again, the group members are asked to share their feedback and talk about the impact of ineffective versus effective responses in meeting the goals of the session.

This is followed by eliciting descriptions of social situations from group members for behavioral rehearsal role plays. Each group member is asked to provide an example of a personally relevant social situation, the same as or similar to the topic of the session, that he or she either has experienced recently or expects to encounter in the near future. It should be a situation that the client feels is not only difficult or challenging, but also personally meaningful to him/her. The therapist can then ask the client in an open-ended manner about the link between the described situation and higher risk of drinking (e.g., "In the past, when you've had a hard day at work dealing with your customers, how did it affect your drinking? What changes can you recall?"). With this guidance most clients understand the relationship between difficult interpersonal situations and increased urges to drink and/or increased drinking. Not only do such questions provide a powerful reminder to clients about the association between these situations and their drinking, but they also help reinforce clients' motivation to engage in the role plays.

Next, each client role-plays the situation with another group member, followed by feedback and suggestions from the rest of the group and the therapist on ways to enhance their responses based on the skills guidelines. True to form, we use the "positive feedback sandwich" technique when giving feedback to clients: (1) praise and recognition of positive aspects of the responses during the role play; (2) constructive feedback on improving the role-play responses, focusing on the one or two most essential and important aspects; and (3) reinforcement for doing the role play and encouragement to repeat it. We cannot overemphasize how vital it is that the behavioral rehearsal role plays be conducted in a nonjudgmental, supportive, and encouraging environment. The burden is on the therapist to ensure that positive communication and constructive criticism are maintained across all group members.

It is not uncommon for some group members (and the occasional therapist!) to experience some performance anxiety before and during the role plays. While validating these feelings of embarrassment or discomfort, the therapist should nonetheless encourage group members to engage in the role plays and inform them that, with time and practice, using the communication skills will be easier and feel more natural. These encouragements are frequently reinforced after clients begin to apply the skills in real-life situations effectively and with positive outcomes. Along these same lines, the therapist should be positive and supportive, giving praise to participants about specific, well-executed, aspects of their performance, and then acknowledge areas that need more practice and attention, so that clients will feel more optimistic about their skills abilities and remain motivated to continue practicing skills in the role plays. This also serves to create a productive, communicative group process, wherein all participants feel secure and supported by the therapist and their fellow group members.

The outline for conducting the behavioral rehearsal role plays is as follows:

1. The therapist briefly summarizes the client's description of the situation to be role-played, reminds the role players to refer to the skills guidelines written on the board during the role play, and instructs them to stay in the role play for 2–5 minutes, until the client has applied the skills.

2. The therapist inquires about the role players' own thoughts, feelings, and reactions to their performance in applying the skills guidelines, giving them the opportunity to voice their opinions about areas of improvement first, which in turn can help increase their sense of control and self-efficacy.

3. The therapist asks the rest of the group for feedback—first, on what they thought worked well, and second, on what observed behaviors needed strengthening. The therapist reminds the group members to be specific about their feedback, for example, "I liked how you maintained eye contact and didn't raise your voice during the role play" is more helpful than "I liked your manner and how you came across," which is too general.

4. After soliciting feedback from the group, the therapist provides constructive feedback on both the positive aspects of the role play and areas that need improvement. Because the therapist asks for the group's feedback first, this is often a brief recapitulation of the main points.

5. The therapist asks the role players to repeat the role play in order to hone their skills and incorporate the feedback.

6. As a final point, the therapist sets the pace for both the session and the role plays. To ensure that sufficient time is spent on the role plays, the therapist should take care to stick to a time frame and avoid lengthy discussions about problem situations, and similarly, focus on only one or two primary areas for improvement.

7. In certain cases, a client may either insist that he or she already uses the skills and does not need to practice them, or that the session module does not apply to him or her. For instance, one of our clients once reported that all of his interpersonal relationships were "excellent" and conflicts rarely, if ever, arose in his life. In our experience conducting communication skills training, clients who report this are usually overestimating their skills level and ability, often without fully realizing it. Rather than try to convince the client otherwise, a better strategy is to simply state, "Yes, there are some skills that perhaps you're already using effectively, and that's great. We believe that even for those of us who are most skilled and comfortable in handling these situations, there is always room for improvement."

Overview of Session Modules

Initially, we developed 13 different topics commonly associated with high-risk situations for drinking into session modules. The reality of managed care makes it increasingly less likely that all modules can be offered to clients, so we have selected eight modules of higher priority, with five additional modules if time allows. The order in which the modules are covered is flexible, depending on the specific issues that clients bring up and/or the level of group functioning. These eight modules are (1) Drink Refusal Skills, (2) Giving Positive Feedback, (3) Giving Criticism, (4) Receiving Criticism about Drinking/Drug Use, (5) Listening Skills, (6) Conversation Skills, (7) Developing Sober Supports, and (8) Conflict Resolution Skills. Time permitting, the other five modules include (1) Nonverbal Communication, (2) Expressing Feelings, (3) Introduction to Assertiveness, (4) Refusing Requests, and (5) Receiving Criticism in General. We describe here the major elements of the rationale and skills guidelines for the first eight modules. At the beginning of the first session, clients are given a brief orientation to the CSST approach, covering the following topics: (1) ground rules such as attendance, policy on abstinence, confidentiality, and dealing with slips and relapses; (2) introduction to CSST; (3) rationale for CSST and its goals; and (4) brief discussion of difficult interpersonal situations and their relationship to relapse for clients. Table 12.1 contains a description and rationale for each module, which the therapist can use to introduce each module. Table 12.2 lists the eight primary modules and their respective skills guidelines. Readers are encouraged to refer to our book (Monti et al., 1989) for complete and detailed descriptions of the session modules and practice exercises.

Cue Exposure with Urge-Specific Coping Skills

Overview

Cue exposure treatment (CET), in its more recent iterations, involves several sessions of clients holding and smelling their preferred and usual alcoholic beverage. The ultimate goal of CET is both to promote clients' habituation to urges to drink and to incorporate coping skills to deal with urges via *in vivo* exposure to alcohol without drinking. Our CET with urge-coping skills consists of 6–10 individual sessions. We have conducted CET in a group format as well, based on data from Pead and colleagues (1993), suggesting that sustained group exposure to alcohol makes the sessions more comparable to real-life alcohol exposure (e.g., sitting at a bar with others present, being at a social gathering, etc.). The aims of most CET approaches are (1) identification of high-risk situations (drinking triggers) that lead to increased urges to drink, (2) exposure to high-risk situations in a controlled environment until the urge to drink diminishes, (3) learning cognitive-behavioral coping skills to manage urges to drink in such situations.

Each session begins for the client with a trial of intensive exposure to his or her favorite, most frequently consumed beverage, served the same way that he or she typically drinks it. Then the therapist conducts one to two trials of imaginal exposure to other drinking triggers, identified during the Drinking Triggers Interview. Clients are instructed to look at the beverage during the exposures and to hold it in their hands as a way to maximize their urges to drink. Clients are instructed to use the new, urge-specific coping skill they learn at each session during the ensuing imaginal exposure to decrease urge to drink. The end of the session is spent reviewing clients' reactions during the exposures and helping to reduce any remaining urge to drink. Finally, clients are

TABLE 12.1. CSST Module Rationales Provided to Clients

Module	Rationale
Drink Refusal Skills	1. A common high-risk situation is being offered a drink or being pressured to drink by others. 2. It takes more than willpower to turn down a drink effectively—it takes assertiveness skills. 3. Because alcohol is so prevalent in our society, it is nearly impossible to avoid all situations involving alcohol. 4. Restaurants, family gatherings, and holidays are common situations involving alcohol. 5. The key is to turn down drink offers quickly and efficiently, without resorting to anger or confrontation.
Giving Positive Feedback	1. Relationships are rewarding and satisfying when we can share positive experiences as well as work on solving problems and issues together. 2. Giving positive feedback is important in nearly all relationships—spouses, children, family, friends, coworkers, supervisors, neighbors, etc. 3. People often fail to give positive feedback. 4. Some people may take others for granted, think others already know how they feel, or be uncomfortable expressing feelings. 5. People with drinking problems often have relationship problems. 6. As problems increase, the positive aspects of the relationship can get overlooked—learning how to give positive feedback can help improve the quality of the relationship.
Giving Criticism	1. It is important to be able to tell people about disagreeable or objectionable behaviors without hurting their feelings or creating an argument. 2. Giving criticism can be difficult for people who have experienced much *destructive*, not constructive, criticism in their lives. 3. To avoid giving constructive feedback to others may make people feel upset, tense, angry, and/or frustrated. 4. These feelings can build up and create an uncomfortable, tense relationship. 5. One might explode at the person or drink to cope with these negative feelings. 6. Giving constructive criticism early on helps to decrease the risk of such events happening and to strengthen the relationship.
Receiving Criticism about Drinking/Drug Use	1. No one likes to receive criticism. 2. However, it can be helpful and enlightening to understand how our behavior might be affecting others and our relationships. 3. By gracefully receiving criticism, we can avoid unnecessary arguments and hurt feelings. 4. This in turn makes getting into larger, more serious conflicts less likely. 5. Serious conflicts are common, high-risk situations for drinking, so learning this skill helps to lessen that risk. 6. With a history of problem drinking, a person is often more susceptible to receiving criticism about past deeds and events related to drinking/drug use. 7. While there is nothing we can do to change the past, there is much we can do in the present and the future to avoid such events. 8. When we acknowledge criticism about past behaviors and drinking, others know that we are trying to address those issues to prevent them from recurring.

(continued)

TABLE 12.1. (continued)

Module	Rationale
Listening Skills	1. Good listening skills allow us to get to know people, feel close to others, and work out problems. 2. Many drinkers report that it was difficult for them to listen effectively while they were drinking—drinking impairs concentration and memory. 3. Practicing these skills in sobriety will help to sharpen them. 4. Many drinkers report feeling lonely; some people drink to cope with loneliness, and others feel lonely because drinking has isolated them from friends and family. 5. Listening skills diminish our loneliness as we repair old relationships and develop new ones.
Conversation Skills	1. Conversation enables us to develop casual as well as more intimate relationships. 2. Because some people drink to feel comfortable socializing, it is key to practice conversation skills without drinking so that we become more comfortable doing it naturally. 3. Others avoid socializing because of difficulty in making conversation, which can lead to high-risk situations such as loneliness, isolation, and boredom. 4. Many people who stop drinking feel lonely and miss socializing with friends who also drink. 5. By building conversation skills, we can begin to meet new people and make friends in sobriety.
Developing Sober Supports	1. Social supports are people in our lives—family, friends, sponsors, acquaintances—who provide moral support and help us cope with problems. 2. These relationships are reciprocal—we, in turn, provide moral and emotional support to those individuals in our lives. 3. People experiencing stressful events do better if they have social support. 4. There are many stresses associated with problem drinking. Chances of successfully coping with these high-risk situations without drinking are improved with a strong social support network. 5. People may be shy about requesting support or may have found that their support networks have dissolved due to their drinking. 6. Building social supports helps us to maintain our sobriety by increasing the network of people we can count on when dealing with stressful events.
Conflict Resolution Skills	1. Many people find it harder to deal with conflicts in close relationships than with acquaintances or strangers. 2. Open and effective communication in close/intimate relationships strengthens that bond, allows for deeper understanding, and makes it less likely that resentment will fester and become a high-risk situation for drinking. 3. Conflict resolution skills draw on all the social skills. 4. The critical ingredient of conflict resolution skills is addressing conflicts and problems quickly, while they are still small.

TABLE 12.2. CSST Skills Guidelines

Module	Skills Guidelines
Drink Refusal Skills	1. Say "no" in a clear, firm, unhesitating voice. 2. Make eye contact with the person. 3. Suggest an alternative activity/food/beverage. 4. Change the subject after saying "no." 5. Avoid excuses or vague answers that don't sound serious, or that suggest that you might change your mind and accept a drink later. 6. Ask the person to stop pressuring you to drink if he or she repeatedly persists in offering you alcohol.
Giving Positive Feedback	1. State your own feelings rather than facts. 2. Be sincere and specific about your feedback—that way, the person knows exactly what you mean, which makes it more likely that he or she will continue to do the behavior or action that you liked again. 3. Don't reject or minimize positive feedback that you receive. 4. Give positive feedback to the person when he or she is not busy or preoccupied, so that he or she can fully appreciate your remarks.
Giving Criticism	1. Wait until you have calmed down first before speaking. 2. State how you feel about the behavior; don't use facts or absolutes. 3. Criticize the behavior, not the person. 4. Use a firm, clear, and nonangry tone of voice. 5. Request a specific behavior change. 6. Be open to compromise. 7. Start and finish on a positive note. 8. Give criticism that is intended to help, not hurt, the person.
Receiving Criticism about Drinking/Drug Use	1. Don't debate, counterattack, or get defensive. 2. Find something to agree with in the criticism. 3. Restate directly and clarify the criticism. 4. Propose a compromise.
Listening Skills	1. Rather than simply waiting for your turn to talk, active listening requires you to attend to the other person *actively* and *purposively*, and try to understand what he or she is saying. 2. Use nonverbal behaviors to demonstrate your interest (maintain eye contact, nod, lean slightly forward). 3. Observe the nonverbal behaviors of the other person, particularly emotional/facial expressions. 4. Ask questions, add comments, and paraphrase. 5. After the other person has completed his or her train of thought, share similar experiences or feelings.
Conversation Skills	1. Listen to and observe the other person, so that you have some ideas about topics of discussion. 2. Choose a time to start a conversation when there is a pause in the person's talk or activity. 3. Use small talk (about weather, sports, current events, hobbies, movies) as a means to get to know others. 4. Conversation is a two-way street—allow the person to speak. 5. It is fine to talk about yourself—you give the other person the chance to learn about you and ask you questions. 6. Use open-ended questions to prompt a response. 7. Observe the other person's nonverbal behaviors and reactions (e.g., looking at watch, shifting weight, looking around the room). 8. If the conversation is winding down, end it gracefully.

(continued)

TABLE 12.2. (continued)

Module	Skills Guidelines
Developing Sober Supports	1. Consider who might be helpful to you in your sobriety. 2. Consider what type of support you need (moral support, problem solving, resources, sharing tasks or responsibilities, etc.). 3. Consider how to get the support you need (asking for help, adding new social supports, giving your support to others, giving feedback about the type of support you need, etc.).
Conflict Resolution Skills	1. You aren't a mind reader—don't expect others to be, either. 2. When something upsets or bothers you, express it directly. 3. Although you are dealing with conflict, it is still essential that you also express positive feelings about your partner. 4. Don't let things build up and fester inside you. 5. It is far easier to resolve smaller problems than a large explosion. 6. Don't "kitchen sink" by stating a laundry list of all the problems or issues. 7. Stick to one point at a time, so that neither of you feels overwhelmed or helpless to solve the problem.

encouraged to practice their new urge-coping skills between sessions when urges to drink arise.

Introduction and Rationale

It can be confusing for clients in treatment programs to participate in CET, when the treatment program personnel are telling them to avoid being near alcohol during their treatment. That is why it is of utmost importance for therapists to explain clearly to clients the rationale for CET. The following major points should be highlighted to clients:

"Many people who have problems with alcohol experience strong urges to drink in high-risk situations. What happens to many people once they begin treatment is that their urges to drink are very low, due to avoidance of trigger situations. While that is a wise strategy in sobriety, you may find that once you leave treatment, your urges to drink become stronger when you encounter high-risk situations. Although planning to avoid trigger situations and drinking settings is best, no one can completely avoid all drinking triggers. For example, you could be out socializing with friends or eating at a restaurant and be offered a drink. Turning on the TV or reading a magazine, you can see advertisements for alcohol any day of the week. In this treatment you will learn to identify your physical and emotional responses to drinking trigger situations. In doing so, you will also learn how to deal with your reactions in trigger situations, so that you don't drink. You will also learn to apply coping skills to deal with urges to drink, in order to manage urges more quickly and effectively.

"We will begin each session with exposure to your drinking triggers, and you will be asked to experience your urges fully, until you feel them diminish and go away. By learning how to cope with urges to drink while you are in treatment, in a safe and secure environment, where you can get help and support, you'll be well equipped to handle urges once you leave. However, don't practice exposing yourself to your drinking triggers on your own. We encourage you to avoid as many trigger situations as you can in your environment, especially early on in sobriety. Having urges to drink does not mean that you are not motivated for treatment or for maintaining your sobriety. Experiencing urges to drink is natural and to be expected. Allow yourself to experience your urges to drink when they do happen, so that you can learn to identify your physical and emotional reactions associated with your urges and learn how to apply coping skills to manage them. It's much easier to cope with urges when you are more aware of them."

Following the rationale, the therapist defines "urge" as to thirst, wish for, desire, or crave an alcoholic beverage. Clients are informed that they will indicate their urge levels on a 0–10 scale throughout the session exposures (0 = "No urge or desire to drink," 10 = "As strong as it gets").

Beverage Exposure

During Cue Reactivity Assessment, the therapist should collect information on the client's preferred and primary alcoholic beverage, how it is prepared, and how it is consumed. For example, if the client's primary alcoholic beverage is a screwdriver, the therapist should ask for the specific brands of vodka and orange juice that he or she uses, the size of the glass used, whether he or she uses ice, whether the glass is chilled, and whether anything else is put in the drink (e.g., straw, fruit garnish, etc.). Although many clients report drinking directly from a bottle or can, we still ask them to pour the drink into a glass during exposure in order to increase the smell of alcohol in the room and to provide important visual cues of alcohol.

Each beverage exposure trial begins with the client pouring and mixing the drink in the glass half to three-fourths full to prevent spillage. The client is asked to give an urge rating on the 0–10 scale. We generally encourage clients to hold the glass, in addition to looking at the beverage and sniffing it, if they report that it increases their urge. The therapist asks clients to concentrate on the aspects of the beverage that give rise to increased urge levels, to focus on their feelings and reactions, and to allow themselves to experience the urges fully. Not uncommonly, some clients report after several sessions that their urges actually decrease when they sniff the alcohol and that the smell of the beverage has become aversive to them. This phenomenon underlines the importance of the therapist asking clients about their urges during each session and instructing them appropriately during the exposures in order to maximize urge levels.

Imaginal Scene Exposure

The therapist should bring the Drinking Triggers Interview hierarchy to each session and add new client-reported trigger situations. The first trigger used is always the highest ranked one, in order for the client to get the greatest amount of practice on the most difficult and salient trigger. To maximize generalization, cover all of the triggers over the sessions.

Prior to the first imaginal exposure, the therapist asks the client to provide more details about aspects of the scene that would increase his or her urge. The client is then asked to imagine the scene clearly and vividly while concentrating on his or her urge to drink:

"Imagine that you're actually in that situation. Pay attention to what you're seeing, hearing, and feeling—everything about the situation. Think about your urge to drink, and tell me your urge level each time it changes. What is your urge to drink now?"

If a client reports either no change in urge levels or increasing urge after applying coping skills, the therapist should ask what he or she was thinking and provide appropriate corrective feedback. If a client states that he or she does not want to think about the trigger situation because it either causes too much distress or makes him or her afraid of experiencing urges to drink, the therapist should gently stress the importance of experiencing an urge in the safe and secure setting of treatment. If the issue is a client's difficulty using imagery, the therapist can use guided imagery during the exposure. This option should only be used in individual-format CET.

Employing Urge-Coping Skills

Before beginning the imaginal exposure trial, the therapist reviews a new coping skill and asks clients to provide examples of each skill that is personally meaningful to them. It is helpful to give clients a sheet listing each coping skill, with several blank lines under each one for clients to fill in relevant examples. For instance, under the heading for the coping skill "Alternative Behaviors," the client might jot down "call a supportive friend," "go for a walk," "listen to music to help me relax," and so on.

Then, when instructed by the therapist, the client imagines using the coping skill while in the high-risk situation. After all of the coping skills have been reviewed over several CET sessions, the client should be encouraged to use any skill or combination thereof to reduce his or her urges to drink. This helps to increase skills generalization and clients' mastery in applying the skills. Clients are reminded by the therapist to use the coping skills between sessions to manage any urges to drink and to anticipate trigger situations that may come up before the next session. The therapist and client thus have an opportunity to identify coping skills to deal with possible urges.

When the urge has gone as high as the client and therapist think it will go, the therapist prompts the client to apply the coping skills learned earlier in the session (or a combination of coping skills in later sessions) to reduce the urge. It is key that the client continue to imagine him- or herself in the scene when using the coping skill. After urge levels reach 2 or less on the 0–10 rating scale, the therapist ends the scene and asks the client to recount what he or she imagined, urges, and the effectiveness of the coping skill in diminishing urges. On average, it takes 3–6 minutes for urges to peak during exposure, and 12 minutes or less to decrease to low levels (Monti et al., 1993a).

Urge-Coping Skills

We teach eight main urge-coping skills in our version of CET: (1) passive delay and delay as a cognitive strategy tool; (2) negative consequences of drinking; (3) positive consequences of sobriety; (4) urge reduction imagery; (5) alternative food or drink; (6) alternative behaviors; (7) cognitive mastery statements; and (8) cognitive distraction. Two strategies that we neither teach nor recommend are *escape* and *avoidance*. While we applaud a client's efforts to avoid alcohol and high-risk situations, particularly early on in treatment, we explain that CET helps him or her to prepare for unexpected urges, and urges that occur in situations in which escape or avoidance may be difficult. Therefore, the client is encouraged to practice the following active coping skills in order to build up his or her repertoire of skills to use now and in the future:

1. *Passive delay and delay as a cognitive strategy tool ("waiting it out")*. The client is instructed during the first session simply to wait out the urge, without using any other

strategy. He or she can then experience time-limited urges, which is often novel information: "I'm really surprised my urge went down so low just by sitting here doing nothing." Clients frequently state that, in the past, they usually drank soon after having an urge and had not thought or believed that the urges would go away on their own, without their drinking. In later sessions, the beverage exposure trials can actually induce boredom in some clients; the therapist can explain how boredom demonstrates habituation to urges as a result of waiting it out.

2. *Negative consequences of drinking.* After thinking about all of the bad things that could happen if he or she drank in that situation, the client should generate a list of more immediate and personally relevant consequences for now or the near future (as opposed to past negative consequences from drinking).

3. *Positive consequences of sobriety.* In contrast to item 2, the client thinks about all of the good things that will happen if he or she remains sober in the situation and does not drink. To highlight the positives, we ask the client to focus on immediate consequences and not simply the converse of negative consequences. "Feeling clearheaded and refreshed in the morning" is therefore preferable to "not waking up with a hangover."

4. *Urge reduction imagery.* Marlatt and Gordon (1985) have written extensively on urge reduction imagery, and our use of this urge-coping skill is based on their work. The therapist instructs the client to transform his or her mental urge into a physical object that he or she can overcome, crush, or destroy. Active images include stomping on, kicking, or hitting the urge, as if it were a ball; passive images include surfing on an urge, as if it were a wave that crests and falls.

5. *Alternative food or drink.* The client lists things that he or she enjoys eating or drinking (nonalcoholic, of course) and imagines consuming them in the situation.

6. *Alternative behaviors.* The client imagines doing another activity in the situation instead of drinking. Preferably, these should be activities that the client finds pleasurable, relatively easy, and that help to distract him or her from the urge. Common examples include taking a walk, calling a friend, working out, listening to music, reading, cooking, and so on.

7. *Cognitive mastery statements.* The client is taught to repeat and rehearse mastery self-statements to reduce urges (e.g., "I can get through this urge because I'm stronger than it is," "I can do it," "Urges can't hurt me, and they go away eventually," and so on.

8. *Cognitive distraction.* The client practices imagining him- or herself in a pleasant scene while in a high-risk situation.

In general, most clients learn the aforementioned urge-coping skills easily and become proficient in them. Typically, clients report that they resonate with and rely on one or two specific coping skills out of the eight that they learn. This further justifies teaching the entire array of skills so that clients can test out which skills work best for them.

GENERAL CONSIDERATIONS IN COPING AND SOCIAL SKILLS TRAINING

Comorbidity with Personality Disorders

Dealing with clients who exhibit severe personality disorders can be difficult for therapists, particularly in a group setting. However, two studies have shown CSST to be more effective than interactional group therapy for clients with sociopathy or psychopathology

(Kadden, Cooney, Gerter, & Litt, 1989; Litt, Babor, DelBoca, Kadden, & Cooney, 1992), whereas another study reported similar drinking outcomes for alcoholics with high sociopathy who received either individual cognitive-behavioral treatment or relationship-focused community reinforcement (Kalman, Longabaugh, Clifford, Beattie, & Maisto, 2000). Occasionally, individuals with personality disorders may question or even dismiss the validity of the various coping skills (e.g., "That won't work for me") or challenge the therapist about the effects of alcohol abuse: "I'm more fun to be around when I'm drinking," "I'm only here because of my job—I don't care if I relapse, I like drinking," and so on. Rather than dispute these points with clients, our approach in these situations is twofold:

1. Urge the client to be a consumer and try out the various strategies to see which ones are helpful to him or her personally.
2. Avoid arguments about the validity of the client's assumptions and instead highlight the negative consequences of alcohol abuse.

This is usually followed by asking clients to describe how they can achieve alcohol's positive effects through alternative behaviors:

"Right now you're here because you want to keep your job and you're not interested much in sobriety. However, you do see the connection between your drinking and potentially losing your job permanently. What other activities can you do, besides drinking, that you also like?"

Gender

Although earlier studies have suggested that women and men might differentially benefit from cognitive-behavioral approaches for alcohol problems (Cronkite & Moos, 1984; Lyons, Welte, Brown, Sokolow, & Hynes, 1982), there is little in the current research literature on the relationship between gender and CSST; most studies report no significant gender differences in treatment outcome among individuals receiving CSST. In a recent study from our own lab, there were no gender differences in outcomes for men and women receiving cocaine-specific coping skills training based in part on CSST (Rohsenow, Monti, Martin, et al., 2000). Project Match did find gender differences, in that men had fewer abstinent days than did women, but have not yet reported any interaction effects between gender and treatment (Project Match Research Group, 1997).

Race and Ethnicity

There is a dearth of information in the research literature on the impact of race and ethnicity on CSST outcomes. While most reports indicate no gender differences in outcomes as a function of race or ethnicity, most individuals participating in these clinical research trials are white, thus limiting the generalizability of findings. One recent, interesting finding of an ongoing clinical trial indicates that at pretreatment, black Americans appear to utilize more coping skills independently to avoid drinking than do their white counterparts (Conigliaro et al., 2000). Clearly, inclusion of ethnic/minority individuals should be a priority for further research efforts in CSST and in alcohol treatment as a whole.

EFFECTIVENESS

Coping and Social Skills Training for Alcohol Problems

CSST is one of the most effective treatments for alcohol problems (Miller et al., 1995). Numerous studies have shown CSST programs to result in decreased alcohol consumption rates at follow-up (Chaney et al., 1978; Cooney, Kadden, Litt, & Gerter, 1991; Eriksen, Bjornstad, & Gotestam, 1986; Ferrell & Galassi, 1981; Greenwald et al., 1980; Kadden et al., 1989; Monti et al., 1990; Oei & Jackson, 1980, 1982; Rohsenow, Smith, & Johnson, 1985). For example, Monti and colleagues (1990) reported that CSST for alcohol dependence has resulted in significant reductions in number of drinks per drinking day at follow-up, while Maisto and colleagues (Maisto, Connors, & Zywiak, 2000) reported that coping skills significantly predicted 12-month alcohol use outcomes.

Cue Exposure Treatment

Increased interest in the application of CET for alcohol dependence has been fueled by the results of a few promising empirical studies. Monti and colleagues (1993b) found that compared to patients in a contrast condition, those receiving CET were significantly more likely to have a higher percentage of abstinent days during the second 3 months after treatment. In this study, patients in the CET condition reported significantly greater use of urge-coping skills during follow-up. Because use of coping skills was also associated with decreased rates of alcohol consumption, these results suggest the long-term effectiveness of urge coping skills in relapse prevention. McCusker and Brown (1995) reported that CET resulted in significant reductions in heart rate and salivation at post-treatment but did not manifest reductions in self-reported craving or anxiety levels. In another investigation of CET, clients who received the CET condition versus a relaxation control treatment reported significantly less alcohol consumption and increased latency to heavy drinking at 6-month follow-up (Drummond & Glautier, 1994).

CONCLUSIONS AND FUTURE DIRECTIONS

Coping and social skills training stands as one of the most empirically supported psychological treatments for alcohol abuse and dependence, having been used in Project Match (Project Match Research Group, 1997) and in Project Combine, a current multisite study funded by the National Institute on Alcohol Abuse and Alcoholism (NIAAA). Its foundations in social learning theory contribute to its focus on the complex interplay of inter- and intrapersonal factors in the initiation, maintenance, and resolution of alcohol-related problems.

Nevertheless, continued research is needed, particularly since the mechanisms through which CSST works have recently been challenged (Morgenstern & Longabaugh, 2000). Better understanding of treatment mechanisms is a top priority for alcoholism researchers (McCaul & Monti, in press), and given CSST's prominence in the field, it is important that it be explored more completely.

In spite of the recent proliferation of medications being developed and used for addictions, psychologically based interventions will most likely continue to enjoy widespread popularity and use. Medications for addictions tend to be most effective when combined with a psychosocial intervention such as coping skills training (Goldstein & Niaura, 1998; O'Malley et al., 1992; Schmitz, Stotts, Rhoades, & Grabowski, 2001).

Indeed, naltrexone, one of the most widely studied medications in current use for treating alcoholism, works optimally when combined with systematic skills training (Monti, Rohsenow, et al., 1999; O'Malley et al., 1992). Naltrexone has not only been shown to decrease urges to drink and drinking in clinical trials (Monti et al., 2001; O'Malley et al., 1992), but it has also been shown to decrease elicited reactions to alcohol stimuli, such as urge to drink during laboratory-measured cue reactivity (Monti, Rohsenow, et al., 1999; Rohsenow, Monti, Hutchison, et al., 2000). Combined with coping skills, it may permit improved learning during skills training, enhanced treatment compliance, and development of healthy, reinforcing alternative skills in order to maintain treatment gains. As new pharmacological interventions are developed for the treatment of alcoholism, it is likely that CSST will continue to enhance their effectiveness. It is especially important that skills be in place when medications are discontinued and that the mechanisms through which both biological and psychological interventions work are clearly delineated. Only through such understanding will treatment effectiveness for alcoholism be maximized.

ACKNOWLEDGMENTS

This work was supported by Grant No. 2 R01 AA07850; by a Merit Review grant from the Medical Research Service Office of Research and Development, Department of Veterans Affairs; and by a Department of Veterans Affairs Career Research Scientist Award to Peter M. Monti.

REFERENCES

Abrams, D. B. (1983). Assessment of alcohol–stress interactions. In L. Pohorecky & J. Brick (Eds.), *Stress and alcohol use* (pp. 61–86). New York: Elsevier–North Holland.

Abrams, D. B., Binkoff, J. A., Zwick, W. R., Liepman, M. R., Nirenberg, T. D., Munroe, S. M., & Monti, P. M. (1991). Alcohol abusers' and social drinkers' responses to alcohol-relevant and general situations. *Journal of Studies on Alcohol, 52*, 409–414.

Abrams, D. B., & Niaura, R. S. (1987). Social learning theory. In H. T. Blane & K. E. Leonard (Eds.), *Psychological theories of drinking and alcoholism* (pp. 131–178). New York: Guilford Press.

Abrams, D. B., Rohsenow, D. J., Niaura, R. S., Pedraza, M., Longabaugh, R., Beattie, M. C., Binkoff, J., Noel, N. E., & Monti, P. M. (1992). Smoking and treatment outcomes for alcoholics: Effects on coping skills, urge to drink, and drinking rates. *Behavior Therapy, 23*, 283–297.

Allen, D. N., Goldstein, G., & Seaton, B. E. (1997). Cognitive rehabilitation of chronic alcohol abusers. *Neuropsychology Review, 7*, 21–29.

Bandura, A. (1977). *Social learning theory.* New York: Prentice-Hall.

Botvin, G. J., Baker, E., Dusenbury, L., Tortu, S., & Botvin, E. (1990). Preventing adolescent drug abuse through a multimodal cognitive-behavioral approach: Results of a 3-year study. *Journal of Consulting and Clinical Psychology, 58*, 437–446.

Brown, S. A., Vik, P. W., Patterson, T. L., Grant, I., & Schuckit, M. A. (1995). Stress, vulnerability and adult alcohol relapse. *Journal of Studies on Alcohol, 56*, 538–545.

Chaney, E. F., O'Leary, M. R., & Marlatt, G. A. (1978). Skill training with alcoholics. *Journal of Consulting and Clinical Psychology, 46*, 1092–1104.

Colby, S. M., Monti, P. M., & Rohsenow, D. J. (1997, October). *Self-reported craving during high-risk situations for alcohol relapse.* Paper presented at National Institute on Alcohol Abuse and Alcoholism Workshop on Treatment and Alcohol Craving, Washington, DC.

Conigliaro, J., Maisto, S. A., McNeil, M., Kraemer, K., Kelley, M. E., Conigliaro, R., & O'Connor,

M. (2000). Does race make a difference among primary care patients with alcohol problems who agree to enroll in a study of brief interventions? *American Journal on Addictions, 9,* 321–330.

Cooney, N. L., Kadden, R. M., Litt, M. D., & Gerter, H. (1991). Matching alcoholics to coping skills or interactional therapies: Two-year follow-up results. *Journal of Consulting and Clinical Psychology, 59,* 598–601.

Cronkite, R. C., & Moos, R. H. (1984). Sex and marital status in relation to the treatment and outcome of alcoholic patients. *Sex Roles, 11,* 93–112.

Drummond, D. C., & Glautier, S. P. (1994). A controlled trial of cue exposure treatment in alcohol dependence. *Journal of Consulting and Clinical Psychology, 62,* 809–817.

Epstein, E. E., & McCrady, B. S. (1998). Behavioral couples treatment of alcohol and drug use disorders: Current status and innovations. *Clinical Psychology Review, 18,* 689–711.

Eriksen, L., Bjornstad, S., & Gotestam, K. G. (1986). Social skills training in groups for alcoholics: One year treatment outcome for groups and individuals. *Addictive Behaviors, 11,* 309–329.

Ferrell, W. L., & Galassi, J. P. (1981). Assertion training and human relations training in the treatment of chronic alcoholics. *International Journal of the Addictions, 16,* 959–968.

Goldstein, M., & Niaura, R. S. (1998). Smoking. In E. J. Topol (Ed.), *Textbook of cardiovascular medicine* (p. 145). Philadelphia: Lippincott Raven.

Graham, K., Annis, H. M., Brett, P. J., & Venesoen, P. (1996). A controlled field trial of group versus individual cognitive-behavioural training for relapse prevention. *Addiction, 91,* 1127–1139.

Greenwald, M. A., Kloss, J. P., Kovaleski, M. E., Greenwald, D. P., Twentyman, G. T., & Zibung-Hoffman, P. (1980). Drink refusal and social skills training with hospitalized alcoholics. *Addictive Behaviors, 5,* 227–256.

Jones, S. L., & Lanyon, R. I. (1981). Relationship between adaptive skills and outcome of alcoholism treatment. *Journal of Studies on Alcohol, 42,* 521–525.

Kadden, R. M., Cooney, N. L., Gerter, H., & Litt, M. D. (1989). Matching alcoholics to coping skills or interactional therapies: Post-treatment results. *Journal of Consulting and Clinical Psychology, 57,* 698–704.

Kadden, R. M., Litt, M. D., Cooney, N. L., & Busher, D. A. (1992). Relationship between role-play measures of coping skills and alcoholism treatment outcome. *Addictive Behaviors, 17,* 425–437.

Kalman, D., Longabaugh, R., Clifford, P. R., Beattie, M., & Maisto, A. A. (2000). Matching alcoholics to treatment: Failure to replicate findings of an earlier study. *Journal of Substance Abuse Treatment, 19,* 183–187.

Litt, M. D., Babor, T. F., DelBoca, F. K., Kadden, R. M., & Cooney, N. L. (1992). Types of alcoholics: II. Application of an empirically derived typology to treatment matching. *Archives of General Psychiatry, 49,* 609–614.

Lyons, J. P., Welte, J. W., Brown, J., Sokolow, L., & Hynes, G. (1982). Variation in alcoholism treatment orientations: Differential impact upon specific subpopulations. *Alcoholism: Clinical and Experimental Research, 6,* 333–343.

Maisto, S. A., Connors, G. J., & Zywiak, W. H. (2000). Alcohol treatment, changes in coping skills, self-efficacy, and levels of alcohol use and related problems 1 year following treatment initiation. *Psychology of Addictive Behaviors, 14,* 257–266.

Mann, K., Gunther, A., Stetter, F., & Ackermann, K. (1999). Rapid recovery from cognitive deficits in abstinent alcoholics: A controlled test–retest study. *Alcohol and Alcoholism, 34,* 567–574.

Marlatt, G. A., & Gordon, J. R. (Eds.). (1985). *Relapse prevention: Maintenance strategies in the treatment of addictive behaviors.* New York: Guilford Press.

McCaul, M. E. & Monti, P. M. (in press). Developments in alcoholism. In M. Galanter (Ed.), *Recent developments in alcoholism research on alcoholism treatment.* New York: Plenum Press.

McCrady, B. S., Stout, R., Noel, N., Abrams, D., & Nelson, H. F. (1991). Effectiveness of three types of spouse-involved behavioral alcoholism treatment. *British Journal of Addictions, 86,* 1415–1424.

McCusker, C. G., & Brown, K. (1995). Cue-exposure to alcohol-associated stimuli reduces autonomic reactivity, but not craving and anxiety, in dependent drinkers. *Alcohol and Alcoholism, 30,* 319–327.

Miller, W. R., Brown, J. M., Simpson, T. L., Handmaker, N. S., Bien, T. H., Luckie, L. F., Montgomery, H. A., Hester, R. K., & Tonigan, J. S. (1995). What works?: A methodological analysis of the alcohol treatment outcome literature. In W.R. Miller & R.K. Hester (Eds.), *Handbook of alcoholism treatment approaches* (2nd ed., pp. 12–44). New York: Allyn & Bacon.

Miller, W. R., & Sovereign, R. G. (1989). The check-up: A model for early intervention in addictive behaviors. In T. Loberg, W. R. Miller, et al. (Eds.), *Addictive behaviors, prevention and early intervention* (pp. 219–231). Amsterdam/Lisse: Swets & Zeitlinger.

Monti, P. M., Abrams, D. B., Binkoff, J. A., Zwick, W. R. Liepman, M. R., Nirenberg, T. D., & Rohsenow, D. J. (1990). Communication skills training, communication skills training with family and cognitive behavioral mood management training for alcoholics. *Journal of Studies on Alcohol, 51,* 263–270.

Monti, P. M., Abrams, D. B., Kadden, R. M., & Cooney, N. L. (1989). *Treating alcohol dependence: A coping skills training guide.* New York: Guilford Press.

Monti, P. M., Binkoff, J. A., Abrams, D. B., Zwick, W. R., Nirenberg, T. D., & Liepman, M. R. (1987). Reactivity of alcoholics and nonalcoholics to drinking cues. *Journal of Abnormal Psychology, 96,* 122–126.

Monti, P. M., Colby, S. M., Barnett, N. P., Spirito, A., Rohsenow, D. J., Myers, M., Woolard, R., & Lewander, W. (1999). Brief intervention for harm reduction with alcohol-positive older adolescents in a hospital emergency department. *Journal of Consulting and Clinical Psychology, 67,* 989–994.

Monti, P. M., Corriveau, D. P., & Curran, J. P. (1982). Social skills training for psychiatric patients: Treatment and outcome. In J. P. Curran & P. M. Monti (Eds.), *Social skills training: A practical handbook for assessment and treatment* (pp. 185–223). New York: Guilford Press.

Monti, P. M., & Kolko, D. (1985). A review and programmatic model of group social skills training for psychiatric patients. In D. Upper & S. M. Ross (Eds.), *Handbook of behavioral group therapy* (pp. 25–62). New York: Plenum Press.

Monti, P. M., & Rohsenow, D. J. (1999). Coping skills training and cue-exposure therapy in the treatment of alcoholism. *Alcohol Research and Health, 23,* 107–115.

Monti, P. M., Rohsenow, D. J., Abrams, D. B., Zwick, W. R., Binkoff, J. A., Munroe, S. M., Fingeret, A. L., Nirenberg, T. D., Liepman, M. R., Pedraza, M., Kadden, R. M., & Cooney, N. (1993). Development of a behavior analytically derived alcohol-specific role-play assessment instrument. *Journal of Studies on Alcohol, 54,* 710–721.

Monti, P. M., Rohsenow, D. J., Colby, S. M., & Abrams, D. B. (1995a). Smoking among alcoholics during and after treatment: Implications for models, treatment strategies, and policy. In J. B. Fertig (Ed.), *Alcohol and tobacco: From basic science to policy* (Research Monograph No. 30). Bethesda, MD: National Institute on Alcohol Abuse and Alcoholism.

Monti, P. M., Rohsenow, D. J., Colby, S. M., & Abrams, D. B. (1995b). Coping and social skills training. In R. K. Hester & W. R. Miller (Eds.), *Handbook of alcoholism treatment approaches* (2nd ed., pp. 221–241). New York: Allyn & Bacon.

Monti, P. M., Rohsenow, D. J., Hutchison, K. E., Swift, R. M., Mueller, T. I., Colby, S. M., Brown, R. A., Gulliver, S. B., Gordon, A., & Abrams, D. B. (1999). Naltrexone's effect on cue-elicited craving among alcoholics in treatment. *Alcoholism: Clinical and Experimental Research, 23,* 1386–1394.

Monti, P. M., Rohsenow, D. J., Michalec, E., Martin, R. A., & Abrams, D. B. (1997). Brief coping skills treatment for cocaine abuse: Substance use outcomes at 3 months. *Addiction, 92,* 1717–1728.

Monti, P. M., Rohsenow, D. J., Rubonis, A. V., Niaura, R. S, Sirota, A. D., Colby, S. M., &

Abrams, D. B. (1993a). Alcohol cue reactivity: Effects of detoxification and extended exposure. *Journal of Studies on Alcohol, 54*, 235–245.

Monti, P. M., Rohsenow, D. J., Rubonis, A. V., Niaura, R. S., Sirota, A. D., Colby, S. M., Goddard, P., & Abrams, D. B. (1993b). Cue exposure with coping skills treatment for male alcoholics: A preliminary investigation. *Journal of Consulting and Clinical Psychology, 61*, 1011–1019.

Monti, P. M., Rohsenow, D. J., Swift, R. M., Gulliver, S. B., Colby, S. M., Mueller, T. I., Brown, R. A., Gordon, A., Abrams, D. B., Niaura, R. S., & Asher, M. K. (2001). Naltrexone, cue exposure with coping skills training, and communication skills training for alcoholics: Treatment process and one-year outcomes. *Alcoholism: Clinical and Experimental Research, 25*, 1634–1647.

Morgenstern, J., & Longabaugh, R. (2000). Cognitive-behavioral treatment for alcohol dependence: A review of evidence for its hypothesized mechanisms of action. *Addiction, 95*, 1475–1490.

Niaura, R. S., Rohsenow, D. J., Binkoff, J. A., Monti, P. M., Pedraza, M., & Abrams, D. B. (1988). The relevance of cue reactivity to understanding alcohol and smoking relapse. *Journal of Abnormal Psychology, 97*, 133–152.

Oei, T. P. S., & Jackson, P.R. (1980). Long term effects of group and individual social skills training with alcoholics. *Addictive Behaviors, 5*, 129–136.

Oei, T. P. S., & Jackson, P. R. (1982). Social skills and cognitive behavioural approaches to the treatment of problem drinking. *Journal of Studies on Alcohol, 43*, 532–547.

O'Farrell, T. J. (1994). Marital therapy and spouse-involved treatment with alcoholic patients. *Behavior Therapy, 25*, 391–406.

O'Farrell, T. J., Choquette, K. A., & Cutter, H. S. (1998). Couples relapse prevention sessions after behavioral marital therapy for male alcoholics: Outcomes during the three years after starting treatment. *Journal of Studies on Alcohol, 59*, 357–370.

O'Farrell, T. J., Choquette, K. A., Cutter, H. S., Brown, E. D., & McCourt, W. F. (1993). Behavioral marital therapy with and without additional couples relapse prevention sessions for alcoholics and their wives. *Journal of Studies on Alcohol, 54*, 652–666.

O'Malley, S. S., Jaffe, A. J., Chang, G., Schottenfeld, R. S., Meyer, R. E., & Rounsaville, B. (1992). Naltrexone and coping skills therapy for alcohol dependence: A controlled study. *Archives of General Psychiatry, 49*, 881–887.

Pead, J., Greeley, J., Ritter, A., Murray, T., Felstead, B., Mattick, R., & Heather, N. (1993, June). *A clinical trial of cue exposure combined with cognitive-behavioral treatment for alcohol dependence.* Paper presented at the 55th Meeting of the College on Problems of Drug Dependency, Toronto, Canada.

Project Match Research Group. (1997). Matching alcoholism treatments to client heterogeneity: Project MATCH posttreatment drinking outcomes. *Journal of Studies on Alcohol, 58*, 7–29.

Rohsenow, D. J., Monti, P. M., Abrams, D. B., Rubonis, A. V., Niaura, R. S., Sirota, A. D., & Colby, S. M. (1992). Cue elicited urge to drink and salivation in alcoholics: Relationship to individual differences. *Advances in Behaviour Research and Therapy, 14*, 195–210.

Rohsenow, D. J., Monti, P. M., Binkoff, J. A., & Liepman, M. R. (1991). Patient–treatment matching for alcoholic men in communication skills versus cognitive-behavioral mood management training. *Addictive Behaviors, 16*, 63–69.

Rohsenow, D. J., Monti, P. M., Hutchison, K. E., Swift, R. M., Colby, S. M., & Kaplan, G. B. (2000). Naltrexone's effects on reactivity to alcohol cues among alcoholic men. *Journal of Abnormal Psychology, 109*, 738–742.

Rohsenow, D. J., Monti, P. M., Martin, R. A., Michalec, E., & Abrams, D. B. (2000). Brief coping skills treatment for cocaine abuse: 12-month substance use outcomes. *Journal of Consulting and Clinical Psychology, 68*, 515–520.

Rohsenow, D. J., Monti, P. M., Rubonis A. V., Sirota, A. D., Niaura, R. S., Colby, S. M., Wunschel, S. M., & Abrams, D. B. (1994). Cue reactivity as a predictor of drinking among male alcoholics. *Journal of Consulting and Clinical Psychology, 62*, 620–626.

Rohsenow, D. J., Niaura, R. S., Childress, A. R., Abrams, D. B., & Monti, P. M. (1990). Cue reactivity in addictive behaviors: Theoretical and treatment implications. *International Journal of the Addictions, 25*(7A & 8A), 957–993.

Rohsenow, D. J., Smith, R. E., & Johnson, S. (1985). Stress management training as a prevention program for heavy social drinkers: Cognitions, affect, drinking, and individual differences. *Addictive Behaviors, 10,* 45–54.

Schafer, K., Butters, N., Smith, T., Irwin, M., Brown, S., Hanger, P., Grant, I., & Schuckit, M. (1991). Cognitive performance of alcoholics: A longitudinal evaluation of the role of drinking history, depression, liver function, nutrition, and family history. *Alcoholism: Clinical and Experimental Research, 15,* 653–660.

Schmitz, J. M., Stotts, A. L., Rhoades, H. M., & Grabowski, J. (2001). Naltrexone and relapse prevention treatment for cocaine-dependent patients. *Addictive Behaviors, 26,* 167–180.

Smith, D. E., & McCrady, B. S. (1991). Cognitive impairment among alcoholics: Impact on drink refusal skill acquisition and treatment outcome. *Addictive Behaviors, 16,* 265–274.

13

Twelve-Step Facilitation Therapy for Alcohol Problems

Joseph Nowinski

This chapter presents an overview of twelve-step facilitation (TSF; Nowinski & Baker, 1998; Nowinski, Baker, & Carroll, 1992). TSF is a structured, time-limited treatment whose goal is to facilitate active involvement in and use of 12-step fellowships such as Alcoholics Anonymous (AA) and Narcotics Anonymous (NA) as a means of overcoming problematic alcohol or drug use.

EFFICACY AND APPLICABILITY OF TWELVE-STEP FACILITATION

Studies of AA have suggested that active involvement in the fellowship is associated with recovery from alcohol abuse (Emrick, Tonigan, Montgomery, & Little, 1993). In one major treatment outcome study, TSF, which is informed by and consistent with what is more generally known as the Minnesota Model of substance abuse treatment (Anderson, 1981; Spicer, 1993), has been found to result in significant and sustained reductions in drinking in a major clinical trial (Project MATCH Research Group, 1997). Compared to cognitive-behavioral therapy and motivational enhancement therapy, TSF was more effective among subjects who measured lower in overall psychopathology. No gender differences in treatment effectiveness were found. A longer-term (3-year) follow-up of subjects treated in Project MATCH (Longabaugh, Wirtz, Zweben, & Stout, 1998) found TSF to be significantly more effective than motivational enhancement therapy among patients whose social environments tended to support drinking. These findings are consistent with one of the major goals of TSF, which is to alter drinkers' lifestyles, including their social environments.

Laundergan (1982) reported follow-up self-report data from 3,638 clients who received treatment at the Hazelden Foundation between 1973 and 1975. Hazelden staff were consulted on the development of TSF and found it compatible with the model of treatment applied there. Based on a 12-month posttreatment response rate of 56%, Laundergan reported that 50% of that group reported abstinence from alcohol use. It is not known what percentage of that group reported significant decreases in drinking short of complete abstinence.

In other studies of the Minnesota Model, Gilmore (1985) followed 1,531 clients who received treatment at Hazelden in 1978, 1980, and 1983, and reported a 12-month response rate of 75%; of this group, 89% reported *either* abstinence or reduced drinking after treatment. Higgins, Baeumler, Fisher, and Johnson (1991), who reported on the outcome of 1,655 clients treated at Hazelden in 1985–1986, found a 66% abstinence rate at 12-month follow-up, based on a return rate of 72%. Finally, Stinchfield and Owen (1998) reported a 71% response rate in a cohort of 1,083 male (68% of sample) and female clients treated at Hazelden for psychoactive substance use disorders between 1989 and 1991. This study, which looked separately at abstinence and reduced consumption, reported an abstinence rate of 53%, with an additional 35% reportedly reducing their use of alcohol and/or drugs. Data were not reported separately for male and female clients.

In Project MATCH, the effectiveness of TSF was not mediated by drinking severity (Project MATCH Research Group, 1997), suggesting that TSF may be applied to mild and moderate drinkers, as well as those traditionally thought of as alcoholics. In addition, several studies on the effectiveness of the Minnesota Model report reduced drinking or drug use as an outcome for a significant portion of the treated populations. However, although it would appear that patients need not necessarily be dependent on alcohol in order to benefit from TSF, and that outcomes for the Minnesota Model range from reduced use to abstinence, the reader should be aware that AA itself advocates abstinence, as opposed to controlled use of alcohol, as the desired long-term goal for those men and women whose drinking experience is marked by a series of failures to moderate use effectively.

THEORETICAL BASIS OF TWELVE-STEP FACILITATION

We admitted we were powerless over alcohol—that our lives had become unmanageable. (Alcoholics Anonymous, 1976, p. 59)

This first "step" of AA acknowledges that a person's life can become increasingly "unmanageable" as a direct result of drinking. AA and its 12-step sister fellowships were founded by and exist for the benefit of those whose experience has shown that, try as they may, they cannot reliably control their use of alcohol (Alcoholics Anonymous, 1976, pp. 21, 24, 30–31). In its "Big Book" (Alcoholics Anonymous, 1976) AA delineates some of the means that the eventual alcoholic may employ in an effort to moderate use:

> Here are some of the methods we have tried: Drinking beer only, limiting the number of drinks, never drinking alone, never drinking in the morning, drinking only at home, never having it in the house, never drinking during business hours, drinking only at parties. ... (p. 31)

From this, it is clear that AA and its 12-step program for recovery is typically not the first avenue taken by the men or women who find the quality of their lives and health suffering on account of drinking.

The Disease Model

The American Medical Association (AMA Committee on Alcoholism, 1956), the American Psychiatric Association (1994), and the World Health Organization (WHO Expert Committee on Mental Health, 1952) have all identified alcoholism as a disease. However, the exact definition of a "disease" remains controversial. Although most people think of a disease as a malaise of biological etiology that is not the result of volitional acts, we know that lifestyle factors such as diet and exercise, which are most certainly volitional, as well as nonbiological factors such as environment and stress, exert strong influences on the development and course of many illnesses.

Alcoholism could be said to be a disease to the extent that it satisfies the following criteria:

- *Identifiable signs and symptoms.* The American Psychiatric Association's (1994, p. 181) *Diagnostic and Statistical Manual of Mental Disorders* identifies a number of specific and observable symptoms of alcoholism, including tolerance, withdrawal symptoms, preoccupation, and inability to moderate use.
- *Biological vulnerability.* Although it is doubtful that alcoholism or drug addiction will prove to be attributable to a single gene, studies of twins consistently find a higher concordance rate for addiction among identical than fraternal twins, even when reared in different families. This effect, moreover, appears to be stronger among males than females (Hesselbrock, 1995; Kendler & Prescott, 1998; Tsuang, 1998; Van den Bree, Johnson, Neale, & Pickens, 1998). Such studies suggest that heredity plays at least some role in vulnerability to addiction.
- *Predictable course.* Surveys of alcohol and drug use patterns consistently find that substance use peaks in young adulthood (U.S. Department of Health and Human Services, 1999). Clearly, not everyone who uses alcohol or drugs progresses to alcoholism or addiction. On the other hand, studies of individuals who start out as heavy drinkers and do so progress tend to find a common pattern, marked by sporadic and unsuccessful efforts to stop or limit use, which continues despite progressively more serious consequences associated with use (Schuckit, Anthenelli, Bucholz, Hesselbrock, & Tipp, 1995; Vaillant, 1983).

The AA View

Although medicine and psychiatry have labeled alcoholism a disease, and while a spirited debate continues regarding the relative contributions of environment, heredity, and lifestyle in the etiology of all diseases, in its own official publications, AA itself does not discuss the disease concept in any detail. The following is typical of what AA has to say about the etiology of alcoholism:

> Opinions vary considerably as to why the alcoholic reacts differently [to alcohol] from normal people. We are not sure why, once a certain point is reached, little can be done for him. We cannot answer the riddle. (Alcoholics Anonymous, 1976, p. 22)

With respect to the diagnosis of alcoholism, AA relies on a single determining factor—loss of control—and puts it this way:

> We know that while the alcoholic keeps away from drink, as he may do for months or years, he reacts much like other men. We are equally positive that once he takes any

alcohol whatever into his system, something happens, both in the bodily and mental sense, which makes it virtually impossible for him to stop. (1976, p. 22)

AA relies on such empirical definitions to define alcoholism. It even invites readers to render their own diagnosis based on experience:

We do not like to pronounce any individual as alcoholic, but you can quickly diagnose yourself. Step over to the nearest barroom and try some controlled drinking. Try to drink and stop abruptly. Try it more than once. It will not take long for you to decide, if you are honest with yourself about it. (1976, p. 31)

Thus, although AA identifies alcoholism as an "illness" in its writings (1976, p. 18), it does not venture far into the debate over its etiology and instead relies on the principle of "attraction" (1952, p. 180) to appeal to those who at some point reach the conclusion, however reluctantly, that they cannot successfully control their drinking and are therefore wiser to pursue a goal of abstinence. Furthermore, in its approach to recovery from alcoholism, the AA model is not medical, but rather relies on changes in the social, spiritual, and psychological realms of day-to-day living.

STRUCTURE AND CONTENT OF TWELVE-STEP FACILITATION

TSF includes a range of interventions that are organized into a "core" or basic program, an "elective" or advanced program, and a brief "conjoint" program for use with the alcohol user and a significant other. Interventions in the TSF core program are most appropriate for what could be termed the "early" or initial stage of recovery from alcohol or drug dependence. By early recovery, we generally mean that stage of change in which an individual takes the initial steps from active substance abuse toward abstinence. The interventions included in the TSF core program could also be said to be directed primarily at the first four stages of change as described by the transtheoretical model of change (Prochaska, DiClemente, & Norcross, 1992; Saunders, Wilkinson, & Towers, 1996): *precontemplation*, referring to a relative unawareness of any need to change one's behavior at all; *contemplation*, meaning the process of coming to a decision to change; *preparation*, or marshaling resources for change; and *action*. These stages of the change process are typically marked by ambivalence, or by what is commonly referred to as *denial* in the recovery field. The primary focus of this chapter is the TSF core program.

TSF also includes a set of interventions that can be brought to bear when working with patients who have moved to the *maintenance* stage of change (Prochaska et al., 1992, p. 1101). In recovery terms, these men and women have shown some sustained sobriety as well as some evidence of having bonded to a 12-step fellowship. Some of the topics included in the advanced program of TSF may also be useful with patients who have relapsed after some period of sobriety.

The conjoint program, which is the third component of TSF, may be used with patients at any stage of change. It is intended to enlist the help of significant others in the change process by teaching them the Al-Anon concepts of *enabling* and *caring detachment* (Al-Anon Family Groups, 1985).

Finally, TSF includes a structured termination session, the goals of which are to assess progress to date and to develop a posttreatment follow-up plan of action.

The various topics that comprise TSF are grouped as follows:

Core (Basic) Program

Introduction and Assessment

The goals of this TSF program module are to provide an overview of treatment, to assess the client's level of substance abuse, and to initiate the process of assigning *recovery tasks*, which include journaling, attending meetings, and reading.

Acceptance

In this module, the therapist introduces and discusses the first step of AA and the concept of *acceptance*: admitting that one has psychological and/or physical symptoms of dependence on alcohol or drugs.

People, Places, and Routines

The focus of this module is the development of a *lifestyle contract* in which the client constructs an inventory of people, places, and routines that would support recovery, and simultaneously identifies those people, places, and routines that represent a risk for relapse.

Surrender

The concept of *surrender* is complex and includes cognitive (belief in the possibility of recovery) as well as behavioral elements (accepting the support and guidance of others who are trying to stay clean and sober).

Getting Active

The final module of the TSF core program seeks to facilitate active participation in AA and/or NA via *telephone therapy*, *sponsorship*, and *service* commitments.

Elective (Advanced) Program

Genograms

In this module, the therapist and client trace substance abuse and its consequences across generations, helping to identify and elucidate vulnerability to addiction and its effects.

Enabling

Enabling refers to the ways in which significant others unintentionally allow the addictive process to continue. The *enabling inventory* is a list of attitudes and behaviors that the addict has systematically encouraged in others to support his or her addiction, and which would need to change in the interests of recovery.

Emotions

In this module, therapist and client explore the role that emotions play in both the initiation of substance abuse and relapse, and alternative ways of coping with emotions such as anxiety, anger, and grief.

Moral Inventories

Steps 4 and 5 of the AA program ask alcoholics or addicts to conduct a *moral inventory* in order to accept personal responsibility for the negative impact that their addiction has had on their significant relationships. To the extent that it is appropriate, recovering persons are then guided toward making amends for their acts of commission or omission.

Relationships

In this module, client and therapist continue the exploration of healing damaged relationships. Specific topics for discussion include communication, conflict resolution, intimacy, and sexuality.

Conjoint Program

This program is used whenever possible when the client has a significant other who is willing to participate. It consists of the following two modules:

Enabling

The first conjoint module covers the subject of enabling, as described earlier. However, in this case, the significant other participates in the construction of the enabling inventory and is helped to identify his or her motives for enabling.

Detaching

Following on the discussion of enabling, the therapist helps the client and significant other identify alternative behaviors and attitudes that will not unintentionally support addiction.

TSF was intended to be implemented as a time-limited (12- to 15-session) intervention. Initially developed as an individual treatment, it has been adapted for use with groups (Maude-Griffin, 1998; Seraganian, Brown, Tremblay, & Annies, 1998). In either format, TSF is a highly structured intervention following a prescribed format. Each begins with a review of the patient's *recovery week*, including any 12-step meetings attended and reactions to them, episodes of drinking (vs. "sober days"), urges to drink, reactions to any readings completed, and any journaling that the patient has done.

The second part of each session consists of presenting new material drawn from the core, elective, or conjoint programs. Each session ends with a wrap-up, including the assignment of *recovery tasks*: readings, meetings to be attended, and other prorecovery behavioral work that the patient agrees to undertake between sessions. This structure is intended to create a degree of momentum in therapy, such that each session begins where the last left off.

PRINCIPLES OF TWELVE-STEP FACILITATION

TSF seeks to be both philosophically and pragmatically compatible with the 12 steps of AA. It is, accordingly, based on certain principles and concepts that follow from the steps and traditions of AA and need to be understood if the intervention is to achieve this desired compatibility.

Early Recovery

Broadly speaking early recovery can be broken down into two phases: *acceptance* and *surrender*. Acceptance refers to the process in which the individual overcomes "denial." Denial refers to the personal belief that one either does not have a drinking problem at all, and/or that one can effectively and reliably control drinking despite negative consequences. In motivational terms, acceptance represents a series of vital insights that are succinctly captured in the first step and begin with the idea that one has in fact lost the ability to control drinking effectively. Acceptance then proceeds to a recognition that drinking is making one's life unmanageable. Finally, it implies a recognition that individual willpower alone is an insufficient force for creating sustained sobriety and restoring manageability to one's life.

Given the realizations that acceptance represents, the only sane alternative to continued chaos and personal failure is to admit defeat (of one's efforts to control use), to embrace the need for abstinence as an alternative to controlled use, and to abandon personal willpower in favor of some "higher" power in order to achieve sobriety. This is the phenomenon commonly referred to as "surrender."

Surrender basically means a willingness to take action and, specifically, to follow the 12 steps as a guide for recovery and spiritual renewal. AA is as much a program of action as a program of insight. Surrender logically follows acceptance and represents the individual's commitment to making whatever changes in lifestyle, attitude, and outlook are necessary in order to sustain recovery. With respect to action, this means frequently attending AA meetings, becoming active in meetings, reading AA literature, getting a sponsor, making AA friends, and giving up people, places, and routines that have become associated with drinking and therefore represent a threat to recovery.

In TSF the action and commitment that are the hallmarks of surrender are guided to some extent by the facilitator, but they are also heavily influenced by individuals whom the patient encounters, and with whom he or she begins to form relationships within AA. One especially significant relationship that TSF actively advocates in early recovery is that with a *sponsor*.

Involvement in AA will inevitably expose both the patient and the therapist alike to a number of key 12-step traditions and concepts, such as the concept of a *Higher Power* (Alcoholics Anonymous, 1976, p. 50), the advocacy of fellowship over professionalism (1952, p. 166), and the concepts of *group conscience* and *spiritual awakening* (1952, pp. 106, 132). Because these concepts and traditions are so central to 12-step fellowships and their philosophy of recovery, the practitioner must not only be familiar with them but also should be prepared to discuss them and their implications for action. Effective assignment of recovery tasks does not require that the therapist be in recovery; on the other hand, it demands familiarity with the culture and traditions of 12-step fellowships. For this reason, therapists who have no personal knowledge of 12-step fellowships are encouraged, as a minimum, to familiarize themselves with their basic AA texts, such as *Alcoholics Anonymous* (1976), *Twelve Steps and Twelve Traditions* (1952), and *Living Sober* (1975). Therapists who are naive about 12-step fellowships are also encouraged to attend several open AA and/or Al-Anon meetings prior to implementing TSF.

Locus of Change

TSF, like AA, considers that the primary locus of change with respect to patients' drinking behavior lies less in the hands of the therapist or the patient's willpower, and more in the hands of the fellowship of AA. Accordingly, the goal in TSF is active participation and involvement in AA. TSF relies on bonding with other recovering alcoholics as the key to sustained sobriety. This is not to say that either the therapist or the therapeutic relationship is insignificant. To the contrary, the TSF "facilitator," a highly skilled professional, must possess not only good psychotherapeutic skills but also a working knowledge of 12-step fellowships and how they operate. In TSF, the therapist guides the patient into recovery, but without allowing therapy itself to become the patient's recovery program. In order to accomplish this, the facilitator must develop considerable skill in knowing when to provide advice and support personally versus when to encourage the patient to seek these things through AA. Such a therapeutic stance places the responsibility for recovery squarely on the shoulders of the patient and defines the therapist–patient role as one of collaboration to achieve the goal of involvement in AA.

Motivation

From its inception, AA has characterized itself as a fellowship "based on attraction rather than promotion" (Alcoholics Anonymous, 1952, p. 180). Through this statement, AA established a tradition of not seeking to attract members through overt advertising or promotion, much less through coercive techniques of any kind. AA's historic rate of growth is such that it has been likened to a "social movement" (Room, 1993). This growth in turn has relied in great part on the notion of identification and attraction, and also on the 12th step, which states: *Having had a spiritual awakening as the result of these steps, we tried to carry this message to alcoholics, and to practice these principles in all our affairs* (Alcoholics Anonymous, 1952, p. 106).

AA assumed from the outset that if an alcoholic attended meetings, listened to the stories of others and identified with them, and spent time with fellow alcoholics who were also trying to stay sober, then sooner or later he or she would be motivated to try the program laid out in the 12 steps. The 12th step, meanwhile, formed the foundation for the institution of sponsorship, in which individuals who have succeeded in sustaining recovery through AA over a period of years, and who have remained active in the fellowship, will take newcomers under their wing for a period of time. They do so in order to support the newcomer and to educate him or her about AA traditions and etiquette (e.g., no "cross-talking" at meetings) that have evolved over the years.

The AA philosophy of attraction also has implications for the therapist who wishes to use TSF. TSF eschews a heavily confrontational approach in favor of what could perhaps be called "care-frontation." This latter approach is more similar to what a newcomer to AA will likely encounter at meetings. Typically, newcomers are welcomed warmly. However, when trying to attract newcomers, there is no "hard sell" here, but instead a low-key, welcoming approach that emphasizes "giving it a try" and "keeping an open mind."

The effectiveness of more coercive approaches at achieving sustained sobriety has not been thoroughly tested. Although some have argued cogently that most people who seek help are pressured to do so in some way or other (Anderson, 1981), in TSF, as in AA, we prefer a shaping approach that emphasizes positive reinforcement of any and all progress made toward recovery. This includes, among other things, recognizing each and every sober day the patient has and expecting "progress rather than perfection" when it comes to abstinence.

Spirituality

One aspect of 12-step recovery that clearly separates it from other models of intervention is its active promotion of spirituality. The guiding books of AA—*Alcoholics Anonymous* (1976) and *Twelve Steps and Twelve Traditions* (1952)—are replete with references to the importance of spirituality to recovery, and the 12th step asserts that following the program of personal growth as outlined in the 12 steps will lead in the end to a spiritual "awakening."

Here are some examples of the way that 12-step fellowships speak of spirituality:

> We have learned that whatever the human frailties of various faiths, those faiths have given purpose and direction to millions. People of faith have a logical idea of what life is all about. Actually, we used to have no reasonable conception whatever. (Alcoholics Anonymous, 1976, p. 49)

> On one proposition . . . these men and women [alcoholics] are strikingly agreed. Every one of them has gained access to, and believes in, a Power greater than himself. (1976, p. 50).

> When a man or a woman has had a spiritual awakening, the most important meaning of it is that he has now become able to do, feel, and believe that which he could not do before on his unaided strength and resources alone. He has been granted a gift which amounts to a new state of consciousness and being. (1952, pp. 106–107)

AA regards spirituality as a force that provides direction and meaning to one's life, and it equates spiritual awakening with a realignment of personal goals, specifically a movement away from radical individualism and the pursuit of the material, toward community and the pursuit of serenity as core values.

What is the source of the spiritual awakening that AA believes can be the ultimate result of thoroughly following its 12 steps? An examination of the 12 steps reveals a strong emphasis on an ongoing process of self-examination and honesty with one's self and others. The 12-step program encourages humility in the sense of a willingness to acknowledge personal shortcomings. It advocates strength of fellowship over ego as an overall approach to life.

When conducting TSF, the clinician should be prepared to discuss the issue of spirituality. At several different points in treatment (Nowinski & Baker, 1998, pp. 73–81; Nowinski et al., 1992, pp. 2, 4, 47–48) the therapist is asked to engage the patient in a discussion of his or her spiritual beliefs. Guidelines provided for these discussions generally focus around the issues of willpower, powerlessness, and faith, as well as personal values and goals.

Pragmatism

Although many people, whose knowledge of AA is limited to a reading of the 12 steps, think of it as strictly a spiritually based program, historically, pragmatism has been as important a theme in AA as spirituality. One official AA publication, *Living Sober* (1975), is subtitled *Some Methods AA Members Have Used For Not Drinking*. This book contains a wealth of practical advice—much of it very compatible with cognitive-behavioral therapies—for avoiding "taking the first drink." Consider the following sampling from its Table of Contents:

> Using the 24-Hour Plan
> Changing Old Routines
> Making Use of "Telephone Therapy"
> Getting Plenty of Rest
> Fending Off Loneliness
> Letting Go of Old Ideas

TSF incorporates this pragmatic aspect of 12-step recovery, particularly in the *recovery tasks* assigned at the end of each session. Through these tasks, the facilitator attempts to educate the patient with respect to some practical methods for staying sober and to create systematically a steady stream of behavioral change, consistently admonishing the patient to focus on "one day at a time," reinforcing progress made, making specific suggestions about additional behavioral changes, and encouraging the patient to solicit and follow practical advice from fellow AA members and a sponsor on issues that range from the best ways to deal with difficult situations to how to cope with cravings, to what to do after a slip, and so on. One of the core topics in TSF involves the creation of a Lifestyle Contract that specifies the kinds of changes the client needs to make in order to support his or her recovery (Nowinski & Baker, 1998, pp. 117–120).

Collaboration and Flexibility

In setting a tone for TSF, the therapist should take an approach that is best described as collaborative. He or she consistently strives to engage the patient in a constructive collaboration toward achieving the goal of sobriety. As an example, the recovery tasks that are decided on at the end of each session are best approached collaboratively as opposed to being purely the therapist's idea. Every core and advanced topic within TSF contains many suggested recovery tasks, but exactly which are "assigned" depends on the particular client.

Regardless of why the client is in treatment (e.g., whether voluntarily or not), the therapist should also keep in mind, as a foundation for the client–therapist relationship, the third tradition of AA, which states: *The only requirement for AA membership is a desire to stop drinking* (Alcoholics Anonymous, 1952, p. 139). This tradition is deliberate in its wording. It means that it is not essential that the patient embrace each and every tenet of AA, or adopt a particular spiritual philosophy. This attitude is supported by the following statement:

> Alcoholics Anonymous does not demand that you believe anything. All of its Twelve Steps are but suggestions. (Alcoholics Anonymous, 1952, p. 26)

Consistent with this, TSF encourages therapists to be flexible within the broad guideline of establishing a collaborative relationship with the patient toward the end of helping him or her stop drinking or using. Confrontation in TSF is common, but it never takes the form of threat. For example, the 12-step facilitator will never terminate treatment because a patient drinks between sessions, or even if he or she shows up intoxicated (although action is necessary in this case to ensure that the client does not drive or otherwise endanger him- or herself or others). On the other hand, the therapist should consistently confront the patient about drinking and its connection to denial and attempt to move the patient through the process of acceptance and surrender. The therapist is asked to advocate "90 meetings in 90 days" as the best strategy for the person in early recovery, and to continue to ask for and encourage frequent attendance at meetings; but he or she never makes compliance with this suggestion a condition of treatment. Similarly, the 12-step facilitator will point out clients' statements that reflect denial and talk frankly but nonjudgmentally with the client about any "slips" that he or she has. The therapist, however, recognizes addiction as a "cunning and clever" illness, and therefore expects both denial and relapse (at least in early recovery) as natural parts of the overall recovery process. Again, the therapist seeks to be a *shaper* of behavior, relying heavily on rapport and reinforcement to achieve the goals of TSF.

TWELVE-STEP FACILITATION IN PRACTICE

Assessment

TSF begins much the way any good treatment should begin: with a thorough assessment. The specific approach to assessment employed in TSF has been described in detail elsewhere (Nowinski & Baker, 1998; Nowinski et al., 1992) and for reasons of space is described only briefly here.

Assessment is important for two reasons. The first and most obvious objective of the assessment is for the therapist to determine the extent of the patient's drinking problem. In reality, however, research has established that both problem drinkers and true alcoholics can benefit from TSF (Project MATCH Research Group, 1997). Therefore, the use of TSF is not necessarily limited to "severe" or "end-stage" alcoholics.

A second objective of the assessment has to do with the issue of motivation. Part of the purpose of taking a thorough alcohol history, as well as a careful inventory of consequences related to drinking, is to establish a collaborative therapeutic relationship with the patient. One way to do this is by reaching a *consensus* regarding the diagnosis and the need for treatment. The process of building rapport and motivating the patient may require the therapist to refer back in later sessions to data collected during the assessment. Therefore, it is important that the clinician keep good records of information gathered. Toward this end, it is recommended that the patient be given a copy of the assessment and be asked to review it as one of his or her first *recovery tasks*.

An alcohol history is graphical representation of chronological changes in the type and amount of alcohol used by the patient, along with correlated events and effects. This is best done using a chart such as that shown in Table 13.1.

In this hypothetical example, the patient reported first use of alcohol at age 11. At that time, he sipped from his father's supply of beer, primarily on weekends. Drinking made him feel "silly," and sometimes it made him sick. He reported that his mother and father fought often at about the same time. By age 13, his use of alcohol had increased to three or four beers, 3 to 4 times a week. This made him feel "high," suggesting that

TABLE 13.1. Alcohol History

Age	Type of alcohol	Frequency	Amount	Effects	Significant (pos./neg.) events
11	Beer	Weekends	1–2	"Silly" "Sick"	Parental conflict
13	Beer	3–4 ×/week	3–4	"High"	Parental divorce
17	Beer/vodka	6–7 ×/week	5–10	"Drunk"	DWI, dropout

he was experiencing some pleasurable affect as a consequence of his drinking, and was using alcohol primarily for its euphoric effects. At about this same time, his parents divorced.

Between the ages of 13 and 17, our hypothetical patient's drinking progressed to the point that he was drinking both beer and vodka almost daily. He also experienced two significant consequences related to his drinking: He was arrested for driving while intoxicated, and he dropped out of school. By this point, most of the euphoric effects of drinking had worn off, and the patient simply felt "drunk" much of the time.

Although Table 13.1 is necessarily brief for purposes of illustration, in practice, the therapist should try to fill it in as completely as possible, adding as much detail as the patient offers. Again, the objective is to engage the patient in a collaborative effort in the creation of this drinking autobiography, most especially to document the *progression* of substance use over time, and the significant events correlated with it.

After the alcohol–drug history is completed, the patient should be given a copy and asked to look it over between sessions. At the next session, the therapist should review it again with the patient, filling in any additional details that the patient recalls as a result of this recovery task.

The second major part of the assessment is an inventory of *consequences* of alcohol and drug use. Again, both for purposes of clarity and to enhance motivation, this is best done chronologically. The therapist can introduce this part of the assessment with an opening statement similar to the following:

"Let's take some time to examine some of the issues, conflicts, and problems that you've experienced over your life and see if any of them are connected in any way to your use of alcohol or drugs."

Negative consequences of alcohol use should be explored both chronologically and categorically. Be sure not to leave out (or allow the patient to avoid) examining each of the following areas.

Physical Consequences

Included here (especially for older patients) are the physical consequences of long-term alcohol abuse, including hypertension, gastrointestinal problems, sleep disorders, weight loss, alcohol- or drug-related injuries and accidents, emergency room visits, blackouts, heart problems, liver disease, and kidney disease. Keep in mind that it is estimated that approximately 50% of all general hospital beds in the United States are occupied with patients whose medical illnesses are alcohol or drug related (National Institute on Alcohol Abuse and Alcoholism, 1990).

Legal Consequences

Alcohol abuse often leads to legal troubles such as DWI (driving while intoxicated) arrests, arrests for disorderly conduct, and so on.

Social Consequences

Social consequences of alcohol abuse include strained relationships, lost relationships, and job conflicts. Substance abusers often alienate their partners, perform progressively more poorly at work, and are dysfunctional as parents. They may lose marriages, jobs, and friends. It is important to do a thorough inventory of such losses, in chronological order, and to connect them to the patients' alcohol history as appropriate.

Psychological Consequences

Habitual use of alcohol, even in the absence of clear signs of dependence, typically leads to negative psychological consequences, such as anxiety and depression, poor anger control, sleep and eating disorders, irritability, and even confused thinking. As habitual use gives way to dependence, and as negative consequences accrue, severe depression, suicidal thinking, and suicide attempts are not uncommon.

Sexual Consequences

Not only is alcohol abuse associated with sexual dysfunction in both males and females (Powell, 1984), but alcohol abuse and dependence are also often correlated with sexual victimization and exploitation. The therapist should explore the patient's sexual history to determine if sexual dysfunction, victimization, or exploitation are present, and, if so, whether they are correlated with substance abuse. Frank discussion of sexuality is often omitted from assessment even though it is often a potential motivator for recovery. Guidelines for conducting substance abuse–related sexual histories have been published elsewhere (Nowinski & Baker, 1998).

Financial Consequences

It is a good idea to have the patient estimate how much money he or she has spent on alcohol in the 2 years prior to the assessment, including not only the cost of the alcohol itself but also the costs due to consequences. The latter include the costs of traffic tickets, legal defense or representation, and lost income.

When both the alcohol history and the inventory of consequences have been completed, the assessment itself ends, with the facilitator sharing a diagnosis and treatment plan. Obviously, this should come as no surprise to the patient if the assessment process has truly been a collaborative venture. Still, the patient and clinician may disagree, especially if the clinician thinks the patient is addicted but the patient does not. What is important for the clinician to note is that it is not essential for the patient to acknowledge alcoholism in order to proceed with TSF.

Acceptance

The first step in AA asks problem drinkers to acknowledge that drinking has made their lives unmanageable and that they are "powerless" over alcohol. Although many individuals take issue with the word "powerless," it is important that clinicians who wish to use TSF not overgeneralize. AA speaks of powerlessness only in the context of alcohol use. Furthermore, more in-depth discussions make it clear that this step refers to the repeated failure of individual to stop or control drinking. It does not in any way imply any kind of generalized powerlessness.

In essence, then, taking the first "step" (i.e., acceptance) represents a statement of humility. It reflects an acceptance of personal limitation—that life has become *unmanageable* as the result of drinking, and that willpower alone has not been enough to change that. Philosophically, the first step (and AA itself) has been characterized as a challenge to the radical individualism that has long been a core theme in American culture (Room, 1993).

In discussing Step 1 with patients it is extremely useful for the therapist to have the alcohol history and the chronology of consequences at hand. The focus of this dialogue should be on the *progressive pattern of unmanageability in the patient's life and the limitations of personal willpower*. If the history and chronology do not make a case for total loss of control, they should at least show a pattern of growing unmanageability that the therapist can point out. The therapist can also encourage the patient to describe some of the methods he or she has used in the past to limit or stop his or her use of alcohol.

People, Places, and Routines

From acceptance, which roughly corresponds to the *contemplation* stage of change (Prochaska et al., 1992), TSF moves on to help the patient *prepare* for change. The vehicle for this, the Lifestyle Contract, is shown in Table 13.2. It is based on the notion that addiction evolves into a virtual lifestyle that is supported by a range of "people, places, and routines." In order to support recovery once the decision has been made to pursue abstinence as a long-term goal, the substance abuser must be prepared to make changes in each of these areas. The Lifestyle Contract, which is developed collaboratively by the patient and therapist, becomes a blueprint for these changes.

Implicit in the design of the Lifestyle Contract is the idea that simply "giving up" certain people, places, and routines will not in and of itself be a successful strategy for change in the long run. People, places, and routines that are supportive of recovery must be substituted for those that pose a threat to recovery. Viewed another way, the Lifestyle Contract describes two alternative lifestyles: one that supports drinking, and an alternative one that supports sobriety.

TABLE 13.2. Lifestyle Contract

	Dangerous to recovery	Supportive of recovery
People	Drinking friends	AA members Nondrinking friends
Places	Bars, casinos	AA meetings Nondrinking friends' homes
Routines	Drinks after work	Meeting AA friends Exercise

Surrender

In TSF, a discussion of surrender follows acceptance and the development of the Lifestyle Contract. Conceptually, surrender represents *action*; specifically, it represents the patient's decision to seek outside help and to abandon personal willpower as a means of controlling or stopping drinking in favor of reaching out to others for guidance and support. Like acceptance, surrender is typically more a process than an event and, again, is one that can evoke intense emotions. It is reflected in Steps 2 and 3 of AA:

> We came to believe that a Power greater than ourselves could restore us to sanity.
> We made a decision to turn our will and our lives over to the care of God *as we understood Him.* (1976, p. 59)

The italics at the end of the third step appear in the original text and are emphasized in order to point out that the AA view of God or a Higher Power is a pluralistic one. There is neither an organized priesthood nor a specific dogma within AA; rather, these are deliberately decentralized fellowships. The closest thing to a dogma are the 12 steps themselves, which are deliberately framed not as dogma but as suggestions. In addition, from its inception, AA has remained intentionally nonprofessional, with leadership roles determined by the individual groups (Alcoholics Anonymous, 1952, pp. 146–154, 166–171).

AA has a long spiritual tradition, to the extent that the 12 steps invite alcoholics to believe in a center of power that is greater than their individual wills. Substituting faith in the group (or some other higher power) for faith in personal willpower has been construed as a form of spiritual conversion or awakening:

> Faith is a dynamic process of construal and commitment in which persons find and give meaning to their lives through trust in and loyalty to shared centers of value, images and realities of power, and core stories. Conversion in AA perspective begins when one reaches and acknowledges a state of helpless desperation in the effort to maintain the false self and the illusion that one can manage one's drinking. Gradually it comes to mean making a commitment to enter into the 12 steps and become part of the 12 traditions of Alcoholics Anonymous. (Fowler, 1993, p. 114)

If Step 1 involves *accepting the problem* (alcoholism or addiction), then Steps 2 and 3 can be thought of as *accepting the solution*, which requires the alcoholic to let go of egotism and hopelessness, to come to believe that he or she can overcome a drinking problem, and to reach out to others in order to do so. Despite its potential to evoke strong emotional responses, Step 1 basically represents a change in cognition—in the way one views his or her drinking. In contrast, Steps 2 and 3 represent more of a spiritual shift. Within 12-step fellowships, this is commonly referred to as "surrender" or "turning it over": moving away from self-centeredness and an excessive belief in individual willpower toward faith and a willingness to reach out and to accept the strength of fellowship. This is more than an abstract notion: In treatment, it will be directly reflected in patients' *hope for recovery*, in their *willingness to become active in the fellowship*, and in their *openness to advice*. When an individual begins to surrender in this fashion, he or she begins to appreciate that accepting powerlessness over alcohol does not in any way imply either helplessness or hopelessness.

When implementing TSF, the clinician should be prepared to engage the patient in a specific and ongoing dialogue about issues such as the limits of willpower, faith, and surrender. It is suggested that at least one entire session be devoted to reading Steps 2 and 3, and discussing the patient's reactions to them. This sort of dialogue is more than a purely intellectual exercise. It is central to introducing the patient to the spiritual foundation of 12-step fellowships. Not all therapists may be comfortable engaging patients in this sort of dialogue. All therapists, however, would be wise to ponder such questions themselves before entering into this kind of dialogue. In the end, it can be very productive to venture down this road, since it represents a highly effective route to working through patients' resistances to becoming active in AA and making full use of the fellowship's social and spiritual resources.

Getting Active

The final component of the TSF core program builds on the work done earlier in constructing the Lifestyle Contract and centers around facilitating the patient's ongoing active participation in AA. Becoming active, in 12-step parlance, means "working" the steps. AA puts it this way:

> Just stopping drinking is not enough. Just not drinking is a negative, sterile thing. That is clearly demonstrated by our experience. To stay stopped, we've found we need to put in place of the drinking a positive program of action. (1975, p. 13)

A popular meditation book expresses similar sentiments in this way:

> Work and prayer are the two forces which are gradually making a better world. We must work for the betterment of ourselves and other people. Faith without works is dead. (Alcoholics Anonymous, 1975, p. 83)

The message here is clear: Recovery requires faith, but it also requires action. Steps 1 and 2 in particular can be thought of as necessary but not sufficient conditions for staying clean or sober. To facilitate recovery, the clinician must be prepared to work continually with the patient toward the goal of active involvement (as opposed to passive participation) in AA. This includes going to meetings frequently and speaking as well as listening, getting phone numbers and using them to establish a support network, seeking a home group and taking on a responsibility, seeking out a sponsor, and reading AA material.

One valuable resource for getting active is the AA publication, *Living Sober* (1975). This book offers a range of specific suggestions with which clinicians who favor a cognitive-behavioral approach should find themselves most comfortable. In describing its purpose, *Living Sober* states:

> Our drinking was connected with many habits—big and little. Some of them were thinking habits, or things we felt inside ourselves. Others were doing habits—things we did, actions we took. In getting used to not drinking, we have found that we needed new habits to take the place of those old ones. (p. 1)

The *recovery tasks* assigned at the end of each session are a useful vehicle for pursuing the goal of getting active within the therapeutic context. These are not unlike the "homework" often employed in cognitive-behavioral therapy, which, like TSF, relies heavily on patient–therapist collaboration and active work on the part of the patient between sessions. In TSF, the clinician ends each session with a series of specific recovery tasks and begins each session with a review of the patient's "recovery week," including progress made on those recovery tasks.

Termination

If TSF has been successful, then termination essentially consists of "turning over" the patient to the care of the AA fellowship. The more successfully the patient and therapist have collaborated toward this end, the more likely it is that the patient will continue his or her progress toward lasting sobriety. This prediction is based in part on AA member surveys, which show that the best predictor of future sobriety is current active participation in AA (Alcoholics Anonymous General Services Office, 1990). In addition, the contribution of AA/NA meeting attendance to maintaining abstinence has received empirical support (Fiorentine, 1999).

Because the overarching goal of TSF is involvement in AA, termination should in part consist of an honest appraisal of how much progress has been made toward that end and what, if any, plans the patient has for furthering that involvement in the future.

Advanced Work

This chapter has focused on a structured, time-limited intervention for what has been called "early" recovery. It is unlikely that any more ground than what has been described here could reasonably be covered in brief therapy. Indeed, the goals of TSF are ambitious. In general, it is not recommended that therapists attempt to do more advanced work with patients until they have a minimum of 6 months of uninterrupted sobriety and have satisfied all goals of the core program.

TSF does include an advanced or "elective" program (Nowinski & Baker, 1998, pp. 95–154; Nowinski et al., 1992, pp. 59–96) that provides therapist guidelines for covering the following topics: genograms, enabling, emotions, moral inventories, and relationships. A discussion of this material is beyond the scope of this chapter; however, parts of the elective program may be considered appropriate for patients who have consolidated their early recovery and are ready to begin the process of "hardening" their recovery, for example, by working on Steps 4 and 5 (the so-called "moral inventory"), or who are ready to begin the process of healing wounded relationships.

REFERENCES

Al-Anon Family Groups. (1985). *Al-anon faces alcoholism*. New York: Al-Anon Family Group Headquarters.

Alcoholics Anonymous. (1952). *Twelve steps and twelve traditions*. New York: Alcoholics Anonymous World Services.

Alcoholics Anonymous. (1975). *Living sober: Some methods A.A. members have used for not drinking*. New York: Alcoholics Anonymous World Services.

Alcoholics Anonymous. (1976). *Alcoholics Anonymous: The story of how many thousands of men and women have recovered from alcoholism* (3rd ed.). New York: Alcoholics Anonymous World Services.

Alcoholics Anonymous. (1990). *Comments on A.A.'s triennial surveys*. New York: Alcoholics Anonymous World Services.

AMA Committee on Alcoholism. (1956). Hospitalization of patients with alcoholism. *Journal of the American Medical Association, 162,* 750–757.

American Psychiatric Association. (1994). *Diagnostic and statistical manual of mental disorders.* (4th ed.). Washington, DC: Author.

Anderson, D. J. (1981). *Perspectives on treatment: The Minnesota experience.* Center City, MN: Hazelden.

Emrick, C. D., Tonigan, J. S., Montgomery, H., & Little, L. (1993). Alcoholics Anonymous: What is currently known? In B.S. McCrady & W.R. Miller (Eds.), *Research on Alcoholics Anonymous: Opportunities and alternatives,* (pp. 41–76). New Brunswick, NJ: Rutgers University Press.

Fiorentine, R. (1999). After drug treatment: Are 12-step programs effective in maintaining abstinence? *American Journal of Drug and Alcohol Abuse, 25*(1), 93–116.

Fowler, J. W. (1993). Alcoholics Anonymous and faith development. In B. S. McCrady & W. R. Miller (Eds.), *Research on Alcoholics Anonymous: Opportunities and alternatives* (pp. 113–135). New Brunswick, NJ: Rutgers University Press.

Gilmore, K. (1985). *Hazelden Primary Residential Treatment Program: 1985 profile and patient outcome.* Center City, MN: Hazelden.

Hesselbrock, V. (1995). The genetic epidemiology of alcoholism. In H. Begleiter & B. Kissin (Eds.), *The genetics of alcoholism* (pp. 40–69). New York: Oxford University Press.

Higgins, P., Baeumler, R., Fisher, J., & Johnson, V. (1991). Treatment outcomes for Minnesota model programs. In J. Spicer (Ed.), *Does your program measure up?: An addiction professional's guide to evaluating treatment effectiveness* (pp. 97–121). Center City, MN: Hazelden.

Kendler, K., & Prescott, C. (1998). Cannabis use, abuse, and dependence in a population-based sample of female twins. *American Journal of Psychiatry, 155*(8), 1016–1022.

Laundergan, J. C. (1982). *Easy does it: Alcoholism treatment outcomes, Hazelden, and the Minnesota model.* Center City, MN: Hazelden.

Longabaugh, R., Wirtz, P., Zweben, A., & Stout, R. (1998). Network support for drinking: Alcoholics Anonymous and long-term matching effects. *Addiction, 93*(9), 1313–1333.

Maude-Griffin, P. M. (1998). Superior efficacy of cognitive-behavioral therapy for urban crack cocaine users: Main and matching effects. *Journal of Consulting and Clinical Psychology, 66*(5), 832–837.

National Institute on Drug Abuse. (1990). *Alcohol and health.* Rockville, MD: Author.

Nowinski, J., & Baker, S. (1998). *The twelve-step facilitation handbook: A systematic approach to early recovery from alcoholism and addiction.* San Francisco: Jossey-Bass.

Nowinski, J., Baker, S., & Carroll, K. (1992). *Twelve-step facilitation therapy manual: A clinical research guide for therapists treating individuals with alcohol abuse and dependence* (Project MATCH Monograph Series, Vol. 1). Rockville, MD: National Institute on Alcohol Abuse and Alcoholism.

Powell, D. (1984). *Alcoholism and sexual dysfunction.* New York: Haworth.

Prochaska, J. O., DiClemente, C. C., & Norcross, J. C. (1992). In search of how people change: Applications to addictive behaviors. *American Psychologist, 47,* 1102–1114.

Project MATCH Research Group. (1997) . Matching alcoholism treatments to client heterogeneity: Project MATCH Posttreatment drinking outcomes. *Journal of Studies on Alcohol, 58,* 7–29.

Room, R. (1993). Alcoholics Anonymous as a social movement. In B. S. McCrady & W. R. Miller (Eds.), *Research on Alcoholics Anonymous: Opportunities and alternatives* (pp. 167–187). New Brunswick, NJ: Rutgers University Press.

Saunders, B., Wilkinson, C., & Towers, T. (1996). Motivation and addictive behaviors: Theoretical perspectives. In F. Rotgers, D. S. Keller, & J. Morgenstern (Eds.), *Treating substance abuse: Theory and technique* (pp. 83–93). New York: Guilford Press.

Schuckit, M. A., Anthenelli, R. M., Bucholz, K. K., Hesselbrock, V. M., & Tipp, J. (1995). The time course of development of alcohol-related problems in men and women. *Journal of Studies on Alcohol, 56,* 218–225.

Seraganian, P., Brown, T. G., Tremblay, J., & Annies, H. M. (1998). *Experimental manipulation of treatment aftercare regimes for the substance abuser.* (National Health Research and Development Program [Canada] Project #6605-4392-404). Unpublished manuscript, Concordia University, Montreal, Canada.

Spicer, J. (1993). *The Minnesota model.* Center City, MN: Hazelden.

Stinchfield, R., & Owen, P. (1998). Hazelden's model of treatment and its outcome. *Addictive Behaviors, 23*(5), 669–683.

Tsuang, M. (1998). Co-occurrence of abuse of different drugs in men. *Archives of General Psychiatry, 55,* 967–972.

U.S. Department of Health and Human Services, Substance Abuse and Mental Health Services Administration. (1999). *National household survey on drug abuse series: H-10* (Summary of findings from the 1998 National Household Survey on Drug Abuse, DHHS Pub. No. [SMA] 99-3328). Washington, DC: Author.

Vaillant, G. E. (1983). *The natural history of alcoholism.* Cambridge, MA: Harvard University Press.

Van den Bree, M., Johnson, E., Neale, M., & Pickens, R. (1998). Genetic and environmental influences on drug use and abuse/dependence in male and female twins. *Drug and Alcohol Dependence, 52*(3), 231–241.

World Health Organization Expert Committee on Mental Health. (1952). *Report of the first session of the Alcoholism Subcommittee* (WHO Technical Report Series, No. 42). Geneva: Author.

14

Couple Treatment for Alcohol Abuse
A Systemic Family-Consultation Model

MICHAEL J. ROHRBAUGH
VARDA SHOHAM

Recent reviews of empirically supported psychosocial treatments indicate that the best efficacy evidence so far available for outpatient alcohol treatment comes from approaches that include spouses or significant others (Baucom, Shoham, Mueser, Daiuto, & Stickle, 1998; McCrady et al., 1986; O'Farrell, Chuquette, & Cutter, 1998). This chapter describes an integrative systemic/strategic couple therapy that (1) focuses on the relational context of drinking, not solely on the individual who drinks; (2) assumes that drinking problems are maintained by ongoing cycles of social interaction; (3) adapts treatment to the client or family's worldview; and (4) accommodates reluctance to change (Rohrbaugh, Shoham, Spungen, & Steinglass, 1995). We developed this approach in the early 1990s for a research project investigating differential indications for couple alcoholism treatments based on cognitive-behavioral versus family systems principles.[1] Although the overall outcomes of the two treatments were not substantially different, the systemic approach appeared better suited than the more confrontational cognitive-behavioral therapy for cases in which alcohol abuse occurred in the context of a difficult couple relationship—particularly one involving demand–withdraw interaction (Rohrbaugh, Shoham, & Racioppo, 2002; Shoham, Rohrbaugh, Stickle, & Jacob, 1998). We therefore suspect that this treatment, or components thereof, has more relevance for some alcohol-involved couples than for others.

Our chapter has three sections: The first describes the background, rationale, and research context associated with treatment development. The second section then outlines the manualized treatment itself, with a flow chart schematizing its major components and implementation choice points. In the final section, we summarize lessons learned from treating 39 couples during the course of the research project, as well as some findings relevant to the model's applicability.

BACKGROUND AND RATIONALE

In developing this systemic/strategic treatment, we attempted to integrate key ideas and techniques from leading family therapy approaches to alcoholism. Thus, from the alcoholic family model of Steinglass, Bennett, Wolin, and Reiss (1987), we drew the concepts of family-level detoxification, couple identity, and alcohol as an external "invader" of family life; from the brief strategic therapy of the Palo Alto (Mental Research Institute) group came the idea of interrupting ironic problem–solution loops and framing suggestions for change in terms consistent with clients' preferred views or "position" (Fisch, 1986; Fisch, Weakland, & Segal, 1982); and from the solution-focused approach of Berg, de Shazer, Miller, and colleagues we adapted techniques that call attention to client strengths and resources (Berg & Miller, 1992). Also important was the key concept of neutrality, applied to alcohol treatment by Lewis (1987) and Borwick (1991), the technique of circular questioning[2] (Flueridas, Nelson, & Rosenthal, 1986; Penn, 1985), and the use of a brief family genogram to illuminate the broader patterns and loyalties across generations (McGoldrick & Gerson, 1985). Finally, we borrowed White and Epston's (1990) externalization tactics to build couple collaboration against alcohol as an external invader, and relied heavily on structural and strategic family therapy techniques to counter resistance and restabilize the system later in therapy (Bepko & Krestan, 1985; Elkin, 1984; Treadway, 1989).

Our aim in integrating these diverse ideas and techniques was to construct an internally consistent therapy faithful to a "systemic" view of alcohol problems and treatment. A central assumption regards alcohol abuse as inextricably interwoven with the family and social context in which it occurs. While not discounting history, our systems model assumes that drinking problems, like other problems, persist primarily as an aspect of current, ongoing interaction between the drinker and his or her significant others (Weakland, Watzlawick, Fisch, & Bodin, 1974). Because the variables crucial to treatment reside not so much within people as between them, the primary focus of alcohol treatment from this perspective is not the individual drinker but the system of relationships in which his or her drinking is embedded.

Nevertheless, despite their common emphasis on the relational context of drinking, the models from which we drew have a number of theoretical and technical incompatibilities. For example, some systems therapists find useful the idea that alcohol abuse can serve temporarily adaptive functions for families (Steinglass et al., 1987), while others clearly do not (Berg & Miller, 1992; Fisch et al., 1982). And some therapists prefer to educate clients about dysfunctional family patterns or teach alternative coping skills, while others work within the clients' own belief system, with the goal of helping them to construct a more workable reality. To avoid procedural confusion, we attempted to specify guidelines for what to do when, and developed rationales for emphasizing some principles and procedures while deemphasizing others. As it turned out, some of the rough spots we encountered in implementing the treatment manual concerned such tensions of integration. In any case, the resulting integration reflects our own theoretical preferences and biases. Ours is but one version of an integrative systemic treatment approach, and by no means the only one possible.

Another consideration in developing a systemic treatment for alcohol abuse was to distinguish it from more established treatment approaches, such as the 12-step model of Alcoholics Anonymous. In contrast to traditional alcohol treatment, we intended the systemic approach to emphasize (1) current interactional determinants of drinking problems rather than personality deficits and copathologies resulting from past experience in a "dysfunctional family"; (2) understanding and using the clients' own language or reality rather than teaching a new belief system; (3) not confronting "denial" directly but using neutrality to build collaboration, shift responsibility to the clients, and avoid "more of the same" solution; and (4) family therapy as collaborative and conjoint rather than "separate and equal." A Q-sort study comparing traditional and systemic views of alcohol treatment generally supported these distinctions (Rohrbaugh et al., 1995).[3]

The research protocol in which we implemented the systemic treatment required that couples participate in up to 20 therapy sessions over a 6- to 9-month period. The first six sessions were typically held on a weekly or biweekly basis, with subsequent sessions scheduled at varying and increasing intervals, depending on the couple's progress. A criterion for entering the project was that one partner in the couple (usually the male) meet DSM-III-R criteria for moderate to severe alcohol dependence. The presence of other problems or comorbid conditions—including severe marital dysfunction—did not exclude a couple from participating as long as drinking was a primary complaint and the partners were married or in a committed relationship.

TREATMENT IMPLEMENTATION

Ideally, therapy occurs in three phases as schematized in Figure 14.1: In an initial *consultation phase* (Sessions 1–6), the therapist conducts a systemic assessment, begins to intervene indirectly using circular- and solution-focused questioning, and offers the couple "treatment" while remaining neutral about whether the spouses should choose it. If both spouses accept, the *treatment phase* consists of "family detoxification" and therapist-initiated intervention to alter couple interaction patterns that help to maintain drinking. The final, *restabilization phase* aims to restabilize the family system without alcohol and to prevent relapse. Throughout therapy, a key principle is to avoid confronting resistance or denial directly. Thus, if resistance arises during the treatment phase—or if the couple does not choose treatment in the first place—intervention shifts to strategic and structural tactics (framed as *continuing consultation*), such as prescribing a controlled drinking experiment, intensifying the restraint-from-change stance, seeing the spouse alone, or involving other family members or friends. The main goal of these tactics is to lead the couple back to family detoxification, or failing that, to provoke change directly.

Phase I: Consultation

In the consultation phase, the therapist not only makes a thorough assessment of the extent and consequences of drinking and (especially) of the family interaction patterns in which drinking is embedded, since these are assumed to play a critical role in problem maintenance, but also solicits details about exceptions to problems, such as how the couple manages to make things go well or keep them from getting worse. The goal is to understand not only what clients *do* but also how they *view* themselves and their situation (e.g., what drinking means in their relationship and in the broader familial/cultural context). Throughout this phase, the therapist attempts to establish an empathetic, collaborative relationship with the clients *as a couple* and to maintain a posture of neutrality by not aligning with either partner against the other and not directly advocating sobriety or change.

In the pivotal sixth session, the therapist gives the couple detailed feedback in the form of an "opinion" formulated by the consultation team (the supervisor and other

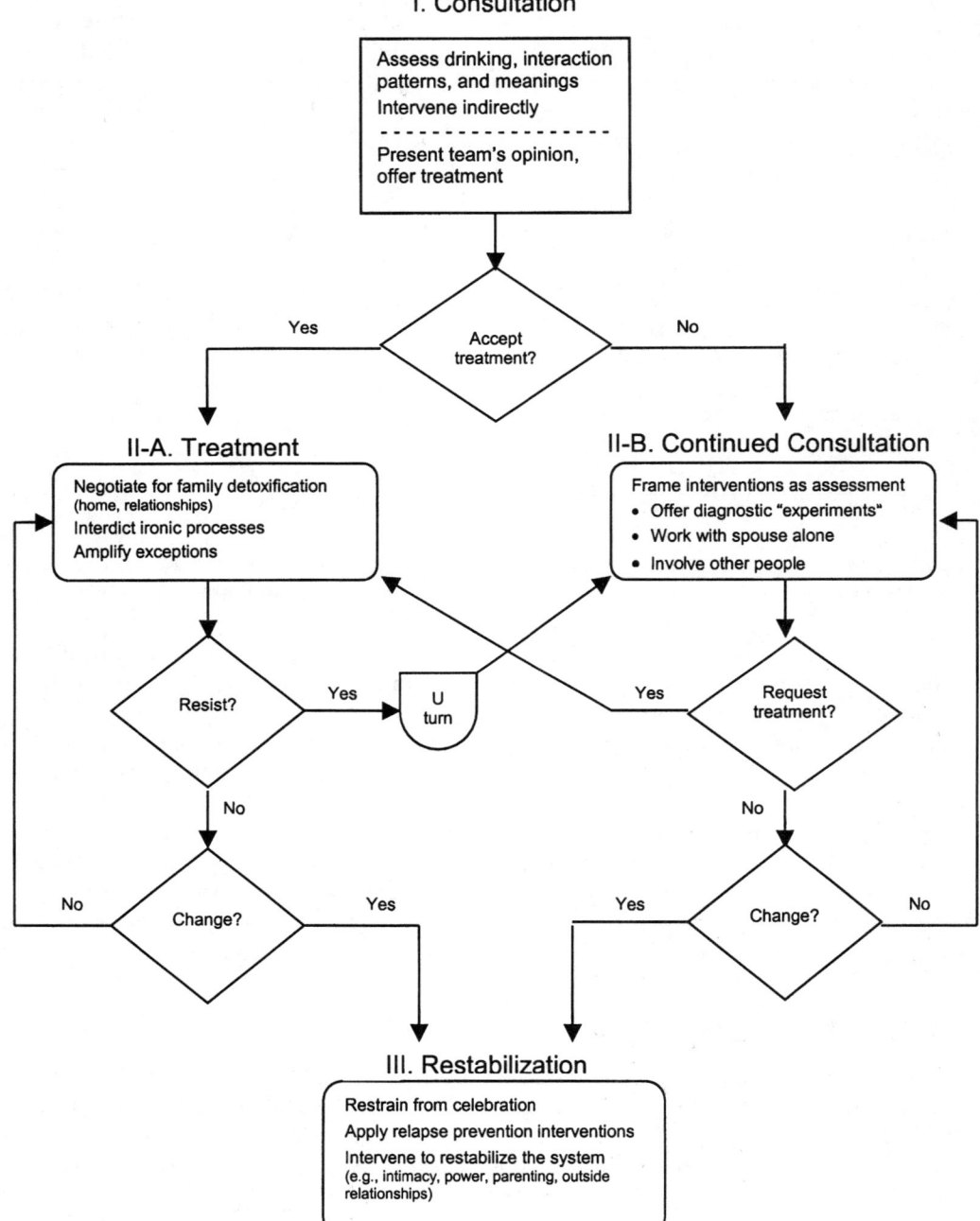

FIGURE 14.1. A systemic therapy for alcohol abuse.

project therapists) and offers the opportunity to participate in what we explicitly call "treatment." This opinion (1) compliments the couple for dealing with a difficult situation, (2) highlights the specific and serious ways in which alcohol has invaded the partners' family life, and (3) predicts that changing this will be difficult, perhaps even entailing unforeseen problems, but possible, if the partners work together in the treatment framework we offer. To proceed, the partners must then actively *choose* treatment, which requires choosing to work toward changing their relationship with alcohol and probably giving it up altogether. If one or both spouses are ambivalent about treatment or unwilling to make a clear commitment, the therapist is careful not to push or sell recovery. Instead, he or she respects the clients' ambivalence and proposes further study of the issue, thus setting the stage for indirect intervention framed as "continued consultation."

Because guidelines for the consultation phase are more specific than those for later phases, we can summarize them on a session-to-session basis:

Session 1: Problems and Solutions

The first meeting begins with a brief orientation to the project, in which the therapist explains the format of therapy (e.g., the scheduling of sessions, confidentiality, missed-appointment policies, and the distinction between "consultation" and "treatment"). This accomplished, the therapist asks in a general way what brought the clients to therapy at this particular time, and eventually queries each spouse specifically about how he or she sees the drinking problem—and whether in his or her view there *is* a problem—without expecting or pressing them to agree. If the spouses mention other complaints related to their marriage, we make clear to them that while our primary focus is problems related to alcohol, we try to address other problems too.

To understand complaints in concrete behavioral terms, the therapist asks for specific examples and seeks to understand where, when, and for how long complaint behaviors have occurred. For example, a complaining but defensive husband might be asked, "What did your wife *do* when she criticized your drinking last week? What happened then? How did you get her to stop?" An important guideline is for the therapist to have enough details to know what the problem might look like on film: "If we had a video of this, what would I see?" Similarly illuminating are questions about what improvement will look like, for example, "What will he (or she, or the two of you) be doing differently that will let you know this problem is taking a turn for the better?"

The therapist then explores each partner's experience with alcohol and other substances in some detail, clarifying what, where, when, how much, and with whom each spouse drinks, and inquiring as well about the severity of drinking (e.g., blackouts, morning drinking, job problems) and use of other substances such as marijuana and cocaine. The therapist also asks about history—for example, when the drinking became a problem for them, who was the first to notice, how drinking patterns have changed over time. However, history is generally less important than what the clients are doing now. Throughout, the therapist pays close attention to the specific ways alcohol has invaded or disrupted the couple's marriage and family relationships, yet is careful to maintain neutrality, because the aim here is not to advocate change but to gather evidence supporting the "alcohol-as-external-invader" metaphor to be used later in the team opinion.

After clarifying the major complaints, the therapist investigates patterns of interaction that help to maintain those complaints. Following Fisch, Weakland, and the Palo Alto group (Fisch et al., 1982), we assume that the most relevant interaction sequences revolve around persistent and well-intentioned attempts to deal with a complaint. Thus, an important strategic goal is for the therapist to identify—and ultimately interrupt—the ironic problem-maintaining solutions applied by the couple, and sometimes by others with whom the partners interact (Rohrbaugh & Shoham, 2001). The most direct way to investigate problem–solution loops is to ask what each spouse has been doing to deal with various complaints, especially those related to drinking, and in this way identify specific interaction sequences in which "more of the same" solution leads to more of the problem, leading to more of the solution, and so on. If there are multiple complaints, it may be necessary to track solution patterns for each spouse separately, though there will often be a common theme or basic thrust to what people are doing (e.g., nagging, attempting to control, talking or not talking about the problem). In any case, the therapist's objective here is simply to recognize problem-maintaining solution patterns—it is neither necessary or helpful at this stage to point them out to the couple.

Although ironic problem-maintaining solution patterns in alcoholism typically involve someone doing something (e.g., one spouse pressuring the other to change), what someone *does not* do (solutions of omission) can be important as well. For example, a wife who early in the marriage had taken a hard line with her husband about not drinking to intoxication later reversed this stance because she did not want to be controlling. As the alcohol problem worsened, she dealt with it less and less directly, busying herself in other activities and, when home, retreating to her study to meditate. Careful inquiry revealed that the former approach, though distasteful, had actually worked—when the wife had set limits, the husband had controlled his drinking. A key intervention in this case involved relabeling the wife's former hard-line stance as "caring" and "reassuring" to the husband (which she wanted it to be), and with this frame, the therapist helped her set limits again in ways that broke the problem cycle.

Although the main reason for tracking interaction sequences is to identify and interrupt ironic problem–solution loops, we also pay attention to differences between "wet" sequences, when someone has been drinking, and "dry" sequences, when he or she has been sober (Leipman, Silvia, & Nirenberg, 1989). These differences often suggest hypotheses about possible adaptive consequences of drinking for the couple, such as increasing or decreasing intimacy or affect (Steinglass, 1981). This construct, recently referred to as "symptom–system fit" (Rohrbaugh, Shoham, & Racioppo, 2002; Rohrbaugh et al., 2001), is relevant to planning for both the balanced Session-6 opinion and for the later restabilization phase, when the couple will be working to establish a satisfactory, alcohol-free relationship.

In addition to understanding what clients are doing, it is important for several reasons to grasp how they *view* themselves, each other, the problem, and therapy. First, intervening to change problem-maintaining interaction patterns will depend on framing therapeutic tasks and suggestions in terms compatible with clients' preferred views (Fisch et al., 1982). Second, the partners' views of the advantages—and especially the disadvantages—of giving up alcohol will be important in preparing the Session-6 opinion. Third, meanings and metaphors are key ingredients in reinforcing the clients' identity as a couple and helping them join together against alcohol, the external invader of their relationship. To lay groundwork for this central therapeutic metaphor, the therapist asks repeatedly about the partners' view of the extent to which they *control* alcohol's intrusion in their lives, as opposed to it controlling them. Finally, some of the most important client views concern their customership for therapy and readiness for change. In addition to present considerations, it is helpful to understand how (if at all) the clients sought help in the past, what they found helpful or unhelpful, how the helper(s) viewed their problems, and how the therapy ended. We are especially interested in their experiences with alcohol treatment programs, including Alcoholics Anonymous and Al-Anon.

Toward the end of Session 1, the therapist explores *exceptions* to problems. The objective in this solution-focused phase of the interview is to ask questions in a way that highlights for the couple possible resources and solutions to the dilemma—for example, "What's different about the times when the two of you enjoy life without alcohol? How do you get that to happen?" (Berg & Miller, 1992). We also ask a solution-focused "miracle question" to orient clients toward a time in the future when the problem no longer exists:

> Suppose that one night, while you are asleep, there is a miracle and the problem that brought you into therapy is solved. However, because you are asleep you don't know that the miracle has already happened. When you wake up in the morning, what will be different that will tell you that this miracle has taken place? What else? (Berg & Miller, 1992, p.13)

To make the prospect of a healthy, alcohol-free future more vivid, the therapist presses for details (e.g., "What will you be doing that is different? What else?"). How clients answer such questions is often less important than how they are asked, since the purpose is less to gather information than to seed ideas about possible change. The session closes with the following solution-focused homework assignment:

> "Between now and our next meeting, pay attention to what it is about your relationship you would like to continue or preserve. In other words, what would you like *not* to change?"

The partners may or may not discuss this with each other as they wish, but the therapist will want to know what they came up with at the next session.

Session 2: The Clients as a Couple

The main purpose of Session 2 is to understand and reinforce the clients' relationship *as a couple*. A simple, specific guideline underscoring this point is that the therapist uses the phrase "you as a couple" as much as possible. The session begins with follow-up on the homework assignment, which can proceed to additional solution-focused questioning about the couple's strengths and resources. In addition to clarifying unfinished business from Session 1, the therapist's options include a semistructured *oral history interview* (Buehlman, Gottman, & Katz, 1992) that traces the evolution of the couple's relationship, a *couple identity exercise* that builds on the positive set established by the solution-focused homework task and brings into focus how the clients view themselves as a couple, or an experiential *sculpting exercise* that further illuminates the couple's problem-maintaining solution patterns at a symbolic or metaphorical level (Papp, 1983) and sets the stage for later interventions aimed at externalizing alcohol as an unwelcome third party in the couple's relationship.

Session 3: Individual Sessions with Each Partner

Here, the therapist meets with the husband and wife separately to assess (1) each partner's commitment to the relationship, (2) whether one spouse feels intimidated by the other, and (3) whether there is actual or potential physical abuse. These meetings can also be used to clarify complaints, patterns of problem maintenance, and each client's position on issues relevant to therapy. The therapist begins by asking if there is anything that the spouses would like to add to what has been discussed, or if there is anything the therapist should know that might be easier to talk about alone. If either spouse asks that a disclosure be treated confidentially, the therapist explains that, although preferring not to share confidences, he or she must preserve the freedom to do what is in the best interest of the couple and each spouse. Depending on what is revealed, the therapist may ask a spouse who is ambivalent about staying in a marriage to give it an honest try, at least for the duration of therapy. If there are concerns about intimidation or the wife's safety, the therapist may discusses with her the possibility of raising these issues later in therapy, when the couple begins to negotiate for change. Of course, the therapist acts much sooner if the husband's active drinking in the consultation phase poses a clear and present danger to the wife or someone else.

Session 4: The Broader System

This session expands the consultation lens to encompass the couple's family and social network. The main objective is to understand how the couple's drinking and relationship problems "fit" the broader system; a second objective is to conduct further indirect intervention through circular questioning.

The couple and therapist first construct a family genogram covering at least three generations, from the partners' grandparents to their own children and grandchildren (McGoldrick & Gerson, 1985). After defining the cast of characters (including important nonrelatives), the therapist asks a series of questions about network relationships and individual-member functioning:

> "Of all the people we've talked about, are any of them especially close or not on speaking terms? Whose opinions do you respect most? Where do they stand on drinking? Who in the family is having problems these days? Where do they turn for advice? Has anyone had a problem with drinking? How was the problem resolved?"

This information has specific applications in later phases of treatment. For example, knowing who is influential in the broader network will have implications for whom the couple should later notify of their commitment to change.

Additional "circular" questions can then be used to explore systemic hypotheses about how the couple's difficulties with drinking fit the larger system and, by implication, to challenge indirectly the couple's problem-supporting premises or suggest avenues of change (Flueridas et al., 1986; Penn, 1985). While some circular questions may be asked of all couples (e.g., "How would your relationship be different if John stopped drinking? If the drinking continues or gets worse, what will life be like for your family 5 years from now?"), most are case specific (e.g., "Will your parents see more or less of the kids if John stops drinking?"). A crucial guideline for circular questioning is that the therapist remain neutral by not taking sides on any issue and not directly advocating sobriety or change.

Session 5: Loose Ends and Clarification

Here, the therapist continues circular questioning, investigates the couple's daily routines and family rituals, and clarifies whatever may still be unclear in preparation for Session

6. He or she reviews the partners' activities on a typical day, from the time they get up until the time they go to bed, and inquires about how they get together with family and friends to socialize and to celebrate special occasions and holidays. In the team's opinion, information about how alcohol disrupts or invades these routines and rituals is useful and highlights patterns to address in working toward family detoxification (Steinglass et al., 1987).

After Session 5, the therapist, supervisor, and other staff meet to (1) review and evaluate the assessment data; (2) outline a carefully constructed feedback message (opinion) for Session 6; and (3) plan tentative strategies for the treatment phase.

Session 6: Presenting the Opinion and Offering Treatment

In the final consultation session, the therapist presents the team's opinion and offers treatment. The opinion is carefully balanced, documenting specific ways in which alcohol has invaded the couple's family life, while acknowledging the many difficulties likely to be associated with sobriety and change. Above all, the therapist avoids taking sides about whether the couple should change. Although "treatment" will be offered, whether to participate can only be decided by the couple. If both spouses do choose treatment, family detoxification in the form of negotiating to change their relationship with alcohol begins right away, in this same session.

The opinion begins with a compliment acknowledging some specific way(s) the spouses have coped effectively with their difficult situation. The main body of the opinion then consists of three interwoven messages:

1. *"Alcohol appears to be a major player invading your family life in ways that are causing serious difficulties."*
2. *"Changing this situation will be very difficult for you as a couple and may have unforeseen negative consequences."*
3. *"Yet we see clear advantages to quitting."*

Each of these messages is carefully documented with information the clients have provided and framed in ways that make use of their own language. In presenting the first message, the therapist develops and extends the metaphor of alcohol as an external invader that seems more in control of the couple's life than vice versa. He or she documents the "invasion" with specific examples and portrays this as a problem for the clients as a couple, not as just the drinker's problem:

> "What I mean when I say that alcohol is a major player in your life is, for example, the time that you said you wanted to spend a certain kind of vacation together and it turned out very differently because of the drinking . . . or that the two of you never seem to be able to have sex together unless Joe has been drinking . . . or that you are in hot water at work because you don't seem to be able to concentrate after you've been drinking."

The second message—that change will be difficult and may entail certain hazards—concerns the future and cannot be documented as specifically as the first (invasion) message. In rendering the opinion, the therapist nonetheless comments on what is likely to be especially difficult for the couple, and notes that giving up alcohol is often difficult for couples generally, if for no other reason than the unpredictability involved.

If one or both spouses are ambivalent about treatment or unwilling to make a clear commitment, the therapist avoids taking sides and does not push or try to sell recovery. Instead, he or she maintains a posture of nonblaming curiosity, trying to understand what the clients themselves are proposing to do about the drinking, and why. If they persist in their ambivalence or opposition to treatment, the therapist respects their position and proposes further study of the issue. At this point, therapy moves to Phase II-B—strategic intervention framed as continued consultation.

Phase II-A: Treatment

Treatment consists of "family detoxification" (a term for therapists, not clients) supplemented by strategic interdiction of problem–solution loops and solution-focused amplification of exceptions to problems. When the couple chooses treatment, the therapist shifts from a neutral stance to align with the clients against alcohol (the invader) and begins helping them negotiate a series of agreements aimed at detoxifying their home environment and, ultimately, their outside social relationships. To this end, we usually recommend that the problem drinker abstain completely from alcohol and that the family establish a completely alcohol-free home. We are willing to be flexible, however, and entertain certain exceptions if the spouses are united in believing such an arrangement is best for them and willing to demonstrate they can handle it responsibly. In any case, the minimum requirement for "treatment" is that the clients, as a couple, have a clear and meaningful goal for change. Ideally, they leave Session 6 with an agreed-upon quitting date and a clear plan for beginning the family detoxification process.

Because our systems therapy places so much emphasis upon clients' explicitly choosing (or not choosing) treatment, it is important to be clear with them that being in treatment means that they, as a couple, have the goal of changing their relationship with alcohol. It also means that they are actively working toward that goal. Being clear about this definition—and whether or not the therapist and clients are doing "treatment" at a given point in therapy—helps to keep change goals more sharply in focus. This is why we are careful to distinguish "consultation" from "treatment," and why we continue or return to "consultation" when customership is lacking.

Family Detoxification

The term "family detoxification" (Steinglass, 1992; Steinglass et al., 1987) refers to a process through which the problem drinker in the family stops drinking and his or her environment becomes alcohol-free. This does not necessarily mean that drinkers will show withdrawal symptoms or other signs of physiological addiction—though they may. It is important to define detoxification as a process that will affect, and be affected by, the drinker's family. Because both spouses have a vital stake in the outcome, they should plan and negotiate as a couple how this process will unfold.

Family detoxification involves both doing and viewing. On the "doing" side, the therapist helps the partners negotiate a series of detailed agreements about how they will deal with alcohol. At the same time, he or she works to help the clients revise the meaning that drinking holds for them as a couple. Important concepts here are "collaboration" and "externalization." The therapist collaborates with the couple in order to help them collaborate with each other in a coalition against alcohol. Externalization refers to interventions designed to help the partners redefine drinking as alien to their relationship and join together against alcohol as an external invader of family life.

Procedurally, the objective is first to detoxify the drinker and the family's daily routines, then to ensure that their external boundaries are protected from any new invasion by alcohol. In this way, the partners move into the outside world with a clear plan that, like a protective bubble, helps them stay alcohol-free (Steinglass, 1992). The therapist helps the partners formulate specific steps they will take in dealing with alcohol, including who will do what and when. As the plan develops, the therapist encourages them to anticipate what might go wrong and to realize that what they propose to do will be difficult. At the next session, he or she inquires in detail about how the plan was implemented, framing noncompliance as partial success and/or understandable reluctance to change. Since family detoxification is a multistep process, a more or less complete plan will usually take a number of sessions to develop and implement. And by that time, it is likely that the couple will be struggling to adjust to fundamental—and potentially very difficult—changes in the relationship. For this reason, the therapist cautions the couple to go slow, suggesting that it is better to achieve change slowly and steadily than to promote rapid change that may not last.

An important principle is that the steps clients take toward family detoxification not be "more of the same" in the sense of recapitulating problem–solution loops. A better aim is to block or reverse interaction sequences revolving around well-intended spousal "solutions" to the problem, especially the specific ways the spouse has attempted to get the drinker to quit alcohol (Weakland & Fisch, 1992). Thus, if the wife tries actively to prevent the drinking (e.g., by hiding bottles), we would prefer that the husband—not the wife—physically remove the alcohol from the home. Conversely, if the wife typically avoids dealing with the alcohol, having her take an active role in removing it would make sense as "less of the same." The point here is simply that family detoxification should be done in a way that alters rather than reinforces typical interaction sequences. In presenting suggestions for change, it is also important to avoid the implication that the drinking is somehow the wife's (or husband's) fault, and to frame suggestions in a manner consistent with her (or his) own views or position (Fisch et al., 1982).

Family detoxification also deals with how alcohol may impinge on the couple's extended family, social network, and work environments. Here, the therapist typically helps the partners rehearse how they will deal with specific, high-risk situations in order to protect their alcohol-free identity. Similarly, if other people (children, family, friends) live in the couple's household or are frequently present, we pay attention to how they will accommodate to the changes the couple is making. It is useful for the therapist to meet these people and, with the couple, seek their collaboration. Another important step in solidifying therapeutic gains is for the couple to notify key family members and associates of their commitment to change. To promote this, the therapist helps the partners decide whom they should notify; what the specific content of the message should be; and how, when, and by whom the notification should be given. Because problem drinkers are often reluctant to let other people know they have a problem, even when they are doing something about it, notification is framed as a crucial but difficult step the couple should take when they are ready.

When family detoxification falters due to noncompliance or partial compliance with the terms of an agreement, we address client reluctance in a nonadversarial, nonblaming way. While the therapist clearly indicates when what the couple does (or does not do) is incompatible with the goal of an alcohol-free home (e.g., the basement is still a part of the house and cooking sherry is still alcohol), it is equally important that he or she acknowledge whatever happened as understandable and, without reprimanding the couple, work toward keeping family detoxification on track. Thus, if the couple follows through on only *some* of an agreement, the therapist might frame this as partial success or take the solution-focused tack by asking how the partners managed to do what they did do. He or she may also take a one-down position—for example, by blaming him- or herself for going too fast or not being clear. And if an agreement collapses altogether, the therapist may frame this as an understandable response to the couple's frustrating situation. The goal of these reframing–supporting tactics is to encourage the couple to try again. If noncompliance continues, however, the therapist makes a U-turn and moves to Phase II-B: intervention framed as "continued consultation." Here, the therapist begins to work more strategically, attempting to address one or both spouse's complaints in the framework of further consultation about whether changing their relationship with alcohol would indeed be worthwhile.

Interdicting Problem–Solution Loops and Finding Exceptions

The second major component of the treatment phase involves interrupting problem-maintaining interaction patterns and amplifying exceptions to problem drinking. To do this, the therapist uses strategies and techniques from both problem-focused (Fisch et al., 1982; Rohrbaugh et al., 2001) and solution-focused brief therapy (Berg & Miller, 1992). These tactics supplement the process of family detoxification and often provide a vehicle for addressing problem patterns more directly, albeit by less direct means.

As noted earlier, an important assessment goal is to identify problem–solution loops in which more of clients' well-intentioned solutions lead to more complaints, which lead to more of the solution, and so on. As problem-maintaining solution patterns become clear, the therapist and team can begin to formulate what less of the same might look like. The key question is this: What behavior, by whom, in what situation, would suffice to reverse the problem-maintaining solution? Pursuing such a "strategic objective" (a term for therapists, not clients) and thus promoting "less of the same" is central to our therapy, regardless of whether the couple formally chooses treatment.

Identifying specific situations in which a problem–solution sequence typically occurs is especially relevant to planning an intervention. In one case, for example, a couple's complaints concerned both the unemployed husband's urge to drink while the wife was at work and a general lack of trust in the relationship. The therapist learned that a predictable interaction sequence ensued when the wife arrived home from work: As she kissed him hello, the husband appeared despondent and sometimes smelled of alcohol; the wife asked what was wrong, got little response, but continued to repeat the question in one form or another until the husband said he did not think she really loved him and that she probably found the men at work more attractive. The wife denied this, but the denial seemed only to confirm the husband's suspicions and an accusation–denial cycle escalated until one of the spouses became angry and left the room. An important series of interventions in this case focused on changing what happened when the wife arrived home from work. The therapist was able to interdict two well-intentioned solutions in this situation with carefully framed suggestions that the wife do things *other* than ask the husband what was wrong, then defend herself in the face of his accusations, especially when he had been drinking.

While focused solution interdiction attends primarily to what people *do* about their complaints, complementary solution-focused tactics attempt to shift how people *view* their situation in order to mobilize resources for change. To accentuate exceptions to complaints, the therapist asks questions such as "How did you manage to do that?", "What did you do differently?", and "What will have to happen for her to do that more often?" The therapist highlights interactional exceptions with questions such as "What do you suppose you do differently when he doesn't drink?" and "What do you imagine she notices is different about you when you don't drink?" Also, because the miracle question introduced in Session 1 provides a useful jumping-off point for exploring exceptions, we often reintroduce it in the treatment phase. (Berg and Miller [1992] describe these and other useful solution-focused strategies for problem drinkers in detail.) While the purpose of solution-focused questioning is to accentuate the positive, we are careful to avoid premature celebration of change; cautious optimism is more characteristic of the therapist's general stance.

Phase II-B: Intervention Framed as "Continued Consultation"

If the couple does not choose treatment, or if treatment reaches the point of a U-turn, therapy continues in the form of strategic and structural interventions framed as further consultation about the advisability of change (see Figure 14.1). The goal of such "continued consultation" is to return the couple to the treatment (family detoxification) track or, failing that, to provoke change less directly. Activities in this phase usually involve one or several of the following: (1) using diagnostic "experiments" designed to challenge the drinker, to show that he or she can control drinking, or the partners, to show they can tolerate change; (2) seeing the spouse alone, especially when he or she is a customer for change and the drinker is not; or (3) involving other people beyond the couple, such as family members, friends, or other helpers.

U-Turns

When family detoxification falters and reframing interventions fail to encourage the clients to try again, therapy moves to Phase II-B, with the announcement of a "U-turn." After consulting with the team, the therapist presents the U-turn decision dramatically and apologetically:

> "We now recognize that we failed to appreciate sufficiently the possible dangers of change, though, in retrospect, the clues were there; let us slow down and consider again the choices you have as a couple, including the choice of living with the drinking."

Reframes that cast the choice not to change in terms of loyalty to a (distasteful) family tradition are sometimes very powerful here. In any case, the therapist usually maintains a restraint from change position unless or until the clients actively request treatment.

Controlled Drinking Experiments

Intervention in the form of a "controlled drinking experiment" (Treadway, 1989) may be useful when one or both spouses indicate, either directly or indirectly, that they believe drinking is not a problem and it is really under control. The main objective of this intervention is to create a situation that challenges the drinker (and couple) to either demonstrate control or request help. The therapist, taking the position that although the drinking may indeed be controllable, it is important to find out just how controllable it is, asks the drinker how many drinks a day he or she can handle responsibly, and seeks to define a level of consumption beyond which both spouses would agree there is a problem.

The therapist then challenges the drinker to observe that limit. We also try to set up the experiment in a way that interdicts the spouse's problem-maintaining solutions. Thus, the spouse may be asked to help by carefully but unobtrusively observing the drinker's behavior—and most important, by suspending usual ways of trying to prevent or stop the drinking (e.g., pleading, lecturing, investigating) so as not to contaminate our observations. The therapist follows up the controlled drinking experiment by framing failure or noncompliance with task as evidence that there probably *is* a problem with controlling drinking—and the couple may then be more amenable to treatment.

Seeing the Spouse Alone

Many of our "continued consultation" strategies involve seeing the spouse alone. This format is most indicated when the spouse is a customer and the drinker is not, or when there is evidence of a coercive relationship in which the wife is in some way intimidated by the drinker (i.e., when she is reluctant to assert herself or take a stand about the drinker's behavior for fear he may be violent, hurt himself, or abandon her). Individual meetings are helpful because they afford better opportunity to help the spouse take a stand or reverse her usual stance in relation to the drinking. For example, a straightforward coaching strategy might help her detach from the problem and avoid the "responsibility trap" (Bepko & Krestan, 1985); structural empowerment strategies might be used to build or reinforce coalitions that would help the spouse take a stand (e.g., "Who best understands your predicament? How about bringing her in next time?"); and rehearsal of specific responses (e.g., leaving home, asking the drinker's friends or relatives to look in on him) may be necessary when there is a possibility of violence or self-destructive behavior. Referral to a support group helps in some cases, but this should supplement, not supplant, direct intervention by the therapist.

The therapist can also use individual sessions for brief therapy interventions aimed at interdicting specific problem-maintaining solutions. Here, we usually frame suggestions in terms of assessment (e.g., Let's try this "to see what we're up against" or "to see how being less reactive fits you") rather than as interventions intended to change things. Another indirect strategy is to ask circular questions about the consequences of the spouse acting or not acting in various ways relative not only to herself but also to various family relationships (e.g., "What would your mother think about you putting your foot down with John? Has she ever done that with your dad?"). Individual meetings with the spouse are framed to be as nonthreatening as possible to the drinker (e.g., I want to try to help her with the problem *she* is having with this), but resistance should be expected and the therapist must not be intimidated. In some cases, individual sessions with the spouse can be interspersed with conjoint and/or individual sessions with the drinker; in other cases, it makes sense to exclude him from the therapy (at least temporarily) and work with the spouse alone.

Finally, we follow Treadway's (1989) maxim: "When stuck, add people." This could involve a relative, friend, employer, or AA sponsor and, depending on the dynamics of a case, such "convening" interventions could be used to mobilize influence, build cotherapeutic coalitions, mark generation boundaries, or detriangulate other family members from the couple's relationship.

Phase III: Restabilization and Relapse Prevention

When the partner stops drinking and the couple's household and social relationships become alcohol-free, the therapist positions him- or herself to help the partners deal with the predictably difficult consequences of sobriety and change. Because the partners' relationship will probably have been organized around alcohol—and because the drinking probably had adaptive, stabilizing consequences for them, in addition to the more obvious negative effects—they are likely to experience alcohol-free family life as *de*stabilizing, at least initially. Our goals for the restabilization phase of therapy are purposefully modest: We do not attempt to resolve deep underlying issues or create fundamental changes in family relationships. In the few sessions available, we aim only to identify possible areas of difficulty and address *some* of them with structural or strategic interventions. (It is reassuring to know that, with alcohol removed, some couples and families will *naturally* restabilize in a more satisfactory way, without our help or intervention.) We also employ specific reframing and rehearsal interventions designed to make relapse less likely and less catastrophic.

The boundaries and procedures of Phase III are necessarily less precise than those for Phases I and II due to the great variability in how couples progress to this point. Although Phase III ideally begins around Session 13 (following the "acute treatment" phase), when the drinking has stopped and family detoxification is complete, some couples are well ahead of this schedule and others are well behind it. Phase boundaries are further clouded by the fact that both restabilization and relapse prevention interventions are likely to have been introduced much earlier in therapy—for example, "restraint from celebration" is applied whenever clients suggest that drinking is behind them and the battle is over (which can occur as early as the first session). The relapse prevention technique of anticipating and planning for high-risk situations is an important element of family detoxification.[4]

APPLICABILITY AND LESSONS LEARNED

Of 39 couples who entered the systemic treatment in our research project,[5] 23 (or 59%) completed the full 20-session regimen and had at least moderately positive drinking and relationship outcomes at termination and follow-up. The primary therapists, trained by the authors, were master's level clinicians with at least a year's experience working with substance abuse clients. Analyses of case records and videotaped therapy sessions indicated that therapists' adherence to the manual and successful implementation of its main components predicted positive outcomes. After the consultation phase, however, distinctions between Phases II-A (treatment) and II-B (continuing consultation) were sometimes difficult to maintain, and few cases went explicitly back to the former from the latter. (One successful couple, in fact, refused the family detoxification component of treatment when it was initially offered, but then did it on their own 2 months later and informed the therapist after the fact!) In general, clients seemed less responsive to the straightforward, step-by-step requirements of family detoxification than to strategic and solution-focused interventions targeting drinking and relationship patterns.

Other lessons we learned highlight limitations of our integrative approach to treatment development. Because the models we drew upon call attention to different clinical phenomena (e.g., hypotheses about adaptive consequences of drinking vs. descriptions of problem–solution loops) and prescribe different therapeutic actions (e.g., neutrality vs. strategic intervention), often for the same clinical situation, we tried to specify rules governing which concepts and techniques to invoke in which circumstances. This effort was only partly successful, however, because therapists sometimes found our what-to-do-when guidelines difficult to apply. It was also clear that therapists implemented some components of the integrative model more effectively than others, and the accessibility of familiar and/or well-specified procedures (e.g., doing a genogram or contracting for family detoxification) sometimes seemed to undermine effective implementation of other, more central or exacting components (e.g., tracking and interrupting ironic problem-solution loops).

In terms of client characteristics, we found no evidence that the severity or chronicity of either drinking or relationship problems limits the model's applicability. What does appear important, however, is that the clients have some degree of commitment to their relationship as a couple, and that at least one of them is concerned about the drinking. Our most difficult and least successful cases involved clients who entered therapy with their "coupleness" in doubt, either because it had not been established, or because one of the partners was thinking about leaving the relationship. Under these circumstances, an approach based on empowering clients *as a couple* would probably not be indicated. In addition, although the treatment's conjoint focus on "you as a couple" was helpful in most cases, we encountered several enmeshed couples for whom "you as an individual" might have constituted a better "less of the same" emphasis.

More systematic evidence concerning the applicability of this approach comes from comparing it to another manualized treatment for alcohol abuse—a cognitive-behavioral therapy (Wakefield, Williams, Yost, & Patterson, 1996) developed for the same project. The design, methodology, and results of this work is described elsewhere (Rohrbaugh et al., 2002; Shoham et al., 1998). Suffice it to say here that, in this randomized trial, we compared family systems therapy and cognitive-behavioral therapy to each other rather than to a control group, in order to test hypotheses relevant to client–treatment matching—namely, that the two treatments would be differentially effective depending on certain client and couple relationship characteristics assessed before therapy began. Although both treatments were conducted in a couple format, they differed dramatically in relative (individual vs. system) focus and especially in the level of demand placed on clients for abstinence and change. Wakefield and colleagues' (1996) highly structured cognitive-behavioral therapy focused primarily on the individual drinker in the context of high demand for abstinence and change (e.g., using Breathalyzer tests to ensure compliance). The systemic therapy was more permissive in this respect, using indirect strategies to work with client resistance and promote change.

Particularly striking were results for two pretreatment markers of a troubled couple relationship: (1) *demand–withdraw interaction*, a common pattern in alcohol-involved couples, in which one partner pursues, criticizes, nags, or demands, while the other distances, defends, avoids, or withdraws (Christensen & Heavey, 1993), and (2) *negative couple affect*, here defined as the ratio of negative to positive partner exchanges (Gottman, 1994). For couples in cognitive-behavioral therapy, high demand–withdraw and negative affect predicted poorer outcome in terms of both retention (dropout) and later abstinence from alcohol, yet for couples in family systems therapy these variables made little difference. In other words, the systemic therapy appeared to be a substantially better fit than cognitive-behavioral therapy for alcoholics in difficult, troubled relationships—and a better hedge against dropout all around. More specific analyses of the wife-demand–husband-withdraw pattern suggested that an alcoholic husband may withdraw from a high-demand therapy in the same way he withdraws from a demanding wife (Shoham et al., 1998). The low-demand "consultation" stance of systemic therapy probably helps to avoid this ironic dynamic.[6]

A more general lesson from this research is that attributes of couple and family relationships can predict differential response to clearly distinctive couple treatments for alcohol abuse. We believe such findings provide a useful counterpoint to recent skepticism about matching individual alcoholic clients to individual treatments (Project MATCH Research Group, 1997). Although the psychotherapy and substance abuse fields have been slow to look beyond the individual client when offering guidelines for selecting different treatments, family-oriented clinicians and researchers will not be surprised by evidence that context matters.

NOTES

1. The Couples Alcoholism Treatment project, based at the University of California, Santa Barbara, was supported by National Institute of Alcoholism and Alcohol Abuse Grant No. R01-AA08970 awarded to Larry Beutler (principal investigator), and Theodore Jacob and Varda Shoham (principal investigators). A discussion of the project's original rationale can be found in Beutler and colleagues (1993).
2. Family therapists use "circular questions" both to assess systemic relationship dynamics (e.g., "Who in the family is most/least concerned about John's drinking? When Dad stopped drinking, did the relationship between Mom and the kids become closer or more distant?") and to intervene indirectly—for example, with questions that challenge problem-maintaining premises or imply possible avenues to change. (For a useful taxonomy of circular questions, see Flueridas et al., 1986).
3. In the Q-sort study described by Rohrbaugh and colleagues (1995), a diverse sample of alcohol treatment professionals sorted 50 opinion statements about the nature of alcoholism and approaches to treatment into eight categories along a continuum from "Least agree" to "Most agree." The item sample included statements intended to represent family systems, 12-step, and cognitive-behavioral viewpoints, as well as other issues in the field. When the Q sorts were factor-analyzed, three main factors emerged, corresponding as expected to the three viewpoints. By comparing the items ranked high and low on each factor viewpoint, it was possible to identify similarities and differences between them.
4. Rohrbaugh and colleagues (1995) provide a more detailed description of the various options available to therapists in Phase III, including approaches to dealing with issues concerning intimacy, parenting, power and control, and outside relationships.
5. In 33 of these couples, the identified alcoholic was the husband. The results reported in Shoham and colleagues (1998) and Rohrbaugh and colleagues (2002) are for male-alcoholic couples only.
6. Although cognitive behavioral and family systems therapy were clearly distinct from each other in this study, it is less clear how similar these approaches are to other treatments carrying a cognitive-behavioral or family systems label. Other alcohol treatments based on behavioral principles, for example, may be less demanding or more relationship-focused than Wakefield and colleagues' (1996) approach and treatments incorporating family systems principles (e.g., Liepman, Nirenberg, & Begin, 1989); Wegscheider's (1976) approach can be much more confrontational than our own brand of family systems therapy (Rohrbaugh et al., 1995). Given the well-documented efficacy of behaviorally oriented couple treatments developed by McCrady and colleagues (1986) and by O'Farrell and colleagues (1998), it may be especially important to understand similarities and differences between these approaches and Wakefield and colleagues' cognitive-behavioral therapy. For a discussion of this, see Shoham and colleagues (1998, pp. 573–574).

REFERENCES

Baucom, D. H., Shoham, V., Meuser, K. T., Daiuto, A. D., & Stickle, T. R. (1998). Empirically supported couple and family interventions for marital distress and adult mental health problems. *Journal of Consulting and Clinical Psychology, 65,* 53–88.

Bepko, C., & Krestan, J. (1985). *The responsibility trap: A blueprint for treating the alcoholic family.* New York: Free Press.

Berg, I. K., & Miller, S. D. (1992). *Working with the problem drinker: A solution-focused approach.* New York: Norton.

Beutler, L. E., Patterson, K., Jacob, T., Shoham, V., Yost, L., & Rohrbaugh, M. J. (1983). Matching treatment to alcoholism subtypes. *Psychotherapy, 30,* 463–472.

Borwick, B. (1991). The co-created world of alcoholism. *Journal of Strategic and Systemic Therapies, 10,* 3–19.

Buehlman, K., Gottman, J. M., & Katz, L. (1992). How a couple views their past predicts their future: Predicting divorce from an oral history interview. *Journal of Family Psychology, 5,* 295–318.

Christensen, A., & Heavey, C. L. (1993). Gender differences in marital conflict: The demand/withdraw interaction pattern. In S. Oskamp & M. Costanzo (Eds.), *Gender issues in contemporary society* (pp. 113–141). Newbury Park, CA: Sage.

Elkin, M. (1984). *Families under the influence.* New York: Norton.

Fisch, R. (1986). The brief treatment of alcoholism. *Journal of Strategic and Systemic Therapies, 5,* 40–49.

Fisch, R., Weakland, J. H., & Segal, L. (1982). *The tactics of change.* San Francisco: Jossey-Bass.

Fleuridas, C., Nelson, T. I., & Rosenthal, D. (1986). The evolution of circular questions: Training family therapists. *Journal of Marital and Family Therapy, 12,* 113–127.

Gottman, J. M. (1994). *What predicts divorce? The relationship between marital processes and marital outcome.* Hillsdale, NJ: Erlbaum.

Leipman, M., Silvia, L., & Nirenberg, T. (1989). The use of behavior loop mapping for substance abuse. *Family Relations, 38,* 282–287.

Leipman, M. R., Nirenberg, T. D., & Begin, A. M. (1989). Evaluation of a program designed to help family and significant others to motivate resistant alcoholics into recovery. *American Journal of Drug and Alcohol Abuse, 15,* 209–221.

Lewis, B. (1987). Cybernetics and the treatment of alcoholism: Thoughts on a model. *Alcoholism Treatment Quarterly, 4,* 127–139.

McCrady, B. S., Noel, N. E., Abrams, D. B., Stout, R. L., Nelson, H. G., & Hay, W. M. (1986). Comparitive effectiveness of three types of spouse involvement in outpatient behavioral alchohlism treatment. *Journal of Studies on Alcohol, 47,* 459–467.

McGoldrick, M., & Gerson, R. (1985). *Genograms in family assessment.* New York: Norton.

O'Farrell, T. J., Choquette, K. A., & Cutter, H. S. G. (1998). Couples relapse prevention sessions after behavioral marital therapy for alcoholics and their wives: Outcomes during three years after starting treatment. *Journal of Studies on Alcohol, 59,* 357–370.

Papp, P. (1983). *The process of change.* New York: Guilford Press.

Penn, P. (1985). Feed forward: Future questions, future maps. *Family Process, 24,* 299–311.

Project MATCH Research Group. (1997). Matching alcoholism treatments to client heterogeneity: Project MATCH post-treatment drinking outcome. *Journal of Studies on Alcohol, 58,* 7–29.

Rohrbaugh, M. J., & Shoham, V. (2001). Brief therapy based on interrupting ironic processes: The Palo Alto model. *Clinical Psychology: Science and Practice, 8,* 66–81.

Rohrbaugh, M. J., Shoham, V., & Racioppo, M. W. (2002). Toward family-level attribute × treatment interaction research. In H. A. Liddle, D. A. Santisteban, R. F. Levant, & J. H. Bray (Eds.), *Family psychology: Science-based interventions* (pp. 215–238). Washington, DC: American Psychological Association.

Rohrbaugh, M. J., Shoham, V., Spungen, C., & Steinglass, P. (1995). Family systems therapy in practice: A systemic couples therapy for problem drinking. In B. Bongar & L. E. Beutler (Eds.), *Comprehensive textbook of psychotherapy: Theory and practice* (pp. 228–253). New York: Oxford University Press.

Rohrbaugh, M. J., Shoham, V., Trost, S., Muramoto, M., Cate, R. M., & Leischow, S. (2001). Couple dynamics of change-resistant smoking: Toward a family-consultation model. *Family Process, 40,* 15–31.

Shoham, V., Rohrbaugh, M. J., Stickle, T.R., & Jacob, T. (1998). Demand–withdraw couple interaction moderates retention in cognitive-behavioral vs. family-systems treatments for alcoholism. *Journal of Family Psychology, 12,* 557–577.

Steinglass, P. (1981). The alcoholic family at home: Patterns of interaction in dry, wet and transitional stages of alcoholism. *Archives of General Psychiatry, 38,* 578–584.

Steinglass, P. (1992, October). *Family-level detoxification: What it is and why it works.* Paper presented at the American Association of Marital and Family Therapy Workshop, Miami, FL.

Steinglass, P., Bennett, L., Wolin, S., & Reiss, D. (1987). *The alcoholic family.* New York: Basic Books.

Treadway, D. C. (1989). *Before it's too late: Working with substance abuse in the family.* New York: Norton.

Wakefield, P., Williams, R. E., Yost, E., & Patterson, K. M. (1996). *Couples therapy for alcoholism: A cognitive-behavioral treatment manual.* New York: Guilford Press.

Weakland, J. H., & Fisch, R. (1992). Brief therapy—MRI style. In S. H. Budman, M. F. Hoyt, & S. Friedman (Eds.), *The first session in brief therapy* (pp. 306–323). New York: Guilford Press.

Weakland, J. H., Watzlawick, P., Fisch, R., & Bodin, A. (1974). Brief therapy: Focused problem resolution. *Family Process, 13,* 141–168.

Wegscheider, S. (1976). *The family trap: No one escapes from a chemically dependent family.* Minneapolis: Johnson Institute.

White, M., & Epston, D. (1990). *Narrative means to therapeutic ends.* New York: Norton.

15

Psychosocial Treatment for Cocaine Dependence

The Community Reinforcement plus Vouchers Approach

Stephen T. Higgins
Stacey C. Sigmon
Alan J. Budney

Cocaine dependence remains a serious public health problem in the United States and abroad. The prevalence of current cocaine use (i.e., within the past month) in the United States, for example, has decreased from a peak of approximately 5.7 million in the mid-1980s to about 1.8 million today, but heavy use (i.e., weekly or more frequently) has remained stable at approximately 600,000 throughout that same period. Of course, it is this relatively recalcitrant practice of heavy cocaine use that contributes most to the public health problem that cocaine dependence represents. While more prevalent in the United States, cocaine abuse is a public health problem in many parts of the world and has become an increasing problem in Europe (see, e.g., Barrio, De la Fuente, Royuela, Diaz, & Rodriguez-Artalejo, 1998; Hunter, Donoghoe, & Stimson, 1995).

Significant scientific advances have been made in understanding cocaine's myriad effects during the past 15 years, including the development of efficacious treatments for cocaine dependence (Higgins, 2000), including the Community Reinforcement Approach plus vouchers, which is the focus of this chapter (Budney & Higgins, 1998). This treatment combines therapy based on an adaptation of the Community Reinforcement Approach (CRA), originally developed as a treatment for severe alcohol dependence (Hunt & Azrin, 1973), with a voucher-based incentive program derived from prior contingency-management interventions used with heroin and other forms of drug abuse (see Higgins & Silverman, 1999). Relapse prevention therapy is another efficacious treatment for cocaine dependence (Carroll, 1998). Some key elements of relapse prevention are included in CRA as well and are reviewed here, but interested readers should consult the therapist manual on relapse prevention for details on the content and implementation of that treatment (Carroll, 1998).

There are no controlled trials supporting the efficacy of inpatient care for cocaine dependence, and the few available comparisons of outpatient versus inpatient treatment have revealed higher costs and no outcome advantage for the latter (Alterman et al., 1994). Thus, the focus of this chapter is outpatient care, with a focus on behavioral interventions, since there is not yet a reliably efficacious pharmacotherapy for cocaine dependence. One exception is disulfiram therapy for patients who abuse cocaine and alcohol, which is discussed here. Although this chapter focuses on the CRA plus vouchers model, we have attempted at least to mention all available information regarding efficacious treatment practices for cocaine dependence.

CONCEPTUAL FRAMEWORK

The CRA plus vouchers treatment is based on concepts and principles of operant conditioning, social learning theory, and behavioral pharmacology. Within this conceptual framework, cocaine use is considered a learned behavior that is maintained through the reinforcing effects of the pharmacological actions of cocaine in combination with social and other reinforcement derived from the cocaine-abusing lifestyle (Higgins & Katz, 1998).

Reliable empirical observations with humans and laboratory animals provide compelling evidence that cocaine produces robust reinforcing effects (Griffiths, Bigelow, & Henningfield, 1980; Higgins, 1997); that is, normal laboratory animals will readily work to earn the opportunity to ingest cocaine, which is the case with many of the other drugs that humans abuse as well (e.g., morphine, amphetamine). These drugs function as primary, unconditioned reinforcers for these laboratory animals in much the same way that food, water, and sex operate. This is an important scientific observation, because it suggests that the reinforcing effects of these drugs are based on biologically normal processes. As such, most physically intact humans can be assumed to possess the necessary neurobiological systems to experience cocaine-produced reinforcement and hence the potential to develop patterns of cocaine use, abuse, and dependence.

Scientific evidence also clearly reveals that cocaine use, abuse, and dependence have multiple determinants (Higgins & Katz, 1998). Genetic, individual, familial, and macroenvironmental factors affect the probability of human cocaine use, abuse, and dependence (i.e., they are risk factors). For example, supporting a genetic contribution, monozygotic twins are significantly more likely to be concordant for cocaine dependence than are dizygotic twins (Kendler & Prescott, 1998; Tsuang et al., 1996). As an example of an individual characteristic affecting the probability of cocaine use, unemployment is associated with a higher prevalence of cocaine use (Substance Abuse and Mental Health Services Administration, 2000). As for family influence, the degree of parental monitoring of youth is inversely associated with the probability of their initiating the use of cocaine or other illicit drugs (Chilcoat & Anthony, 1996). As an example of still other macroenvironmental risk factors, children from more disadvantaged neighborhoods are at greater risk for being offered the opportunity to use cocaine (Crum, Lillie-Blanton, & Anthony, 1996). Also supporting the influence of neighborhood, putative race/ethnicity differences in the prevalence of crack cocaine use are significantly reduced by controlling for the presence of other crack users in the neighborhood (Chilcoat & Schütz, 1995; Lillie-Blanton, Anthony, & Schuster, 1993).

CRA PLUS VOUCHERS TREATMENT

The CRA plus vouchers treatment attempts to impact those risk factors over which one can exert control, namely, individual skills and the physical and social environments of the user. The overarching goal of this treatment is systematically to weaken the influence of reinforcement derived from cocaine use and the cocaine-abusing lifestyle, and to increase the frequency of reinforcement derived from healthier alternative activities, especially those that are incompatible with continued cocaine use and abuse.

The clinic in which we have conducted most of our research on the use of CRA plus vouchers to treat cocaine dependence is a university-based outpatient center that specializes in the treatment of adults. All initial clinic contacts are handled by a trained staff member who establishes that the treatment seeker reports problems related to cocaine use, is at least 18 years of age, and resides within the county in which the clinic is located. We restrict treatment to adults, anticipating that adolescents will likely need other services, and we restrict participation to individuals who reside within the same county because of the intensity of the treatment, which requires multiple clinic visits per week. Those not meeting these criteria are referred elsewhere for treatment.

For those who meet these inclusion criteria, we offer an intake appointment within 24 hours of clinic contact. A rapid intake procedure significantly reduces the relatively high attrition rate between the initial clinic contact and intake interview that is commonly observed with the cocaine-dependent population (Festinger, Lamb, Kirby, & Marlowe, 1996). When clients cannot come to the clinic within 24 hours, a secondary goal is to have them come in within 72 hours.

Intake Assessment

The intake assessment for this treatment takes about 3 hours to complete. While a longer assessment might produce additional useful information, we try to get treatment underway as expeditiously as possible in order to reduce early treatment dropout. The assessment is focused on collecting detailed information on current and past cocaine and other substance use, employment/vocational status, recreational interests, social supports, family and social problems, legal issues, treatment readiness, and psychiatric functioning. We use a semistructured drug history interview that we developed to collect details about cocaine and other drug use. We use the Addiction Severity Index (ASI; McLellan et al., 1985) to obtain a quantitative, time-based assessment of problem severity regarding alcohol use; drug use; and employment, medical, legal, family, social, and psychological functioning. We use the Cocaine Dependency Self-Test (Washton, Stone, & Hendrickson, 1988) to obtain specific information regarding the type of adverse effects of cocaine use that clients have experienced. The Michigan Alcoholism Screening Test (MAST; Selzer, 1971) is one of several instruments used to assess alcohol problems. The Beck Depression Inventory (BDI; Beck, Ward, Mendelson, Mock, & Erbaugh, 1961) is used to assess depressive symptomatology, and the Symptom Checklist 90—Revised (SCL-90-R; Derogatis, 1983) screens for psychiatric symptomatology more generally. The Stages of Change Readiness and Treatment Eagerness Scale (SOCRATES; Miller & Tonigan, 1996) is used to assess clients' perception of the severity of their cocaine and other drug use, and their readiness to reduce drug use. We developed a Practical Needs Assessment questionnaire to assess immediate problems that could interfere with initial treatment engagement (e.g., housing, legal, transportation, or child care). Finally, we use the DSM Checklist to make substance use diagnoses (Hudziack et al., 1993).

Prior to leaving the intake interview, clients always meet at least briefly with a therapist, so that they depart this initial session feeling that treatment has begun, and, very importantly, with concrete plans for how they will abstain from cocaine use until their next clinic visit.

CRA Therapy Sessions

The recommended duration of treatment in this model is 24 weeks, followed by 6 months of aftercare. The influence of duration of this treatment has not been systematically assessed for cocaine dependence. The shortest duration that has been tested and shown to be efficacious is 12 weeks (Higgins et al., 1991). Therapy is delivered by master's level therapists in individual sessions (1.0–1.5 hours each) scheduled at least twice weekly during the initial 12 weeks, and once weekly during the final 12 weeks of treatment.

The primary goal of this treatment is to promote cocaine abstinence, which is communicated clearly to clients. A variety of other problems are addressed in treatment as well, but only if they are judged by the clinical staff to be related to the client's likelihood of immediate or longer-term success in achieving cocaine abstinence. Staff work hard at keeping treatment focused on resolving the problem of cocaine use, and against being sidetracked by other pressing problems that may have no direct or indirect bearing on the presenting problem of cocaine dependence. Patients with problems in need of professional attention but deemed unrelated to cocaine dependence are referred out.

Therapy sessions focus on the following six general topics, depending on the needs of the individual client. First, clients are instructed in how to functionally analyze their cocaine use; that is, how to recognize antecedents and consequences of their cocaine use. They are instructed in how to use that information to reduce the probability of future cocaine use. A twofold message is conveyed to the client: (1) Cocaine use is orderly behavior that is more likely to occur under certain circumstances than others; (2) by learning to identify the circumstances that affect one's cocaine use, plans can be developed and implemented to reduce the likelihood of future cocaine use. These methods are based on those initially developed for functional analysis of alcohol use (see McCrady, 1986, 2001; Miller & Muñoz, 1982).

Using the information gleaned from the functional analyses, clients are taught to restructure their daily activities in order to minimize contact with known antecedents of cocaine use, to find alternatives to the positive consequences of cocaine use, and to make explicit the negative consequences of cocaine use. Most clients are also taught cocaine-refusal skills, since despite their best efforts to avoid risky situations, most are likely to be offered opportunities to use cocaine at some point in the future. This is approached as a special case of assertiveness training using procedures developed by McCrady (1986) and Sisson and Azrin (1989) for drink refusal training. Results from at least one clinical trial have supported the efficacy of these procedures in reducing cocaine use (Monti, Rohsenow, Michalec, Martin, & Abrams, 1997). Therapists explain the rationale for cocaine-refusal skills training, engage the client in a detailed discussion of the key elements of effective refusal, assist the client in formulating his or her own refusal style (incorporating the key elements), and role-play potential scenarios wherein the client may be offered cocaine.

Second, developing a new social network that will support a healthier lifestyle and getting involved with recreational activities that are enjoyable and do not involve cocaine or other drug use is addressed with all clients. Systematically developing and maintaining contacts with "safe" social networks and participation in "safe" recreational activities remain a high priority throughout treatment for the vast majority of clients. Specific treatment goals are set and weekly progress on specific goals is monitored. We often have clients complete a leisure-interest inventory (Rosenthal & Rosenthal, 1985) to prompt ideas about activities that they might have liked previously or otherwise might want to explore. We encourage clients to sample new activities even if they are unsure whether they will find them enjoyable. Clinic staff monitor the local press for upcoming events that are appropriate, bring them to the attention of clients, and sometimes accompany clients to the events, if necessary.

Third, various other forms of individualized skills training are provided, usually to address some specific skills deficit that may directly or indirectly influence a client's risk for cocaine use (e.g., time management, problem solving, assertiveness training, social skills training, and mood management). For example, some level of time-management skills is essential to success with the social/recreational goals discussed earlier. All clients are given daily planners to facilitate scheduling. Because patients lose or forget their planners, providing photocopies to cover the next week of treatment is a good strategy. Time management in some form is typically stressed throughout treatment. The importance of writing down a schedule of activities that explicitly promote cocaine abstinence between therapy sessions is emphasized in each session. Planning for "high risk" times is particularly emphasized. Use of "to do" lists, daily planning, and prioritizing activities is addressed as well.

As other examples of skills training, we implement the protocol found in *Control Your Depression* (Lewinsohn, Muñoz, Youngren, & Zeiss, 1986) with those patients whose depressive symptomatology continues after they discontinue cocaine use. We sometimes implement social skills and relaxation training with individuals who report social anxiety about meeting new people, dating, and so forth (see Goldfried & Davison, 1994). For persistent problems with insomnia following discontinuation of cocaine and other drug use, we implement a protocol based on those developed by Lacks (1987) and Morin (1993). We often work with clients regarding money management. This might simply involve helping some clients arrange direct deposit for their paycheck, so that they are not tempted to use due to having a large sum of cash on hand. For others, this might involve a plan to get out of debt, which can help to reduce stress.

Fourth, unemployed participants are offered Job Club, which is an efficacious method for assisting chronically unemployed individuals to obtain employment (see the Job Club manual; Azrin & Besalel, 1980). Because the majority of patients who seek treatment for cocaine dependence at our clinic are unemployed, this is a service that we offer many of our clients. We assist others in pursuing educational goals or new career paths. A meaningful vocation is assumed to be fundamental to a healthy lifestyle, and we recommend goals directed toward vocational enhancement for all clients.

Fifth, participants with non-drug-abusing romantic partners are offered reciprocal relationship counseling, which is an intervention designed to teach couples positive communication skills and how to negotiate reciprocal contracts for desired changes in each other's behavior (see, e.g., Azrin, Naster, & Jones, 1973). We attempt to deliver relationship counseling across eight sessions, with the first four sessions delivered across consecutive weeks, and the next four delivered on alternating weeks.

Sixth, HIV/AIDS education is provided to all participants in the early stages of treatment, along with counseling directed at addressing any specific needs or risky behavior of the individual client. Clients are given information about and are encouraged to get tested for HIV antibodies and hepatitis B and C. Those interested in testing are assisted by clinic staff in scheduling an appointment.

Seventh, all who meet diagnostic criteria for alcohol dependence or report that alcohol use is involved in their use of cocaine are offered disulfiram therapy, which is an integral part of the CRA treatment for alcoholism (Meyers & Smith, 1995; Sisson & Azrin, 1989). Participants generally ingest a 250 mg/day dose under clinic staff observation on urinalysis test days, and, when possible, under the observation of a significant other on the other days.

Use of substances other than tobacco and caffeine is discouraged as well via CRA therapy. Anyone who meets criteria for opiate dependence is referred to an adjoining service located within our clinic for opioid replacement therapy (see Bickel, Amass, Higgins, Badger, & Esch, 1997). We recommend marijuana abstinence because of the problems associated with its abuse but have found no evidence that marijuana use or dependence adversely affects treatment for cocaine dependence (Budney, Higgins, & Wong, 1996). Importantly, we never dismiss or refuse to treat a client due to other drug use. We recommend cessation of tobacco use but usually not during the course of treatment for cocaine dependence. That practice may change should research demonstrate that smoking cessation can be successfully integrated into simultaneous treatment for other substance abuse or dependence disorders.

Upon completion of the 24-week treatment, participants are encouraged to participate in 6 months of aftercare in our clinic, which at minimum involves a once-monthly brief therapy session and a urine toxicology screen. More frequent clinic contact is recommended if the therapist or client deems it necessary. These clinic visits might be considered booster sessions. They are used not only to monitor progress and to address problems with cocaine use or other aspects of the lifestyle changes initiated during treatment but also to allow for a gradual rather than abrupt termination of the client's involvement with the clinic.

Voucher Program

The goal of the voucher program, an incentive program designed to increase retention and cocaine abstinence, is that this program play a major role during the initial 12 weeks of treatment, during which time CRA therapy is ongoing as well. The voucher program is discontinued at the end of 12 weeks. CRA is used to assist clients in restructuring their lifestyles, so that naturalistic reinforcers are in place to sustain cocaine abstinence once the vouchers are discontinued.

The voucher program is implemented in conjunction with a rigorous urinalysis-monitoring program. Urine specimens are collected from all participants according to a Monday, Wednesday, and Friday schedule during weeks 1–12, and a Monday and Thursday schedule during weeks 13–24 of treatment. Specimens are collected under the observation of a same-sex staff member and screened immediately via an onsite Enzyme Multiplied Immunoassay Technique (EMIT, Syva Corp., San Jose, CA) to minimize delays in delivering reinforcement for cocaine-negative specimens. All specimens are screened for benzoylecgonine, a cocaine metabolite, and one randomly selected specimen each week also is screened for the presence of other abused drugs. Failure to submit a scheduled specimen is treated as a cocaine-positive. Breath alcohol levels (BALs) are assessed during clinic visits for urine specimen collection. Clients are informed of their urinalysis and BAL results within several minutes after submitting specimens.

Points earned for urine specimens collected during weeks 1–12 that test negative for benzoylecgonine are recorded on vouchers and given to participants. Points are worth the equivalent of $0.25 each. Money is never provided directly to subjects. Instead, points are used to purchase retail items in the community. A staff member makes all purchases. The first negative specimen is worth 10 points at $0.25/point, or $2.50. The value of vouchers for each subsequent, consecutive negative specimen increases by 5 points (e.g., second = 15 points, third = 20 points, etc). To further increase the likelihood of continuous cocaine abstinence, the equivalent of a $10 bonus is earned for each three consecutive negative specimens. Specimens that are cocaine-positive or failure to submit a scheduled specimen reset the value of vouchers back to the initial $2.50 value, from which they can escalate again according to the same schedule. Submission of five consecutive cocaine-negative specimens following submission of a positive specimen returns the value of the voucher back to where it was prior to the reset.

SUPPORTING RESEARCH

A series of controlled clinical trials support the efficacy of the CRA plus vouchers treatment (Higgins et al., 1991, 1993, 1994, 1995; Higgins, Wong, Badger, Haug Ogden, & Dantona, 2000). The initial two trials conducted with this treatment involved comparisons with drug abuse counseling based on the disease model approach (Higgins et al., 1991, 1993). In both trials, CRA plus vouchers promoted better retention and greater cocaine abstinence than drug abuse counseling, demonstrating the efficacy of the intervention. One of those trials also included posttreatment assessments supporting the efficacy of CRA plus vouchers through 6-month follow-up (Higgins et al., 1995).

Next, we implemented a dismantling strategy. Assessing the efficacy of the voucher component was the first step. Patients were randomly assigned to receive CRA with ($n = 20$) or without ($n = 20$) vouchers (Higgins et al., 1994). Vouchers significantly improved client retention and cocaine abstinence during the 6-month outpatient treatment. During the 6-month posttreatment follow-up, those treated with CRA plus vouchers reported greater reductions in cocaine use, and only the CRA plus vouchers group showed significant reductions in psychiatric symptomatology on the ASI (McLellan et al., 1985). A more recent trial conducted with 70 cocaine-dependent outpatients demonstrated the contribution of the voucher program to increased cocaine abstinence rates through 1 year of posttreatment follow-up (Higgins et al., 2000).

The efficacy of monitored disulfiram therapy in decreasing alcohol and cocaine use in patients who abuse both substances has been confirmed in several studies, including a well-conducted randomized trial (Carroll, Nich, Ball, McCance, & Rounsaville, 1998).

Because much of the aforementioned work was completed in Vermont, the generality of these findings to inner-city, cocaine-dependent patients was examined. The studies by Carroll and colleagues demonstrated the generality of the disulfiram component of CRA to an inner-city population, and a number of well-controlled trials have also demonstrated the efficacy of the voucher component in inner-city populations (Kirby, Marlowe, Festinger, Lamb, & Platt, 1998; Piotrowski & Hall, 1999; Silverman et al., 1996). Moreover, the positive results with vouchers are consistent with still other findings supporting the efficacy of other contingency–management interventions in reducing cocaine use, even among severely dependent groups such as homeless (Milby et al., 1996) and schizophrenic (Shaner et al., 1997) cocaine-dependent individuals. To our knowledge, the entire CRA plus vouchers intervention has not yet been studied in an inner-city population.

Other findings from the literature on treatment of cocaine dependence have also influenced our clinical practices. As noted earlier, several randomized clinical trials have demonstrated the efficacy of relapse prevention therapy in the treatment of cocaine dependence (e.g., Carroll et al., 1994; Maude-Griffin et al., 1998), and at least one trial has supported the efficacy of coping skills training (Monti et al., 1997). Those two interventions have substantive overlap with the skills training component of CRA (functional analysis of drug use, drug avoidance and refusal training, problem solving, etc.) and thus support the efficacy of those practices. At least one trial demonstrates that couple therapy can reduce relapse among male illicit-drug abusers, including cocaine abusers (Fals-Stewart, Birchler, & O'Farrell, 1996), which supports our practice of offering relationship counseling.

Prevalence rates of a broad array of non-substance-related psychiatric disorders are greater in the cocaine-dependent than in the general population (Rounsaville et al., 1991; Wasserman, Havassy, & Boles, 1997). However, there is no evidence that these problems adversely affect outcome with CRA plus vouchers, relapse prevention, or other psychosocial treatments for cocaine dependence (e.g., Tidey, Mehl-Madrona, Higgins, & Badger, 1998). More severe forms of psychopathology (e.g., schizophrenia) in the cocaine-dependent population have not been well studied and may adversely affect outcomes.

IMPLEMENTING THE CRA PLUS VOUCHERS TREATMENT: A CASE EXAMPLE

The purpose of the following case illustration is to demonstrate the various steps involved in implementing the CRA plus vouchers treatment. This case also illustrates the multifaceted problems with which cocaine-dependent patients present.

Bill, a 32-year-old, divorced Caucasian male, was self-referred to the clinic for cocaine dependence. At the time of intake, Bill lived alone but shared custody of his 9-year-old son with his ex-wife. A high school graduate, Bill reported a history of seasonal employment as a painter but was currently unemployed. He reported that most of his friends and associates abused alcohol, cannabis, or cocaine. Although Bill reported a prior history of engaging in healthy social/recreational activities, he had not done so with regularity for a number of years.

Bill reported a history of involvement with the criminal justice system, including one prior conviction for drug possession and a second conviction for driving while intoxicated. He was incarcerated for a total of 4 months related to these charges. Bill was not under criminal justice supervision at the time he sought treatment.

Presenting Complaint

Bill reported an increased frequency of cocaine use during the month prior to intake and wanted help with discontinuing cocaine use before it escalated further. He reported numerous prior attempts to stop using cocaine on his own, as well as one prior formal treatment episode for cocaine dependence, each associated with minimal success. At intake, Bill expressed concern that his continued cocaine use would jeopardize his partial custody of his son; he also reported financial problems related to his drug use.

Assessment

Cocaine Use

Bill met DSM-IV criteria for cocaine dependence. His first cocaine use occurred at age 17, and he reported using cocaine intranasally once per month with friends for the next 10 years. Bill's cocaine use had increased to almost weekly in the past 5 years, during which time he also began smoking cocaine. During the past month, he was using several times weekly, his most recent use being 1 day prior to treatment intake, when he smoked 6 g of cocaine with his friends at a bar and then at home. He reported this to be his typical pattern of use. Bill also reported experiencing numerous adverse consequences related to cocaine use, including losing his job (also related to alcohol use), spending his savings on cocaine, a strained relationship with his ex-wife, depression, anxiety, and violent impulses. He reported that his one previous treatment episode for cocaine dependence had occurred approximately 5 years earlier and was a brief, 10-day inpatient stay, after which he was abstinent from cocaine use for approximately 1 month. That represented his longest period of abstinence since becoming a regular cocaine user.

Other Drug Use

Bill also met DSM-IV criteria for alcohol and nicotine dependence at intake. He reported drinking 12 days out of the past 30, usually ingesting 6–8 beers and several shots of hard liquor per occasion. He reported smoking approximately 25 cigarettes per day, which increased to 40 cigarettes on days that he used cocaine. He also reported occasional marijuana use but did not meet criteria for marijuana abuse or dependence.

Other Psychiatric Problems

Bill reported a history of depression, anxiety, and suicidal ideation. He also noted that he had experienced problems controlling violent behavior, for which he had previously received counseling. At treatment intake, Bill reported depressive symptoms (BDI score was 21), but no current suicidal ideation.

Motivation to Change

Bill's scores on the SOCRATES at intake indicated a strong commitment to cocaine abstinence. He also expressed a commitment to alcohol abstinence and agreed to initiate disulfiram therapy but noted that he planned to return to social drinking after completing treatment. He was not interested in discontinuing marijuana or tobacco use.

Conceptualization of the Case

Bill reported a history of erratic employment, particularly during the past 5 years when he worked as a house painter. His work schedule depended greatly on the weather. He worked long hours when the weather was good and then erratically, or not at all, when the weather was poor. He noted that this erratic work schedule left little time to pursue regular recreational activities during the better weather, then provided little or no structure during times when the weather was bad. Bill reported not making plans for recreation or socializing in advance. Instead, his leisure time was typically spent hanging out with friends, the majority of whom also used alcohol, marijuana, or cocaine. His time with these friends usually involved going to a local bar, where heavy drinking and cocaine use were common.

Bill noted that he refrained from hanging out with friends or using drugs on those weekends when his son visited with him. However, of late, Bill was missing visitation opportunities with his son due either to his work schedule or his escalating pattern of cocaine use.

In this case, Bill's erratic job schedule, lack of planning for times when not at work, absence of involvement in healthy recreational activities, association with other substance abusers, and irregular visitation with his son seriously restricted the potential for alternative sources of reinforcement to compete with cocaine use. Over time, this dynamic situation unfolded in such a way that cocaine and alcohol use were gaining increased control over Bill's behavior. The treatment plan was designed to alter this pattern.

Treatment Plan

Cocaine abstinence was our first priority in Bill's treatment plan. Second, we recommended alcohol abstinence because of the close relationship between his cocaine and alcohol use. As mentioned previously, Bill was unwilling to change his marijuana use despite the rationales we provided regarding the benefits of taking a break from marijuana use as well as the potential adverse consequences of continuing to smoke. Therefore, our clinical approach was to look for opportunities during the course of treatment to reinforce any movement toward reducing or discontinuing marijuana use, but not to make Bill's current reluctance to change this problem behavior a point of contention.

Bill's other explicit treatment goals were reestablishing a regular pattern of visitation with his son and involvement in healthy recreation, including some activities that could be done on weekends or other high-risk times for cocaine and alcohol use. We provided to Bill the following rationale as to why we deemed participation in these activities a high priority:

"Many times, when cocaine or other drugs become a regular part of someone's life, the person stops doing many of the healthy activities that he used to enjoy. He also spends less time with friends and family who do not abuse drugs, and ignores family responsibilities. That seems to be true in your case. While you used to engage in a lot of healthy recreational activities, you have gotten away from many of those activities since becoming involved with cocaine, and more recently, you're starting to ignore weekends with your son—weekends with someone you love dearly, but also someone with whom you remain sober.

Healthy family, social and recreational activities are very important in people's lives. They provide meaning, something to look forward to, a way to decrease boredom or to feel healthy, and a chance to be with people you genuinely love and care about. All these things can play a big part in helping you to initiate and sustain cocaine abstinence; that is, cocaine has a serious grip on your behavior these days, as does alcohol. To succeed in breaking that grip, you need to have things going on in your life that provide something positive to look forward to, that can bring you into contact with the benefits of abstaining from drug use, that can be done at those times when you used to head off to the bar. You need meaningful alternatives. If the things you do are not satisfying or enjoyable, or if you don't do anything but sit around and feel lonely or bored, then you are more likely to resume drug use. This is why we will work with you in developing a detailed treatment plan to help you develop a regular schedule of healthy social and recreational activities, and generally healthy lifestyle. To begin with, take out the daily planner we gave you and think of some activities that will help you to abstain from cocaine and alcohol use between today and your next clinic visit. We're going to pay special attention to Saturday night, because that is the day that you've said is particularly high risk for cocaine use."

Also of high priority was to assist Bill in finding employment that would provide a stable work schedule. Toward this end, we recommended that Bill participate in Job Club activities, which are described in greater detail later in this chapter. In an effort to increase Bill's social contacts with people who did not use drugs or alcohol, we sought to help him plan activities with his son and several other safe people whom he knew but had not spent time with during the past few years. Regarding psychiatric problems, we decided to monitor Bill's BDI scores weekly to see if they followed the precipitous decline that typically occurs with cocaine-dependent patients within a couple weeks after entering treatment. We also noted that if Bill's problems controlling violent behavior had not subsided with a period of cocaine and alcohol abstinence, we would include anger management training in the treatment plan.

The treatment plan is implemented and adjusted as we deem necessary based on client progress or lack thereof during the course of treatment. Here, we outline the progress made in implementing this treatment plan.

Cocaine Abstinence

Contingent vouchers, the primary intervention for promoting initial abstinence, were made available to Bill according to our standard 12-week protocol. Functional analysis was also initiated with Bill, beginning in Sessions 1 and 2. Circumstances that increased the likelihood that Bill would use cocaine included being at a bar with friends, using alcohol, and being bored or depressed, especially during a period of unemployment. Bill identified spending time with his son, going hunting or fishing, and visiting other family members as circumstances that decreased his likelihood of using cocaine. This information was updated and used throughout Bill's course of treatment in both self-management and social and recreational activities planning.

Shown in Figure 15.1 is a cumulative record of Bill's cocaine urinalysis results during the 24-week course of treatment. His only relapse to cocaine use occurred approximately halfway through treatment. While at home on a Saturday morning, Bill received a call from some friends with whom he had used cocaine in the past, who asked him to join them at a local bar to watch a football game on television. Rather than visiting his parents that afternoon as he had planned, he met his friends at the bar to watch the game. Bill began using cocaine at the bar and then continued using at a friend's house later that night and the following day. As a result of this binge, Bill missed the scheduled visitation with his son on Sunday morning and did not go to work on Monday. When he came to the clinic on Monday for his scheduled appointment and provided a sample that tested positive for recent cocaine use, Bill's therapist asked him to review the weekend's events. In functionally analyzing Bill's use, his therapist reviewed the circumstances that had led to his using cocaine, as well as the negative consequences of the binge (i.e., missing the scheduled visitation with his son, missing work). His therapist also took this opportunity to note how Bill's sudden change in plans on Saturday had increased his vulnerability for problems. He helped Bill to outline a strategy for making plans that would be more difficult to break, including scheduling activities earlier in the day, so that the plans would have less chance to become derailed, and scheduling visitation with

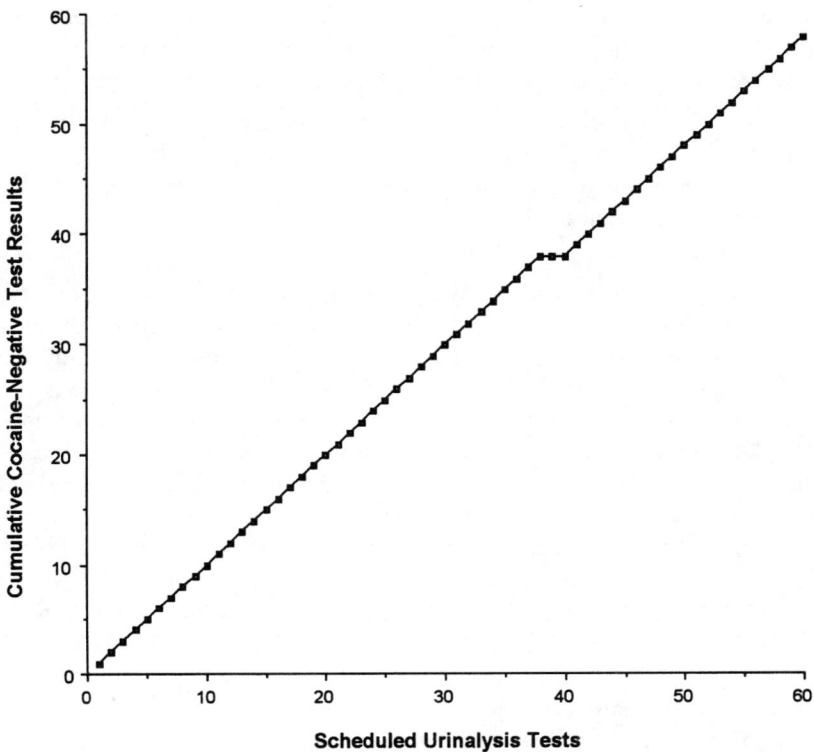

FIGURE 15.1. A cumulative record of Bill's urinalysis test results (y axis) across 60 consecutive urinalysis tests (x axis) conducted during 24 weeks of treatment. Negative tests are represented by vertical rightward lines, and the two positive tests (tests 39 and 40) by horizontal rightward lines.

his son for high-risk days, such as Saturdays, rather than Sundays. Bill's therapist also noted that continued contact with drug-using friends would continue to put him at risk. To this end, he helped Bill to refine his plans for minimizing contact with bars and drug users, and to increase the time he spent with "safe" people, such as his son. Finally, the therapist reminded Bill that his voucher level would return to the previous value after five consecutive negative urine samples, and they discussed potential ways of using Bill's vouchers to facilitate healthy activities with his son during the upcoming weekend.

Bill and the therapist continued to implement the treatment plan with the few modifications mentioned. Although Bill's sample on the Wednesday following his binge remained positive from that weekend use, his sample on Friday tested negative for cocaine, and there were no further instances of cocaine use during Bill's 24-week treatment. His record of documented cocaine abstinence was excellent.

Alcohol Abstinence

During the first session, the therapist discussed with Bill the rationale for disulfiram therapy:

THERAPIST: Bill, I'd like to go over a few reasons for you to give disulfiram therapy and alcohol abstinence a try. First, your history indicates that if you drink, you are more likely to use cocaine. You're not alone in that regard. The scientific evidence is very clear that, for many individuals who seek treatment for cocaine dependence, alcohol and cocaine use are closely linked.

BILL: But I don't even want to get drunk any more. I just want to be able to have a few drinks. Is that a problem too?

THERAPIST: Use of even modest doses of alcohol, even just a few drinks, can significantly decrease your chances of successfully abstaining from cocaine use. In our experience, and the experience of other clinics around the country, you can make greater progress with cocaine abstinence by using disulfiram and abstaining from alcohol use than if you continue to drink. The second thing I want to emphasize is that you've also reported a history of depression and suicidal ideation. Substance use, particularly alcohol use, can worsen depressive symptoms and increase suicide risk. A period of abstinence may help a lot with those problems. And still another point to consider is that agreeing to disulfiram therapy represents a concrete demonstration of your commitment to abstinence and substantial lifestyle changes. This would be beneficial in general, but it could also help ease some of the strain in your relationship with your ex-wife and your concerns about how continued alcohol and drug use could jeopardize custody of your son.

Bill agreed to disulfiram therapy for the duration of treatment. A schedule was set up for Bill to ingest a 250 mg dose three times per week under the observation of clinic staff. For disulfiram therapy to be effective, there must be a plan for monitoring compliance with the medication regimen. In addition to disulfiram therapy, the therapist worked with Bill to functionally analyze his alcohol use, similar to the process for cocaine. They reviewed specific circumstances under which Bill was more likely to drink, less likely to drink, and listed the negative consequences he had previously experienced with his alcohol use. The therapist and patient developed a plan for finding alternative ways to relax that did not involve the bar or drinking.

Bill was compliant with disulfiram therapy throughout treatment. When the end of the 24 weeks of treatment approached, Bill expressed a desire to "be able to have a drink if he wanted" and requested to discontinue disulfiram therapy as planned. His therapist expressed concerns about this jeopardizing the substantial progress Bill had made and reviewed the past negative consequences that Bill had experienced from drinking, as well as his history of alcohol use increasing his likelihood of using cocaine. When it was clear that Bill would not consider continuing disulfiram therapy, his therapist worked with him to determine what he could do to minimize his risk for problem drinking and, subsequently, cocaine use (i.e., setting goals for frequency of drinking, amount consumed per occasion, where and with whom he drank). This was done using Miller and Muñoz's (1982) *How to Control Your Drinking* manual.

Other Drug Use

Bill continued the same pattern of marijuana use that he reported in the intake interview. He repeatedly asserted that marijuana use was not interfering with his other treatment goals. In turn, his therapist provided rationales for stopping or reducing marijuana use on numerous occasions but was unsuccessful in initiating abstinence.

Family/Social Support

Bill's therapist helped him to plan a regular schedule of visitation with his son and also assisted him in planning activities during those visits. He also assisted Bill in reinitiating contact with several safe friends with whom he had stopped interacting. Bill met a woman who was not a substance abuser while attending the gym as part of the regular recreational activities described here and began dating regularly.

Recreational Activities

After discussing the importance of developing recreational activities that would compete with cocaine use, Bill and his therapist decided on a goal of participating in three of these activities per week and sampling one new activity per month. Bill used the vouchers he earned for cocaine abstinence to pay for many of these activities. During treatment, Bill consistently met his goal of three recreational activities per week, including going to the local gym to work out, fishing, and taking his son to the movies.

Employment/Education

Bill participated in Job Club, during which he came to the clinic three times per week, reviewed local employment classifieds, completed a resume and cover letters with the help of clinic staff, filled out job applications, and rehearsed for job interviews. Bill successfully obtained a full-time job painting homes that allowed him to work consistently throughout the year. The vocational goal then was modified to help him avoid excessive hours, which could hinder his ability to balance work and recreational activities.

Psychiatric Monitoring

Recall that Bill's BDI score at intake was 21, which is well into the clinical range. By the second week in treatment and, not incidentally, after an initial period of cocaine abstinence, Bill's BDI score dropped precipitously to a 6. Such substantial and rapid decreases in depressive symptomatology are the norm rather than the exception with cocaine-dependent patients. We continued to monitor his symptoms throughout treatment. No further problems were evident; thus, no additional treatment for depression was indicated. Bill reported no problems with anger management during treatment, so that problem was not addressed further.

Summary of Treatment Progress

During treatment, Bill made substantial progress toward establishing a stable record of cocaine abstinence, eliminating problem drinking, and increasing involvement in social and recreational activities. He also obtained employment, which provided a consistent work schedule, and experienced a reduction in depressive symptoms and problems with anger management. The one area in which we were unable to make progress was Bill's use of marijuana.

Follow-Up

Following completion of the 24-week treatment protocol, Bill participated in 6 months of aftercare and follow-up assessments. Thus, we have a relatively good picture of his continued progress with cocaine abstinence and related treatment goals. Bill reported no instances of cocaine use during the follow-up period and his urinalyses results supported those reports. He also stated that he continued to minimize frequency of drinking, particularly by avoiding bars and high-risk people. Regular marijuana use continued during follow-up, as it had during treatment, and the client remained uninterested in changing that behavior.

Bill was able to maintain partial custody of his son and reported that his relationship with both his son and ex-wife had improved as a function of his cocaine abstinence and reduced drinking. He continued to express satisfaction with his current employment and reported engaging in social and recreational activities regularly. Bill also reported minimal depressive symptomatology at the follow-up assessments, and there was no indication of problems with anger management.

SUMMARY AND CONCLUSIONS

The CRA plus vouchers treatment is an efficacious intervention for outpatient management of cocaine dependence. The intervention is based on current scientific understanding of cocaine dependence and its related risk factors. This chapter provides for readers an introduction to this treatment approach, with an emphasis on the more practical aspects of implementing the treatment. The case study particularly emphasizes how this treatment is implemented. In describing the treatment, we have tried at least to mention what has been learned from our own research and that of others about effective practices for outpatient treatment of cocaine dependence. Of course, a chapter in a book cannot provide readers with all of the necessary information for effective treatment implementation, and this one is no exception. Readers seeking more detailed information on implementation of efficacious treatments for cocaine dependence should consult the therapist manuals on this treatment (Budney & Higgins, 1998) and relapse prevention (Carroll, 1998).

ACKNOWLEDGMENTS

Preparation of this chapter was supported in part by Research Grant Nos. DA09378 and DA08076 and Training Grant No. DA07242 from the National Institute on Drug Abuse.

REFERENCES

Alterman, A., O'Brien, C. P., McLellan, A. T., August, D. S., Snider, E. C., Droba, M., Cornish, J. W., & Hall, C. P. (1994). Effectiveness and costs of inpatient versus day hospital cocaine rehabilitation. *Journal of Nervous and Mental Disease, 182,* 157–163.

Azrin, N. H., & Besalel, V. A. (1980). *Job Club Counselor's manual*. Baltimore: University Park Press.

Azrin, N. H., Naster, B. J., & Jones, R. (1973). Reciprocity counseling: A rapid learning based procedure for marital counseling. *Behaviour Research and Therapy, 11,* 364–382.

Barrio, G., De la Fuente, L., Royuela, L., Diaz, A., & Rodriguez-Artalejo, F. (1998). Cocaine use among heroin users in Spain: The diffusion of crack and cocaine smoking. *Journal of Epidemiology and Community Health, 52,* 172–180.

Beck, A. T., Ward, C. H., Mendelson, M., Mock, J., & Erbaugh, J. (1961). An inventory for measuring depression. *Archives of General Psychiatry, 4*, 561–571.

Bickel, W. K., Amass, L., Higgins, S. T., Badger, G. J., & Esch, R. A. (1997). Effects of adding behavioral treatment to opioid detoxification with buprenorphine. *Journal of Consulting and Clinical Psychology, 65*, 803–810.

Budney, A. J., & Higgins, S. T. (1998). *The community reinforcement plus vouchers approach: Manual 2: National Institute on Drug Abuse therapy manuals for drug addiction* (NIH Publication No. 98-4308). Rockville, MD: National Institute on Drug Abuse.

Budney, A. J., Higgins, S. T., & Wong, C. J. (1996). Marijuana use and treatment outcome in cocaine-dependent patients. *Journal of Experimental and Clinical Psychopharmacology, 4*, 1–8.

Carroll, K. M. (1998). *A cognitive-behavioral approach: Treating cocaine addiction. Manual 1: National Institute on Drug Abuse therapy manuals for drug addiction* (NIH Publication No. 98-4309). Rockville, MD: National Institute on Drug Abuse.

Carroll, K. M., Nich, C., Ball, S. A., McCance, E., & Rounsaville, B. J. (1998). Treatment of cocaine and alcohol dependence with psychotherapy and disulfiram. *Addiction, 93*, 713–727.

Carroll, K. M., Rounsaville, B. J., Nich, C., Gordon, L. T., Wirtz, P. W., & Gawin, F. H. (1994). One-year follow-up of psychotherapy and pharmacotherapy for cocaine dependence: Delayed emergence of psychotherapy effects. *Archives of General Psychiatry, 51*, 989–997.

Chilcoat, H. D., & Anthony, J. (1996). Impact of parent monitoring on initiation of drug use through late childhood. *Journal of the American Academy of Child and Adolescent Psychiatry, 35*, 91–100.

Chilcoat, H. D., & Schütz, C. (1995). Racial/ethnic and age differences in crack use within neighborhoods. *Addiction Research, 3*, 103–111.

Crum, R., Lillie-Blanton, M., & Anthony, J. (1996). Neighborhood environment and opportunity to use cocaine in late childhood and early adolescence. *Drug and Alcohol Dependence, 43*, 155–161.

Derogatis, L. R. (1983). *SCL-90-R: Administration, scoring and procedures manual–II*. Towson, MD: Clinical Psychometric Research.

Fals-Stewart, W., Birchler, G. R., & O'Farrell, T. J. (1996). Behavioral couples therapy for male substance abusing patients: Effects on relationship adjustment and drug-using behavior. *Journal of Consulting and Clinical Psychology, 64*, 959–972.

Festinger, D. S., Lamb, R. J., Kirby, K. C., & Marlowe, D. B. (1996). The accelerated intake: A method for increasing initial attendance to outpatient cocaine treatment. *Journal of Applied Behavior Analysis, 29*, 387–389.

Goldfried, M. R., & Davison, G. C. (1994). *Clinical behavior therapy* (2nd ed.). New York: Wiley.

Griffiths, R. R., Bigelow, G. E., & Henningfield, J. E. (1980). Similarities in animal and human drug taking behavior. In N. K. Mello (Ed.), *Advances in substance abuse: Behavioral and biological research* (pp. 1–90). Greenwich, CT: JAI Press.

Higgins, S. T. (1997). The influence of alternative reinforcers on cocaine use and abuse: A brief review. *Pharmacology Biochemistry and Behavior, 57*, 419–427.

Higgins, S. T., Budney, A. J., Bickel, W. K., Badger, G. J., Foerg, F. E., & Ogden, D. (1995). Outpatient behavioral treatment for cocaine dependence: One-year outcome. *Experimental and Clinical Psychopharmacology, 3*, 205–212.

Higgins, S. T., Budney, A. J., Bickel, W. K., Foerg, F. E., Donham, R., & Badger, G. (1994). Incentives improve outcome in outpatient behavioral treatment of cocaine dependence. *Archives of General Psychiatry, 51*, 568–576.

Higgins, S. T., Budney, A. J., Bickel, W. K., Hughes, J. R., Foerg, F., & Badger, G. (1993). Achieving cocaine abstinence with a behavioral approach. *American Journal of Psychiatry, 150*, 763–769.

Higgins, S. T., Delaney, D. D., Budney, A. J., Bickel, W. K., Hughes, J. R., Foerg, F., & Fenwick,

J. (1991). A behavioral approach to achieving initial cocaine abstinence. *American Journal of Psychiatry, 148,* 1218–1224.

Higgins, S. T., & Katz, J. L. (Eds.). (1998). *Cocaine abuse: Behavior, pharmacology, and clinical applications.* San Diego, CA: Academic Press.

Higgins, S. T., & Silverman, K. (Eds.). (1999). *Motivating behavior change among illicit-drug abusers: Research on contingency-management interventions.* Washington, DC: American Psychological Association.

Higgins, S. T., Wong, C. J., Badger, G. J., Haug Ogden, D. E., & Dantona, R. L. (2000). Contingent reinforcement increases cocaine abstinence during outpatient treatment and one year of follow-up. *Journal of Consulting and Clinical Psychology, 68,* 64–72.

Hudziak, J., Helzer, J. E., Wetzel, M. W., Kessel, K. B., McGee, B., Janca, A., & Przybeck, P. (1993). The use of DSM-III-R checklist for initial diagnostic assessments. *Comprehensive Psychiatry, 34,* 375–383.

Hunt, G. M., & Azrin, N. H. (1973). A community-reinforcement approach to alcoholism. *Behaviour Research and Therapy, 11,* 91–104.

Hunter, G. M., Donoghoe, M. C., & Stimson, G. V. (1995). Crack use and injection on the increase among injecting drug users in London. *Addiction, 90,* 1397–1400.

Kendler, K. S., & Prescott, C. A. (1998). Cocaine use, abuse and dependence in a population-based sample of female twins. *British Journal of Psychiatry, 173,* 345–350.

Kirby, K. C., Marlowe, D. B., Festinger, D. S., Lamb, R. J., & Platt, J. J. (1998). Schedule of voucher delivery influences initiation of cocaine abstinence. *Journal of Consulting and Clinical Psychology, 66,* 761–767.

Lacks, P. (1987). *Behavioral treatment of persistent insomnia.* New York: Pergamon Press.

Lewinsohn, P. M., Muñoz, R. F., Youngren, M. A., & Zeiss, A. M. (1986). *Control your depression.* New York: Simon & Schuster.

Lillie-Blanton, M., Anthony, J. C., & Schuster, C. R. (1993). Probing the meaning of racial/ethnic group comparisons in crack-cocaine smoking. *Journal of the American Medical Association, 269,* 993–997.

Maude-Griffin, P. M., Hohenstein, J. M., Humfleet, G. L., Reilly, P. M., Tusel, D. J., & Hall, S. M. (1998). Superior efficacy of cognitive-behavioral therapy for urban crack cocaine abusers: Main and matching effects. *Journal of Consulting and Clinical Psychology, 66,* 832–837.

McCrady, B. S. (1986). *Behavioral marital therapy for alcohol dependence.* Unpublished treatment manual, Rutgers University, New Brunswick, NJ.

McCrady, B. S. (2001). Alcohol use disorders. In D. H. Barlow (Ed.), *Clinical handbook of psychological disorders: A step-by-step treatment manual* (3rd ed., pp. 376–433). New York: Guilford Press.

McLellan, A. T., Luborsky, L., Cacciola, J., Griffith, J., Evans, F., Barr, H. L., & O'Brien, C. P. (1985). New data from the Addiction Severity Index. *Journal of Nervous and Mental Disease, 173,* 412–423.

Meyers, R. J., & Smith, J. E. (1995). *Clinical guide to alcohol treatment: The community reinforcement approach.* New York: Guilford Press.

Milby, J. B., Schumacher, J. E., Raczynski, J. M., Caldwell, E., Engle, M., Michael, M., & Carr, J. (1996). Sufficient conditions for effective treatment of substance abusing homeless. *Drug and Alcohol Dependence, 43,* 39–47.

Miller, W. R., & Muñoz, R. F. (1982). *How to control your drinking.* Albuquerque: University of New Mexico Press.

Miller, W. R., & Tonigan, J. S. (1996). Assessing drinkers' motivation for change: The Stages of Change Readiness and Treatment Eagerness Scale (SOCRATES). *Psychology of Addictive Behaviors, 10,* 81–89.

Monti, P. M., Rohsenow, D. J., Michalec, E., Martin, R. A., & Abrams, D. B. (1997). Brief coping skills treatment for cocaine abuse: Substance use outcomes at three months. *Addiction, 92,* 1717–1728.

Morin, C. M. (1993). *Insomnia: Psychological assessment and management.* New York: Guilford Press.

Piotrowski, N. A., & Hall, S. M. (1999). Treatment of multiple drug abuse in the methadone clinic. In S. T. Higgins & K. Silverman (Eds.), *Motivating behavior change among illicit-drug abusers: Research on contingency-management interventions* (pp. 183–202). Washington, DC: American Psychological Association.

Rosenthal, T. L., & Rosenthal, R. H. (1985). Clinical stress management. In D. H. Barlow (Ed.), *Clinical handbook of psychological disorders* (pp. 145–205). New York: Guilford Press.

Rounsaville, B. J., Anton, S. F., Carroll, K., Budde, D., Prusoff, B. A., & Gawin, F. (1991). Psychiatric diagnoses of treatment-seeking cocaine abusers. *Archives of General Psychiatry, 39,* 161–166.

Selzer, M. L. (1971). The Michigan Alcoholism Screening Test. *American Journal of Psychiatry, 127,* 89–94.

Shaner, A., Roberts, L. J., Eckman, T. A., Tucker, D. E., Tsuang, J. W., Wilkens, J. N., & Mintz, J. (1997). Monetary reinforcement of abstinence from cocaine among mentally ill patients with cocaine dependence. *Psychiatric Services, 48,* 807–810.

Silverman, K., Higgins, S. T., Brooner, R. K., Montoya, I. D., Cone, E. J., Schuster, C. R., & Preston, K. L. (1996). Sustained cocaine abstinence in methadone maintenance patients through voucher-based reinforcement therapy. *Archives of General Psychiatry, 53,* 409–415.

Sisson, R., & Azrin, N. H. (1989). The community reinforcement approach. In R. K. Hester & W. R. Miller (Eds.), *Handbook of alcoholism treatment approaches: Effective alternatives* (pp. 242–258). New York: Pergamon Press.

Substance Abuse and Mental Health Services Administration (2000). *Summary of Findings from the 1999 National Household Survey on Drug Abuse.* Rockville, MD: National Clearinghouse for Alcohol and Drug Information.

Tidey, J. W., Mehl-Madrona, L., Higgins, S. T., & Badger, G. J. (1998). Psychiatric symptom severity in cocaine-dependent outpatients: Demographics, drug use characteristics and treatment outcome. *Drug and Alcohol Dependence, 50,* 9–17.

Tsuang, M. T., Lyons, M. J., Eisen, S. A., Goldberg, J., True, W., Lin, N., Meyer, J. M., Toomey, R., Faraone, S. V., & Eaves, L. (1996). Genetic influences on DSM-III-R drug abuse and dependence: A study of 3,372 twin pairs. *American Journal of Medical Genetics, 67,* 473–477.

Washton, A. M., Stone, N. S., & Hendrickson, E. C. (1988). Cocaine abuse. In D. M. Donovan & G. A. Marlatt (Eds.), *Assessment of addictive behaviors* (pp. 364–389). New York: Guilford Press.

Wasserman, D. A., Havassy, B. E., & Boles, S. (1997). Traumatic events and post-traumatic stress disorder in cocaine users entering private treatment. *Drug and Alcohol Dependence, 46,* 1–8.

IV

Psychological Treatments for Severe Personality Disorders

Our current diagnostic system (DSM-IV) defines a personality disorder as "an enduring pattern of inner experience and behavior that deviates markedly from the expectations of the individual's culture, is pervasive and inflexible, has an onset in adolescence or early adulthood, is stable over time, and leads to distress and impairment" (American Psychiatric Association, 1994, p. 629). Due to the pervasive and inflexible nature of the problem, personality disorders are listed on a separate axis because "they might be otherwise overlooked when attention is directed to the usually more florid Axis I disorders" (p. 26).

Personality disorders fall into three clusters: Cluster A (paranoid, schizoid, and schizotypal personality disorders), cluster B (antisocial, borderline, histrionic, and narcissistic personality disorders), and cluster C (avoidant, dependent, and obsessive–compulsive personality disorders). The classification of individuals into these categories has been controversial, and future diagnostic systems are likely to adopt a more dimensional view toward personality problems. Moreover, the distinction between "florid" Axis I disorders and "pervasive" Axis II psychopathology is not without controversy. As the following chapters demonstrate, there are now a number of psychological strategies available to modify, change, and even eliminate such inflexible and pervasive problems. These strategies include cognitive-behavioral intervention, interpersonal therapy, and psychodynamic approaches. All of these treatment orientations typically conceptualize personality disorders as maladaptive responses to environmental stress. The goal of these interventions is to help patients develop and utilize more effective coping strategies. The therapist's response to the patient's problem behavior typically plays a crucial role because it reflects the general interpersonal problems the patient has with other people, including friends, coworkers, and family members. Not surprisingly, this makes personality disorders particularly difficult to treat.

Some of the most severe and challenging problems a therapist encounters when treating a patient with a personality disorder includes suicide, emotional dysregulation (as in borderline personality disorder), and aggressive behaviors (as in antisocial personality disorder and conduct disorder in adolescents). For this reason, we have decided to focus primarily on Cluster B personality disorders. As presented in Chapter 16 by Kelly

Koerner and Marsha Linehan, dialectical behavior therapy (DBT), is an effective technique to modify emotional dysregulation and suicidality in patients with borderline personality disorders. Unlike conventional cognitive-behavioral therapy, in which the therapist challenges problematic beliefs through hypothesis-testing experiments, the DBT therapist creates the experience of the contradictions inherent in the patient's own position. DBT is one of the most well-supported treatment protocols for borderline personality disorder. Another form of intervention for this disorder with less empirical support—but promising preliminary results—is the multiple family group treatment for borderline personality disorder (discussed in Chapter 17 by Teresa Whitehurst, Maria Elena Ridolfi, and John Gunderson). As the name implies, this treatment is conducted in a group format that provides the opportunity to practice new ways of solving interpersonal problems during the treatment session. Aside from problems due to emotional dysregulation, antisocial behaviors represent some of the greatest treatment challenges. Chapter 18 (Elizabeth Letourneau, Phillippe Cunningham, and Scott Henggeler) describes multisystemic treatment of antisocial behavior in adolescents, which is an empirically supported treatment for chronic juvenile offenders and juveniles with substance use disorders. The goal of this treatment is to identify and modify various risk factors for delinquent behavior across different social systems (school, home, friends, etc.). The chapter provides a very nice and detailed case example of this treatment approach. Finally, Arthur Freeman (Chapter 19) and Nathaniel Kuhn and Leigh McCullough (Chapter 20) illustrate some general cognitive and psychodynamic techniques for treating personality disorders.

REFERENCE

American Psychiatric Association. (1994). *Diagnostic and statistical manual of mental disorders* (4th ed.). Washington, DC: Author.

16

Dialectical Behavior Therapy for Borderline Personality Disorder

KELLY KOERNER
MARSHA M. LINEHAN

Dialectical behavior therapy (DBT) is a cognitive-behavioral treatment originally developed as a treatment for chronically suicidal individuals who met criteria for borderline personality disorder (BPD). In the past, public mental health outpatient services have addressed the needs of patients with schizophrenia and bipolar disorder (Rascati, 1990; Swigar, Astrachan, Levine, Mayfield, & Radovich, 1991) but not specifically those of patients with BPD. Addressing the needs of individuals with BPD poses several challenges. First, BPD is associated with worse outcomes across several Axis I diagnoses (Ames-Frankel et al., 1992; Baer et al., 1992; Coker, Vize, Wade, & Cooper, 1993; Kosten, Kosten, & Rounsaville, 1989; Phillips & Nierenberg, 1994), indicating that standard treatments may be less effective with this patient group. Furthermore, individuals with BPD typically need treatment for multiple complex and severe Axis I problems, often in the context of unrelenting crises and the management of high-risk suicidal behavior. Legal and ethical concerns about patient suicide make it difficult to limit hospital use (Fine & Sansone, 1990; Rissmiller, Steer, Ranieri, Rissmiller, & Hogate, 1994) even when "revolving door" use of involuntary inpatient facilities may inadvertently be iatrogenic. Additionally, suicide attempts, threats of suicide attempts, and anger are among the factors reported by psychotherapists as extreme stressors (Hellman, Morrison, & Abramowitz, 1986). Helping is made more difficult still by the patients' exquisite emotional sensitivity and the involvement of multiple treatment providers.

Consequently, as DBT was developed, the nature of the patients' problems led to modifications of standard cognitive-behavioral therapy, from addition of therapeutic strategies that balanced and complemented the cognitive-behavioral change strategies to ways of structuring the treatment and the setting. The resulting treatment manuals (Linehan, 1993a, 1993b) organize these strategies into protocols that can be flexibly used to provide comprehensive treatment with multidisorder, severely impaired individuals. DBT has been perceived as a way to improve services for BPD patients, who consume a disproportionate number of mental health dollars but often have not had specific services designed to treat their problems (Swenson, 2000). The option of outpatient DBT has been discussed as an ethical alternative to involuntary commitment for chronically suicidal patients (Behnke & Saks, 1998), and the data suggest that it is an efficacious treatment for severely impaired individuals.

DATA ON CLINICAL EFFICACY AND COST-EFFECTIVENESS

Despite its public health significance, there is little research available on the psychosocial treatment of suicidal behavior (Linehan, 2000b) and less still on the treatment of suicidal behavior and other severe dysfunctional behavior among patients meeting criteria for BPD (Linehan, Rizvi, Shaw Welch, & Page, 2000). Clinical lore and literature about effective treatment of BPD is vast, whereas the empirical literature is sparse. Other than a promising 18-month partial hospital program (Bateman & Fonagy, 1999, 2000), DBT is the only treatment with demonstrated efficacy for reducing parasuicide among chronically suicidal, multidisorder patients with BPD. (Parasuicide is any acute, intentional, self-injury that causes tissues damage, with or without the intent to die.) Researchers have investigated the efficacy of comprehensive DBT, and components and adaptations of DBT (cf. Koerner & Dimeff, 2000; Koerner & Linehan, 2000, for comprehensive reviews). To date, the evidence from randomized controlled trials on the comprehensive treatment suggests that comprehensive DBT is more effective than treatment as usual in reducing targeted problem behaviors. In the more severely impaired populations of individuals with BPD, DBT was shown to reduce parasuicidal behavior and substance abuse, increase treatment retention, and improve global functioning (Linehan, Armstrong, Suarez, Allmon, & Heard, 1991; Linehan et al., 1999, in press; Linehan & Heard, 1993; Linehan, Tutek, Heard, & Armstrong, 1994). With a less severely disordered population of patients with BPD, DBT produced specific improvements in suicidal ideation, depression, and hopelessness, even compared with a treatment-as-usual condition that also produced clinically significant changes in depression (Koons et al., 2001). Similar results were found in a matched control trial (Stanley, Ivanoff, Brodsky, Oppenheim, & Mann, 1998) and in a randomized controlled trial comparing DBT-oriented treatment to client-centered supportive treatment (Turner, 2000). Of the limited follow-up data available, outcomes appear to hold up to 1 year after treatment (Linehan, Heard, & Armstrong, 1993). Participants in research trials have been similar to those served by community mental health services in that, in addition to meeting criteria for BPD, they have had high rates of comorbid mood and anxiety disorder, substance abuse, eating disorders, and other Axis II disorders.

Although DBT was developed for the treatment of patients with suicidal behavior, adaptations have been created for other historically difficult-to-treat populations with a high treatment dropout rate, who are multidiagnostic and have problem behaviors that can be reasonably linked to difficulties regulating emotions (Linehan, 2000a). In addition to successful adaptation to treat patients with BPD and comorbid substance abuse (Linehan & Dimeff, 1997), others have extended DBT to other patient populations and disorders (eating disorders: Safer, Telch, & Agras, 2001; Telch, Agras, & Linehan, 2000; suicidal adolescents: Rathus & Miller, in press; juvenile and adult mentally ill offenders: McCann, Ball, & Ivanoff, 2000; Trupin, Stewart, Beach, & Boesky, in press; depressed elderly persons: Lynch, 2000). Conceptual papers have described DBT adapted to treat domestic violence (Fruzzetti & Levensky, 2000) in couples and families in which a member meets criteria for BPD (Hoffman, Fruzzetti, & Swenson, 1999), and integrated into exposure therapy for patients with posttraumatic stress disorder (Melia & Wagner, 2000; Zafert & Black, 2000).

From available data on DBT's cost-effectiveness, Heard (2000) found that 1-year treatment costs for DBT were no more expensive than treatment as usual in total mental health care costs: DBT mean total health care costs were $9,856 (median $8,093) versus treatment as usual costs of $19,745 (median $13,917). DBT had significantly less variability, an important point for health care economists, meaning that, on average, costs were more predictable and predictably lower for DBT. Costs were allocated differently in DBT than treatment as usual, with more costs shifted to outpatient psychotherapy and less to psychiatric hospitalization and emergency services. Similar findings were obtained by the Mental Health Center of Greater Manchester in New Hampshire, which was awarded the 1998 Gold Achievement Award by the American Psychiatric Association (1998) for the excellence of their small community-based DBT program. In data collected on 14 clients who completed their DBT program over a 12-month period, they found a 77% decrease in hospital days (from 479 to 85 days); a 76% decrease in partial hospital days (from 173 to 42 days); a 56% decrease in crisis beds (from 170 to 73 days); and an 80% decrease in emergency services (from 61 to 12 days). Hospital costs were decreased from $483,000 to $83,000 by shifting some of these dollars to outpatient costs (from $49,000 to $141,000), resulting in an overall decrease in total treatment costs from $645,000 to $273,000.

Further research is needed to determine the components of DBT that are responsible for its efficacy, to examine its clinical and cost-effectiveness in routine mental health care settings, and to investigate its efficacy with other patient populations. There is obviously a tension between the adoption of a promising treatment for a difficult-to-treat patient group and careful consideration of the extent of evidence to support it. While the evidence regarding DBT's efficacy is stronger than that for any other treatment approach for this patient population, the lack of component analysis studies means that it is premature to conclude which element(s) of DBT may be responsible for clinical outcomes, or whether the comprehensive treatment is required. For example, DBT may have its effects because any organized, systematic approach guided by consistent case formulation and treated by a team that shares fundamental assumptions will be more effective than treatment as usual. Or DBT may have its effects to the extent that it harnesses basic cognitive-behavioral techniques and actively treats suicidal behavior as a form of maladaptive problem solving. Or it may be that pervasive modeling and strengthening of the client's valid responses alone or in combination with cognitive-behavioral interventions may create conditions for client change. Or DBT may owe its effectiveness to the influence of dialectical philosophy and strategies. Individuals who meet criteria for BPD tend toward dichotomous, rigid thinking, and behavior and emotional extremes, as do their treatment teams at times. Dialectics may offer a means of creating a synthesis from polar opposites to find a balanced middle path. We discuss each of these in turn but begin with several important concepts from dialectical philosophy that permeate all other aspects of the treatment.

DIALECTICAL PHILOSOPHY

Dialectical philosophy has been influential across the sciences. In DBT, it provides the practical means for both the therapist and the client to retain flexibility and balance. Dialectics is a method of persuasion and a worldview, or set of assumptions about the nature of reality. An essential idea in both is that each thesis or statement of a position contains its own antithesis or opposite position. For example, suicidal patients often want simultaneously to live and to die. Saying aloud to the therapist, "I want to die" rather than killing oneself in secrecy contains within it the opposite position, that of wanting to live. However, it is not that wanting to live is "more true" than wanting to die. The person genuinely does not want to live life as it currently is—few of us would trade places with our BPD clients. Nor does the low lethality of a suicide attempt mean that the person did not truly want to die. The client simultaneously holds both opposing positions. Opposing truths stand side by side. Dialectical change or progress comes from the resolution of these opposing positions into a synthesis. The entire dialogue of therapy constructs new positions in which the quality of one's life does not give rise to the desire to die. Suicide is one option out of an unbearable life. However, building a life that is genuinely worth living is an equally valid position.

Cognitive modification strategies in DBT are based on dialectical persuasion. The therapist challenges problematic beliefs not with reason or hypothesis testing experiments, but through conversations that create the experience of the contradictions inherent in the client's own position. For example, a client who experiences immediate relief from intense emotional pain when she burns her arms with cigarettes is reticent to give it up because none of the skills work as well or as quickly as parasuicide. As the therapist begins to assess the factors that led up to this incident of parasuicide, the client nonchalantly says, "The burn really wasn't that bad this time."

THERAPIST: So what you're saying is that if you saw a person in a lot of emotional pain, say, your little niece, and she was feeling as devastated as you were that night you burned your arm, you'd burn her arm with a cigarette to help her feel better.

CLIENT: No, I wouldn't.

THERAPIST: Why not?

CLIENT: I just wouldn't.

THERAPIST: I believe you wouldn't, but why not?

CLIENT: I'd comfort her or do something else to help her feel better.

THERAPIST: But what if she was inconsolable and nothing you did made her feel better? Besides, you wouldn't burn her that badly.

CLIENT: I just wouldn't do it. It's not right. I'd do something but not that.

THERAPIST: That's interesting, don't you think?

The client simultaneously believes that one should not burn another under any circumstances and that burning herself to get relief is insignificant. In dialectical persuasion, the therapist highlights the inconsistencies among the client's own actions, beliefs, and values. The dialogue focuses on helping the client reach a viewpoint that is more whole and internally consistent with her own values.

A dialectical worldview permeates DBT. A dialectical perspective holds that one cannot make sense of the parts without considering the whole, that the nature of reality is holistic even if it appears that one can talk meaningfully about an element or part independently. This has a number of implications. Clinicians never have a "whole" perspective on a client. Rather, therapists are like the blind wise men each touching a part of an elephant, and each being certain that the whole is exactly like the part he is touching: "An elephant is big and floppy," "No, long and round and thin," "No, solid like a wall." The therapist who interacts with the patient in a one-to-one supportive relationship sees incremental progress. The nurse whose sole contact consists of arguments declining demands for additional anxiolytics, the crisis worker who sees the person over and over only at her worst, and the group leader who has to repair the damage of the person's sarcastic comments to another group member have alternative perspectives. Each true, but each also partial.

Applying a dialectical perspective further implies that it is natural and to be expected that these differing and partial perspectives be in radical opposition. The existence of "yes" gives rise to "no"; "all" to "nothing." Whether it is the nature of reality or simply the nature of human perception or language, this process of oppositional elements in tension with each other regularly occurs. As soon as someone on the inpatient unit thinks the patient can be reasonably discharged, someone else on the team will bring forward the reasons why that is not a good idea. One person voices the position of holding a hard line on program rules, which elicits someone else's description of why, in this case, an exception to the rule should be made. Both opposing positions may be true or contain elements of the truth (e.g., there are valid reasons to discharge and to delay discharge). From this point of view, polarized, divergent opinions should be expected when a client has complex problems that generate strong emotional reactions in his or her helpers.

A related idea is that one cannot make sense of elements without reference to the whole, which is to say that identity is relational. The only reason he looks old is because she looks younger; the only reason I look rigid is because you are flexible. Furthermore, the way we might identify or define a part changes and is changed by alterations in other parts of the whole. The client we have all come to think of as "the critic" in a skills training group, who is constantly pointing out how unhelpful the skills and skills trainer are, suddenly becomes a joy when a new member joins the group. They share the same blend of humor and skepticism, but where the one is caustic, the other is wry—their chemistry together takes the sting out of the criticism and creates a lighter but still pointed feedback loop for the lead skills trainer. The group leader, released from the siege mentality and genuinely seeing the critic's humor now, becomes more creative and likable. Taking a dialectical perspective means that words such as "good" or "bad" or "dysfunctional" are snapshots of the person in context, not inherent qualities. It also draws one into considering a web of causation rather than a linear model of causation. This idea translates into a clinical understanding that everything is caused and could not be otherwise, even if the causes are not apparent at the moment. From a dialectical perspective, the attention is not on the client alone but is rather on the relationships among the client, the client's community, the therapist, and the therapist's community.

Taken together, these views lead to the stance that truth evolves. On a treatment team, this means that no one person has a lock on the truth, and any understanding is likely partial and likely to leave out something important. Therefore, DBT puts a great emphasis on dialogues that lead to synthesis rather than individual reasoning from immutable facts.

FUNCTIONS OF COMPREHENSIVE TREATMENT AND MODES OF SERVICE DELIVERY

Services for multidisorder patients with severe and chronic problems can be structured to provide either comprehensive treatment to address all of the patients' problems or treatment for only a subset of problems (Linehan, 1999). Standard outpatient DBT is a comprehensive treatment that typically delivers services through the modes of individual psychotherapy, skills training (either in a group or individually), as-needed phone consultation to the patient, and a consultation team for therapists. However, because treatment settings differ widely in their modes of service delivery, it is useful to think of the functions that must be accomplished to address a patient's problems comprehensively, independent of the mode of service delivery. First, comprehensive treatment must enhance the client's capabilities; that is, the treatment should help clients acquire and integrate the repertoires they need to be effective. This can be done via skills training, psychoeducation, self-help handouts and readings, and pharmacotherapy. Second, comprehensive treatment must improve motivation by strengthening clinical progress and reducing factors that inhibit and or interfere with progress (e.g., emotions/physiological responses; cognitions/cognitive style; overt behavior patterns, environmental events). This can be accomplished in psychotherapy or the milieu through contingent reinforcement, aversive consequences, extinction, exposure–response prevention procedures, and cognitive modification. Third, comprehensive treatment ensures generalization so that the skillful responses learned in therapy transfer and are integrated for effective responses within a changing natural environment. This can be accomplished through after-hours and crisis phone coaching, milieu treatments, therapeutic communities, and *in vivo* interventions (e.g., case management). Fourth, comprehensive treatment enhances therapist capabilities and motivation. In essence, a comprehensive treatment must "treat" the therapist so that therapists, like clients, acquire, integrate, and generalize the response repertoires they need to do effective treatment and are motivated to use them. This can be accomplished through supervision, therapist consultation meetings, continuing education, treatment manuals, adherence and competency monitoring, and staff incentives. Finally, comprehensive treatment structures the environment for both client and therapist to increase the chance of treatment success through contingency management within both the treatment program as a whole and the community. This is usually accomplished through the role of clinic director or administrative interactions, case management, and family and marital interventions.

In standard outpatient DBT, these five functions are delegated across modes of service delivery. Specific duties and roles are assigned, and each mode has specific targets it is responsible for treating. For example, the individual psychotherapist is assigned the role of treatment planning, ensuring that progress is made on all DBT targets, helping integrate other modes of therapy, consulting to the patient on effective behaviors with other providers, and management of crises and life-threatening behaviors. This allows the primary therapist, often the person who knows the client's capabilities best, to teach, strengthen, and generalize new skills to crises, without reinforcing dysfunctional behavior. The skills trainer's role is to ensure that the client acquires new skills. To maximize learning and keep roles from conflicting, he or she only minimally targets behaviors that interfere with skills training (e.g., dissociating in group, coming late), referring the client back to the primary individual therapist to work on the bulk of those problems. Similarly, in suicidal and other crises, the skills trainer refers the client back to the individual therapist after requisite suicide risk assessment, but only the minimal intervention needed to get the client in contact with the primary therapist. In addition to weekly sessions of individual psychotherapy and skills training, the client also has access to as-needed telephone coaching calls to assist generalization of skills. The therapist also has a weekly consultation meeting with peers to ensure that he or she has the skills and motivation needed to be effective.

Its setting-specific treatment aims and length of stay determine the comprehensiveness of treatment offered by a particular mode of service delivery. For example, acute inpatient and short-term outpatient settings treat a limited number of focused targets consistent with short length of stay, but it is outside the scope of their mission to offer comprehensive treatment. Comprehensive treatment may not be appropriate or required in each mode of service delivery, but the idea is that somewhere in the system, each of the five functions will be addressed. If any one of these functions is missing, one might expect the client to make some, but not sustained, progress. For example, skills may be taught but no one is helping to motivate the client to apply them to specific situations or generalize them across situations. Or the individual therapist who has insufficient time to help the client acquire needed skills, or who lacks adequate support and training, fails to sustain the treatment plan with a client in perpetual crisis. Treatments with multidisorder patients may fail when there is a lack of comprehensive treatment with clearly assigned roles, targets, and structure.

Standard DBT had been modified to fit different treatment settings. For example, comprehensive DBT program implementation has been described in a partial hospital program (Simpson et al., 1998), inpatient (Bohus, et al., 2000; Swenson, Sanderson, Dulit, & Linehan, 2001), standard community mental health center (Mental Health Center of Greater Manchester, 1998) and Veterans Administration clinic settings (Koons et al., 2001), and within an Assertive Community Treatment program (Cunningham, Wolbert, & Lillie, in press). However, often the treatment goals and resources of a setting may create pressure to modify standard comprehensive DBT, so that only a subset of modes/functions of the comprehensive treatment are provided. While some modifications may be logical and prove effective, others, while sensible, may not. In the absence of tightly controlled component analysis research, therefore, the suggested course is to implement DBT as closely to protocol as possible, making changes systematically, and collecting data in the particular setting. For example, in our own training of teams to implement DBT in their settings, we encourage an adoption of DBT that is as close to protocol as possible first, and require those in training to evaluate their implementation as part of training.

Although a setting may vary in the functions and modes adopted, key DBT concepts and treatment strategies are constant across variations. We use clinical case examples that are composites of multiple actual clients to illustrate principles and strategies. We turn now to the basic ideas of DBT case conceptualization.

DIALECTICAL BEHAVIOR THERAPY AS FRAME

A number of elements of DBT provide a structure or conceptual frame within which to work. DBT organizes case conceptualization based on biosocial theory and level of disorder. These in turn translate into both a basic collaborative therapeutic stance and treatment goals and targets that are hierarchically organized according to importance.

Borderline Personality Disorder as a Pervasive Disorder of the Emotion Regulation System

In DBT, conceptualization of the primary problem of BPD as a pervasive disorder of the emotion regulation system not only guides all treatment interventions but also provides a psychoeducational frame so that client and therapist share a common understanding of problems and interventions. From this perspective, BPD criterion behaviors function to regulate emotions (e.g., parasuicide) or are a consequence of failed emotion regulation (e.g., dissociative symptoms or transient psychotic symptoms). Emotion dysregulation both interferes with problem solving and creates problems in its own right. For example, a client comes into session after having been fired from her job because she lost her temper with a customer. When the therapist asks what happened, the client becomes overwhelmed with shame and withdraws to the point of curling into a fetal position, mute, in the chair. This disrupts the help the therapist might have provided and creates a new situation about which the client feels shame (how she acted in therapy). After leaving the session, the feeling of shame becomes unbearable and the client repeatedly slams her head against her bedroom wall. Maladaptive behaviors, including extreme behaviors such as parasuicide, function to solve problems, and in particular, dysfunctional behaviors solve the problem of painful emotional states by providing relief.

The etiology of BPD has yet to be established. Childhood maltreatment, particularly childhood sexual abuse, may play a role given the observed correlation among BPD, suicidal behavior, and reports of childhood sexual abuse (e.g., Wagner & Linehan, 1994). However, not all persons who have been maltreated meet criteria for BPD, nor do all who meet criteria for BPD have histories of childhood maltreatment. Consequently, DBT interventions are guided by a general biosocial theory that explains how BPD develops and is maintained (Linehan, 1993a).

The biosocial theory holds that this pervasive difficulty regulating emotion comes from biologically based emotion vulnerability in transaction with particular environmental circumstances. Biologically, the person who develops BPD behavioral patterns is thought to be predisposed to have three characteristics: (1) high sensitivity to emotional cues (immediate reactions, low threshold for emotional reaction); (2) high reactivity (extreme reactions and the subsequent dysregulated cognitive processing that high arousal produces); and (3) a slow return to baseline (long-lasting reactions, which contribute to sensitivity to the next stimulus). The vulnerable person also is thought to have deficits in emotion regulation (e.g., problems decreasing or increasing physiological arousal, reorienting attention, inhibiting mood-dependent action, and organizing behavior in the service of external non-mood-dependent goals).

Environmentally, invalidation of thoughts, feelings, and behavior, independent of the actual validity of the behavior, is thought to contribute to the development of emotion regulation problems. Examples of invalidating responses include rejecting self-descriptions as inaccurate, dismissing, disregarding, or directly criticizing or punishing valid behavior, pathologizing normative responses, and rejecting valid responses and instead attributing them to socially unacceptable characteristics (e.g., overreactive emotions, manipulative intent, lack of motivation). Pervasive and consistent invalidation leads to learning maladaptive behavior or failing to learn adaptive behavior. For example, when others indiscriminately reject a person's communication of private experiences, the individual consequently fails to learn to trust his or her own experiences as valid response to events, and to effectively regulate emotions. Instead, the person learns to actively self-invalidate and to search the social environment for cues about how to respond. When others punish emotional displays and intermittently reinforce emotional escalation, the person does not learn to express emotions accurately or communicate pain effectively, but instead learns to oscillate between emotional inhibition and extreme emotional experience and expression. When others oversimplify the ease of problem solving and meeting goals, the individual does not learn to tolerate distress, to solve difficult problems in living, or to use shaping and other strategies to self-regulate effectively. Instead, the person learns to respond with high negative arousal to failure, form unrealistic goals and expectations, and hold perfectionistic standards.

The transactional nature of this model implies that individuals may develop BPD patterns of behavior in different ways: Even moderate vulnerability to emotion dysregulation may produce BPD patterns in a sufficiently invalidating environment. Even a "normal" level of invalidation may be sufficient to create BPD patterns for those who are highly vulnerable to emotion dysregulation. Over time, as an emotionally dysregulated person lives in an invalidating environment, he learns to respond to himself in the same manner that others have, invalidating his emotional experiences and dismissing pain and difficulty, oversimplifying the ease of solving problems, and holding unrealistic expectations. Repeated failures to regulate emotion and consequent interpersonal and achievement problems also generate self-directed hate and contempt. Over time, the person, who despite his best efforts is unable to regulate emotions, learns to despair of ever being "normal," which leads to a sense of emotional agony, of perpetually falling into the abyss and losing control. The task of changing seems impossible and the person can become resigned to the trauma of being a chronic mental patient or living an excruciatingly painful life.

Therefore, DBT targets reduction of painful emotions and solutions to problems that give rise to painful emotions. Therapy must simultaneously help the patient build a life that is worth living and replace maladaptive problem solving with adaptive, skillful problem solving. However, because it takes time to improve life circumstances so that there is less emotion to regulate, the first goal is to develop means of regulating the dysfunctional action tendencies associated with emotions, no matter how emotionally dysregulated one feels.

DBT uses the biosocial theory for psychoeducational purposes, along with matter-of-fact education about diagnosis to orient clients to the treatment rationale and how treatment will address their particular problems.

Levels of Disorder and Stages, Goals, and Targets of Treatment

In DBT, the goals and targets of treatment are determined by the extent of disorder in a commonsense fashion. For example, consider the differences between two clients. One uses heroine, has temporarily lost custody of her children, has no regular residence, and has been kicked out of methadone treatment programs due to problems with anger. She made a near-lethal suicide attempt when her children were taken away. The other, a nurse, is also addicted to opiates and has had his license suspended for stealing drugs from work. He, however, has a stable living situation, supportive family, a hopeful attitude about the drug treatment program offered through his employee assistance program, and an employer who is willing to take him back when he is clean. Many of the interventions for addiction will be the same, but the first person will need additional interventions to create a chance of success (or even placement) in a drug treatment program. Treating some of her behaviors (e.g., suicide attempts) will take precedence over others, and multiple problems may need to be solved simultaneously with the drug abuse. In a commonsense way, the severity of behavioral dyscontrol determines the goals and targets of treatment.

Consequently, DBT has four stages of treatment determined by level of disorder (Linehan, 1993a, 1999). The first stage of DBT is for the most severe level of disorder.

Stage 1 of therapy targets behaviors needed to achieve reasonable (immediate) life expectancy, control of action, and sufficient connection to treatment and behavioral capabilities to achieve these goals. To reach these goals, treatment time is allocated to give priority to targets in the following order of importance: (1) suicidal/homicidal or other imminently life-threatening behavior; (2) therapy-interfering behavior of the therapist or client; (3) behavior that severely compromises the client's quality of life; and (4) deficits in behavioral capabilities needed to make life changes. For a suicidal client, life-threatening behaviors include suicide crises behaviors (behaviors that convince the therapist or others that the patient is at high risk for imminent suicide, such as credible threats and suicide planning or preparations), parasuicidal acts, and suicidal ideation and communication (targeted only when new or unexpected, intense or aversive, or if it interferes with skillful problem solving). Therapy-interfering behaviors of the client include not attending therapy, noncollaboration, noncompliance, behaviors that interfere with other patients, and behaviors that burn out the therapist, push therapist limits, or reduce motivation to treat the client. Therapy-interfering behaviors of the therapist include actions that unbalance therapy, such as being extremely accepting or change-focused, too flexible or rigid, too nurturing or withholding, too vulnerable or irreverent in one's style, as well as being disrespectful. Behaviors that interfere with quality of life include mental-health-related dysfunctional response patterns, such as those found in DSM Axes I and IV; high-risk or unprotected sexual behaviors; extreme financial difficulties; criminal behaviors; seriously dysfunctional interpersonal behaviors; serious problems related to employment, school, illness, and housing.

DBT targets specific skills deficits as particularly relevant to BPD and provides training to help clients (1) regulate emotions; (2) tolerate distress; (3) respond skillfully to interpersonal conflict; (4) observe, describe, and participate without judging, with awareness and a focus on effectiveness; and (5) manage their own behavior with strategies other than self-punishment. These skills are linked to the particular BPD criterion behaviors, with mindfulness intended to decrease identity confusion, emptiness, and cognitive dysregulation; with interpersonal effectiveness that addresses interpersonal chaos and fears of abandonment; with emotion regulation skills intended to reduce labile affect and excessive anger; and with distress tolerance to help reduce impulsive behaviors, suicide threats, and parasuicide. Targets from these four areas (life-threatening, treatment interfering, quality of life interfering, and skills deficits) are monitored and provide the main agenda for individual therapy sessions.

Even (or especially) when the client is in Stage 1, the therapist takes care to articulate the further stages of therapy. It is important to communicate that the goals of therapy are not simply to suppress severe dysfunctional behavior, but rather to build a life that any reasonable person would consider worth living. When working with patients who have been in the system for a long time, it is important to communicate that the goal is to get them not only out of hell but also into a life that is actually worth living—a life that is so good that thoughts of suicide do not arise. DBT is not a palliative treatment. It is meant to be curative in the sense that, although a person will likely continue to be more emotionally sensitive than the average person, he or she no longer meets criteria for BPD and has a quality of life and set of skills that make this emotional vulnerability tolerable. Many clients who are not out of control still experience tremendous emotional pain due either to posttraumatic stress responses or other painful emotional experiences that leave them alienated or isolated from meaningful connections to people or vocation. They suffer lives of quiet desperation, in which their emotional experiencing is either too intense (although behavioral control is maintained) or they are numbed out. Therefore, with these clients, the goals of therapy in Stage 2 are to have nontraumatizing emotional experience and connection to the environment. In Stage 3, clients synthesize what has been learned, increase their self-respect and an abiding sense of connection, and work toward resolving problem in living. Targets here are self-respect, mastery, self-efficacy, a sense of morality, and an acceptable quality of life. Stage 4 (Linehan, 1999) focuses on the sense of incompleteness that many individuals experience even after problems in living are essentially resolved. For many, this will fall outside the realm of therapy and within a spiritual practice that gives rise to the capacity for sustained joy and expanded awareness of self, past to present, self to other, and peak experiences, flow, or spiritual fulfillment.

Although the stages of therapy are presented linearly, progress is often not linear and the stages overlap. When problems arise, it is not uncommon to return to discussions such as those in pretreatment, in an attempt to regain commitment to the treatment goals or methods. At termination or before breaks, especially if not well prepared, the client may resume Stage 1 behaviors. The transition from Stages 1 to 2 is also difficult for many, because exposure work can lead to intensely painful emotions and consequent behavioral dyscontrol. Like other trauma approaches (e.g., Cloire, 1998; Keane, Fisher, Krinsley, & Niles, 1994; Najavits, Weiss, Shaw, & Muenz, 1998), DBT encourages acquisition of skills to a sufficient level that one has a reasonable quality of life/stability of behavior control prior to systematic exposure to the cues associated with past traumas.

Level of disorder and stages of treatment have implications for service delivery. Many clinics have different levels of care contingent on severity of behavioral dyscontrol. What is required is to have reinforcers (e.g., more and more in-depth services) available and contingent on progress rather than on continuation of maladaptive behavior. For example, if someone can only get individual therapy by being completely out of control, or if that client loses access to an individual therapist as soon as he or she is out of crisis, then the contingencies favor lack of progress and continued crises.

DIALECTICAL BEHAVIOR THERAPY AS PROBLEM SOLVING: BEHAVIORAL PRINCIPLES, BEHAVIORAL ASSESSMENT, AND PROBLEM-SOLVING PROCEDURES

DBT is a cognitive-behavioral therapy and uses empirically supported behavior therapy protocols to treat Axis I problems. As do other cognitive-behavioral approaches, it emphasizes use of behavioral principles and assessment to determine the controlling variables for problem behaviors. It uses standard cognitive-behavioral interventions (e.g., self-monitoring, behavioral and solution analyses, didactic and orienting strategies, contingency management, cognitive restructuring, skills training and exposure procedures). Rather than describe cognitive-behavioral interventions in depth, we assume the reader is familiar with them and we instead highlight interventions uniquely emphasized in DBT. For example, all cognitive-behavioral approaches include psychoeducation and place a strong emphasis on orienting the client to the treatment rationale and methods. However, because emotional arousal often interferes with processing and collaboration, the DBT therapist frequently must do what could be called micro-orienting, instructing the client specifically about what to do in the particular treatment task at hand. Similarly, when cognitive-behavioral therapists generate solutions, they typically also preemptively assess what would prevent the use of the solution or troubleshoot. In DBT, this troubleshooting takes on added emphasis because the client often has severe, mood-dependent behaviors and one cannot assume generalization in the same way one would with a less mood-dependent person. DBT modifies use of standard cognitive-behavioral therapy to adapt to the patient's multiple, serious chronic problems.

As with other cognitive-behavioral approaches, Stage 1 of DBT begins with thorough assessment, discussion, and agreement to the goals of treatment and the means that will be used to achieve them. In the first several sessions, the primary therapist gathers the history needed to assess suicide risk accurately, to begin to identify situations that evoke parasuicide and suicidal ideation, and to manage suicidal crises. In particular, the therapist identifies the conditions associated with near-lethal suicide attempts, parasuicide acts with high intent to die, and other medically serious parasuicidal behavior.

Also, as with other cognitive-behavioral approaches, the client and therapist explicitly and collaboratively agree to the essential goals and methods of treatment. While it is not important to have a written contract, it is important to have a mutual, verbal commitment to treatment agreements. Because DBT requires voluntary rather than coerced consent, both the client and the therapist must have the choice between DBT and other treatment options.

During these initial sessions, DBT emphasizes strategies that help clients strengthen their commitment to change. For example, when a client has an extensive history of psychiatric hospitalization, the therapist and client discuss the pros and cons of this and its compatibility with the client's ultimate goal of a life worth living. In one case, the client described how hospitalization had derailed important life goals. Her last relationship ended after she went into the hospital "because he didn't want to be with a mental patient." During the series of hospitalizations before that, she missed so much time in community college that it was impossible to make up the work, so she withdrew from classes. She also had exhausted her parents' medical benefits and they refused to pay out of pocket, so she sought disability status, which she found both a relief and a humiliation. After thorough consideration of the pros and cons, both the client and therapist knew the advantages and disadvantages of using and not using psychiatric hospitalization. In the following excerpt, the client has just said she wants to stop going into the hospital, but she is afraid—in the past going in the hospital has seemed like the only way to avoid killing herself.

THERAPIST: So, when you have thoughts of killing yourself, it is a huge relief to go into the hospital—there is close monitoring and structure, less demand on you, and all of that makes you less worried you will kill yourself. But the problem has been that going into the hospital did not help you get better at keeping yourself alive or do anything to solve the problems that were making you suicidal.

CLIENT: Right, things actually got worse, Bobby left me. I lost school.

THERAPIST: It's a tough situation. The hospital is a short-term break, like a vacation from your life, but the same problems are there when you get out and sometimes they get worse. But I can imagine it could be difficult for you to give up the hospital at this point in your life. You have medical assistance that helps now with the hospital bills and it sounds like the hospital staff care about you when you go in. Staying a mental patient is the line of least resistance.

CLIENT: I hate myself like this. I hate my life.

THERAPIST: It's as if things you want are on the other side of rough waters, but when the waters get rough, we pull you out and put you in an indoor swimming pool. You find your stroke again, but as soon as you are back in the "real thing" and overwhelmed, your mind says "Get out, you can't do this." It's almost automatic now to go into the hospital. In this therapy, we could make it a goal to help you solve the problems that are making you suicidal, without going in the hospital, so that you learn how to get through difficult situations. We need to find a way for you to be able to stay in rough waters, swimming, but with enough help so you don't drown and can keep swimming to where you want to go. Is that of interest, finding a way to solve your life problems without going in the hospital?

CLIENT: Yes. I just don't think I can do it. Going in the hospital is the only thing that kept me from killing myself.

THERAPIST: Would you like to get so you can keep yourself from killing yourself without going in the hospital?

CLIENT: Yes.

THERAPIST: It is going to be really hard. You sure you want to do this?

CLIENT: I don't have a choice. I am going to end up dead if this doesn't change.

THERAPIST: Why not be dead?

CLIENT: If it comes to it, I will. But if I have got one chance, I want to take it.

THERAPIST: Then one thing we could agree to is that you will not go into the hospital at all this year, so we can put all of our energy into solving the problems that make you suicidal and finding ways for you to get through the roughest parts but still be able to keep yourself alive.

CLIENT: The whole year! But what if I get suicidal?

THERAPIST: You will get suicidal, or at least let's hope you do, because it is going to take us a lot of practice before we get you swimming well.

CLIENT: I can't do it. Going in the hospital is the only thing that's kept me alive.

THERAPIST: You have a perfect right to seek out whatever help you need, and going in the hospital when you get suicidal is certainly an option. From what you said, though, that means that you give up your goals for completing school and find a partner who does not mind that you occasionally go in the hospital.

CLIENT: (*Silent.*)

THERAPIST: When you say you want a "normal life," I think you can get there, but the hospital seems incompatible with your goals. Therapy won't work unless you and I have the same goals and game plan for how we will get there. Do you want to work with me to find a way for you to handle these very difficult situations without going in the hospital?

CLIENT: I want to do it. I'm scared I can't.

THERAPIST: Let me tell you a little more about the treatment program, because the combination of the skills training group and the phone coaching may give you some of the help and structure you found helpful in the hospital, so you may be able to do more than you think you can.

In this excerpt, the therapist summarized the problem with going in the hospital and oriented the client to an alternative treatment plan to reach her long-term goals. The therapist played the devil's advocate, at times articulating why the status quo of using the hospital is preferable. This allowed the client to voice the reasons why change is important (and avoided a polarized discussion, with the therapist presenting reasons for change, while the client counters with those for the status quo because she is scared). The therapist also highlighted the freedom to choose and the lack of alternatives in a way that helped the client reckon with the unavoidably painful aspects of failing to change. The therapist asked for small changes to which the client could easily agree (foot in the door), as well as large changes beyond what the client could imagine (door in the face), both strategies that help the client move toward a greater commitment to changing behaviors she wants to change. The therapist also encouraged the client and affirmed her ability to change. Commitment strategies such as these are woven into any discussions in which the client's commitment to change could use strengthening. So, for example, when this client calls to say she is considering going to the emergency room, the therapist might quickly recap the pros and cons to help her regain motivation for finding alternatives to hospitalization before turning to the problems giving rise to the use for hospitalization.

After the client and therapist develop their goals and agreements, the client, using a diary card, begins to monitor those behaviors they have agreed to target. Whenever one of the targeted problem behaviors occur, the therapist and client conduct an in-depth analysis of events and situational factors before, during, and after that particular instance (or set of instances) of the targeted behavior. The chain analysis yields an accurate and reasonably complete account of the behavioral and environmental events associated with the problem behavior. First, they clearly define the problem behavior. Second, they identify both general vulnerability factors (the context that gives precipitating events influence, e.g., physical illness, sleep deprivation, and other conditions that influence emotional reactivity) and specific precipitating events that began the chain of events leading to the problem behavior. Third, they identify each link between the precipitating event and the problematic behavior to yield a detailed account of each thought, feeling, action, and event that moved the client from point A to point B, as well as determine what consequences occurred after the behavior.

For example, say the problem behavior was a suicide preparation in which the client gathered a potentially lethal overdose of medications. The vulnerability factors included quitting her job due to conflict with a manager 2 weeks earlier and difficulty getting a new job. On Mother's Day, she had called her mother to wish her well and to ask to borrow money for her rent. During the call, her mother interrupted her to take a call on the other line. After several minutes she came back on the line to say she wanted to get off the telephone with the client so she could talk to the brother and his children. Feeling hurt, the client said sarcastically, "Who wants to talk to a pathetic daughter when you have a son like him," and hung up abruptly. After she hung up, she kicked the kitchen table so hard that it rattled the windows and she slammed out of the room.

The precipitating event was that unbeknownst to the client, her roommate had been in the living room with her boyfriend and was extremely embarrassed that her boyfriend left because of the incident. Later, the roommate said she did not appreciate her "throwing a tantrum," and that it was too hard living with her moodiness. The argument escalated and the roommate ended it by saying the client should start looking for someplace else to live.

There were then a number of dysfunctional links that led to the client's preparing for suicide. Her anger at her roommate faded as the client remembered how out of control she was after the call. She felt humiliated and decided she had to move rather than face the roommate or her boyfriend. She then felt trapped because she could not afford to move without help from her mother, now ruled out because the phone call went poorly. She began to dwell on thoughts about how "pathetic" she was and had no one to blame but herself; her shame intensified. These feelings were made worse by the client's feeling hurt and rejected by her mother, who preferred to talk to her brother. Then, the image of everyone at her funeral, sad but relieved that she was gone and no longer a burden, came into her mind and she felt calm and at peace. She thought of pills she had stockpiled in a chest in the basement. The client heard her roommate preparing to leave, and feeling very calm, she stuck her head out to apologize for embarrassing her roommate earlier and to say she was not feeling well, so was going to bed early. She then wrote her mother a good-bye note for 2 hours before going to the basement to get the pills. Her roommate, who had gone out to dinner, felt badly about arguing after the client's heartfelt apology and instead of staying over at her boyfriend's as usual, came home unexpectedly, in part to apologize herself. She walked into the client's room, saw and read the note, and was waiting for the client when she came back with the pills in her hand. They had an emotional conversation in which the roommate said she had no idea things were so bad and that she would cover the rent until the client got a job. The roommate's support and offer to help greatly alleviated the client's emotional distress.

As the therapist and client discussed this chain of events over several sessions, the therapist highlighted dysfunctional behavior, focusing on emotions, and helped the client gain insight by recognizing the patterns between this and other instances of problem behavior. They identified each juncture at which an alternative, more skillful response might have produced positive change, so that suicide preparation was unnecessary. In particular, the therapist assessed alternative behavior that would have been more adaptive and skillful, and why that more skillful alternative did not happen. This process of identifying the problem and analyzing the moment-to-moment chain of events over time to determine which variables control/influence the behavior occurs for each targeted problem behavior as it occurs. In generating solutions, the therapist suggests DBT skills.

THERAPIST: So, at that point, when you have the conversation with your mom, you feel hurt, unloved, angry, and guilty about being a burden to her, and right before you kick the table—right there, what could you do to help yourself? What was the main emotion right there?
CLIENT: I was frustrated with her and myself, and hurt.
THERAPIST: Okay, which would you rather work on first, the hurt or the anger at her, or at yourself?
CLIENT: Feeling frustrated with myself was the worst.
THERAPIST: Let's go through some options there. Are you better off by accepting how angry you are at yourself or by trying to change it? Accepting it? Okay. So what skills could you use right there?

As in other cognitive-behavioral approaches, the absence of adaptive behavior is considered due to one of four factors linked to behavior therapy change procedures. First, the client may have a capability deficit (i.e., does not have the necessary skills in her repertoire). DBT views specific skills deficits as particularly relevant to BPD; therefore, the therapist assesses whether clients can (1) regulate emotions; (2) tolerate distress; (3) respond skillfully to interpersonal conflict; (4) observe, describe, and participate without judging, with awareness and a focus on effectiveness; and (5) manage their own behavior with strategies other than self-punishment. When clients lack these skills, skills training is appropriate. In this case, for example, the client lacked skills in regulating the action tendencies associated with anger, particularly when anger was secondary to feeling hurt or guilty. For her, an important skill was tolerating the distress of feeling hurt and guilty while inhibiting sarcasm and other angry actions that made the situation worse.

The second possible reason for the lack of skilled performance is that circumstances reinforce dysfunctional behavior in that problem behavior may lead to positive or preferred outcomes, or create an opportunity for other preferred behaviors or emotional states. In this instance, suicide planning and imagery were associated with a sense of calm and peace. The third possibility is that conditioned emotional responses block more skillful responding. Effective behaviors may be inhibited or disorganized by intense or out-of-control emotions. In this example, anger and embarrassment interfered with the client immediately apologizing to her roommate, and shame and guilt at being a burden interfered with solving the problems with both her mother and roommate. If this is the case, then some version of exposure-based treatment is indicated. The fourth possibility is that effective behaviors are inhibited by faulty beliefs or assumptions. If the problems are identified here, then cognitive modification strategies are appropriate. For example, the client had a number of unrealistic beliefs about the effect that her suicide would have, associating it with a sense of calm and peace.

DBT also puts strong emphasis on treating dysfunctional behaviors that are common across target areas or that occur in-session and interfere with therapy or mirror areas in the client's life outside of therapy. For example, a client described the chain of events that ended in his using heroin, and the one key link appeared to be a dysphoric mood and the thought "It doesn't matter, nothing matters." This same link had been key when he had quit past therapies and jobs. As he recounted the situation, he began to experience this same mood in-session. When the therapist turned the conversation to consider how the client might handle the situation differently next time, the client said in a quiet, defeated voice, "What's the point?"

THERAPIST: What just happened? You just finished telling me about this and I say, okay, let's see what we can do about it. Then what happened? What are you feeling?
CLIENT: Nothing is going to help. Why go through all this?
THERAPIST: That is the thought. What is the emotion you are feeling?
CLIENT: (*Silent, therapist waiting.*) I don't know.
THERAPIST: My guess is it's despair and fear, but maybe also fatigue and feeling overwhelmed.
CLIENT: (*Silent.*)
THERAPIST: This is life and death. (*Leans forward, quiet but intense.*) This is what gets you every time, not just with using but also when you want to kill yourself. You have got to find a way to get active in this conversation so we can figure it out. Think for a minute, I say 'Let's do something about this' and you feel what?
CLIENT: It's not worth it, I'm not worth it.
THERAPIST: You look very sad when you say that. Is this feeling like how you felt before you used? What would it take when you feel like this to get yourself not to use, not to give up?
CLIENT: I would have to feel good about myself, like all of this is worth it.
THERAPIST: All right. What makes it worth it? What can you feel good about?
CLIENT: I don't know.
THERAPIST: When you get to this point, you have to find something to feel good about. It has to be genuine and something you really believe. Take a deep breath. Ask

"What can I feel good about?" and listen for the answer. Don't make one up, just listen for the answer.

In this case, the therapist stayed with the task until the client generated several things he genuinely felt good about that shifted his in-session mood. Then, together they thought about how the client could do this in his life outside therapy (e.g., what would cue him to remember to fight off the despair rather than give in to the mood?).

DIALECTICAL BEHAVIOR THERAPY AS VALIDATION

DBT shares elements with other supportive treatment approaches. Exquisite emotional sensitivity, proneness to emotional dysregulation, and a history of failed attempts to change either intense emotionality or the problem behaviors associated with it make supportive treatment elements important. DBT validation strategies are meant to communicate not only empathetic understanding but also the validity of the client's emotions, thoughts, and actions. These strategies in DBT are important in and of themselves, as well as in combination with change strategies.

For example, under stress, Marie hears voices. She has tried a number of antipsychotic medications but has never experienced them as helpful. She works in a copy shop where there are occasionally high-pressure deadlines. Under stress, the usual low-level murmuring becomes so intrusive that she starts talking aloud to herself, stops sleeping, and becomes disheveled, thereby increasing the cues from others that provoke paranoia of being watched and criticized. The voices spiral into yet more intense criticism and negative commentary. Marie went twice to vocational school in order to learn skills for another, less stressful job, but each time the stresses of school set off the same sequence of events and she quit. Choosing not to work and instead to go on disability would be humiliating for her, but her family, who have been supporting her during periods of unemployment, encouraged it. In the following conversation, Marie has just finished explaining to her therapist the difficulties she currently has at work coping with increasingly intrusive and critical voices.

THERAPIST: Well, maybe you might discuss adjusting medications with your psychiatrist.
CLIENT: Medications have never helped. It's stupid to keep wasting his and my time with this.
THERAPIST: I know you have tried a number of them, but maybe you never really had an adequate trial. The last one you discontinued after only a week because of side effects.
CLIENT: I can't tolerate the side effects.
THERAPIST: Right, but maybe there's a way of managing the side effects a bit better.
CLIENT: I already told him about the side effects and he didn't do anything. You call him.
THERAPIST: Oh, so you already spoke with him? What was said? (*Wants to get the facts and also to assess whether there is a communication problem interfering with the client getting what she needs.*)
CLIENT: You don't get it, do you? (*Stands up, begins to pace the room angrily.*) You've never taken antipsychotic medications, have you? You can't think! You can't function! I feel like a zombie. Why go through that, lose my job again because I'm so

out of it? (*Stops and leans against a wall with her eyes closed.*) I'm tired of trying and getting my hopes up.
THERAPIST: Okay. (*Flustered, pauses.*) You want to rule out medication then as a solution?
CLIENT: (*Begins to lightly hit the back of her head against the wall.*) I can't stand this. I would rather be dead than have to fight like this just to get through a day.

In this instance, assessing whether the medication could be adjusted or the side effects better managed is experienced as a tremendous oversimplification of the problem, and not solving the problem is destroying Marie's life. The threat that the therapist will offer only solutions that have already been tried and therefore leave Marie trapped in a painful cycle of trying medications that will ultimately fail to solve the problem sets off her anger, despair, and thoughts of suicide. Aspects of Marie's response are extreme—she has a low threshold for emotional cues, and her emotional reactions are intense. But the emotional arousal itself is simultaneously a normative and predictable process given the importance of solving the problem and the interpretation of the therapist's comments.

It is a normal psychological process for emotional arousal to occur when significant goals are blocked and important self-constructs are disconfirmed. For example, a person with a learning disability that seriously impairs his ability to read will prefer an instructor of a course with heavy reading to say "You probably are not going to make it in this class," rather than "You are a smart person and a hard worker. I expect you will do fine." When feedback is inconsistent with important self-constructs, the consequent arousal and the sense of being out of control result in both failure to process new information and intense effort to gain control. If the instructor were to persist in reassuring him about his competence, the student's emotional arousal would increase and he would try harder to make the professor understand how debilitating a reading disability is. People prefer feedback, even if negative, that is consistent with important self-constructs, a process called self-verification (Swann, 1997).

Many therapeutic tasks, however, require just such a process of invalidating important self-constructs. When the client says "I can't stand this emotional pain," the therapist's interventions are versions of "Yes, you can," disagreeing with the client's perspective. One can expect the client to feel more emotional, out of control, and less collaborative. To help the client change requires intervening in a manner that modulates the emotional arousal so that work on the therapeutic task continues. With clients who are highly sensitive to emotional cues (e.g., who tend to respond in an angry or extremely despairing manner to perceived threat), the therapist may become more and more careful in what he or she says in order to avoid setting off the client's reaction. But this means that the client does not change. In fact, emotional sensitivity and intensity (e.g., anger or despair) are inadvertently made more likely (negatively reinforced) as the therapist withdraws a focus on change. The therapist must simultaneously align with the client's goals and self-constructs, without reinforcing dysfunctional behavior, without evoking such emotional reactivity that the therapeutic task is derailed, and without dropping a focus on needed change.

In other words, the therapist must respond differentially to what is valid and what is invalid in the client's responses. The term "valid" is meant in three ways (Linehan, 1997b, 1997c). A response is valid if it is (1) relevant and meaningful, (2) well-grounded or justifiable in terms of facts or authority, or (3) an appropriate or effective means to obtain one's ends. For example, a case manager who has ignored repeated requests by a client to become his own payee, because the client typically injudiciously spends the money, hears the request but responds as if it is irrelevant. Yet the desire to be more independent is valid. The same behavior, however, can be both valid and invalid. The case manager's ignoring requests is valid in the sense of being justifiable based on the client's mishandling of money, but it is invalid to the extent that it ignores the client's normative desire to control his own money.

When a client says she hates herself, hatred might be a justifiable response if the person violated her own important values (e.g., deliberately harmed another person out of anger). The response of self-hatred may be justifiable but at the same time ineffective because it is incompatible with the balanced problem solving required to keep oneself from doing the hateful behavior again. Even patently invalid behavior may be valid in terms of being effective. Cutting one's arms in response to overwhelming emotional distress makes sense given that it often produces relief from unbearable emotions: It is an effective emotion regulation strategy. From this perspective, all behavior is valid in some way. Even extreme dysfunctional behavior may be valid in terms of historically making sense—all of the factors needed for the behavior to develop have occurred; therefore, how could the behavior be other than it is?

Therefore, aside from relying on empathy alone, DBT has emphasized validation. To validate means to confirm, authenticate, corroborate, substantiate, strengthen, ratify, or verify. To validate, the therapist actively seeks out and communicates to the client how a response makes sense by being relevant, meaningful, justifiable, or effective. Validating an emotion, thought, or action requires empathy, an understanding of the particular or unique significance of the context from the other person's perspective. However, validation adds to this the communication that the emotion, thought, or action is a valid response. Were the client to ask, "Can this be true?", empathy would be understanding the "this," whereas validation would be communicating "yes." Validation strategies help the therapist simultaneously align with the client's goals and self-constructs, without reinforcing dysfunctional behavior, without evoking such emotional reactivity that the therapeutic task is derailed, and without dropping a focus on needed change. Validation is a therapeutic "yes, but . . . " when combined with change strategies, so that the therapist simultaneously communicates why something could not be otherwise yet must change.

This ability to communicate the validity of the client's responses is sometimes essential for the success of change-oriented strategies. Unless the client believes that the therapist truly understands the dilemma ("You've never taken antipsychotic medications. You've never had to talk to your pharmacotherapist as a BPD person who is instantly suspect"), he or she will not trust that the therapist's solutions are appropriate or adequate, and there will be no collaboration and no new learning. In nearly all situations, the therapist may usefully validate that the client's problems are important, that a task is difficult, that emotional pain or a sense of being out of control is justifiable, and that there is wisdom in the client's ultimate goals, even if not by the particular means he or she is currently using.

In the first level of validation, the therapist communicates that the client's responses are valid by listening without prejudging. So, for example, the case manager hears the client's request to become his own payee without construing it solely in terms of the mismanagement of money. In the second level of validation, paraphrasing, the therapist communicates understanding by repeating or rephrasing, using words close to the client's own without added interpretation. The third level is mind reading, or the ability to understand what is meant without the client having to explain things. Particularly with clients at high risk for suicide, it is important for the therapist to be able to imagine what it might be like to walk down the hall after an appointment, alone, in order to troubleshoot any crisis plans adequately.

The fourth level of validation is to communicate that something makes sense in terms of past learning or past biology. For example, to a client who constantly seeks reassurance that therapy "is going okay," the therapist might validate this response by saying, "Given the shifting from foster care placement to placement, it makes sense to have the feeling of waiting for the other shoe to drop." This is in contrast to the fifth level of validation, in which the therapist communicates how a response makes sense in the current situation. Using the same example, the therapist might search for ways that he or she is communicating ambivalence or in some other way cueing the client's response, so that seeking reassurance is sensible. DBT favors finding the ways a response is currently valid whenever possible. This can be difficult. For example, a client who was a phlebotomist left vials of blood in her pharmacotherapist's office mailbox when she was furious with him. The therapist might say,

"I understand it drives you crazy when you don't feel listened to, but on the other hand we have to get you more skillful, so that you don't have to act so weird in order to get someone's attention. I understand the intense anger and urge to get some revenge given how powerless you feel, but this is not going to work out if you want to be taken seriously."

The sixth level of validation is radical genuineness. One aspect of this is not fragilizing the patient but rather responding to the client as a person deserving of equal respect or, said differently, playing to the person's strengths rather than vulnerability. So, for example, if a colleague entered a room to talk about a problem and then curled up in a fetal position on the floor, the average person would be surprised and confront the behavior. With BPD clients, however, fragility is often assumed, resulting in use of the kind of high-pitched, singsong voice one uses with children: "Do you think you could sit up?" DBT advocates a matter-of-fact but nonjudgmental "What are you doing? You are suffering too much here for us to let you act like a nut case about it, and it's hard to have a conversation with you on the floor like that." Nongenuineness prevents the free flow of confrontation, self-involving self-disclosure, irreverence, and other therapist responses that are important information for the client to help him or her change and accurately read the social situation.

Returning to the example of Marie, the therapist's questions are reasonable, but Marie's extreme sensitivity makes it necessary for him to provide more validation.

THERAPIST: Marie. Marie. Listen, sit down for a second. I can't think when you are pacing around like that. No, I have not taken antipsychotics, but the way I see it is that you are being tortured. Doing a good job at work and supporting yourself are incredibly important. I know you have tried a million things before, but you are going to be dead if we cannot find some way to have you be able to work, yet not have to fight like hell just to get through a day. We've got to find a solution to this.
CLIENT: I'm tired of this. I'm tried of getting my hopes up.
THERAPIST: Who said anything about getting your hopes up? If this was easy, you and your past doctors would have solved it. What I am asking is that you work with me. It may take us a long time to figure this out. It's like being an athlete with arthritis. The more you do your sport, the worse it hurts; the less you do your sport, the more it hurts. You can't do things the old way, and you don't know another

way. You have a chronic problem with these voices and we have to find some way for you to get what you want without so much suffering. Are you willing to work with me on this?

CLIENT: Okay.

THERAPIST: I mean will you work with me on this even when you are tired and exhausted and having side effects? Where we keep trying to find the right combination or balance of medication and work stress that really makes you satisfied with your life? Okay. But I have to understand the facts so I can help. Let me ask the question again and don't bite my head off: What exactly have you talked about with your doctor about the side effects and what can be done to minimize them?

It is likely that if Marie could stay engaged in problem solving, they might find a number of ways out of her dilemma. Although the task of finding a genuinely workable balance between medication and stress level is very difficult, it is necessary for a reasonable quality of life. It could be that by better regulating other elements of Marie's life, she could in fact tolerate the stress level of occasional deadlines without switching jobs. More social support, a different role in the production process at work, a less perfectionistic evaluation of her own performance, more acceptance of having a brain that responds with psychotic symptoms under stress—any of these might be the outcome of their conversation. But the therapist must in some way communicate to Marie that he understands and sees what is valid in her response to reduce emotion dysregulation to open the possibility for collaboration.

PRINCIPLE-DRIVEN USE OF PROTOCOLS FOR SEVERE AND CHRONIC, MULTIDIAGNOSTIC, DIFFICULT-TO-TREAT PATIENTS: DIALECTICAL BEHAVIOR THERAPY AS JAZZ

Treating patients with multiple severe and chronic disorders requires the therapist not only to know treatment protocols for specific disorders but also to have some cohesive way of integrating them to treat an ever-changing clinical picture. The complexity of the task is further complicated because of the work one must do to establish and keep a collaborative and productive therapeutic relationship. One could treat the presenting or major problem first, see what resolves, and then proceed to treat the multiple other Axis I disorders sequentially. However, even if one had enough time (and enough insurance coverage) to do so, between one session and the next, a typically dysregulated client has had a major life crisis. For example, last week a client was assigned readings to orient her to treatment for panic disorder. The therapist came to the session ready to discuss the treatment rationale. However, in the intervening week the client had a fight with her boyfriend, who left her living on the street and staying in a homeless shelter for the past 2 days. While at the shelter, she was sexually harassed, setting off nightmares and some dissociative symptoms. Because of the chaos, she skipped skills training group and doubts she can make it to group this week either. Living on the street, she ran into some of her old drug buddies and used heroin. She describes the week in a matter-of-fact tone of voice, yet her diary card shows high ratings on misery and suicidal ideation, and when the therapist assesses suicidality, she discovers the client has her preferred means in her car. As the session continues, the client dissociates to the point that she is not talking.

DBT was developed for people with multiple disorders who are often in crises. DBT interventions hierarchically target behaviors, so that the immediate focus is to assess and treat suicide risk. However, in addition to getting rid of the immediate means and addressing the problems associated with suicidal behavior, the therapist may also need to address the problem of housing, going to skills group, not using heroin again, managing the dissociative symptoms, and processing the end of the romantic relationship. This requires the therapist to apply mini-interventions drawn from effective behavioral protocols to problems as they arise. The required improvisation is akin to jazz—built upon sound mastery of one's instrument and understanding of music but tightly linked to the exact moment and players. This flexible application of strategies results from overlearning behavior therapy protocols and also from applying dialectical philosophy and strategies that help at therapeutic impasses.

In addition to the mastery of behavior therapy protocols, a number of strategies are included in DBT that function to keep polarized positions from remaining polarized. The first of these is that core strategies are used to balance acceptance and change. For example, DBT requires the therapist to have a balanced communication style. On the acceptance side is use of a responsive style, in which the patient's agenda is taken seriously and responded to directly rather than interpreted for its latent meaning. For example, if a client asks something personal about the therapist, the therapist is more likely to use self-disclosure, warm engagement, and genuineness either to answer the question or matter-of-factly decline to answer based on personal limits.

However, this style alone, or an imbalance toward this style, can lead to impasse. When the glum client who has told the same story of grievance many times has a therapist who simply paraphrases in the same monotone as the client, the probability is that the client's mood will stay the same or worsen. Consequently, reciprocal communication is balanced by irreverence that jolts the patient off track to allow him or her to resume the therapeutic task at hand. For example, the therapist might use an unorthodox, offbeat manner. The therapist, who has been just as engaged as the client in a power struggle, suddenly shifts tone and laughs, "You know, this moment is just not as black and white as I had hoped." Similarly, the therapist may plunge in where angels fear to tread. For example, he might say matter-of-factly to the woman whose major precipitant to suicidal crisis is the threat of losing her husband, "Look, cutting yourself and leaving blood all over the bathroom is destroying any hope of having a real relationship with your husband." Or to a new client, "Given that you've assaulted two of your last three therapists, let's start off with what led up to that and how it's not going to happen with me. I'm going to be of no use to you if I'm afraid of you." Using an irreverent style of communication includes using a confrontational tone, oscillating intensity, or at times expressing omnipotence and impotence in the face of the client's problems.

Another way that DBT balances acceptance and change is in case management strategies. Individuals who meet criteria for BPD often have multiple treatment providers; consequently, a number of strategies have been developed to help the client–therapist dyad manage the relationships with other clinicians and family members. DBT is weighted toward a consultation-to-the-patient strategy that emphasizes change. The DBT therapist consults with the patient about how to handle relationships with other treatment providers and family members, rather than consulting with other treatment providers and family members about how to deal with the patient. So, for example, this means that the therapist does not meet with other professionals about the patient, but rather that the patient is present at treatment planning meetings (preferably has set them up him- or herself). Rather than meet with another provider without the client present, a conference call might be scheduled during an individual session. If the therapist has to meet without the client present for some practical reason, the conversation is discussed in advance and shared with the client. This same principle holds for conversations with the patient's family. Even in a crisis, the spirit of consulting to the patient is maintained whenever possible. If the emergency room's triage nurse or resident-on-call contacts the therapist to ask what he or she would like done, the DBT therapist is likely to first ask to speak with the patient in order to discuss how going in the hospital does and does not coincide with the client's long-term goals and their agreed-upon treatment plan. The therapist might then coach the patient on how to interact skillfully with the emergency room staff or have the patient communicate the plan to the staff and then simply have the staff confirm that with the therapist, if that is required for credibility. If the hospital staff were concerned about suicide risk and were reluctant to release the person, the DBT therapist would not "tell" the hospital staff to release the patient, but instead might coach the patient on what was needed to decrease the legitimate worries of the staff.

The DBT therapist intervenes in the environment on the patient's behalf when the short-term gain is worth the long-term loss in learning, when the patient is unable to act on his or her own and outcome is very important, when the environment is intransigent and high in power, to save the life of the patient or avoid substantial risk to others, and when it is the humane thing to do and will cause no harm or when the patient is a minor. In these cases, the therapist may provide information, advocate, or enter the environment to give assistance. However, the usual role is of one of consultant to help the patient become more skillful in personal and professional relationships.

Other dialectical strategies include using metaphor or playing the devil's advocate in order to prevent polarization. The therapist may call a patient's bluff or use extending; for example, when a client on an inpatient unit threatens suicide, the therapist might say, "Listen, this is really serious. We should go right now and make your room safe and get you into a suicide gown." Informed by dialectical philosophy, the therapist and treatment team assume that their case formulations are partial and therefore move to assess what is left out when there is an impasse (dialectical assessment). The therapist may view a discouraging event as an opportunity to practice distress tolerance (making lemonade out of lemons) or allow rather than prevent natural change (such as a group leader leaving and being replaced), knowing that this, too, is an opportunity to practice acceptance of reality as it is.

CONCLUSIONS

The essence of the dialectical perspective is that truth evolves. DBT offers the strongest empirically based approach for helping individuals with BPD whose severe and chronic problems create tremendous suffering. Although many aspects of its frame are likely to remain intact, the change and acceptance strategies, and in particular, the specific modes and functions of the treatment required to produce positive outcomes, are intended to become refined or replaced to integrate new scientific findings, so that DBT will evolve and continually incorporate new efficacious elements as they are developed.

REFERENCES

Ames-Frankel, J., Devlin, M. J., Walsh, T., Strasser, T. J., Sadik, C., Oldham, J. M., & Roose, S. P. (1992). Personality disorder diagnoses in patients with bulimia nervosa: Clinical correlates and changes with treatment. *Journal of Clinical Psychiatry, 53,* 90–96.

Baer, L., Jenike, M. A., Black, D. W., Treece, C., Rosenfeld, R., & Greist, J. (1992). Effect of Axis II diagnoses on treatment outcome with clomipramine in 55 patients with obsessive–compulsive disorder. *Archives of General Psychiatry, 49*, 862–866.

Bateman, A., & Fonagy, P. (1999). Effectiveness of partial hospitalization in the treatment of borderline personality disorder: A randomized controlled trial. *American Journal of Psychiatry, 156*, 1312–1321.

Bateman, A., & Fonagy, P. (2000). Treatment of borderline personality disorder with psychoanalytically oriented partial hospitalization: An 18-month follow-up *British Journal of Psychiatry, 177*, 107–111.

Behnke, S. H., & Saks, E. R. (1998). Therapeutic jurisprudence: Informed consent as a clinical indication for the chronically suicidal patient with borderline personality disorder. *Loyola Law Review, 31*, 945–982.

Bohus, M., Haaf, B., Stiglmayr, C., Pohl, U., Bohme, R., & Linehan, M. (2000). Evaluation of inpatient dialectical behavior therapy for borderline personality disorder—a prospective study. *Behaviour Research and Therapy, 38*, 875–887.

Cloitre, M. (1998). Sexual revictimization risk factors and prevention. In V. M. Follette, J. I. Ruzek, & F. R. Abueg (Eds.), *Cognitive-behavioral therapies for trauma* (pp. 278–304). New York: Guilford Press.

Coker, S., Vize, C., Wade, T., & Cooper, P. J. (1993). Patients with bulimia nervosa who fail to engage in cognitive behavior therapy. *International Journal of Eating Disorders, 13*, 35–40.

Cunningham, K., Wolbert, R., & Lillie, B. (in press). "It's about me solving my problems": Clients' assessments of dialectical behavior therapy. *Cognitive and Behavioral Practice*.

Fine, M. A., & Sansone, R. A. (1990). Dilemmas in the management of suicidal behavior in individuals with borderline personality disorder. *American Journal of Psychotherapy, 44*, 160–171.

Fruzzetti, A. E., & Levensky, E. R. (2000). Dialectical behavior therapy for domestic violence. Rationale and procedures. *Cognitive and Behavioral Practice, 7*, 435–447.

Heard, H. L. (2000). *Cost-effectiveness of DBT in the treatment of BPD*. Unpublished dissertation, University of Washington, Seattle.

Hellman, I. D., Morrison, T. L., & Abramowitz, S. I. (1986). The stresses of psychotherapeutic work: A replication and extension. *Journal of Clinical Psychology, 42*, 197–205.

Hoffman, P. D., Fruzzetti, A. E., & Swenson, C. R. (1999). Dialectical behavior therapy: Family skills training. *Family Process, 38*, 399–414.

Keane, T. M., Fisher, L. M., Krinsley, K. E., & Niles, B. L. (1994). Posttraumatic stress disorder. In M. Hersen & R. T. Ammerman (Eds.), *Handbook of prescriptive treatments for adults* (pp. 237–260). New York: Plenum Press.

Koerner, K., & Dimeff, L. A. (2000). Further research on dialectical behavior therapy. *Clinical Psychology Science and Practice, 7*, 104–112.

Koerner, K., & Linehan, M. M. (2000). Research on dialectical behavior therapy for borderline personality disorder. *Psychiatric Clinics of North America, 23*, 151–167.

Koons, C. R., Robins, C. J., Tweed, J. L., Lynch, T. R., Gonzalez, A. M., Morse, J. Q., Bishop, G. K., Butterfield, M. I., & Bastian, L. A. (2001). Efficacy of dialectical behavior therapy in women veterans with borderline personality disorder. *Behavior Therapy, 32*, 371–390.

Kosten, R. A., Kosten, T. R., & Rounsaville, B. J. (1989). Personality disorders in opiate addicts show prognostic specificity. *Journal of Substance Abuse and Treatment, 6*, 163–168.

Linehan, M. M. (1993a). *Cognitive-behavioral treatment of borderline personality disorder*. New York: Guilford Press.

Linehan, M. M. (1993b). *Skills training manual for treating borderline personality disorder*. New York: Guilford Press.

Linehan, M. M. (1997a). Behavioral treatments of suicidal behaviors: Definitional obfuscation and treatment outcomes. In D. M. Stoff & J. J. Mann (Eds.), *Neurobiology of suicide: From the bench to the clinic* (pp. 302–328). New York: Annals of the New York Academy of Sciences.

Linehan, M. M. (1997b). Self-verification and drug abusers: Implications for treatment. *Psychological Science, 8*, 181–183.

Linehan, M. M. (1997c). Validation and psychotherapy. In A. Bohart & L. Greenberg (Eds.),

Empathy reconsidered: New directions in psychotherapy (pp. 353–392). Washington, DC: American Psychological Association Press.

Linehan, M. M. (1999). Development, evaluation, and dissemination of effective psychosocial treatments: Levels of disorder, stages of care, and stages of treatment research. In M. G. Glantz & C. R. Hartel (Eds.), *Drug abuse: Origins and interventions* (pp. 367–394). Washington, DC: American Psychological Association.

Linehan, M. M. (2000a). Commentary on innovations in dialectical behavior therapy. *Cognitive and Behavioral Therapy, 7,* 478–481.

Linehan, M. M. (2000b). Behavioral treatments of suicidal behaviors: Definitional obfuscation and treatment outcomes. In R. W. Maris, S. S. Canetto, J. L. McIntosh, & M. M. Silverman (Eds.), *Review of suicidology 2000* (pp. 84–111). New York: Guilford Press.

Linehan, M. M. (2000c). The empirical basis of dialectical behavior therapy: Development of new treatments vs. evaluation of existing treatments. *Clinical Psychology: Science and Practice, 7,* 113–119.

Linehan, M. M., Armstrong, H. E., Suarez, A., Allmon, D., & Heard, H. L. (1991). Cognitive-behavioral treatment of chronically parasuicidal borderline patients. *Archives of General Psychiatry, 48,* 1060–1064.

Linehan, M. M., & Dimeff, L. A. (1997). *Dialectical behavior therapy manual of treatment interventions for drug abusers with borderline personality disorder.* Seattle: University of Washington Press.

Linehan, M. M., Dimeff, L. A., Reynolds, S. K., Comtois, K. A., Shaw-Welch, S., Heagerty, P., & Kivlahan, D. R. (in press). Dialectical behavior therapy versus comprehensive validation plus 12-step for the treatment of opioid dependent women meeting criteria for borderline personality disorder. *Drug and Alcohol Dependence.*

Linehan, M. M., & Heard, H. L. (1993). Impact of treatment accessibility on clinical course of parasuicidal patients: Reply. *Archives of General Psychiatry, 50,* 157–158.

Linehan, M. M., Heard, H. L., & Armstrong, H. E. (1993). Naturalistic follow up of a behavioral treatment for chronically parasuicidal borderline patients. *Archives of General Psychiatry, 50,* 971–974.

Linehan, M. M., Rizvi, S. L., Shaw Welch, S., & Page, B. (2000). Psychiatric aspects of suicidal behaviour: Personality disorders. In K. Hawton & K. van Heeringen (Eds.), *International handbook of suicide and attempted suicide* (pp. 147–178). Sussex, UK: Wiley.

Linehan, M. M., Schmidt, H., Dimeff, L. A., Craft, J. C., Kanter, J., & Comtois, K. A. (1999). Dialectical behavior therapy for patients with borderline personality disorder and drug-dependence. *American Journal on Addictions, 8,* 279–292.

Linehan, M. M., Tutek, D. A., Heard, H. L., & Armstrong, H. E. (1994). Interpersonal outcome of cognitive behavioral treatment for chronically suicidal borderline patients. *American Journal of Psychiatry, 151,* 1771–1776.

Lynch, T. R. (2000). Treatment of elderly depression with personality disorder comorbidity using dialectical behavior therapy. *Cognitive Behavioral Practice, 7,* 468–477.

McCann, R. A., Ball, E. M., & Ivanoff, A. (2000). DBT with an inpatient forensic population: The CMHIP forensic model. *Cognitive and Behavioral Practice, 7,* 447–456.

Melia, K., & Wagner, A. W. (2000). The application of dialectical behavior therapy to the treatment of posttraumatic stress disorder. *National Center for Posttraumatic Stress Disorder Clinical Quarterly, 9,* 6–12.

Mental Health Center of Greater Manchester, New Hampshire. (1998). Integrating dialectical behavioral therapy into a community mental health program. *Psychiatric Services, 49,* 1338–1340.

Najavits, L. M., Weiss, R. D., Shaw, S. R., & Muenz, L. R. (1998). "Seeking safety": Outcome of a new cognitive-behavioral psychotherapy for women with posttraumatic stress disorder and substance dependence. *Journal of Traumatic Stress, 11,* 437–456.

Phillips, K. A., & Nierenberg, A. A. (1994). The assessment and treatment of refractory depression. *Journal of Clinical Psychiatry, 55,* 20–26.

Rascati, J. N. (1990). Managed care and the discharge dilemma: Commentary. *Psychiatry, 53,* 124–126.

Rathus, J. H., & Miller, A. L. (in press). Dialectical behavior therapy adapted for suicidal adolescents: A pilot study. *Suicide and Life-Threatening Behavior*.

Rissmiller, D. J., Steer, R., Ranieri, W. F., Rissmiller, F., & Hogate, P. (1994). Factors complicating cost containment in the treatment of suicidal patients. *Hospital and Community Psychiatry, 45*, 782–788.

Safer, D. L., Telch, C. F., & Agras, W. S. (2001). Dialectical behavior therapy for bulimia nervosa. *American Journal of Psychiatry, 158*, 632–634.

Simpson, E. B., Pistorello, J., Begin, A., Costello, E., Levinson, J., Mulberry, S., Pearlstein, T., Rosen, K., & Stevens, M. (1998). Use of dialectical behavior therapy in a partial hospital program for women with borderline personality disorder. *Psychiatric Services, 49*, 669–673.

Stanley, B., Ivanoff, A., Brodsky, B., Oppenheim, S., & Mann, J. (1998). *Comparison of DBT and "treatment as usual" in suicidal and self-mutilating behavior*. Paper presented at the 32nd annual meeting of the Association for the Advancement of Behavior Therapy Convention, Washington, DC.

Swann, W. B. (1997). The trouble with change: Self-verification and allegiance to the self. *Psychological Science, 8*, 177–180.

Swenson, C. R. (2000). How can we account for DBT's widespread popularity? *Clinical Psychology Science and Practice, 7*, 87–91.

Swenson, C. R., Sanderson, C., Dulit, R. A., & Linehan, M. M. (2001). The application of dialectical behavior therapy for patients with borderline personality disorder on inpatient units. *Psychiatric Quarterly, 72*, 307–324.

Swigar, M. E., Astrachan, B. M., Levine, M. A., Mayfield, V., & Radovich, C. (1991). Single and repeated admissions to a mental health center. *International Journal of Social Psychiatry, 37*, 259–266.

Telch, C. F., Agras, W. S., & Linehan, M. M. (2000). Group dialectical behavior therapy for binge-eating disorder: A preliminary, uncontrolled trial. *Behavior Therapy, 31*, 569–582.

Trupin, E. W., Stewart, D. G., Beach, B., & Boesky, L. (in press). Effectiveness of a dialectical behavior therapy program for incarcerated female juvenile offenders. *Child and Adolescent Mental Health*.

Turner, R. M. (2000). Naturalistic evaluation of dialectical behavior therapy-oriented treatment for borderline personality disorder. *Cognitive and Behavioral Practice, 7*, 413–419.

Wagner, A. W., & Linehan, M. M. (1994). Relationship between childhood sexual abuse and topography of parasuicide among women with borderline personality disorder. *Journal of Personality Disorders, 8*, 1–9.

Zayfert, C., & Black, C. (2000). Implementation of empirically supported treatment for PTSD: Obstacles and innovations. *Behavior Therapist, 23*, 161–168.

17

Multiple Family Group Treatment for Borderline Personality Disorder

TERESA WHITEHURST
MARIA ELENA RIDOLFI
JOHN GUNDERSON

Recent shifts in mental health care services place the family in a more prominent role in the treatment of mentally ill patients. With managed care now more widespread, mentally ill persons' access to professional treaters has become strictly regulated by insurance companies. This has resulted in care that is less intensive, increasingly time-limited, and more reliant upon nonprofessionals and noninstitutional settings. Most chronically mentally ill patients must now receive services in community settings that turn to the family, often due to lack of other options, as the primary source of support.

The number of individuals meeting criteria for borderline personality disorder (BPD) is high, approximately 11% of psychiatric outpatients and 20% of psychiatric inpatients (Gunderson, 2001; Widiger & Frances, 1988). This disorder is also chronic; between 57% and 67% of patients continue to meet criteria 4–7 years after the first diagnosis, and up to 44% continue to meet criteria 15 years later. Women borderlines outnumber men by 3 or more to 1 among hospitalized patients (Gunderson, 1984). BPD is more commonly diagnosed among adolescents and young adults than other age groups (McGlashan, 1987). Approximately 10% of patients with BPD die by suicide, but the suicide rate becomes significantly higher among borderline individuals who have attempted suicide or otherwise injured themselves at least once in the past. A number of studies suggest that BPD is linked to impulse or action disorders such as antisocial personality and substance abuse disorders. Two studies found that 13% of hospitalized substance abusers were also diagnosed with BPD (Inman, Bascue, & Skoloda, 1985). The connection between BPD and other impulse disorders suggests an underlying and familial difficulty with impulse control (Ruiz-Sancho & Gunderson, 1997).

Despite the magnitude of the clinical problem represented by patients with BPD, development and research of model programs for the treatment of this disorder are lagging. It is against this backdrop that our multiple family group (MFG) program for families of patients diagnosed with BPD has been developed.

Though only a modest number of medication trials have been conducted, they have largely confirmed the clinical tradition that such treatments have adjunctive and usually modest effects with this population (Soloff, 1993). Less work still has been done on psychosocial modalities (e.g., individual, group, and family psychotherapies, and rehabilitative or milieu therapies. Dialectical behavior therapy, a highly structured, manualized cognitive-behavioral treatment of BPD developed by Marsha Linehan (see Koerner & Linehan, Chapter 16, this volume) is the most significant exception. The effectiveness of this treatment has been demonstrated in a controlled outcome study (Linehan, 1993; Linehan, Armstrong, Suarez, Allmon, & Heard, 1991). Though other research has demonstrated the value of day treatment, interpersonal groups, and psychoanalytic psychotherapies (see Gunderson, 2001), dialectical behavior therapy stands alone as an empirically validated, BPD-relevant psychosocial treatment that has made a significant impact on health care. The need remains for the development of new psychosocial treatments of BPD that can address other aspects of dysfunction and be implemented in a variety of public health care settings.

The current model combines a psychoeducational approach with the format of a MFG. We propose our model in the context of the proliferation of support groups run by mental health care consumers and their families. Such groups, including Alcoholics Anonymous, National Alliance for the Mentally Ill, and the Manic–Depressive and Depressive Association are increasingly popular and clinically effective in improving the course of severe and chronic mental illness. The factors that make them effective may also account for the success of MFGs in the management of mental illness.

The MFG program at McLean Hospital is a structured treatment that contains elements shown to be highly effective tools for achieving change for families with other types of severe chronic psychiatric illnesses. The first of these elements is psychoeducation, an effective treatment for families of patients with schizophrenia. The psychoeducational approach uses didactic lessons to inform families of people with BPD about the nature of the illness, and teaches skills for reducing stresses that affect the course of the illness. The second essential element is the MFG format, which functions to expand the family's social network, reduce the sense of stigma associated with mental illness, and improve the quality of communication in the family (McFarlane, 1990). The treatment reported here has used these elements and made them disorder-relevant (i.e., addresses the handicaps specific to BPD, as well as the factors in the family environment that can affect the course of BPD).

It is expected that such an approach will have value for families of people with BPD given the recurrent clinical observation that the most serious and dangerous behaviors marking this disorder—suicide attempts, self-mutilation, and rage reactions—often occur in response to interactions with the family. By becoming more aware of the patient's sensitivities, parents can develop skills for identifying and addressing the BPD offspring's emotional reactions more effectively. In this process, parents may learn to protect their offspring from stresses that they are unable to tolerate, and may thereby reduce patients' experience of repeated crises and allow for progress toward improved psychosocial functioning.

In order to be replicable and relevant in a variety of treatment settings, a treatment for BPD must fulfill four key requirements. Such a treatment must be (1) teachable and effective in the hands of therapists from diverse training backgrounds, (2) sufficiently structured and well-described to achieve relatively consistent effectiveness, (3) disorder-relevant and geared toward the management of problems that are unique to BPD, and (4) capable of delivering its benefits at less expense than alternative treatments. Our MFG program has been designed to meet these requirements for clinicians working in a variety of settings.

FAMILY-RELEVANT FACTORS IN THE DEVELOPMENT AND MAINTENANCE OF BORDERLINE PERSONALITY DISORDER

Early efforts to understand the etiology of BPD and the factors that maintain it were focused on the theory that pathological forms of parental overinvolvement foster the borderline offspring's dependence and abandonment fears (Shapiro, 1978, 1982; Zinner & Shapiro, 1975). Masterson and Rinsley (1975) considered borderline psychopathology resistant to correction unless changes were made in the person's primary social milieu, which for many patients is the family. As a result of such observations, clinicians undertook family therapies based on identifying conflicts and encouraging the expression of feelings. While it provided a powerful approach that could sometimes prove very useful, most families avoided it because of its focus on intrafamily conflict and a confrontational, authoritarian style. It was especially unsuitable for families that were fragmented, nonverbal, or had minimal interactions with their borderline offspring.

Empirical studies, however, soon made it evident that the overinvolved and separation-resistant families described by Masterson were not the norm; such families were found to represent a minority, perhaps 25% (Gunderson, Kerr, & Englund, 1980). Patients with BPD tend to have family histories in which parents are insufficiently involved (Frank & Paris, 1981; Gunderson et al., 1980; Gunderson & Zanarini, 1989; Links, Steiner, & Huxley, 1988; Soloff & Millward, 1983; Zanarini, 1997) and are either perpetrators or unavailable to help the patient process and recover from traumatic experiences (Gunderson & Sabo, 1993; Links et al., 1990; Links & van Reekum, 1993; Millon, 1987; Paris & Zweig-Frank, 1992).

Other studies suggest that parents of patients with BPD often had serious psychiatric problems themselves, including substance abuse, depression, and BPD (Akiskal et al., 1985; Goldman, D'Angelo, & Demaso, 1993; Links et al., 1988; Loranger, Oldham, & Tulis, 1982; Loranger & Tulis, 1983; Pope, Jonas, & Hudson, 1983; Soloff & Millward, 1983; Zanarini, Gunderson, & Frankenburg, 1990). This bleak and very critical picture of these patients' families discouraged clinicians from involving them in treatment, which was reflected in the virtual absence of any new papers about family therapies during the 1980s or 1990s.

BACKGROUND FOR A PSYCHOEDUCATIONAL APPROACH TO FAMILIES

The emergence during the last decade of a deficit model for BPD to replace the earlier conflict model has encouraged a different approach to families. When the patient is seen as suffering from deficits, expectations are lowered; education about these deficits and how the environment needs to accommodate them becomes available to families. This change in the borderline construct made the research on treating families with a schizophrenic offspring—a better recognized deficit disorder—very relevant to BPD. The psychoeducational treatments were designed to teach families to recognize the signs of schizophrenia as symptoms of an illness, beyond the control of the patient, and also called upon families to create a "designer environment" adapted to the unique needs of the patient with schizophrenia. Emphasis upon the illness model to explain symptomatic behavior provided families with a rationale for changing their responses to the patient with schizophrenia, just as the handicap model provides the rationale for change in the current treatment. Those treatments have consistently lowered the relapse rate of schizophrenia in multiple outcome studies performed with families from a variety of socioeconomic backgrounds (Leff, 1992; McFarlane & Dunne, 1991). The psychoeducational approach for families has had a more powerful effect upon relapse rates than that observed from medications (with which it is synergistic) and surpasses the benefits of other types of psychosocial interventions with schizophrenic and other diagnostic groups (Gabbard et al., 1997).

Before the psychoeducational therapy for schizophrenia was developed, this research had shown that individuals with schizophrenia from families high in expressed emotion (EE)—meaning hostile, critical, and overinvolved—had higher relapse rates than low-EE families (50% vs. 14%), that a psychoeducational approach could reduce EE (the putative stressor), and that this thereby reduced relapse rates (Goldstein, 1990; Leff, 1989; McFarlane, 1990; McFarlane, Link, Dushay, Marchal, & Crilly, 1995). Research using the EE construct has now been initiated for families with a member with BPD. In one of these studies, Hooley and Hofmann (1999) found the surprising result that patients with BPD suffered relapses (i.e., rehospitalizations) more often when they experienced parental underinvolvement, and that relapses were not associated with high levels of criticism and hostility. Thus, with patients with BPD, the stage has been set to use a psychoeducational approach, with different targets than for other diagnostic groups.

While the most feasible format for most practitioners involves individual families, McFarlane has demonstrated advantages of MFGs with families having a member with schizophrenia (McFarlane, 1990; McFarlane et al., 1995). The combination of the psychoeducation and MFG modalities led to a remarkably low relapse rate of 12.5% after 1 year. In a literature review, Fristad, Gavazzi, Centolella, and Soldano (1996) suggested that this modality reduces relapse rates, thereby lowering costs and improving quality of life for adults with schizophrenia and major mood disorders. This research was confirmed by our experience; MFGs involving patients with BPD also appeared to enhance consumer satisfaction, while doubtlessly being cost-effective.

TARGETS FOR FAMILY INTERVENTION

Although the strengths and weaknesses of families of patients with BPD vary, they tend to have in common a "translation" problem, in that (1) the individual with BPD has difficulty communicating clearly his or her emotional state to family and peers, (2) family members fail to hear and/or acknowledge his or her underlying emotional messages, and (3) conversations within the family tend to have an emotional intensity that the patient (and often the family) finds overwhelming.

Individuals with BPD have difficulty expressing their more vulnerable or "unacceptable" feelings in words, relying instead on dramatic acting-out behaviors to signal their distress. It is understandable, then, that communication between parents and their offspring with BPD are fraught with faulty or inadequate signals. An earlier study from McLean Hospital showed that parents of teens with BPD were less aware of their child's feelings and self-image than were parents in a comparison group composed of families with teens having other personality disorders (Young & Gunderson, 1995). For example, whereas in the patient with BPD, suicidality and self-injurious behaviors may signal a desperate need for care and attention, the parents may focus only on the dangerousness to their child. This suggests that the alienation associated with the patients' inability to "get through" to their parents may be a significant risk factor for relapse. Hence, parents' increased insight and acknowledgment of interpersonal needs may diminish the sense of alienation in their children, thus decreasing the recurrence of crises.

In our work with families of patients with BPD, we have observed a tendency for other family members, particularly parents, to gloss over, dismiss, or try to "fix" their borderline member's expressions of negative feelings. This often springs from their fear of making matters worse (i.e., that being supportive when the patient is expressing hopeless or suicidal feelings might "open a can of worms"). When patients' negative feelings are cut short or passed over, however, feelings of insecurity and fear of abandonment are triggered. Family members, particularly parents, must become aware of this dynamic in order to avoid the common traps of "fixing" or ignoring bad feelings in the hope that they will disappear.

GOALS OF TREATMENT

The purpose of the MFG treatment program is to ameliorate factors in the family environment that increase the risk of relapse in the patient with BPD. By "relapse," we refer to the recurrence of self-endangering crises, diminished functioning in school or work, and violence or other behaviors that require intensified psychiatric treatment. MFGs also reduce the sense of stigma and isolation in the family and allow members to benefit from one another's experience. The atmosphere of mutual support makes the intervention and the task of changing more palatable for families that may be reluctant to accept intervention. The previous success of MFGs and peer support groups provides a positive precedent for the use of MFGs in this treatment.

Because many families have participated in therapies for the sake of their child with BPD that were ineffective or unpleasant, clinicians should underscore the novelty of the current treatment. In every encounter with families, the clinician should keep in mind the three primary goals of the MFG:

1. *Educate families about BPD.* Despite often extensive contacts with mental health professionals in the past, many families do not have a solid understanding of the nature, treatment, or course of BPD. Education of families serves to enlighten and reassure them, because they come in with no working model of this disorder and are understandably anxious due to what they perceive as a mysterious and chaotic disorder.

2. *Teach families needed skills.* Family members are provided with guidelines that follow logically from an intellectual understanding of this diagnosis. The problem-solving sessions focus on teaching skills for applying the guidelines to everyday problems. This family-empowering methodology differs from the traditional clinician's role of offering advice for specific problems as they are brought to his or her attention.

3. *Develop a working alliance.* In speaking about this disorder with families, clinicians emphasize the conception of BPD as a disorder with clear deficits requiring new expectations more in line with what the patient is capable of doing, and a family environment that is altered such that those deficits are tapped as rarely as possible. The clinician

should explain that the course of this disorder can be modified by adapting the family environment to the handicaps of the patient. By avoiding a blaming or interpretive stance that would alienate family members, the clinician can become a trustworthy source of support and information for the family.

OVERALL STRUCTURE OF MULTIPLE FAMILY GROUP TREATMENT

Confidentiality

Confidentiality remains an important issue for all concerned. Patients should be told that the MFG leaders are working as members of the patient's treatment team; hence, issues of safety and family dynamics will be discussed with the patient's individual therapist or case manager. Openly stating this condition at the outset will prevent patients and families from splitting staff members by selectively revealing information to different parties. Personal information that is not relevant to safety issues and family functioning is to be treated with the confidentially observed in individual psychotherapy.

Three Phases of Treatment

Treatment occurs in three phases: (1) joining, (2) the didactics prerequisite, and (3) the psychoeducational MFG. Phase I is focused on history taking, problem identification, and calming the family's anxieties while establishing an alliance. Phase II is a 4-week, intensive didactics course designed to provide families immediately with a core of the most essential information they need to better care for and interact with their child, before geographical moves, work schedule changes, or other life changes may result in attrition. Phase III, the MFG itself, involves repetition and practice of material already learned, along with ongoing problem solving, communication, and other special interest topics. This important aspect of the MFG continues for as long as the family attends, but its value is equaled or even overshadowed by the tremendous emotional support the family receives from other families who understand.

Phase III is more directly therapeutic in that the goals therein have to do with ongoing psychological and behavioral changes in family members. The didactic portion of the MFG is presented during the first hour of the 2-hour group. While special topics may be presented (e.g., substance abuse and BPD, handling holidays and vacations, the role of dialectical behavior therapy in the patient's treatment), we have three primary modules that are taught and practiced regularly: problem solving, communication skills, and mirroring.

Information thus presented may be "recycled" in the first hour of other 2-hour sessions throughout the year. This recycling helps families to overlearn the material, so that they can benefit from another MFG activity: active learning and practice, such as role-play and empty-chair techniques. These active, participatory sessions make the new behaviors and thinking patterns more accessible and natural *in vivo*.

Due to the ongoing demand, and because delaying a family's entry often results in disengagement (the family being most interested in getting involved during a crisis), we have changed our previous protocol. Initially, the MFG service was a research program that families could join only after attending a daylong Saturday workshop. These workshops were offered twice yearly and featured a range of professional and lay speakers. As a clinical program with the aim of meeting the needs of families, the MFG is, within limits, now open to new members throughout the year. These limits are (1) completing the joining sessions and 4-week didactics prerequisite, and (2) maintaining group size.

The bimonthly MFG groups are not time-limited, and we have recently added a monthly Saturday workshop to the MFG schedule that features presentations by clinicians with expertise regarding issues (e.g., substance abuse, eating disorders) and treatments (e.g., psychopharmacology, dialectical behavior therapy, group therapies) of interest to families of patients with BPD. The Saturday workshops are open to families unable to attend during the week and to weekday MFG members as an "add-on" educational experience. We encourage as many members of the extended family to attend as possible, for as long as possible, while the patient is receiving treatment. The average time that a family regularly attends this phase is now 12 to 18 months, although many return from time to time after they have terminated, as the need arises. Some return for only a few "booster sessions" at a time, while others rejoin the group on a regular basis.

PHASE I: JOINING

Joining is an individualized family process. The didactics sessions, while preferably containing two or more families, may be held with individual families, if others are not available. When a family drops out due to long-standing improvement or other factors, another family may be carefully introduced into the group. We have found that giving advance notice to the group facilitates this process, and the check-in segment of the first integrated group will necessarily be longer to accommodate telling the new family's story. Families who have been chosen as candidates for this treatment are first invited to attend two or three joining sessions with one of the group leaders. The leader meets with one family at a time, without the patient present. The joining phase serves multiple functions that are central to the success of the treatment.

Joining provides an opportunity to explain the psychoeducational MFG treatment and to clarify how it differs from therapies that families may have tried in the past. This helps families who have been disappointed by failure or negative experiences in previous family treatments. Families should be told that the groups will enable them to function as members of the treatment team by coaching them on methods of creating a customized family environment to meet the needs of their children. In doing so, the families learn about the nature of the alliance and their role in the treatment. Family members who believe that their actions can influence the course of the illness are usually interested in joining the treatment. The following dialogue between the clinician and the fictional Smith family is an example of a conversation during the joining phase.

CLINICIAN: I'm glad you'll be joining our MFG. It's unlike traditional family therapy because there are other families in the room, all of whom are there for the same reasons you are: to learn how to help your family member with BPD, to recognize "triggers" that lead him or her to act out, and to give and receive other family members' support.

MR. SMITH: I certainly hope it's different, because we've gone the family therapy route and it didn't change a thing. Plus I didn't like being a dumping ground for all Sandy's complaints about her life.

MRS. SMITH: Well, I think it did help us to understand her better.

CLINICIAN: I think you'll find the MFG a very different experience. You'll be learning about BPD, listening to other family members' experiences, and developing new strategies for communicating with Sandy. The emphasis will be on getting the support you need, not on accusations or blame.

MR. SMITH: Well, that's a good thing, because I know we weren't perfect parents, but we weren't terrible either. I want to help her, but the "blame game" gets us nowhere.

CLINICIAN: Exactly. You'll find that many family members have come to the same conclusion. In the group, our emphasis will be on what family members can do *today* to help themselves and their relatives with BPD.

MRS. SMITH: I think this is what we need, because, to tell you the truth, I don't know why Sandy gets so enraged at us. Usually it blindsides us, and we have no idea what we could have done differently. At other times, her sudden crying spells worry us terribly, but nothing we say to her seems to help.

CLINICIAN: You've hit on an important point: There's a lot that you can do to help Sandy and your family in relation to her, and this is what you'll learn in the MFG. Nobody can do the work for her—people with BPD are ultimately responsible for their own growth—but you, as family members, can contribute greatly to her progress by tailoring your family environment to her special needs.

MR. SMITH: You mean we have to bend over backwards for her? Because we already stifle what we'd really like to say to avoid getting her upset.

CLINICIAN: What I mean by a tailored environment is more like installing a ramp when someone in your family has to use a wheelchair: By making sensible adjustments to the home, you avoid accidents and help the wheelchair-bound person become more independent. Family members of people with BPD can learn how to make certain key adjustments to make crises less likely and encourage a higher level of functioning.

Because some family members—in common with the patient with BPD—have a high degree of interpersonal sensitivity, a sense of connection with one of the group leaders is very important. As families develop an affective alliance, the group becomes less threatening to them, and this may help them to stay in the group even if initially they do not feel adequately supported. Our experience has been that sensitive family members may drop out of the group due to feeling uncomfortable sharing personal experiences, and the joining sessions can do a lot to prevent this cause of premature termination.

Engaging the Underinvolved Family

When the family has been underinvolved, the initial joining sessions are particularly important. The supportive and educational approach with the family eases wariness and encourages development of an alliance. We have observed that some families have lessened their degree of involvement after becoming discouraged and exhausted by recurrent crises, often over a period of years during which the borderline pathology was not recognized or addressed. Other families avoid initiating contact with their offspring with BPD because they worry that such contact will exacerbate his or her dependence on them. Either way, the patient is usually not improving to any significant degree. This, we think, can be a product of the family's underinvolvement, which repeatedly triggers in the patient feelings of abandonment and disconnection, often leading to desperate searches for reparenting by others, self-destructive behaviors, and rehospitalizations. Clinicians can help family members begin to recognize this pattern by making reflective statements:

- "So your son seemed to be just fine on his own until the suicide attempt?"
- "It sounds like you respond when Jennifer calls you in a crisis, but you try not to call her because, whenever you do, you hear her vulnerability and she seems to really need you. Is that right?"
- "If I understand you correctly, your daughter's crises seem to 'come out of nowhere.' Yet, between hospitalizations, you try to 'leave well enough alone,' because every conversation seems to end with tears or anger. Is this the 'roller coaster' you referred to?"

Reflecting back statements that reveal underinvolvement is often sufficient to help family members recognize the problems inherent in this strategy. Initial joining sessions and the MFG can help structure more predictable, manageable, and non-crisis-oriented contact.

Responding to Exclusion of Family by Offspring with Borderline Personality Disorder

Sometimes the patient is extremely angry at the parents, to the point of forbidding them to speak to his or her clinician and/or of cutting off all contact with the family. This situation may occur when parents have not acknowledged prior abusive behaviors or traumatic experiences. Such parents are more likely to drop out of the family group than others, because of overwhelming feelings of anger, regret, or shame. Our approach is to view them with the same compassion with which we view the patient, in recognition of the tendency for abusive or neglectful behavior to have been passed down intergenerationally. Parents and patient need help in accepting responsibility for their roles in the present relationship, despite the urge to blame one another for their difficulties (Mitton & Links, 1996).

We have observed that those parents who have been participating for 6 months or longer are especially effective in helping other parents express remorse regarding past mistakes. This can be an especially powerful antidote to the patient's sense of being misunderstood and disconnected from the family. When this occurs, even those patients who have been hostile to their parents and suspicious of their involvement in the MFG become grateful for and supportive of their family's involvement.

Various methods of recruiting participants have been used. Most effective is to refer family members to the MFG when they are seeking help, usually during a crisis. The clinicians responsible for the patient's care are especially important here in terms of encouraging the family to get involved. One caveat, however, is that some patients will resist the involvement of their family in this treatment. We have found it helpful to tell the patient that this program can "teach your parent (or others) about your problems, so that they can be more helpful in the future." In the end, however, that patient's endorsement is not required for the family to join this treatment.

History Taking

In order to recruit the patient's family members into active work for his or her benefit and as allies of the treatment team, we begin by listening carefully to the family's concerns. Often, due to the accumulation of frustration, worry, and failed attempts to help the patient, family members have a desperate need to vent feelings to a caring professional whose role is not laden with the anxieties that families, especially parents, may feel regarding the family or individual therapist.

It is wise during the initial two to four sessions of this phase to listen attentively and take notes, even if the clinician already has the history in hand. Family members, especially parents, have a need to describe developmental milestones, early suspicions that something was wrong, and recent disturbing symptomatology. This often helps the clinician begin to formulate a working model of this family, providing information about important incidents relating to the patient, as well as the family's overall emotional tone now and during the patient's developmental years.

Family members also need to communicate their confusion about what is happening now, contrasting this with what they used to see. Parents often emphasize how bright, capable, even "perfect" the child was in earlier years. They need a mental health professional to hear and believe the positive qualities that they remember in their child, because the current focus is so heavily upon problems and deficits.

Listening and empathizing with this historical storytelling is vital for the establishment of an enduring alliance and to elicit the family's commitment to participation in the family groups. In particular, expressing one's understanding of and empathy with the painful sense of "mystification"—the inability to make sense of current events in light of past events—leads not only to more rapid trust and engagement but also begins the process of calming fears and restoring hope.

Problem Identification

As family members begin to wind down, having shared most of what they feel is important for the clinician to know about their loved one with BPD, the clinician should begin the task of listing and categorizing the primary problems that the family is having with the patient. Helping the family shift from expressing emotions and concerns about the patient's psychological state to refocusing on the issues having to do with the family–patient interface often requires considerable clinical skill. The clinician becomes more active at this point in the joining process, gently guiding the family away from questions and fears about the patient's psyche, toward those problems that directly involve the family in some way. This can be difficult. Often the family will press for answers and certainty with regard to the patient's treatment needs and prognosis. Gradually, the clinician should emphasize "what we can do," which is to learn how best to respond to the family member with BPD.

Categorizing problems can be very helpful for families in need of a sense of order. Sifting through worries about the patient's self-esteem, career or marriage potential, likelihood of suicide, and so on, the clinician refocuses the conversation onto problems that the disorder has created for the family. In an initial study of 40 families (Gunderson & Lyoo, 1996), the most common categories of problems were (in order): (1) communication, (2) dealing with hostile or rageful reactions, and (3) fears about suicide. The clinician can then summarize the family's primary problems due to the disorder and offer assurances that the burden created by these and similar problems are familiar to mental health staff and can be significantly reduced to everyone's benefit.

We begin by familiarizing the family with the criteria for BPD, making sure that they are understood. We then evaluate, with the family, how these criteria apply or are observed in the behavior of the relative with BPD. Central to this educational process is emphasizing that patients have deficits—handicaps that can, albeit slowly, be overcome. While some patients and family members will not want to hear the "slow" aspect of this, others find it comforting to know there is no short-term solution. Too often, they have been unrealistically optimistic, resulting in profound disillusionment.

PARENT: I thought Eric was getting the best treatment possible, but now I hear you saying that his progress will take a long time. This isn't what we wanted to hear.

CLINICIAN: No matter how effective the treatment, individuals with BPD do not improve overnight. They have a serious disorder that affects almost every aspect of their lives and has interfered with their functioning and stability for years. Improvement takes time. Family members can often improve the rate of improvement by learning all they can about BPD in general and their relative with BPD in particular, then adapting their interactions to avoid "stepping on" his or her weak areas.

PARENT; I know you're right. I mean, it's obvious that he's got serious problems. It's just that we keep hoping and thinking he'll grow out of this phase soon and get on with his life.

CLINICIAN: The MFG may be very helpful to you in this regard. Most family members have at one time or another assumed that the disturbing symptoms and behaviors were just part of a passing phase. When it doesn't pass, they're very disappointed and don't know where to go from there. Once families accept that improvement will take time, they feel less pressured to "fix the problem." Individuals with BPD feel less pressured, and less a source of disappointment, when their families stop expecting immediate improvement.

During the joining sessions, families should be provided with a copy of the 14 coping guidelines (see Table 17.1). We encourage family members to post these on the refrigerator door or keep them in a wallet or purse for easy reference. Encouraging relatives to read or view educational materials is a good segue to the next visit, because it heralds a shift in orientation toward didactics and active work by clinician and family.

Readiness for Didactics Course

When the joining sessions in the phase of alliance building have been completed, family members are "ready" for the MFG (i.e., they are ready to try to change). Readiness for involvement in the family group is noted by three factors: (1) accepting the borderline diagnosis, or at least the possibility that some or all of the criteria "fit"; (2) reconciling to the long-term course of this disorder; and (3) wanting help in the ways that they relate to the patient. At this point, they are ready for interventions designed to help them improve their communication with the patient.

PHASE II: PREREQUISITE DIDACTICS

The second phase of treatment is more strictly didactic, although always supportive. The families are provided with educational presentations and materials, and become actively engaged in jointly determining learning goals. Family members self-administer checklists or quizzes that function as ongoing assessments of how well they understand the information presented. The material is presented multimodally (e.g., verbally, in written form,

TABLE 17.1. Family Guidelines

Goals: Go slowly

1. Remember that change is difficult to achieve and fraught with fears. Be cautious about suggesting that "great" progress has been made or giving "You can do it" reassurances. "Progress" evokes fears of abandonment.
2. Lower your expectations. Set realistic goals that are attainable. Solve big problems in small steps. Work on one thing at a time. "Big" or long-term goals lead to discouragement and failure.

Family environment: Keep things cool

3. Keep things cool and calm. Appreciation is normal. Tone it down. Disagreement is normal. Tone it down, too.
4. Maintain family routines as much as possible. Stay in touch with family and friends. There's more to life than problems, so don't give up the good times.
5. Find time to talk. Chats about light or neutral matters are helpful. Schedule times for this, if necessary.

Managing crises: Pay attention but stay calm

6. Don't get defensive in the face of accusations and criticisms. However unfair, say little and don't fight. Allow yourself to be hurt. Admit to whatever is true in the criticisms.
7. Self-destructive acts or threats require attention. Don't ignore them. Don't panic. It's good to know. Do not keep secrets about this. Talk openly with your family member and make sure professionals know about it.
8. Listen. People need to have their negative feelings heard. Don't say "It isn't so." Don't try to make the feelings go away. Using words to express fear, loneliness, inadequacy, anger, or needs is good. It's better to use words than to act out on feelings.

Addressing problems: Collaborate and be consistent

9. When solving a family member's problems, *always*:
    a. Involve the family member in identifying what needs to be done.
    b. Ask whether the person can "do" what's needed in the solution.
    c. Ask the person whether he or she wants you to help "do" what's needed.
10. Family members need to act in concert with one another. Parental inconsistencies fuel severe family conflicts. Develop strategies that everyone can stick to.
11. If you have concerns about medications or therapist interventions, make sure that both your family member and his or her therapist/doctor know. If you have financial responsibility, you have the right to address your concerns to the therapist or doctor.

Limit setting: Be direct but careful

12. Set limits by stating the limits of your tolerance. Let your expectations be known in clear, simple language. Everyone needs to know what is expected of them.
13. Do not protect family members from the natural consequences of their actions. Allow them to learn from reality. Bumping into a few walls is usually necessary.
14. Do not tolerate abusive treatment such as tantrums, threats, hitting, and spitting. Walk away and return to discuss the issue later. Be cautious about using threats and ultimatums. They are a last resort. Do not use threats and ultimatums as a means of convincing others to change. Only give them when you can and will carry through. Let others—including professionals—help you decide when to give them.

---

metaphorically [object lessons], and visually [imagery]). This multimodal teaching method is especially helpful for those parents who, due to differences in either their own learning styles and/or overwhelming anxiety regarding ongoing crises, have difficulty understanding lectures or densely written material.

Throughout the four sessions, the clinician encourages family members to express feelings and concerns, and to offer feedback to others. Also emphasized is the clinician's belief that the family is now becoming an important part of the treatment team. The family is thereby provided with a greater sense of control and safety, and many parents find relief from the profound sense of self-blame with which they struggle.

Required Attendance

Once their child with BPD is no longer in crisis, some fathers drop out of the MFG, while their wives continue to participate. Both parents, however, attend the early joining sessions, perhaps due to the gravity of the current crisis. We discovered that another factor allowing both to attend the joining sessions is flexibility: These sessions are set according to both parents' work schedules. For this reason, we have made the 4-week didactics course available to single families, with flexible scheduling, if they cannot meet at the same time as other families who are ready to begin this phase. Making this allowance has enabled us to ask, during the joining sessions, for a commitment from both husband and wife (we also invite other members of the family) to attend all four meetings. We strongly encourage their joint attendance at the subsequent twice-monthly MFG, pointing out the variety of group times available on weekday evenings, as well as Saturdays, to encourage husbands and wives to participate together.

Anecdotally, we have observed faster and more significant improvement in the functioning of offspring with BPD when both parents have attended the MFG, including one case wherein the divorced and remarried parents attended, accompanied by the stepparents. This takes enormous courage and dedication on the part of the parents, and we are quick to praise them for their participation in a context that naturally involves a degree of tension.

Avoiding the "Good Parent" Role

Throughout the MFG treatment, but especially early in the process, it is essential to convey the message that family members are an important ally, not people whose relative's problems confirm their badness or imply poor parenting. Likewise, the clinician should avoid the common trap of unwittingly presenting him- or herself as one who could have easily avoided these problems. Such an attitude is quickly sensed by the family, who may disengage if the clinician presents as the "good parent," with the family thus relegated to the "bad parent" role. Clinicians should take care to avoid any stance that suggests they are potential rivals for the patient's loyalties.

PHASE III: THE PSYCHOEDUCATIONAL MULTIPLE FAMILY GROUP

The 2-hour meetings of this phase that occur after the didactics portion is completed are changed from weekly to twice monthly. Five to seven families are ideal. More does not allow adequate attention for everyone, and less than five families diminishes the diversity of feedback. The first hour involves either practice of material already learned, or a new or recycled topic (didactic module).

The second hour is devoted to check-ins with the families, problem solving, feedback, and support. The therapist functions more as a teacher or leader than as a transference object. Supporting the most distressed family members, encouraging more adequate family boundaries, and helping parents to set limits and minimize miscommunication are all important therapeutic subgoals in the service of reducing the emotional intensity that patients with BPD find overwhelming, and that families find stressful and exhausting.

The multiple family format encourages pattern recognition. A basic human process for handling novelty is the analysis of experiences, so that a pattern can be detected. Once this is accomplished, the individual can effectively cope with what was previously unmanageable chaos. Pattern recognition helps not only to reduce the feelings of stigmatization and isolation that plague families prior to engagement in the group but it also reinforces learning. For example, when a parent hears that other families have observed a behavior pattern in their children with BPD similar to what he or she has observed in his or her own child, a feeling of relief ("My child isn't the only one who locks herself in her room and won't communicate") and greater understanding ("Looking back, I think that my daughter isolates in her room prior to separations, too"). Parents thus becomes more alert to their child's self-destructive patterns and better understand how and why they begin. This enables them to recognize signs of impending trouble, so that destructive acting-out or crises can be prevented.

To encourage socializing and lighter topics at the start and close of every MFG meeting keeps the group informal and reinforces the notion that there is more to life than problems. It is important to ask families about vacation plans or hobbies from time to time, so that they "remember" that they have many pleasures as well as problems. Many family members struggle, particularly in the beginning of their group involvement, with the assumption that as long as their family member is miserable, they should be also.

We encourage the opposite perspective: When family members are empowered with greater insight and skills that are helpful to the patient with BPD, their positive impact will be much greater if they themselves are not exhausted, stressed, or entirely focused on difficulties. Moreover, when clinicians share some of their personal interests, vacation plans, and foibles, this reinforces the idea that the families are being taught, helped and supported, and looked upon as health care consumers and collaborators in a joint venture, not as patients.

Didactic Modules

Problem-Solving Module

In this module, families learn how to solve problems and negotiate conflicts with their family member with BPD. Families first have a go-round in which each lists a discrete problem for which a solution is needed. We encourage families to come up with specific problems rather than general issues. For example, rather than discuss how available families should be for their member with BPD, families are encouraged to limit themselves to specific problems, such as whether they should answer repeated phone calls late at night. The problems are listed on an erasable board that all can see, and the families decide upon one to discuss as a group. This discussion leads to a beneficial process. The leaders take a careful history of the family's situation, thus demonstrating to the group what information is most relevant to the management of the problem.

The group is then asked to brainstorm some possible solutions to this family's problem. No criticism of ideas is allowed at this stage, and even implausible or humorous solutions are written on the board. Also forbidden at this stage is any discussion of the pros and cons of ideas. The group leader explicitly instructs family members in the brainstorming, keeping in mind that many people are unfamiliar with the technique:

- "While we're brainstorming possible solutions, 'the sky's the limit.' All ideas are welcome, no matter how outlandish."
- "Remember, during brainstorming, no criticisms of ideas are allowed."
- "We'll discuss the pros and cons of each idea after we finish brainstorming."
- "I'll write down your ideas as you give them to me, then we'll discuss each."
- "The goal is to become accustomed to coming up with a wide array of possible solutions to problems or conflicts with your child."
- "Nobody has any ideas yet? While you're thinking, I'll get us started with one of my own."

Leaders should be careful here to avoid falling into the advice-giving role. The aim is to get family members involved in generating many possible solutions to the problem.

Next, the pros and cons of each solution are discussed. The leader duly records on the board all advantages and disadvantages offered by family members. The leader is especially alert to any signs that the coping guidelines are being used, or could be brought into the discussion, and takes any opportunity to praise family members:

- "Did anyone notice that Sarah's idea corresponded to guideline 4?"
- "Jim's suggestion goes right along with the guideline about keeping a 'cool' family environment."
- "Great idea! Does anyone know which guideline Cathy's idea supports?"

No criticism of family members' ideas, however outlandish, should be made and, as always in the MFG, interpretation is never offered. Families of the mentally ill are highly sensitive to criticism and may feel more hurt than benefited by such comments. Interpretations are often also unwelcome and can encourage the family's expectation that others have the answers. Over time, as family members experience more problem-solving sessions and are influenced by the models of other group members, as well as positive reinforcement, they usually change unhelpful attitudes.

Finally, the family whose problem is being solved is asked to select a solution that family members prefer to implement. At this point, remaining questions about who will do what are addressed, especially with respect to the words that the family member will use with the patient in implementing the solution. The leader then briefly reviews the chosen solution and the steps for its implementation. Once family members understand and become comfortable, this process is frequently used during the first hour of ongoing MFG sessions.

Communication Module

In this module, family members are taught how to practice "cool" communication with the patient. While this is the ultimate goal, families should be reminded that conflict cannot be swept under the rug. Suppressing conflict results in anger and resentment that is likely to find some form of expression, such as a hostile tone of voice or annoyance over a trivial and unrelated matter. Hence, families are taught the following method for handling the inevitable conflicts and confrontations.

First, the family member is taught to describe the patient's behavior that triggers the conflict by citing observable behavior, without adding comments about the person, which serves only to heighten the tension in the confrontation. Then, the family member is instructed to tell the patient how he or she felt as a result of the behavior. Family members are encouraged to make "I feel..." statements, avoiding criticism and editorial commentary.

Finally, the family member is to explain what specific behavior change he or she would like to see. Leaders can model the positive tone and specificity of this request, again stressing that comments about behavior are less critical in tone than those that get into areas of character, intent, or personality, and thus make the confrontation less stressful. Families are encouraged to offer thanks and appreciation immediately after positive change subsequent to a confrontation. Leaders can help family members better understand this communication method by offering obvious, and sometimes humorous, examples of "what to say" and "what not to say":

- "Notice how your observation of Heather's oversleeping will come across differently if you avoid commenting on her character: 'I've noticed that you overslept several days this week,' versus 'You're being irresponsible lately, oversleeping almost every day.'"
- "Imagine how you'd respond to these two statements: 'You're gambling on your future, and I guarantee you'll get fired if you keep oversleeping,' versus 'I'm worried that the oversleeping could cause you to lose your job.'"
- "When you ask for a behavior change, make sure it's clear and nonpersonal. For example, notice how differently Heather would 'hear' the same request depending on its wording: 'You'd better start getting up on time,' versus 'I'd like you to get up on time because this job has been very good for you. I'm wondering what would help you to start doing this?'"

Mirroring Module

A significant focus in our work with families is on helping family members to hear and to tolerate the seemingly endless negative affect experienced by the patient with BPD during periods of crisis, rather than to gloss over or otherwise try to "extinguish" it by minimizing or refusing to acknowledge it. This is very difficult work for family members who fear lifelong dependence and unhappiness for the patient and are understandably leery of focusing on negative feelings. We help family members understand the value of a more secure connection with the patient with BPD, and teach them how mirroring and acknowledgment can strengthen that connection.

Fonagy and colleagues (1995) observed that young children develop a sense of secure attachment when raised by caregivers who can experience and transform their negative feelings into a tolerable form. To accomplish this transformation, the caregiver mirrors the intolerable affect and sends emotional signals indicating that the affect is "contained." In addition, the caregiver shares valuable coping strategies or information regarding the cause of the distress, thus increasing the child's understanding and reducing helplessness and confusion. The child is thus relieved and learns valuable lessons for managing future distressing events as the current intolerable distress is (1) accurately perceived by the parent, (2) reflected back to him or her ("I can see that it hurts"), and (3) rendered tolerable by soothing parental messages that share adult mastery, as in "Poor thing, I know it hurts, but soon it will stop because, see, it didn't break the skin."

In this module we teach an analogous sequence of responses. The focus is on the impact of early experiences on one's ability to accurately mirror the emotional states of one's offspring. Family members are asked to reflect upon the degree of mirroring that they received as children.

CLINICIAN: Can anyone here remember how well you were "mirrored" as a child?

FAMILY MEMBER 1: *(laughing)* One of my mother's favorite statements when I came in with cuts and bruises was "Stop crying, you're not hurt!"

CLINICIAN: So much for feeling understood!

FAMILY MEMBER 2: My mom was sympathetic when it came to physical injuries like that, but she seemed to back away whenever I felt down. She'd tell me to cheer up and stop feeling sorry for myself.

FAMILY MEMBER 3: Dad told me that boys don't cry. It was as simple as that.

CLINICIAN: I think we're seeing a pattern here. Many of you never received the kind of mirroring you're trying to learn how to give to your own relative with BPD. Your own parents probably didn't receive it, either, nor theirs, and so on. Keep this in mind so that you (1) don't blame yourselves for inadequate "mirroring" in the past, and (2) don't get discouraged when this technique feels a bit awkward or difficult.

Family members are then asked to consider how accurately they have been able to mirror their own child's emotional state. Going through these steps helps family members avoid self-blame, as does the didactic component of the module. In the didactic component, we describe studies such as that of Fonagy and colleagues (1991), which found that parents with a high degree of self-reflection were three or more times more likely to have securely attached children than parents with low reflective capacity. This exercise is highly effective in terms of lessening defensiveness vis-à-vis past failures of empathy with their offspring with BPD, because the logic is relatively straightforward: If parents have never experienced mirroring, they cannot be expected to know how to provide this subtle but critical form of support to their children.

By framing empathetic failure as something that family members themselves lacked in their relationships with their own parents, they can accept rather than defend against their offspring's complaints about not being "heard" or understood. After the discussion, family members practice mirroring with the group leader and other family members, often using real-life examples of conversations with their child that had ended badly. By role playing, failures and successes in mirroring become immediately obvious. These role plays, in which the goal is to provide mirroring, not sympathy or defensiveness or "fixing," elicit from parents a wide range of feelings. Family members are able to realize and express regret, sadness, and the joy of discovering what they have been doing wrong. Parents become eager to learn how better to "mirror" their offspring with BPD once they understand (1) how to improve this skill, and (2) how it benefits their family member.

Group Cohesion

After 2 to 3 months, family members have become comfortable with one another. This group cohesion reflects increased trust and reduced feelings of being stigmatized or blameworthy. Family members can now begin to admit to past mistakes and receive sympathetic "We've been there" feedback from others.

At this point, entry of new members should be allowed judiciously. A new family that has completed the didactics during the joining sessions and shows readiness can be introduced into the group from time to time. However, we have found that too many new people in a given time period can be unsettling to current group members. A good rule of thumb that we have learned from experience is to keep the number generally constant: A new family should enter the group only after one of the families has stopped attending. Avoid the temptation to book a larger room as the number of families increases. Instead, begin a new group.

The format within the meetings now evolves into a predictable brainstorming and problem-solving format during the second hour, in which family members expect to receive suggestions from others and are encouraged to change patterns of response to the patient with BPD. During this hour, the clinician makes frequent reference to the guidelines and underscores the message that change is not easy. As one parent put it, "Change isn't easy for anyone who hasn't signed up for it."

The first half of the meeting consists of a new or "recycled" module from the earlier weekly didactics. Initially, to avoid redundancy, we presented special topics only once, but families vary tremendously in their ability to learn and process new information, particularly when they are worried or involved in an ongoing crisis with the patient. Hence, we now "recycle" important topics during the first half of 2-hour meetings.

As in dialectical behavior therapy groups, members may have been involved in the group long enough to have heard the topic more than once. However, families consistently report that they need this repetition. Many family members have commented that each time they hear the information, they learn something new. They seem cognizant of the difficult nature of this "emotional learning." Because new experiences make different parts of the module more or less salient at any given time, the repetition of the module serves to help families better integrate and generalize what is taught to a variety of situations involving the patient.

Maintenance and Ongoing Support

Families that have been attending the MFG for over a year either decide to terminate or they continue "for the support," which is how many refer to their continuing participation. Overlearning is an objective in our program, because it facilitates automaticity and activates new behaviors without the delay of trying to remember what was taught. This makes for better use of information taught in the family groups *in vivo*, while communicating with the patient with BPD. Hence, repeating modules and continuing to receive and provide feedback to newer families is a plus for the family as well as the group.

The family may signal its discontinuation when things have improved considerably for both patient and family. After a period of not attending, family members may ask to begin coming again, usually when new problems or crises have cropped up, or when good progress has been made and developmental milestones have been reached (such as the patient returning to college or work), that are nonetheless taxing to the patient and thus to the family.

Saturday Workshops

We have now begun to offer a 2-hour Saturday special interest workshop each month for those family members whose schedules do not permit them to attend during the week. This format also encourages attendance of people who are too wary, unmotivated, or are ineligible for our weekday MFGs. In the format for the Saturday sessions, clinicians with expertise in a given area area (e.g, substance abuse, self-harm, medication, dialectical behavior therapy) speak during the first hour, leaving plenty of time for questions and answers. The second hour is then devoted, like our weekday MFGs, to the usual check-in, problem solving, and support. The Saturday groups bring a broad array of clinical experience and wisdom to the families, who greatly appreciate the opportunity to ask specific questions for which they have not yet found answers. We have observed more husbands accompanying their wives on Saturdays than during any weekday groups, which boosts parental learning and consistency at home, and improves morale of the wives and the group as a whole. For this reason, and because of increased demand for Saturday sessions by mostly dual-career couples with offspring with BPD, these workshops may increase in frequency to twice monthly.

SUMMARY AND DISCUSSION

The MFG program at McLean Hospital is a clinical service that has been offered to patients with BPD and their families for the past 4 years. We have described it here in the hope of communicating our enthusiasm and to encourage its use elsewhere. The psychoeducational format has important advantages over other approaches. It helps ally parents who are otherwise alienated. What is taught can affect change more quickly and directly than interventions that require exploration and discovery. Another advantage of psychoeducation is its relatively easy replicability. Others can learn to provide the basics of this approach (i.e., teaching, supporting, and problem solving with only modest training).

We believe that the MFG format has clinical as well as cost–benefit advantages over single-family interventions. MFGs reduce fears that one's family is defective and to blame for all the problems experienced by the patient. With other families in the room, there is a sense that "we're all in this together," that everyone is grappling with similar problems. Hearing stories about BPD individuals in other families is very helpful for family members who, as is so often the case, have assumed that only their child experiences such severe or chronic symptoms and difficulties.

We underscore the need for further research to gain empirical data with regard to clinical practices that will relieve family burden and lower rates of patient crises, especially hospitalizations. The empirical investigation of our psychoeducational MFG involved 11 families who participated for a year. The results indicate that the BPD subjects made desirable changes during the year (i.e., diminished hospitalizations and self-destructive acts). It is not, of course, possible to infer whether the benefits were due to changes made by their families. The level of consumer satisfaction was uniformly high. There is a need for further testing of the continuing development of these interventions. Finally, we need to test the effectiveness of the component modules. A randomized controlled trial will need to be conducted in the future.

Finally, clinicians should continually ask families what has and has not helped. Families and their members with BPD can enrich the clinician's understanding of what is needed and guide the development of the curriculum. Families we have worked with over the years have provided us with important feedback that continues to play a central role in the ongoing development of the MFG program described in this chapter.

REFERENCES

Akiskal, H., Chen, S., Davis, G., Puzantian, V., Kashgarian, M., & Bolinger, J. (1985). Borderline: An adjective in search of a noun. *Journal of Clinical Psychiatry, 46,* 41–48.
Fonagy, P., Steele, M., Steele, H., Leigh, T., Kennedy, R., Mattoon, G., & Target, M. (1995).

Attachment, the reflective self and borderline states: The predictive specificity of the Adult Attachment Interview and pathological emotional development. In S. Goldberg, R. Muir, & J. Kerr (Eds.), *Attachment theory: Social, developmental and clinical perspectives* (pp. 223–278). Hillsdale, NJ: Analytic Press.

Fonagy, P., Steele, M., Moran, G., Steele, H., & Higgitt, A. C. (1991). The capacity for understanding mental states: The reflective self in parent and child and its significance for security of attachment. *Infant Health Journal, 13*, 200–216.

Frank, H., & Paris, J. (1981). Recollections of family experience in borderline patients. *Archives of General Psychiatry, 38*, 1031–1034.

Fristad, M., Gavazzi, S. M., Centolella, D., & Soldano, K. (1996). Psychoeducation: An intervention strategy for families of children with mood disorders. *Contemporary Family Therapy, 18*, 371–383.

Gabbard, G., Lazar, S. G., Hornberger, J., & Spiegel, D. (1997). The economic impact of psychotherapy: A review. *American Journal of Psychiatry, 154*(2), 147–155.

Goldman, J., D'Angelo, E., & Demaso, D. (1993). Psychopathology in the families of children and adolescents with borderline personality disorder. *American Journal of Psychiatry, 150*, 1832–1835.

Goldstein, M. (1990). Psychosocial factors relating to etiology and course of schizophrenia. In M. I. Herz, S. I. Keith, & J. P. Docherty (Eds.), *Handbook of schizophrenia: Vol. 4. Psychosocial treatment of schizophrenia* (pp. 1–23). Amsterdam: Elsevier.

Gunderson, J. (1984). *Borderline personality disorder*. Washington, DC: American Psychiatric Press.

Gunderson, J. (2001). *Borderline personality disorder: A clinical guide*. Washington, DC: American Psychiatric Press.

Gunderson, J., Kerr, J., & Englund, D. (1980). The families of borderlines: A comparative study. *Archives of General Psychiatry, 37*, 227–233.

Gunderson, J., & Lyoo, I. (1996). Family problems and relationships for adults with borderline personality disorder. *Harvard Review of Psychiatry, 4*, 272–278.

Gunderson, J., & Sabo, A. (1993). The phenomenological and conceptual interface between borderline personality disorder and PTSD. *American Journal of Psychiatry, 150*(1), 19–27.

Gunderson, J., & Zanarini, M. (1989). Pathogenesis of borderline personality disorder. In A. Tasman, R. E. Hales, & A. J. Frances (Eds.), *Annual Review of Psychiatry, 8*, 25–42.

Hooley, J. M., & Hoffman, P. D. (1999). Expressed emotion and the clinical outcome in borderline personality disorder. *American Journal of Psychiatry, 156*, 1557–1562.

Inman, D. J., Bascue, L. D., & Skoloda, T. (1985). Identification of borderline personality disorders among substance abuse inpatients. *Journal of Substance Abuse Treatment, 2*(4), 229–232.

Leff, J. (1989). Controversial issues and growing points in research on relatives' expressed emotions. *International Journal of Social Psychiatry, 35*, 133–145.

Leff, J. (1992). Problems of transformation. *International Journal of Social Psychiatry, 38*(1), 16–23.

Linehan, M. M. (1993). *Cognitive-behavioral treatment of borderline personality disorder*. New York: Guilford Press.

Linehan, M., Armstrong, H., Suarez, A., Allmon, d., & Heard, H. (1991). Cognitive-behavioral treatment of chronically parasuicidal borderline patients. *Archives of General Psychiatry, 48*, 1060–1064.

Links, P., Boiago, I., & Huxley, G. (1990). Sexual abuse and biparental failure as etiologic models in BPD. In P. S. Links (Ed.), *Family environment and borderline personality disorder* (pp. 105–120). Washington, DC: American Psychiatric Press.

Links, P., Steiner, M., & Huxley, G. (1988). The occurrence of borderline personality disorder in the families of borderline patients. *Journal of Personality Disorders, 2*, 14–20.

Links, P., & van Reekum, R. (1993). Childhood sexual abuse, parental impairment and the development of borderline personality disorder. *Canadian Journal of Psychiatry, 38*, 472–474.

Loranger, A., & Tulis, E. (1983). Family history of alcoholism in borderline personality disorder. *Archives of General Psychiatry, 42,* 153–157.

Loranger, A., Oldham, J., & Tulis, E. (1982). Familial transmission of DSM-III borderline personality disorder. *Archives of General Psychiatry, 39,* 795–799.

Masterson, J., & Rinsley, D. (1975). The borderline syndrome: The role of the mother in the genesis and psychic structure of the borderline personality. *International Journal of Psycho-Analysis, 56*(2), 163–177.

McFarlane, W. R. (1990). Multiple family groups and the treatment of schizophrenia. In M. I. Herz, S. J. Keith, & J. P. Docherty (Eds.), *Handbook of schizophrenia: Vol. 4. Psychosocial treatment of schizophrenia* (pp. 167–189). Amsterdam: Elsevier.

McFarlane, W. R., & Dunne, E. (1991). Family psychoeducation and multi-family groups in the treatment of schizophrenia. *Directions in Psychiatry, 11*(20), 2–7.

McFarlane, W. R., Link, B., Dushay, R., Marchal, J., & Crilly, J. (1995). Psychoeducational multiple family groups: Four-year relapse outcome in schizophrenia. *Family Process, 34,* 127–144.

McGlashan, T. (1987). BPD: Long-term effects of comorbidity. *Journal of Nervous and Mental Disease, 175,* 457–473.

Millon, T. (1987). On the genesis and prevalence of the borderline personality disorder: A social learning thesis. *Journal of Personality Disorders, 1,* 354–372.

Mitton, J. M., & Links, P. S. (1996). Helping the family: A framework for intervention. In P. S. Links (Ed.), Clinical assessment and management of severe personality disorders [Special issue]. *Clinical Practice, 35,* 195–218.

Paris, J., & Zweig-Frank, H. (1992). A critical review of the role of childhood sexual abuse in the etiology of borderline personality disorder. *Canadian Journal of Psychiatry, 37,* 125–128.

Pope, H., Jonas, J., & Hudson, J. (1983). The validity of DSM-III borderline personality disorder. *Archives of General Psychiatry, 40,* 23–30.

Ruiz-Sancho, A. M., & Gunderson, J. G. (1997). Families of patients with BPD: A review of the literature. In O. F. Kernberg, B. Dulz, & V. Sachsse (Eds.), *Handbook of borderline personality disorder* (pp. 771–792). Stuttgart: Schattauer-Verlag.

Shapiro, E. (1978). The psychodynamics and developmental psychology of the borderline patient: A review of the literature. *American Journal of Psychiatry, 135,* 1305–1315.

Shapiro, E. (1982). On curiosity: Intrapsychic and interpersonal boundary formation in family life. *International Journal of Family Psychiatry, 3,* 69–89.

Soloff, P. (1993). Studying the treatment contract in intensive psychotherapy with borderline patients. *Psychiatry: Interpersonal and Biological Processes, 56*(3), 264–267.

Soloff, P., & Millward, J. (1983). Psychiatric disorders in the families of borderline patients. *Archives of General Psychiatry, 40,* 37–44.

Widiger, T., & Frances, A. (1988). Treating self-defeating personality disorder. *Hospital and Community Psychiatry, 39*(8), 819–821.

Young, D., & Gunderson, J. (1995). Family images of borderline adolescents. *Psychiatry, 58,* 164–172.

Zanarini, M. (1997). Evolving perspectives on the etiology of borderline personality disorder. In M. C. Zanarini (Ed.), *Role of sexual abuse in the etiology of borderline personality disorder* (pp. 1–14). Washington, DC: American Psychiatric Press.

Zanarini, M., Gunderson, J., & Frankenburg, F. (1990). Discriminating borderline personality disorder from other Axis II disorders. *American Journal of Psychiatry, 147*(2), 161–167.

Zinner, J., & Shapiro, E. (1975). Splitting in the families of borderline adolescents. In J. Mack (Ed.), *Borderline states in psychiatry* (pp. 103–122). New York: Grune & Stratton.

18

Multisystemic Treatment of Antisocial Behavior in Adolescents

ELIZABETH J. LETOURNEAU
PHILLIPPE B. CUNNINGHAM
SCOTT W. HENGGELER

Multisystemic therapy (MST) was developed in the late 1970s to address the mental health needs of seriously delinquent youth and their families. Traditional therapeutic approaches had largely failed with juvenile offenders, and the early successes demonstrated by the developers of MST (e.g., Henggeler et al., 1986) led to federal funding for rigorous clinical outcome studies. Today, MST is best known for empirically supported success with chronic juvenile offenders and juveniles with substance use disorders (Borduin et al., 1995; Henggeler, Melton, Smith, Schoenwald, & Hanley, 1997; Henggeler, Pickrel, & Brondino, 1999). These positive results have recently been extended to youth presenting with psychiatric emergencies (e.g., homicidal, suicidal, psychotic) (Henggeler, Rowland, et al., 1999; Rowland et al., 2000; Schoenwald, Ward, Henggeler, & Rowland, 2000), and ongoing randomized clinical trials are examining the efficacy of MST with several other clinical populations (e.g., families in which physical assault has occurred, children with diabetes). In addition, studies are currently in progress examining the effectiveness of MST using various models of service delivery (e.g., continua of care) and delivered in different settings (e.g., school-based) (Henggeler, Schoenwald, Rowland, & Cunningham, in press). Taken together, the data supporting MST with juvenile offenders have led reviewers and national agencies to identify MST as one of the most clinically promising and cost-effective treatments currently available (Elliott, 1998; Farrington & Welsh, 1999; Kazdin & Weisz, 1998; National Institute on Drug Abuse, 1999; Tate, Reppucci, & Mulvey, 1995; U.S. Department of Health and Human Services, 1999, 2001).

The effectiveness of MST with deep-end and chronic users of mental health and juvenile justice services has been linked to several departures made by MST from more traditional child and family treatment programs (Henggeler, 1999b). This chapter reviews these departures and the principles that guide MST implementation, and presents the "next steps" that must be taken to ensure that juvenile delinquents and their families receive effective treatment.

DEPARTURES FROM TRADITIONAL THERAPEUTIC APPROACHES

Theoretical Basis

MST is based on a theory of human behavior (i.e., social ecological theory; Bronfenbrenner, 1979) that is strongly supported by the extant literature. Social ecological theory views individuals as nested within increasingly complex systems (e.g., family, school, neighborhood). Like a drop of water landing in a still pond, the behavior of one person in one system has a "ripple effect" on the behavior of others in the remaining systems. Thus, problem behavior is maintained by problematic interactions within and across the multiple systems in which the child is embedded. The influence of these interactions on a child's delinquent behavior may be direct (e.g., the delinquent peers of a child expect and encourage him to fight classmates) or indirect (e.g., parental work stress impacts monitoring, which leads to association with deviant peers). Conversely, appropriate behaviors can have the same ripple effect, in which positive interactions serve to strengthen and maintain a child's behavioral gains. Thus, the effects of multiple systems are hypothesized to occur conjointly to increase or decrease risk for delinquent behavior.

Importantly, extant correlational and longitudinal research in the areas of delinquency and adolescent substance abuse provide strong support for the theory of social ecology. Adolescent antisocial behavior is multidetermined and has been reliably linked with a consistent set of risk factors across multiple systems within the ecology of youth (Henggeler, 1997; Loeber & Farrington, 1998), including individual factors (e.g., poor verbal skills, attributional bias), family characteristics (e.g., lack of monitoring, low warmth), peer characteristics (e.g., association with deviant peers), school factors (e.g., low achievement, chaotic school environment), and neighborhoods factors (e.g., high mobility, criminal subculture) (Henggeler, Schoenwald, Borduin, Rowland, & Cunningham, 1998). The aggregate of these risk factors, not just the presence of a single factor, places youth at increased risk for aggressive or otherwise delinquent behavior (Garbarino, 2001). These findings suggest, therefore, that optimal interventions should have the capacity to address a comprehensive range of risk factors in the youth and family's social ecology.

Caregivers as Key Agents of Change

A second significant departure from more traditional therapy is the fact that MST views caregivers as the key to altering antisocial behavior patterns and maintaining positive behavioral gains once treatment has ended. In mental health and juvenile justice systems, caregivers are often identified as part of the problem but are not considered an essential part of the solution. Although all systems within which children are embedded are viewed as important sources of behavior maintenance, from the MST perspective, caregivers have the most direct, immediate, and consistent impact on their children's lives and will be present long after therapy has ended. Thus, helping caregivers become the agents of change ensures that adults in the child's life will be available to handle future difficulties that may arise. Moreover, a related goal of MST is to strengthen relationships between caregivers and indigenous resources (e.g., grandparents, neighbors, teachers), recognizing that caregivers will need significant support from other adults as they alter the ways in which they parent.

Home-Based Treatment Delivery Model

A third substantial departure from traditional therapy by MST is the use of the home-based treatment delivery model. Central to the mission of MST is overcoming barriers to treatment access, and the home-based model of service delivery provides several important advantages in this regard. First, home-based treatment avoids potential iatrogenic effects of placing delinquent youth together in treatment groups (Arnold & Hughes, 1999; Dishion, McCord, & Poulin, 1999). Second, home-based treatment helps to overcome common barriers that families of delinquent youth face in getting to appointments (e.g., unreliable transportation, inflexible work schedules, caregiver mental health problems that interfere with appointment keeping). Third, working with families in their homes provides a rich source of ecologically valid information about relationships between youth and their caregivers, and this information is critical in designing effective interventions. Fourth, meeting families at their convenience and in their homes helps to establish rapport and engage them in the therapeutic process. Fifth, the low caseloads that characterize home-based treatment (3 to 6 families) provide therapists with the time resources needed to engage caregivers and deliver intensive services. Finally, therapists are available 24 hours per day, 7 days per week, which allows an immediate response to crises that could lead to out-of-home placements.

Strengths-Based Focus

Many families of seriously troubled youth have long histories of receiving mental health services that focused on personal and family deficits. For most people, relationships built primarily on weaknesses are difficult to maintain (hence, the reluctance of most adults to get annual medical examinations). From the initial assessment through the end of treatment, MST aims to identify the strengths and needs of families in crisis. Strengths are then used as levers for therapeutic change. Wherever possible, the positive is identified and emphasized by the MST team. Disparaging comments or labeling is prohibited from communications between MST therapists and all parties (including other professionals) involved with the family. This is not to suggest that MST therapists take a "Pollyannaish" approach to their clients. Indeed, these youth and families fall well to the right of the psychological distress bell curve. However, all such families possess at least some strengths (e.g., love for their child, ability to maintain employment) that can be used when delivering empirically validated interventions. Like the use of the home-based delivery model, the use of a strength-based treatment is critical for engaging family members in treatment, which is a critical step toward achieving favorable outcomes.

Multisystemic Therapy Quality Assurance

None of the departures from traditional therapy, nor even the effectiveness demonstrated in clinical trials, automatically assures that MST will be effective with a given family. Indeed, the transition from efficacy (i.e., implementation under ideal circumstances) to effectiveness (i.e., implementation in real-world settings) poses an extremely challenging set of problems pertaining to, for example, lack of provider organization accountability for outcome, and referral and funding mechanisms that arbitrarily limit treatment duration and intensity or favor traditional, restrictive placements (Schoenwald & Henggeler, in press). These barriers are not unique to MST. The effective implementation of any evidence-based intervention is likely to require some method of quality assurance that goes beyond prevailing standards (Bickman & Noser, 1999; Mikeson & Shaha, 1996; Sluyter, 1998).

To facilitate positive therapeutic outcome in real-world settings, MST employs a rigorous quality assurance system that provides continuous feedback between families, therapists, supervisors, and consultants (Henggeler & Schoenwald, 1999). This system includes several interrelated components: (1) The assessment and intervention process is manualized and focuses on a set of nine treatment principles that set the playing field for therapist behaviors (described more fully later; Henggeler & Schoenwald, 1998); (2) supervisory and consultation processes are manualized for the on-site MST supervisors and the off-site MST experts who provide weekly support and consultation to MST teams; (3) provider organizations receive extensive organizational consultation to ensure the provision of necessary resources (e.g., funding, low caseloads, interagency collaboration) prior to and following the development of MST programs; and (4) the adherence of therapists and supervisors to MST protocols is monitored continuously through a therapist adherence measure completed by families, and a supervisor adherence measure completed by therapists. Importantly, several studies have recently shown that therapist adherence is associated with positive outcomes, including improved family relations, decreased delinquent peer affiliation, and reduced long-term rates of rearrest and incarceration (Henggeler et al., 1997; Henggeler, Pickrel, & Brondino, 1999; Huey, Henggeler, Brondino, & Pickrel, 2000; Schoenwald, Ward, Henggeler, & Rowland, 2000).

TREATMENT PRINCIPLES OF MULTISYSTEMIC THERAPY

Treatment specification is essential for therapist adherence to a treatment model and for tracking those therapeutic elements most responsible for behavior change. Because of the comprehensive goals of MST (i.e., to impact identified risk factors effectively across social systems), MST treatment is unique to the strengths and needs of each family. This uniqueness precludes creating a session-by-session manual in which all possible methods for impacting all possible systems are outlined. Rather, a manual was developed in which nine MST treatment principles are identified and described to guide treatment implementation (Henggeler et al., 1998). These nine core principles are the essence of MST and, as indicated previously, therapist adherence to these principles predicts positive treatment outcome.

Principle 1: The primary purpose of assessment is to understand the fit between the identified problems and their broader systemic context. Consistent with both social ecological theory and the multidetermined nature of antisocial behavior, MST therapists attempt to discern the "fit" of problem behavior within the youth's social network. A comprehensive assessment is conducted in the home and with other relevant parties (e.g., extended family, school personnel) to identify the circumstances under which identified problems occur and factors that may serve to maintain or attenuate these difficulties. After gathering information from multiple sources, the MST therapist develops hypotheses regarding specific links between different systems and the youth's behavior. A "fit circle" (see Figure 18.1) is created that depicts these hypotheses. The identification of

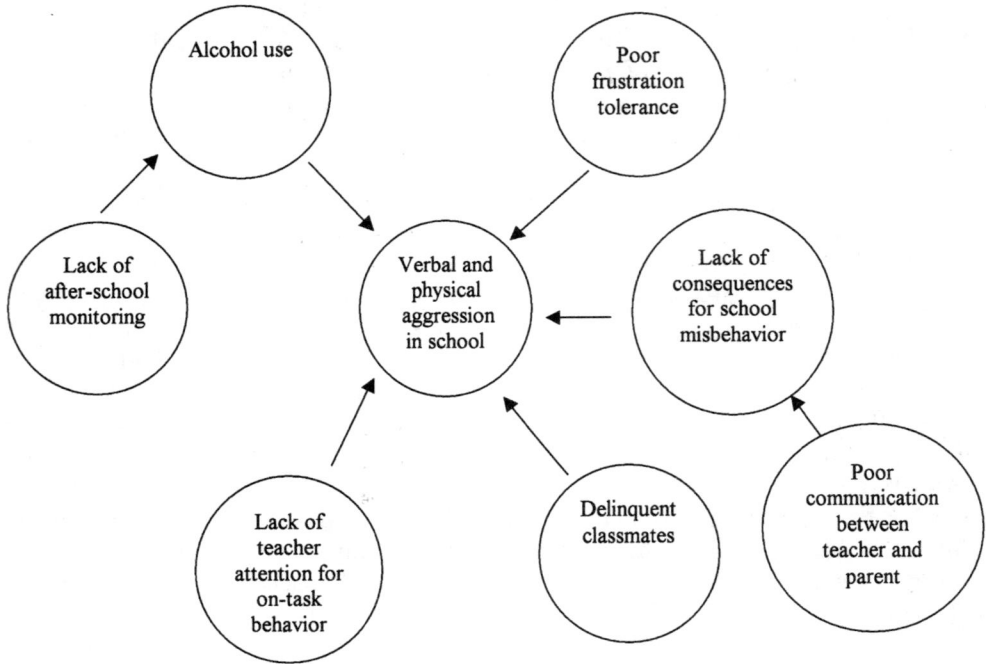

FIGURE 18.1. Sample fit circle for Mike's aggression.

needs and strengths across multiple systems encourages therapists to look beyond the individual and family to find additional factors that must be targeted if change is to occur and be sustained.

As is seen in Figure 18.1, Mike's primary problem behavior (verbal and physical aggression in school) is hypothesized as being maintained by problematic interactions in and between two systems, school and home. Specifically, at the individual level, Mike's use of alcohol and his poor frustration tolerance are thought to increase his risk for verbal and physical aggression. At the school level, delinquent peers approve of and encourage violent behavior, which then often goes unpunished by his teachers. Poor communication between Mike's teachers and his mother also reduce the likelihood of appropriate consequences for inappropriate behaviors being applied at home. Finally, Mike has too much unstructured time, and this increases his risk for getting into trouble after school.

Principle 2: Therapeutic contacts should emphasize the positive and use systemic strengths as levers for change. Clinical change with youth can be effected only to the extent that family members and other important members of the youth's ecology are actively engaged in treatment. To increase engagement and collaboration, the therapist must identify family strengths on which to base the treatment plan. Caregivers often desire change but have prior experiences that present barriers to engagement with the MST therapist. For example, parents might have experienced long-term frustration with their child's behavior, negative interactions with the mental health care system, or problems, such as substance use, that impact their ability to parent effectively. One purpose of focusing on a family's strengths in designing an intervention is to increase the likelihood that therapists and caregivers will work collaboratively. Another purpose is to bolster the confidence of caregivers, which is essential if the caregiver is to participate actively in treatment and maintain positive therapeutic changes once treatment has ended. Several techniques are used for maintaining a strength focus, including use of nonpejorative language in communicating with the family or with others on the family's behalf, providing liberal use of positive reinforcement, and focusing on problem solving (i.e., identifying barriers to treatment progress and developing interventions to target those barriers).

The identification of strengths is also crucial to the design of effective interventions. In almost all cases, more than one method can be used to address a specific problem behavior. For example, when impulsive behavior is targeted, potential solutions include using medication (following appropriate assessment to determine whether a biological component is present), altering contingencies at home to reward reflective behavior, and teaching the child specific strategies for controlling his or her behavior. If a strength of the family is consistent monitoring of the child, teaching caregivers to alter contingencies might be highly effective. Likewise, if the child is cognitively advanced, individual cognitive-behavioral therapy might be an appropriate intervention. By clearly labeling, showcasing, and reinforcing strengths, therapists help engage caregivers and other members of the child's ecology who will need to work diligently to achieve and maintain behavior changes.

Principle 3: Interventions are designed to promote responsible behavior and decrease irresponsible behavior among family members. The purpose of this principle is to cue therapists to specify clearly those behaviors that require change and the strengths on which to base interventions. Rather than providing a diagnosis (e.g., a caregiver has a substance abuse problem), problems should be conceptualized as behaviors that either need to be decreased (e.g., drinking when monitoring one's child) or increased (e.g., remaining abstinent between the hours of 3:00 and 9:00 P.M.). By framing behaviors as either responsible or irresponsible, therapists help caregivers and others see how these problems serve to maintain or attenuate a child's problem behaviors. Also, goals to increase or decrease specific behaviors may seem more realistic than goals to eliminate a psychological disorder.

Principle 4: Interventions are present focused and action oriented, targeting specific and well-defined problems. MST interventions are designed to target those factors hypothesized as most directly linked to problem behaviors. Delinquent youth have often experienced a number of life stressors (e.g., sexual assault, loss of a parent through death or divorce) that may have been relevant early in the development of problem behaviors. However, these more distal factors do not necessarily explain why problem behaviors are maintained. Distal factors are also often static or unchangeable (e.g., divorced parents will not remarry, regardless of their child's behavior). Thus, MST focuses on factors present in the here and now that are directly related to the maintenance of problem behaviors and amenable to intervention.

A second reason for focusing on more proximal factors is that the MST therapist will know quickly whether the intervention plan is having the intended effect. When measurable change is not occurring, the therapist reconceptualizes the fit or identifies barriers to change and modifies the intervention plan. The present-focused, action orientation of MST contrasts therapies that target factors from the distant past and that profess change comes slowly and only after substantial time in treatment. Families of highly antisocial youth do not usually have the luxury of waiting months or years for treatment change. Their children are often at imminent risk for out-of-home placement, expulsion from school, or imprisonment. Furthermore, these families are also likely to be at their wits' end. Families of delinquent youth need to see positive change, and they need to see it quickly, if they are to remain engaged with and committed to the intervention process.

Principle 5: Interventions target sequences of behavior within and between multiple systems that maintain the identified problem. Interactions within systems (e.g., family) and between systems (e.g., family and school) are targeted for intervention when these interactions serve to maintain problem behaviors. Problem behavior is considered the end result of a sequence of such interactions and not a spontaneous event. For example, a teacher is unable to meet with a parent due to scheduling conflicts. The teacher becomes frustrated and does not communicate regularly with the parent, whose child is now truant from school without her knowledge. The child becomes involved with deviant peers while away from school, in part because there are no consequences for the truancy. The MST intervention will target the youth's truancy and inappropriate school behaviors within the context of the sequence(s) that led to this behavior, including helping the child's mother and teacher to facilitate communication, and then setting up a daily monitoring system that includes immediate consequences both for truancy or other misbehavior at school and at home, and for appropriate behaviors.

Regarding between-system interventions, parent–school alliances are frequently strained and often need to be enhanced. This is particularly true when part of the treatment plan is the implementation of a consistent behavioral contingency plan across school and home. In this case, members of both systems must understand and agree on the targeted behaviors and the specific contingencies to be put into place with the child. A meeting involving all relevant parties is arranged by the therapist, who then works with the caregiver and the teacher to improve relations, if necessary. As with interventions within systems, interventions targeting between-systems interactions address both the problem behavior and the sequence of actions that precedes that behavior.

Principle 6: Interventions are developmentally appropriate and fit the developmental needs of the youth. The physical, intellectual, and social needs of youth are considered when designing interventions. Youth have different needs at different times in their lives, and treatment must be sensitive to these needs to be successful. For example, interventions with children, young adolescents, and developmentally delayed older adolescents are carried out primarily through caregivers and give due consideration to youth's developmental needs (e.g., the need for peer socialization in school-age children). On the other hand, interventions with older adolescents, who are more cognitively and developmentally mature, will focus more on preparation for independent living. For example, getting a 17-year-old who has failed school repeatedly to graduate high school may be less important than improving his or her ability to find gainful employment. In particular, contingencies for behavior plans must be suited to the needs and wants of the child. Whereas money may be an appropriate and highly salient reinforcer for teenagers, watching a movie with parents may be more reinforcing for a 10-year-old.

In addition to the developmental capacity of youth, that of caregivers is also considered in treatment design. For example, grandparents may be excellent resources for assistance in child rearing, but may lack the energy needed for full-time parenting and might not, therefore, be appropriate candidates when youth must be placed temporarily outside the home.

Principle 7: Interventions are designed to require daily or weekly effort by family members. Daily or weekly effort by relevant parties helps ensure that measurable changes occur quickly and that barriers to such change are identified. Consequently, once a treatment plan is developed, all participants in the plan are expected to begin work immediately. Efforts may involve daily monitoring of behaviors targeted for change, daily practice of new skills, frequent communication exchanges between newly developed social resources, and so on.

The expectation of daily effort also holds for therapists, who are on call 24 hours a day, 7 days a week. The majority of client contact usually occurs within the first few weeks of treatment and lessens as caregivers improve their ability to manage their children's behavior as indigenous resources are strengthened. To support the flexibility and high energy required of therapists, treatment programs must also make a commitment to the MST model. Most importantly, therapists maintain small caseloads of 3 to 6 families and are not expected to "mix models" (e.g., treat some families with a more traditional 9 to 5 office-based treatment and others with MST).

Principle 8: Intervention effectiveness is evaluated continuously from multiple perspectives with providers assuming accountability for overcoming barriers to successful outcome. The purpose of this principle is to gauge treatment effectiveness on a continuous basis. By including information from multiple sources, MST therapists increase the validity of the data. For example, if a therapist asks a chronic juvenile offender how school is going, a likely response would be "All right." However, if the therapist then asks the teacher, a possible response is "Terrible!" By evaluating information on an ongoing basis, MST therapists quickly recognize when change is not occurring. They then are responsible for identifying and targeting barriers. When barriers appear intractable, MST therapists are encouraged to design creative solutions to get around these barriers rather than to attack repeatedly the same issue with the same strategy, thereby setting up caregivers or others for repeated failure. For example, if a child remains unmonitored after school, when continuous monitoring is the goal, the therapist identifies the barrier (e.g., caregiver drug use) and attempts either to address that barrier (e.g., via interventions to reduce substance use) or to find a way around the barrier (e.g., identify other responsible adults in the natural ecology who can provide supervision) as a short-term solution.

Principle 9: Interventions are designed to promote treatment generalization and long-term maintenance of therapeutic change by empowering caregivers to address family members' needs across multiple systemic contexts. Essentially, MST posits that the focus of treatment should be on empowering caregivers to handle the challenges of raising children effectively and independently (Henggeler, Cunningham, Pickrel, Schoenwald, & Brondino, 1996). For this to occur, MST therapists must refrain from taking care of clients and using their own professional skills to solve clients' problems. Rather, caregivers are supported in effecting desired changes themselves. By providing caregivers with the necessary tools and resources required for managing their children's behavior, and sometimes their own, therapists should eventually become irrelevant and unnecessary for improved behavior. To accomplish the goal of this principle, MST therapists must seek to help caregivers obtain indigenous resources (e.g., friends, family, neighbors) that can be galvanized to support their efforts to take control of their children's behavior. Thus, more formal resources (e.g., case managers) are eschewed in favor of informal resources.

In conclusion, these nine principles guide treatment design and implementation, yet allow for necessary individualization of treatment for each family.

CASE EXAMPLE

To demonstrate the use of the MST principles, a brief clinical case example is provided and relevant principles are identified when applicable.

Presenting Information

Mike, a 13-year-old male African American, was ordered into treatment by a judge after being convicted of arson. He had set his garage on fire, which was the most destructive act in a 2-year history of increasing verbal and physical aggression described by Mike and his mother.

Intake Assessment and History

Mike was living with his mother, a 29-year-old maternal uncle, 19- and 20-year-old brothers, and the 18-year-old, pregnant girlfriend of the 20-year-old brother. During the home-based assessment (Principle 1), the therapist noted that Mike's family lived in a small house, that the surrounding neighborhood consisted of mainly low-income families, and that drug trafficking appeared to be taking place near Mike's home. During the interview with Mike, his mother, and the other members of the household, everyone acknowledged that Mike was easily provoked and frequently argued and cursed but was not physically aggressive at home. The act of arson for which Mike was charged was his first criminal conviction. However, family members described a 2-year history of verbal and physical aggression and other behavioral problems (e.g., clowning around in class) at school. Mike denied substance use. His mother concurred but acknowledged that Mike's 19-year-old brother and his uncle both drank frequently. Furthermore, the family history was significant for substance abuse by Mike's father who was currently in jail and had had no contact with Mike or his mother for many years.

The MST therapist also interviewed Mike's primary teacher and observed his behavior in class (Principle 1). Earlier in the year, Mike had been transferred to a class for children with behavioral problems and was currently being considered for expulsion due to his noncompliant classroom behavior and weekly episodes of physical aggression. Mike acknowledged that he misbehaved in school when encouraged by his friends, and this was confirmed by the therapist during school observation. Mike's teacher reported that he was easily provoked and responded with verbal and physical aggression. The relationship between Mike's teacher and his mother was clearly strained, after several failed attempts to meet. Mike's mother, however, held two jobs and was rarely available to attend such meetings.

Mike's probation officer reported that he was likable and seemed to follow instructions fairly well. However, he noted that he frequently saw Mike in the company of other delinquent teenagers.

Despite these needs, the family had numerous strengths on which to build a treatment plan (Principle 2). Mike was a good-looking, verbally skilled boy who generally got along well with adults. His mother was very committed to his well-being, held two jobs, and was able to meet her family's basic needs. Family members had strong affective bonds, particularly those between Mike and his mother. Mike's uncle and brothers clearly cared for him and expressed their willingness to do "whatever it takes" to get Mike off probation and behaving more appropriately, especially toward his mother.

In addition to these family strengths, there were several school and community strengths as well. Mike's teachers liked him and were willing to give him another chance, especially now that he was actively involved in treatment. At the community level, a nearby neighborhood center provided after-school activities for teenagers (see Table 18.1 for list of strengths and needs).

Safety

Because of Mike's episode of arson, his safety and that of his family members needed to be ensured. Mike indicated to the MST therapist that he had set the fire only as an attention-getting prank and had not intended to burn down the home or harm anyone. This explanation "fit" with the assessment data suggesting Mike's strong need for attention (Principle 1). Nevertheless, it was important to secure the area (i.e., dangerous substances, including gasoline cans, paint thinner, and other highly flammable substances, were removed) and identify whether other contributing factors might help to predict future destructive behavior (e.g., lax monitoring).

After these dangerous substances were removed and a schedule was developed whereby Mike would have adult supervision during after-school hours, he could be maintained safely in the community. Supervision and monitoring were provided by members of Mike's ecology (e.g., his mother, brothers, and uncle; Principles 3 and 9) and by professionals working temporarily with Mike (e.g., MST therapist, probation officer).

Fit Assessment

During the strengths and needs assessment, the MST therapist hypothesized that several fit factors either directly or indirectly influenced Mike's aggressive behaviors (Figure 18.1), including (1) association with deviant peers, who modeled and approved of aggressive behavior; (2) school failure (i.e., poor classroom management by his teachers); (3) weak behavioral contingencies at home (i.e., lack of monitoring after school, poor communication between Mike's teachers and his mother); (4) impulsivity; (5) Mike's desire to be the center of attention; and (6) alcohol use. These correlates to Mike's behavior were then used to developing a well-specified MST treatment plan (Principles 4, 5, and 8).

After observing Mike and his family during the first week of treatment, the MST therapist observed a pattern to his aggressive behavior. Specifically, his verbal and physical aggression at school were correlated with poor supervision the previous evening. On nights that his mother worked late, Mike's uncle or one of his brothers was scheduled to provide supervision. Of the three men, only his oldest brother did so consistently. However, unannounced home visits by the MST therapist revealed that Mike's uncle and his 19-year-old brother were either drinking or absent during those evenings they were supposed to supervise him. Furthermore, Mike was also drinking (the therapist smelled alcohol on his breath) and this consumption appeared to be linked to increased verbal aggressiveness and irritability at home and at school the following day. Thus, one setting

TABLE 18.1. Systemic Strengths and Needs

Strengths	Needs
Individual	
Personable, outgoing, enjoys attention from peers and adults. Self-reliant. Responds well to supervision, structured free time, and behavioral contingencies. Very insightful and honest. Athletic. Only one arrest; physically aggressive behavior limited to school.	Mike is verbally and physically aggressive and often irritable. He exhibits poor frustration tolerance and poor impulse control. He is also a crowd pleaser. Diagnosed substance abuse.
Family	
Mike's mother works hard to provide for her family's basic needs. She is invested in Mike's improvement and values school performance. She and Mike have a very positive relationship. All family members are concerned about Mike's behavior.	Mike's mother lacks assertiveness and is frequently away from home (due to work) during high-risk times for Mike's drinking. There are financial problems. No set household rules and limited structure or supervision for Mike. His mother has minimal support in managing her home even with the presence of other adults. Mike's uncle and one brother abuse alcohol. Crowded living conditions.
Peers	
Mike makes friends easily.	Mike's school friends are all involved in delinquent behavior and peers approve of and goad Mike into physically and verbally aggressive acts at school.
School	
Mike's teacher and the school counselor like him, see potential for high achievement and are invested in seeing him return to mainstream classes.	Mike's special classroom groups all delinquent youth together, thus increasing Mike's exposure to deviant peers. The teacher has poor classroom management skills and inconsistently applies consequences to inappropriate behavior (and almost never provides consequences for appropriate behavior). No after-school programs offered. Strained relationship with Mike's mother.
Community	
Community center is close to home and offers after-school programs.	The family resides in a low-income neighborhood characterized by a criminal subculture.

event for Mike's school misbehavior was his alcohol consumption when left unmonitored.

Family members were aware of the use of alcohol by Mike's brother and uncle but denied concerns about alcohol abuse or dependence, largely because neither man became violent when intoxicated, as had Mike's father when he still resided with the family. Family members were unaware that Mike also drank. Alone in his bedroom, Mike consumed beer and hard liquor that he stole from his brother and uncle.

While Mike's alcohol use appeared to explain his irritability and aggressiveness at home and influence his behavior at school, school observations conducted during the first week of treatment also suggested that his behavior was maintained by positive reinforcement from peers, as well as extra attention from teachers and school administrators.

Negative consequences were effective with Mike but inconsistently applied by his teacher, who was overwhelmed with the behavior problems of 15 other students. In addition, though he frequently engaged in appropriate, on-task behavior and appeared to enjoy most subjects, Mike was rarely reinforced for studying.

Overarching Goals

Mike, his mother, his uncle and brothers, and significant others (e.g., probation officer and teachers) were asked what they wanted to accomplish by the end of treatment. His mother's goals were for Mike to get back into his mainstream class, to stop being physically and verbally aggressive at school and verbally aggressive at home, and to stop drinking. Mike's goals were to have his own bedroom and to get out of the special needs class. His brothers and uncle wanted him to be less irritable and less "easily set-off" at home. Mike's teacher wanted him to stop fighting and cursing at school, and his probation officer wanted to see Mike engage in some appropriate after-school activities with prosocial peers.

Family and Individual Interventions

Several of the overarching goals involved decreasing Mike's verbally aggressive behavior at home. Since it was hypothesized that his verbal aggression was associated with alcohol use, Mike's alcohol consumption and access to alcoholic beverages needed to be monitored. Three interventions were designed to address this fit factor. First, Mike's mother decided to throw out all alcoholic beverages and to forbid the presence of alcohol in the house. Second, a plan was developed whereby Mike would be under adult supervision from the moment he returned home from school until his mother returned home from work. Third, Mike, his mother, and the therapist developed a plan for structuring Mike's free time, thereby giving him less opportunity to obtain alcohol from other sources.

Regarding the first intervention, Mike's mother held a family meeting, during which she stated that alcohol was no longer permitted in the house and explained that this was due to Mike's modeling his older relatives' drinking behavior. She worked with the therapist on developing the assertiveness skills necessary both to hold this meeting and to enforce the new rule.

For the second intervention, a schedule was developed with Mike's oldest brother and his girlfriend to provide supervision two weekdays per week. On the remaining days, Mike was signed up for basketball at the nearby neighborhood center. Rules for appropriate behavior were clearly posted at the center and reviewed with Mike by his new coach.

In the third intervention, a plan structuring Mike's free time was clearly posted on the refrigerator so that Mike and the adults providing supervision were aware of what he should be doing at what time (e.g., homework, chores, play, curfew). In addition, Mike's mother and MST therapist developed a contingency plan that clearly specified inappropriate verbalizations (i.e., curses and threats) and provided clear consequences for those behaviors, such as removal of access to phone and television privileges. Appropriate behavior was rewarded with access to privileges (Principles 3 and 7). Although she could not monitor Mike's behavior at all times, his mother started making random calls to check on his behavior with the adult scheduled to supervise Mike that evening.

The MST therapist used observation and interviews with Mike's family members and his coach to determine whether these interventions were impacting Mike's aggressive behaviors. In addition, the frequency, duration, and intensity of verbal outbursts were tracked daily by Mike's mother or the brother providing supervision, and these were reviewed by the MST therapist.

Individual Interventions

Mike's alcohol use was monitored closely by his mother and family members. In addition, random Breathalyzer tests were employed by the therapist, and eventually by Mike's mother, to assess his alcohol consumption.

School Interventions

Mike's behavior at home improved quickly with these interventions, but he continued to engage in aggressive behavior at school. School observations suggested that Mike was subjected to peer pressure to fight and act out in class, and that his teacher was not consistent in the use of negative consequences with Mike, nor did she reinforce his prosocial behaviors. To address these concerns, a plan was developed, with recommendations from Mike's teacher and the school counselor, that provided emergency consultation with the therapist, same-day response from Mike's mother for any school disruption, and contingency management (Principle 6). In a meeting scheduled by the therapist that included the teacher, school counselor, and Mike's mother, the treatment goals were reviewed and the school was reengaged (i.e., agreed to delay the expulsion decision). In addition, the meeting helped overcome some of the negative attributions held by the teacher toward the mother and vice versa (Principle 5). A daily report card was developed and instituted such that Mike's verbal or physical aggression resulted in response cost and positive practice (e.g., time-out, apologizing publicly for his inappropriate behavior) and aversive consequences at home (e.g., loss of privileges). His appropriate interactions with peers and teachers, on the other hand, were rewarded with praise from the teacher and points to be used toward tangible rewards (e.g., time in the library to listen to music; permission to get involved in extracurricular school activities that Mike thought he would enjoy) and access to privileges at home.

In addition to the daily report card, clear guidelines were laid out by the principal specifying what Mike had to accomplish in order to return to his mainstream classes. Specifically, Mike needed to demonstrate appropriate behavior for 3 weeks, with no verbal or physical assaults. To reduce the influence of negative peers, Mike reviewed with his therapist ways to avoid engaging in fights when provoked, and with his teacher, ways to avoid high-risk situations (e.g., crowded hallways just before and following lunch and free periods).

As with all aspects of the treatment program, the therapist was responsible for tracking each component of the home and school interventions to ensure appropriate implementation and to determine whether the plans were decreasing Mike's inappropriate behaviors (Principle 8).

Outcomes

Mike followed the home and school behavioral plans, eliminated his drinking, and exhibited fewer behavioral problems across contexts. These interventions dramatically reduced Mike's verbal aggression at home and his verbal and physical aggression at school. Unable to reach the 3-week criterion without any infractions, Mike was not returned to his mainstream class by the end of the school year. However, his improvement was such that the school agreed to enroll him in mainstream classes the following year. In addition, Mike continued to play basketball at the community center and, during the school year, became involved in the school newspaper. Mike's mother, with the support of the therapist, was able to maintain household standards such that she was not solely responsible for upkeep and finances. Mike's uncle and 19-year-old brother continued to drink excessively but no longer did so in Mike's presence. Moreover, they were gainfully employed and able to help with household expenses.

In summary, this case illustrates the necessity of developing a team comprising the major stakeholders in a child's social ecology to effect long-term, positive change. The complexity of such treatment is much greater than when dealing only with a child, or only with a family. The ecological validity of the treatment, however, is also greater and likely accounts to some degree for the consistently favorable outcomes.

EMPIRICAL FINDINGS AND EFFECTIVENESS

As recently summarized (Henggeler, 1999a, 1999b), rigorous evaluation has been fundamental to the development of MST. Seven randomized clinical trials and one quasi-experimental trial have been completed with youth presenting serious clinical problems and their families; 14 other studies with varying target populations are underway. The majority of the published trials have been conducted in field settings, and targeted populations including inner-city delinquents (Henggeler et al., 1986), violent and chronic juvenile offenders (Borduin et al., 1995; Henggeler et al., 1997; Henggeler, Melton, & Smith, 1992; Henggeler, Melton, Smith, Schoenwald, & Hanley, 1993), substance abusing or dependent juvenile offenders with high rates of psychiatric comorbidity (Brown, Henggeler, Schoenwald, Brondino, & Pickrel, 1999; Henggeler, Pickrel, & Brondino, 1999; Schoenwald, Ward, Henggeler, Pickrel, & Patel, 1996), youth presenting psychiatric emergencies (i.e., suicidal, homicidal, psychotic) (Henggeler, Rowland, et al., 1999; Schoenwald et al., 2000), maltreating families (Brunk, Henggeler, & Whelan, 1987), and juvenile sexual offenders (Borduin, Henggeler, Blaske, & Stein, 1990). Most of these studies have focused on youth deemed to be at imminent risk for out-of-home placements such as incarceration, residential treatment, or psychiatric hospitalization.

Results support the short- and long-term clinical effectiveness of MST, as well as its potential to produce significant cost savings and capacity to retain families in treatment. In comparison with control groups, and at a cost of approximately $5,000 per family, MST has consistently demonstrated improved family relations and family functioning, improved school attendance, and decreased adolescent drug use (Henggeler et al., 1998). Of importance to policymakers, MST has demonstrated 25–70% decreases in long-term rates of rearrest, and 47–64% decreases in long-term rates of days in institutional placements. These findings led reviewers to conclude that MST is a highly cost-effective treatment model (Aos, Phipps, Barnoski, & Lieb, 1999).

In addition to these clinical outcomes, MST has also been show to be consumer-friendly. Recent studies with substance abusing or dependent juvenile offenders (Henggeler et al., 1996) and youth presenting psychiatric emergencies (Henggeler, Rowland, et al., 1999) have had treatment completion rates of 98% and 97%, respectively. It should also be noted that the positive outcomes achieved by MST have occurred in the context of relatively inclusive participant criteria; that is, in most studies, comorbidity was *not* an exclusion criterion; boys *and* girls participated; and different racial, ethnic, and socioeconomic categories were well represented. Importantly, treatment effectiveness was not impacted as a function of these demographic factors (Borduin et al., 1995; Henggeler et al., 1992). Given these positive outcomes, the adoption of MST by providers who serve juvenile delinquents has increased dramatically in the past several years (Henggeler et al., 1998).

FUTURE DIRECTIONS

Experts across numerous, relevant fields were invited by the U.S. Surgeon General to identify state-of-the-art treatment programs and barriers to service access. Based on their comments, a national action agenda crafted for children's mental health included eight primary goals, with specific "action steps" identified to facilitate the achievement of these goals (U.S. Department of Health and Human Services, 2001). The goals and action steps are very much in line with the theory and practice of MST; in fact, MST was specifically named by several of these experts as one of the most clinically and cost-effective treatments for adolescents with serious behavioral problems. Recommended action steps included implementing evidence-based clinical practice, removing barriers to treatment by providing home-based treatment, specifically targeting youth at risk for entering the juvenile justice system, treating children within the broader context of the family, and providing for quality assurance mechanisms to determine whether treatment actually has the intended effects.

As noted by the Director of the National Institute of Mental Health, numerous barriers remain to the adoption of evidence-based treatment, and there is "a terrifying gap between what we know and how we act" (U.S. Department of Health and Human Services, 2001, p. 15). Thus, the next generation of research must focus on identifying those factors that will (1) increase the adoption of evidence-based treatments by major stakeholders (e.g., federal regulations, funding agencies that require evidence-based treatments), (2) encourage bright and motivated professionals to enter and remain in this challenging field (e.g., competitive base salaries, merit-based raises), and (3) improve and maintain the implementation of evidence-based practices with high fidelity (e.g., therapist training and ongoing supervision, assessment of therapist adherence to the treatment model).

Practitioners have the opportunity and the responsibility to provide the best possible treatment for children and adolescents. Appropriate implementation of evidence-based treatments can change the lives of youth presenting serious clinical problems, many of whom would otherwise end up in prison, or as educational and vocational failures. However, private and public providers must put in place, and funders must support, the resources necessary to allow therapists to address known risk factors and improve protective factors, overcome barriers to treatment access, empower caregivers, use evidence-based interventions, assume accountability for outcomes, and incorporate strong quality assurance systems to promote treatment fidelity.

ACKNOWLEDGMENTS

Writing of this chapter was supported by Grant Nos. RO1 DA10079, RO1 DA13066, and U10-DA13727 from the National Institute on Drug Abuse; Grant Nos. RO1 MH59138, RO1 MH51852, and RO1 MH60663 from the National Institute of Mental Health; Grant No. RO1

AA12202 from the National Institute on Alcohol Abuse and Alcoholism; Grant No. 96.2013 from the Casey Foundation; Grant No. A10535 A from the South Carolina Department of Health and Human Services—Federal Flow Down; and Grant No. PO1 HS10871 from the Agency for Healthcare Research and Quality.

REFERENCES

Aos, S., Phipps, P., Barnoski, R., & Lieb, R. (1999). *The comparative costs and benefits of programs to reduce crime: A review of national research findings with implications for Washington State, Version 3.0.* Olympia, WA: Washington State Institute for Public Policy.

Arnold, M. E., & Hughes, J. N. (1999). First do no harm: Adverse effects of grouping deviant youth for skills training. *Journal of School Psychology, 37*, 99–115.

Bickman, L., & Noser, K. (1999). Meeting the challenges in the delivery of child and adolescent mental health services in the next millennium: The continuous quality improvement approach. *Applied and Preventive Psychology, 8*, 247–255.

Borduin, C. M., Henggeler, S. W., Blaske, D. M., & Stein, R. J. (1990). Multisystemic treatment of adolescent sexual offenders. *International Journal of Offender Therapy and Comparative Criminology, 34*, 105–113.

Borduin, C. M., Mann, B. J., Cone, L. T., Henggeler, S. W., Fucci, B. R., Blaske, D. M., & Williams, R. A. (1995). Multisystemic treatment of serious juvenile offenders: Long-term prevention of criminality and violence. *Journal of Consulting and Clinical Psychology, 63*, 569–578.

Bronfenbrenner, U. (1979). *The ecology of human development: Experiments by nature and design.* Cambridge, MA: Harvard University Press.

Brown, T. L., Henggeler, S. W., Schoenwald, S. K., Brondino, M. J., & Pickrel, S. G. (1999). Multisystemic treatment of substance abusing and dependent juvenile delinquents: Effects on school attendance at posttreatment and 6-month follow-up. *Children's Services: Social Policy, Research, and Practice, 2*, 81–93.

Brunk, M., Henggeler, S. W., & Whelan, J. P. (1987). Comparison of multisystemic therapy and parent training in the brief treatment of child abuse and neglect. *Journal of Consulting and Clinical Psychology, 55*, 171–178.

Dishion, T. J., McCord, J., & Poulin, F. (1999). When interventions harm: Peer groups and problem behavior. *American Psychologist, 54*, 755–764.

Elliott, D. S. (Series Ed.). (1998). *Blueprints for violence prevention* (University of Colorado, Center for the Study of Prevention of Violence). Boulder, CO: Blueprints.

Farrington, D. P., & Welsh, B. C. (1999). Delinquency prevention using family-based interventions. *Children and Society, 13*, 287–303.

Garbarino, J. (2001). Violent children: Where do we point the finger of blame? [Editorial]. *Archives of Pediatric and Adolescent Medicine, 155*, 13–14.

Henggeler, S. W. (1997). The development of effective drug abuse services for youth. In J. A. Egerston, D. M. Fox, & A. I. Leshner (Eds.), *Treating drug abusers effectively* (pp. 253–279). New York: Blackwell.

Henggeler, S. W. (1999a). Multisystemic treatment of serious clinical problems in children and adolescents. *Clinician's Research Digest, 21*, 1–2.

Henggeler, S. W. (1999b). Multisystemic therapy: An overview of clinical procedures, outcomes, and policy implications. *Child Psychology and Psychiatry Review, 4*, 2–10.

Henggeler, S. W., Cunningham, P. B., Pickrel, S. G., Schoenwald, S. K., & Brondino, M. J. (1996). Multisystemic therapy: An effective violence prevention approach for serious juvenile offenders. *Journal of Adolescence, 19*, 47–61.

Henggeler, S. W., Melton, G. B., Brondino, M. J., Schere, D. G., & Hanley, J. H. (1997). Multisystemic therapy with violent and chronic juvenile offenders and their families: The role of treatment fidelity in successful dissemination. *Journal of Consulting and Clinical Psychology, 65*, 821–833.

Henggeler, S. W., Melton, G. B., & Smith, L. A. (1992). Family preservation using multisystemic therapy: An effective alternative to incarcerating serious juvenile offenders. *Journal of Consulting and Clinical Psychology, 60,* 953–961.

Henggeler, S. W., Melton, G. B., Smith, L. A., Schoenwald, S. K., & Hanley, J. H. (1993). Family preservation using multisystemic treatment: Long-term follow-up to a clinical trial with serious juvenile offenders. *Journal of Child and Family Studies, 2,* 283–293.

Henggeler, S. W., Pickrel, S. G., & Brondino, M. J. (1999). Multisystemic treatment of substance abusing and dependent delinquents: Outcomes, treatment fidelity, and transportability. *Mental Health Services Research, 1,* 171–184.

Henggeler, S. W., Rodick, J. D., Borduin, C. M., Hanson, C. L., Watson, S. M., & Urey, J. R. (1986). Multisystemic treatment of juvenile offenders: Effects on adolescent behavior and family interactions. *Developmental Psychology, 22,* 132–141.

Henggeler, S. W., Rowland, M. R., Randall, J., Ward, D., Pickrel, S. G., Cunningham, P. B., Miller, S. L., Edwards, J. E., Zealberg, J., Hand, L., & Santos, A. B. (1999). Home-based multisystemic therapy as an alternative to the hospitalization of youth in psychiatric crisis: Clinical outcomes. *Journal of the American Academy of Child and Adolescent Psychiatry, 38,* 1331–1339.

Henggeler, S. W., Schoenwald, S. K., Rowland, M. R., & Cunningham, P. B. (in press). *Multisystemic treatment of children and adolescents with serious emotional disturbance.* New York: Guildford Press.

Henggeler, S. W., & Schoenwald, S. K. (1998). *Multisystemic therapy supervisory manual.* Charleston, SC: Multisystemic Therapy Institute.

Henggeler, S. W., & Schoenwald, S. K. (1999). The role of quality assurance in achieving outcomes in MST programs. *Journal of Juvenile Justice and Detention Services, 14,* 1–17.

Henggeler, S. W., Schoenwald, S. K., Borduin, C. M., Rowland, M. D., & Cunningham, P. B. (1998). *Multisystemic treatment of antisocial behavior in children and adolescents.* New York: Guilford Press.

Huey, S. J., Henggeler, S. W., Brondino, M. J., & Pickrel, S. G. (2000). Mechanisms of change in multisystemic therapy: Reducing delinquent behavior through therapist adherence and improved family and peer functioning. *Journal of Consulting and Clinical Psychology, 68,* 451–467.

Kazdin, A. E., & Weisz, J. R. (1998). Identifying and developing empirically supported child and adolescent treatments. *Journal of Consulting and Clinical Psychology, 66,* 19–36.

Loeber, R., & Farrington, D. P. (Eds.). (1998). *Serious and violent juvenile offenders: Risk factors and successful interventions.* Thousand Oaks, CA: Sage.

Mikeson, L. D., & Shaha, S. (1996). Improving quality in psychotherapy. *Psychotherapy, 33,* 225–236.

National Institute on Drug Abuse. (1999). *Principles of drug addiction treatment: A research-based guide* (NIH Publication No. 99–4180). Bethesda, MD: National Institutes of Health.

Rowland, M. D., Henggeler, S. W., Gordon, A. M., Pickrel, S. G., Cunningham, P. B., & Edwards, J. E. (2000). Adapting multisystemic therapy to serve youth presenting psychiatric emergencies: Two case studies. *Child Psychology and Psychiatry Review, 5,* 30–43.

Schoenwald, S. K., & Henggeler, S. W. (2002). Services research and family based treatment. In H. Liddle, G. Diamond, R. Levant, & J. Bray (Eds.), *Family psychology intervention science* (pp. 259–282). Washington, DC: American Psychological Association.

Schoenwald, S. K., Henggeler, S. W., Brondino, M. J., & Rowland, M. D. (2000). Multisystemic therapy: Monitoring treatment fidelity. *Family Process, 39,* 83–103.

Schoenwald, S. K., Ward, D. M., Henggeler, S. W., Pickrel, S. G., & Patel, H. (1996). MST treatment of substance abusing or dependent adolescent offenders: Costs of reducing incarceration, inpatient, and residential placement. *Journal of Child and Family Studies, 5,* 431–444.

Schoenwald, S. K., Ward, D. M., Henggeler, S. W., & Rowland, M. D. (2000). MST vs. hospitalization for crisis stabilization of youth: Placement outcomes 4 months post-referral. *Mental Health Services Research, 2,* 3–12.

Sluyter, G. V. (1998). Total quality management in behavioral healthcare. In P. W. Corrigaon & D. F. Gifford (Eds.), *Building teams and programs for effective psychiatric rehabilitation: New directions for mental health services, No. 79* (pp. 35–43). San Francisco: Jossey-Bass.

Tate, D. C., Reppucci, N. D., & Mulvey, E. P. (1995). Violent juvenile delinquents: Treatment effectiveness and implications for future action. *American Psychologist, 50*, 777–781.

U.S. Department of Health and Human Services. (1999). *Mental health: A report of the Surgeon General—executive summary.* Rockville, MD: Author.

U.S. Department of Health and Human Services. (2001). *Report of the Surgeon General's Conference on Children's Mental Health: A national action agenda.* Rockville, MD: Author.

19

Cognitive-Behavioral Therapy for Severe Personality Disorders

Arthur Freeman

Noted psychoanalyst Frieda Fromm-Reichmann taught students that there were two kinds of patients: Those that they helped rather easily, and those that they ultimately learned from. Given Fromm-Reichmann's view, the therapy of patients with various disorders of character or personality are perhaps the most educational experiences in the clinician's caseload. Typically, these patients do not believe that the life problems that confront them are their fault or issue. They see the world, "others," circumstances and situations, the configuration of the stars and the planets, or just bad luck as the cause of their difficulties. Their percepts are generally ego-syntonic, so that they will not usually opt for psychotherapy as a way of coping with life problems. When they do come for therapy, they often do so unwillingly, and then only because of family pressure or legal remand. It is not their first choice for changing their circumstance. The patients with personality disorders are often baffled by the negative responses of others. They may be mystified by the situations in which they seem to find themselves, often seeing difficulties that they encounter in dealing with other people or tasks as external and independent of their behavior. They may have little idea about how they got to be the way they are, how they contribute to their life problems, or, most importantly, how to change. The individuals with personality disorders as part of the clinical picture generally require more work within the session, a longer duration for therapy, and more therapist energy than is expended with and for other non-personality-disordered patients. All of this expenditure of time and energy occurs without the same rate of change and satisfaction for both the therapist and the patient (Beck, Freeman, & Associates, 1990; Costello, 1996; Freeman, Pretzer, Fleming, & Simon, 1990; Gunderson, 2001; Gunderson & Gabbard, 2000; Kernberg, 1984; Stone, 1993).

By definition, the problems that they manifest are "enduring patterns of perceiving, relating to, and thinking about the environment and oneself that are exhibited in a wide range of social and personal contexts" (American Psychiatric Association, 2000, p. 630). When therapists recognize that treatment of an individual involves the treatment of a personality disorder, they often view these patients as especially difficult (Merbaum & Butcher, 1982; Rosenbaum, Horowitz, & Wilner, 1986). In many cases, this view is realistic. It is based not so much on the patient's personality disorder but on the relative severity of the disorder and its degree of impact on the person's life. The greater the severity of the personality disorder, the greater the therapeutic difficulty will likely be.

The goals of working with the patient with an Axis I diagnosis (e.g., depression) and a concomitant personality disorder must be modified from the standard treatment for the Axis I disorder. For the patient with both Axis I and Axis II problems, the Axis I problem(s) will stimulate or activate the Axis II disorder, and the Axis II disorder will serve as a substrate to fuel the Axis I problems. This bidirectional influence makes the treatment far more complex. The therapist must decide where to begin the therapy work, where to focus the therapy, and what reasonable goals to expect for both the Axis I and the Axis II problems. In all cases, the treatment goal is not cure, but rather modification of the patient's behaviors and thoughts. Broadly, the behavior manifested by the individual with a personality disorder is compulsive, inflexible, thoughtless, highly noticeable, negative, maladaptive, extreme, at odds with the general community, energy consuming, ego-syntonic (self-consonant), and interpersonally conflictual. Embedded within each problem or problem area is the suggestion of the treatment focus or direction. For example, the goal of working with the patient whose behavior is compulsive is to increase his or her repertoire of response. When there is inflexibility, the treatment goal is to help the patient to have a greater range of motion. Thought*less* behavior needs a greater thoughtfulness. Highly noticeable and negative behavior needs to be reduced and/or camouflaged so that it is less noticeable. When the behavior is maladaptive and extreme, the therapy must focus on greater adaptation to the demands and expectations of the general community. Essentially, this would involve a modulation or a moderation of the identified behavior(s), thereby moving the patient from the extremes of behavior to more central positions. Given that the behavior is self-consonant, the person may not see a need to change. In the words of the immortal Popeye the Sailor Man, the patient believes that "I y'am what I y'am." The therapy must focus on goals that are perceived as valuable to the patient (e.g., getting more of what the patient wants). Inasmuch as the behavior of the person with a personality disorder is typically interpersonally conflictual, we can expect the interpersonal conflicts to be played out in the therapy. The patient (or therapist) who expects that as a result of therapy the patient will become a totally different person than he or she was prior to therapy will invariably be disappointed. By making small steps toward the desired goals, therapy can move ahead slowly but effectively.

Even when these individuals have strong motivation to change, they are often limited because they are skills deficient. The spirit may be willing but, in some cases, the skills may be weak. To put it simply, the years of not acting in a particular way may have left them skills deficient. They do not have the skills to make the life changes that they, and others, expect of them, so therapy must have a strong psychoeducational (skills building) focus.

THE THERAPEUTIC RELATIONSHIP

The therapeutic relationship will be one of the key ingredients in the treatment of the patient with a personality disorder. It will be a microcosm of the patient's responses to other people and situations in his or her environment. As noted earlier, the lack of interpersonal skills, motivation, or belief that it is important to be interpersonally connected, or the fear of closeness, will all impact the therapeutic relationship. The individual with a personality disorder is frequently exquisitely attuned to the slightest nuance or suggestion within a relationship and, by virtue of that sensitivity, is easily triggered to respond when he or she perceives some slight, challenge, disagreement, or potential loss. For example, being 2 minutes late for a session with a patient with a dependent personality disorder may evoke anxiety about abandonment. The same 2-minute lateness will raise the specter of being taken advantage of in the patient with the paranoid personality disorder, and anger from the patient with a borderline personality disorder. Building and maintaining the trust essential to good therapy is generally imperative.

The collaborative nature of the therapy must be constantly stressed. Therapists must keep in mind that collaboration is not always 50:50. With many patients, the collaboration may be 80:20, or 90:10, with the therapist needing to carry the greater burden, which often brings with it a high level of stress and burnout. Without the therapist's active support, the patient may quickly become frightened and disillusioned, and leave therapy. The collaborative set involves setting mutually acceptable goals for therapy that are reasonable, sequential, realistic, meaningful, proximal, and within the patient's repertoire. The therapist's negative reactions to the patient, often termed countertransference, must be acknowledged and addressed directly by the therapist.

It is essential that the therapist pay careful attention to the content, context, and style of the patient's presentation. Each element can offer clues to the patient's cognitions. Each clue must then be questioned for accuracy. Similarly, the therapist must be keenly attuned to any and all mood shifts, whether positive or negative.

To avoid problems of his or her own misstatement or exaggeration, it is essential for the therapist to take notes for *precise* recollection. Making an approximate statement will for some patients indicate a lack of caring. Related to this is the need for the therapist to be aware of and address any heightened anxiety on his or her own part, or that of the patient.

It is also important for the therapist to be aware that making a statement such as "that was a very good job" may mean that the patient may always expect his or her behavior to be seen positively or feel that the therapist is just "saying" that because that is what therapists are supposed to do. It is important to avoid or try to limit judgmental statements (either positive or negative).

If the therapist is comfortable in doing so, he or she should try to use the patient's language and metaphors as often as possible. If, however, the language or metaphors are uncomfortable for the therapist, then he or she must address the issue with the patient. For example, John's language was designed to shock. Every third word in a sentence was a four-letter expletive. The therapist chose not to mirror this language inasmuch as it was not how the therapist spoke.

The relationship can be influenced by how the therapist self-monitors. For example:

Though an experienced therapist, Alex was unable to keep his personal life out of his sessions. He was distracted by his difficult divorce. He sometimes did not focus on what the patient was saying. When one patient said that Alex did not seem to be listening, it was important that Alex admit the "core" of truth in this patient reaction. Trying to interpret away or turn the perception back on the patient will ultimately backfire. As the punch line on an old joke states, the patient may say, "I'm crazy, not stupid."

The therapist cannot avoid difficult issues. For cluster B patients, the "difficult" issues are often highly charged with emotion, often with anger. These need to be confronted clearly and directly. Intimidation is part of the problem only if the therapist allows him- or herself to be intimidated. The therapist needs to remain calm though empathetic in the face of patient upset. The emotional or difficult issue will often manifest itself when issues are raised with 5 minutes left in the session. The therapy must be particularly aware of time constraints in the individual session or in the therapy in general.

One important relationship-building technique is to ask frequently for patient feedback. This must take place throughout the session and especially at the end. It will be important for the therapist to know what ideas the patient is taking home from each therapy session.

Finally, it is essential for the therapist to maintain limits and boundaries, and be aware of and address negative or positive countertransference.

ASSESSMENT

The initial goal of therapy is an assessment of the problems. Based on the assessment data, the therapist will first develop a conceptualization of the patient's problems and then a realistic, appropriate, and collaborative treatment plan.

The assessment will be both formal and informal. The first goal is to assess whether the problem is mild, moderate, or severe. We recommend that the personality disorder diagnoses be consistent with the DSM coding system used for major depressive disorders. This would involve the following codes: "The fifth digit indicates the following: 1 for Mild severity, 2 for Moderate severity, 3 for Severe without Psychotic Features, 4 for Severe with Psychotic Features, 5 for Partial Remission, 6 for In Full Remission, and 0 if Unspecified" (American Psychiatric Association, 2000, p. 319).

Formal measures include the Millon Clinical Multiaxial Inventory, Third Edition (MCMI-III; Millon, 1994) or Minnesota Multiphasic Personality Inventory–2 (MMPI-2; National Computer Systems, 1989). This revision of the classic MMPI offers a number of scales that identify personality disorders.

There are, however, a number clinical assessment tools that can help the clinician identify persons who have personality disorders.

The chain or functional analysis is a simple and helpful assessment tool that can indicate potential points of intervention. The chain analysis involves the therapist having the patient follow a sequence of experience(s) from start to finish. The goal is to find the "weakest link" that can then offer possibilities for intervention. Figure 19.1 illustrates a simple chain diagram. The question for the therapist to ask the patient is "Then what?" The functional analysis, also useful as a homework tool, can help the patient to think in terms of sequelae and consequences (Figure 19.1).

A second screening for personality disorders emerges from the interview and patient history, and includes the following factors:

1. The chronicity of problem based on a report from the patient or significant others.
2. Frequent resistance or therapeutic noncompliance.
3. Therapy seems to have come to a halt for no apparent reason.
4. The patient is unaware of the effect of his or her behavior on others.
5. There is a question about the patient's motivation for treatment.
6. The patient gives "lip service" to therapy, but there are no observable changes.

386   PSYCHOLOGICAL TREATMENTS FOR SEVERE PERSONALITY DISORDERS

7. The patient views problems as "core" to self.
8. Therapy is a series of "brushfires" or crises.
9. There are extensive previous therapeutic contacts.
10. Self-consonant (ego-syntonic) nature of problems.
11. Poor self-monitoring of affect or action.
12. Poor or impaired monitoring of the reactions of others.

While none of these points is by itself diagnostic, the pattern must lead the therapist to explore the possibility for personality disorder.

The Freeman Diagnostic Profile System (Freeman, 1998) uses the DSM-IV criteria to construct a profile that points to targets for therapy (Figure 19.2).

Using DSM criteria, the clinician reviews the diagnostic criteria *with the patient* and then maps out the targets for therapy, based on the motivation of the patient and the therapist, the skills of the therapist and the patient, the available time, and the stated goals of the therapy. Therapeutic change can then be assessed over the baseline.

We believe that it makes sense to offer and explain the patient's diagnosis. Patients

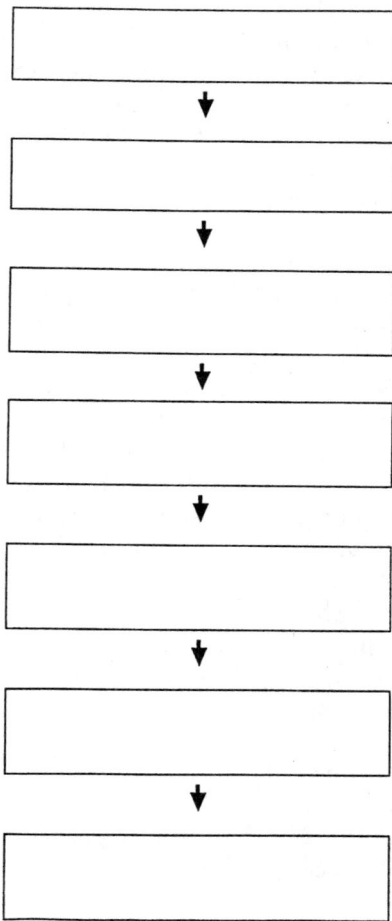

FIGURE 19.1. Chain analysis.

DIAGNOSTIC PROFILING SYSTEM
(© FREEMAN, 1998) REVISED EDITION

Date of Assessment:_____
Session#:____ Evaluator:_____

Patient Name:_____ Patient#:_____ Location:_____

Birthdate:_____ Age:_____ Race:_____ Gender:_____ Birthorder:_____ Marital/Children:_____

Employment:_____ Education:_____ Disability:_____ Medication:_____

Physician:_____ Referral Question:_____

Instructions: Record the diagnosis including the code number. Briefly identify the criteria for the selected diagnosis. Working with the patient either directly or as part of the data gathering of the clinical interview, SCALE the SEVERITY of EACH CRITERION for the patient at the PRESENT TIME. Indicate the level of severity on the grid.

DIAGNOSIS (DSM/ICD) with Code:
Axis I:_____
Axis II:_____
Axis III:_____

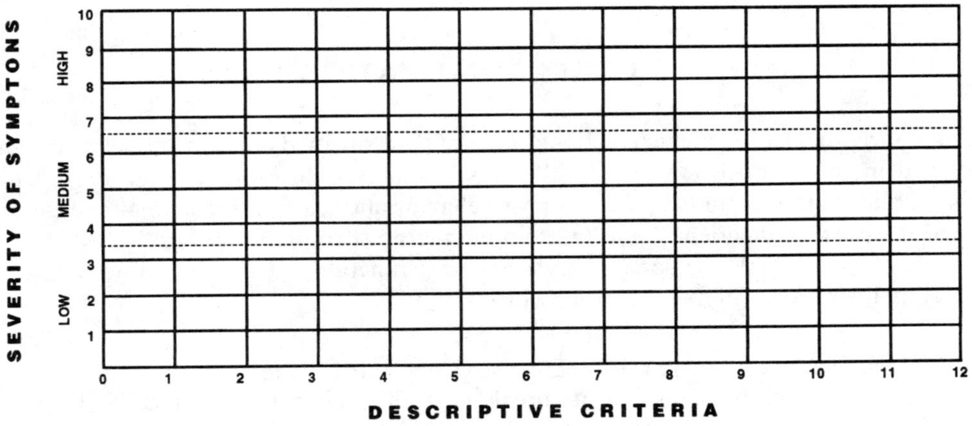

[Grid: SEVERITY OF SYMPTONS (y-axis, 1–10, LOW/MEDIUM/HIGH) vs DESCRIPTIVE CRITERIA (x-axis, 0–12)]

CRITERIA:
1 _____   7 _____
2 _____   8 _____
3 _____   9 _____
4 _____   10 _____
5 _____   11 _____
6 _____   12 _____

Do you believe that the above noted criteria are a reasonably accurate sample of the patient's behavior? **YES or NO**
If **NO**, please indicate why:_____
Are there any reasons to believe that this individual is an imminent danger to himself/herself or others? **YES or NO**
If **YES**, please indicate the danger._____

FIGURE 19.2. Freeman Diagnostic Profiling System.

often have been given diagnoses either directly or indirectly. It is incumbent on the therapist to explain the meaning of those diagnoses. This does not necessarily mean the "official" DSM label (though that may be the case with some patients), but a less pejorative and more easily understandable term. For example, patients with a paranoid personality can be called "cautious." Patients with a schizoid personality can be called "autonomous." Patients with a schizotypal personality can be called "creative in their view of the world." Patients with borderline personality are called "very sensitive." Patients with histrionic personality can be called "dramatic or having a distinctive flair." Patients with a narcissistic personality will readily accept that they are "special." Patients with an antisocial personality can be said to "march to their own drummer." Patients with an avoidant personality will not argue when told the problem is that they are "shy." Patients with a dependent personality will likely see themselves as "people persons." Patients with an obsessive–compulsive personality can be called "careful and structured."

The goal in sharing these terms is not simply to find some euphemism for the "real" term but to use a behavioral descriptor that has relevance for the patient's life and meaning as an explanatory framework for understanding the problems.

CONCEPTUALIZATION

The conceptualization, which is based on the assessment data, is a model that can be viewed in three dimensions. If the therapist's conceptualization is accurate, it will do three things: (1) explain the patient's past behavior and experience, (2) make sense of the patient's present experience, and (3) help the therapist to predict future behavior.

Some individuals' personality style has been functional in life and is not considered an Axis II disorder. Witness the following:

Mark, a 67-year-old cardiothoracic surgeon, had for the past 40 years been up at 4:30 A.M. each morning. He ate breakfast and was in the hospital by 5:00 A.M. and in the surgical suite by 5:30. Mark would often do several procedures in a row. He would have lunch from noon to 1:00 P.M. and then attend meetings, teach, write, or dictate chart notes. He would be home at 6:00 P.M. If there were a need, he would return to the hospital in the evening or sometimes be called in for weekend emergencies that required his particular expertise. Even though he could have more junior staff perform the surgeries, he preferred to do them himself. As a result of his skill and creativity, Mark was quite successful. He had published several surgical texts and monographs, invented or modified surgical instruments, and was now head of the Department of Cardiothoracic Surgery at a large medical center.

The eldest son of immigrant parents who were Holocaust survivors, he knew at a very early age that his goal was medicine. Mark studied hard to get into a good college and won a scholarship. He went on to a prestigious medical school and then sought and was accepted into prized residencies in cardiology and then surgery. Mark had been married to Deborah for 35 years and had two sons. His wife stated that she did not spend much time with him, but that was the "lot of the wife of a surgeon." Deborah described Mark as perfectionistic, demanding, and at, times, insulting. She stated that this was to be "expected" of a surgeon inasmuch as the wives of other surgeons compared notes and all agreed that this was the way that surgeons were and one had to accept it. She believed that underneath his bluster, Mark was warm and loving but could not show it. Likewise, his sons accepted his long hours of work and interpersonal style. It was, after all, the foundation for their financial ease as children, and they both credited their present success to his demandingness. One son was a physician, and the other, an attorney.

Mark had sought therapy at the request/entreaty of his wife. He was, at that point, no longer able to practice surgery due to the advancement of Parkinson's disease. Although he was still head of the department and could teach and write, none of these meant anything to Mark. Now when he arose at 4:30 A.M., he stalked the house with no place to go. He was depressed (Beck Depression Inventory = 42) and suicidal. Having worked so hard and been so successful, financially secure, and a good provider for his family, he was at a loss to explain his depression. He felt himself to be a failure, based on his lack of productivity. The same motivating idea ("You are what you produce") that had driven him to be successful now drove him to despair. Labeled for years as "dedicated" and "caring," his behavior was now seen as part of an obsessive–compulsive personality disorder.

Many Axis II patients are silent about or deny their personality problems as a reflection of the disorders themselves. Whether diagnosed as having personality disorders or not, some patients believe that their personalities are an appropriate focus of treatment, whereas others fear such a focus. The collaborative nature of goal setting is one of the most important features of cognitive therapy. Power struggles over conflicting goals usually impede progress (Foon, 1985).

UNDERSTANDING SCHEMAS

Personality disorders are probably one of the most striking representations of Beck's concept of schema (Beck et al., 1990; Freeman, 1987, 1988; Freeman et al., 1990). Schemas are templates that individuals use to organize and understand their world. Most people, however, are "schema blind" and unaware of the rules and templates they have developed. The goal of therapy is therefore to make the schemas explicit, so that they can be directly addressed. Inasmuch as these rules govern information processing and behavior, they can be classified into a variety of useful categories, such as personal, familial, cultural, religious, gender, or occupational schemas. Schemas can be inferred from behavior or assessed through interview and history taking. The degree to which particular schemas are on the continuum from active to inactive, as well as unchangeable to changeable, is an essential dimension in conceptualizing the patient's problems (Beck et al., 1990; Freeman, 1987, 1988; Freeman et al., 1990).

Active versus Inactive Schemas

The *active schemas* that govern our usual integration of information and everyday behavior have to do with how we integrate other people's behavior and generally relate to people and tasks. *Inactive schemas* are outside awareness and become active when a new situation relevant to the schema occurs. At the point that these schemas become active, they will govern behavior. When the stimulus situation is no longer present, the inactive schemas recede to their previous state of dormancy. For example, the notion of getting on a airliner and flying anywhere in the world became so commonplace that one could arrive 20 minutes before flight time, show a driver's license, and board a plane. One could carry a set of steak knives as a gift, or have a Swiss Army knife on a key chain. There was some vague idea that flying might have hazards, but these were minimal. Subsequent to the horror of September 11, 2001, flying takes on a new dimension. What was dormant ("Flying may be dangerous") now becomes active ("Flying *is* dangerous"). A person may state, "It's silly to be worried about strangers." Now others reinforce that same concern, especially if that stranger looks suspicious. The latent schema related to fear has been activated. When a schema is activated across all situations, whether or not relevant to the specific schema, the schema is said to be active. This activity is particularly prominent in the "neuroses" (Axis I disorders), in which every situation may be interpreted in terms of personal loss or defeat (depression) or danger (anxiety). In the personality disorders, the schemas are often highly charged and global.

Noncompelling versus Compelling Schemas

Schemas may be classified as noncompelling or compelling. A noncompelling schema is one that the individual believes in but can relatively easily challenge and/or surrender. Compelling schemas are not easily challenged and are modified only with great difficulty, or not at all. Historical examples include the religious or political martyrs who chose to die rather than surrender their compelling views. Since Axis II disorder patients are generally governed by long-lasting, habitual schemas, these deeply ingrained rules and beliefs are not easily changed, even when the patient is highly motivated to do so. The chronicity of the personality disorder results from the development of these dysfunctional schemas relatively early in life.

From birth through middle childhood, schemas continuously change through the process of adaptation to the requirements of life. Through the interactive processes of assimilation and accommodation, these schemas facilitate the organization and understanding of the phenomenological world (Freeman & Leaf, 1989; Rosen, 1989). For many reasons, some schemas do not mature and are maintained at an earlier level of development. This is the beginning of an Axis II problem. The schemas that are basically functional in this earlier part of life are being applied during later, more demanding times. While most of these early schemas at one time functioned to help the individual meet changing life/world experiences, they have long since lost their functional value by dint of never having been modified. For example, a 1-year-old child who would like to be picked up conveys this message to a caretaker by lifting his or her arms and grunting or crying. The caretaker responds by picking the child up. As the child matures, the schemas is altered. The schema "I can do for myself" develops, and the child no longer has the schematic worldview that "I need others to take care of me and meet my basic needs." When a child at age 1 demands attention and help, it is often thought of as cute. When that same schema is manifested at age 31, it is not cute, but quite dysfunctional. Often, compelling schemas that a patient often "knows" to be erroneous are hard to change. These schemas become fixed when they are reinforced and/or modeled by parents. Inasmuch as schemas have survival value, the therapist must be aware that even alluding to the need or goal of "giving it up" will arouse anxiety for the patient. After all, these rules are what, in patients' eyes, have allowed them to survive. The therapist must be aware that in working with patients with personality disorders, therapy will evoke anxiety because the individuals are being asked to give up who they are and to step out of their safety zone. It may be uncomfortable, limiting, and lonely in there, but to go out means "I may get hurt, and feel anxious." Beck and Emery (1985), in discussing the treatment of agoraphobia, state, "It is crucial that the patient experience anxiety in order to ensure that the primitive cognitive levels have been activated (since these levels are directly connected to the affects). The repeated, direct, on-the-spot recognition that the danger signals do not lead to catastrophe . . . enhance[s] the responsivity of the primitive level to more realistic inputs from above" (p. 129).

In discussing therapy plans with a patient diagnosed at intake as depressed and having a borderline personality disorder, the patient asked, "Why are you talking about trying to teach me to control my anxiety? I'm depressed. I'm not anxious at all." At that point the therapist told her about the need to master anxiety reduction skills, pointing out that these skills would be an essential factor in successful therapy inasmuch as the discussion of certain issues might be anxiety provoking. The therapist raised the discussion of ways in which the patient had isolated and put herself into an emotional cocoon. The patient responded, "It's good to have that safety and I don't understand why I should ever give it up." Unless the therapist starts to help the patient to cope with the increased anxiety by challenging perceived safety measures, she may leave therapy.

Given the importance of the schematic changes, we must recognize that they are difficult to alter. The schema is held firmly in place by behavioral, cognitive, and affective elements. Changing only one factor will probably not effectively change the schema. The therapeutic approach must take a tripartite approach. To take a cognitive approach and try to argue the patient out of their distortions will not work. Having the patient abreact within the session to fantasies or recollections will not be successful by itself. A therapeutic program that addresses all three areas is essential.

A second factor has to do with the stage of life in which the schemas were developed. For example, let us suppose that a child is born to a schizophrenic mother. The mother may shift in and out of the psychosis. She may at some moments remember the infant, and feed and comfort it. At other times the child is left hungry, cold, uncomforted, and uncomfortable, and will acquire ideas about the world in a sensorimotor mode. The child may have cellular reactions without words or images about the world being ungiving, confusing, arbitrary, and cruel. These "ideas" come from the "cloud" (Layden, Newman, Freeman, & Byers-Morse, 1993). Whether these vague ideas can then be modified using abstract verbal techniques is questionable. These individuals may be the patients that we cannot treat using the present therapeutic technology. Schemas learned early from a credible source and later strongly reinforced will similarly be hard to alter.

Schematic Reconstruction

The goal of the therapy is to help patients to identify the different rules by which they live. The change options can be viewed on a continuum. The first point on the continuum is *schematic restructuring*. This may be likened to urban renewal. Having decided that a structure is unsound, the decision is made to tear down the old structure and build a new one in its place. (This has been a goal of therapy for many years, particularly psychoanalysis.) Whether this restructuring is reasonable is very questionable. An example of schematic restructuring is when a person with a paranoid personality become a fully trusting individual.

Schematic Modification

A second possibility, *schematic modification*, involves smaller changes in the basic manner of responding to the world. This would be akin to modifying a kitchen in your home.

A coat of paint, new refrigerator and stove, and a new floor make the room look very different. There is no major reconstruction. In therapy, the person with a dependent personality disorder could be helped to modify the belief that "I cannot survive without the support of others" to "In almost every situation, I cannot survive without the support of others." This very small modification allows patients some "wiggle" room in his or her beliefs. The patient has moved from an absolute belief to one that is now conditional. Further modification might be "In most situations, I cannot survive without the support of others."

Schematic Reinterpretation

The third possibility, *schematic reinterpretation*, involves helping patients to understand and reinterpret their lifestyle and their schema in more functional ways. Using the example of airport safety, I would hope that the ads for airport security personnel include some reference to their being able to meet criteria for mild paranoid personality disorder. I think that we would all be far more comfortable knowing that the persons in charge of security are suspicious, distrusting, hypervigilant, and question the motives of others.

Schematic Camouflage

A fourth possibility, *schematic camouflage*, involves the patient being willing to self-instruct to deal with acknowledged areas of concern. For example:

> Howard, a psychologist, had grown up in a setting in which he was a favored child in a family of five children. He was called "the little prince." He developed a narcissistic personality disorder consistent with what he learned about being special. Howard also learned that this was not helping him in his career. He was able to camouflage or hide his disorder successfully until there was significant stress, and then the disorder came out very forcefully, but most of the time, he was able to contain the disordered behavior.

The most reasonable goal when working with patients with an Axis II disorder is either to modify or reinterpret the schemas. By schematic reinterpretation, the therapist can find ways for patients to deal with their schema/rules in a more adaptive and functional manner. Given that the rules are not necessarily good or bad, it would depend on how they are interpreted. For example, someone who had a great need to be loved or admired might choose to teach preschool children, who kiss and hug the teacher. For one who wants to be looked up to and respected, earning or buying a title (i.e., Professor, Doctor, or Colonel) can meet the need for status.

TREATMENT OF PERSONALITY DISORDERS

Perhaps the single most important element in treatment is the notion that the therapist must have a clear, strong idea of how the "finished product" of therapy will look. The idea of a free-floating, unstructured, meandering treatment is antithetical to cognitive therapy. The therapist must be able to set treatment goals that are reasonable, sequential, proximal, within the patient's potential repertoire, agreed to by the patient, and seen by the patient as valuable. If the therapist cannot share with the patient the realistic goals of therapy, the therapy cannot proceed. The idea "Let's start the therapy, move along, and see where we go" is not for therapy. That is more of a model for a mystery moonlight cruise. If schemas were all visual, a clear picture of the schema for therapy might show a therapist pointing at maps and pictures of existing and more accurate schemas. A more skillful or experienced therapist might have more maps and pictures than a less skillful one. The patient's vigilance about the details of the figures, and the willingness and ability to recall the images when under stress are important. In addition, in order to maintain trust, it is important for patients to understand in advance that they are on their own when they try to effect changes in their lives, but they can expect encouragement to proceed and moral support from their therapist, whatever their performance and its outcome.

Following the assessment, the therapist must make sure that the patient is educated either directly or indirectly about what cognitive-behavioral therapy involves. The initial therapeutic focus may be on relieving the presenting symptoms (i.e., anxiety or depression). In helping patients to deal with their anxiety or depression, the therapist can teach them the basic cognitive therapy skills necessary in working with the more difficult personality disorder. If the therapist can help the patient become less depressed or anxious, the patient may accept that this therapy may have some value after all, and it may be worthwhile continuing. Some patients with Axis II disorders may, having brought the anxiety and depression under control with fairly standard techniques, choose to leave therapy. One technique that may be helpful with these patients is to differentiate between "symptom therapy" and "schema therapy." By learning about the importance of working on the schemas, the patient may choose to stay in therapy.

The rate and frame of treatment must be discussed. Patients who expect that they will be "cured" in 12–20 sessions must be apprised of the greater severity and chronicity of these personality problems and how these problems will take a longer time to modify. Twelve to 20 months (or more) is a far more reasonable time frame for the treatment of personality disorders. Therapy can be structured in modules of 2–10 sessions. Rather than asking the patient to begin therapy with some vague notion of a time frame, the therapist can offer a series of modules that allow a focus on a particular area, issue, relationship, problem, and skills deficit. This keeps both therapist and patient focused.

The patient's significant others can be valuable allies in the therapeutic endeavor by helping the patient to do homework and test reality, and by offering support in making changes. The significant others can also be important sources of data about the patient's past behaviors. Meeting with the significant others may enable the therapist not only to piece together a family history of problems but also to understand what keeps the patient behaving in the same dysfunctional way. Finally, the significant others might be involved in marital or family therapy with the patient. For example:

> Anna, a 41-year-old woman who was unmarried and lived at home, came to the therapy with her parents. She was employed as a secretary in a law firm, a job that she had since high school. When invited into the office by the therapist, she asked if her parents could come in with her. Rather than create a difficult situation, the therapist agreed. Anna then sat quietly while her parents explained to the therapist the problem (Anna's shyness, her lack of friends, and her poor social skills), discussed Anna's weaknesses (there were, in their view, many), and asked questions of the therapist regarding his experience and credentials. Early in the session, the therapist asked Anna a question. She began to respond, but it appeared that she might disagree with her mother. Her mother turned to Anna and said, "You don't know what you're talking about." Anna said no more in the session. As a result of meeting

with her parents in this first session, it was clear why Anna had developed the way she had. She was shunted aside, even to the point of coming to the initial therapy session and not being either encouraged or allowed to speak for herself.

HOMEWORK

Homework is the "glue" that makes therapy contiguous. It is the between-session connectors that give the flow to therapy. We must recognize that therapy cannot and does not happen an hour a week within the confines of the therapy room. The patient must be socialized to use homework throughout the therapy, starting with the first session. If the patient does not develop a homework "tradition," then when the therapy sessions come to an end, so will the change process. When therapy ends, everything is homework. The homework must be cast as a no-failure experience. If the patient does the homework, the results can be reviewed. If he or she does not do the homework, the therapist can use that as grist for the therapeutic mill regarding what stopped the patient from doing the homework. The homework is not optional but rather is the laboratory part of the therapy.

The homework should grow organically from the session material, so that it is meaningful. It is essential for the therapist to know whether the patient has the time, motivation, and resources to do the homework. (For an excellent description of a range of homework assignments, see Rosenthal, 2000.)

IMPEDIMENTS TO CHANGE

Rather than use terms such as "resistance" or "noncompliance," I prefer the term "impediments to change." These impediments come from four sources: the patient, the therapist, the environment, and the nature of the patient's pathology. As noted earlier, each area of difficulty must be used as a cue for designing and building the treatment. Clearly, not all factors affect every patient, and the therapist can go through the list to identify issues that are relevant for a particular patient.

Patient factors
1. Lack of patient skill to comply.
2. The patient has negative cognitions regarding previous treatment failure.
3. The patient has negative cognitions regarding the consequences of his or her changing on others in his or her world.
4. The patient has secondary gain from maintaining his or her symptoms.
5. The patient has a fear of changing.
6. Lack of patient motivation to change.
7. The patient has a negative set about virtually everything in life, including therapy.
8. Limited or poor self-monitoring.
9. Limited or poor awareness or monitoring of others.
10. The patient has a demanding personal style.
11. The patient is constantly frustrated with lack of treatment progress.
12. The patient has the perception of lowered status by virtue of needing or of being in treatment.

Therapist factors
1. Lack of therapist skill.
2. The patient's and therapist's distortions are congruent.
3. The therapist has not socialized the patient to the therapy.
4. Lack of collaboration and a poor working alliance.
5. The therapist lacks data about the patient.
6. The therapist believes that he or she is far smarter and talented than he or she really is (therapeutic narcissism).
7. Poor timing of interventions.
8. The therapist lacks experience.
9. Therapy goals are unstated, unrealistic, or vague.
10. Lack of explicit contract and agreement with therapy goals.
11. The therapist lacks an understanding of the developmental process.
12. The therapist has unrealistic expectations of the patient.

Environmental factors
1. Environmental stressors preclude changing.
2. Significant others foil or sabotage therapy.
3. Agency reinforcement of pathology and illness allowing the patient to maintain compensation and/or benefits.
4. Cultural issues preclude help seeking.
5. The homeostasis of the family system operates to keep the patient in his or her "role."
6. Ongoing family pathology reinforces and continues to model the pathological behavior.
7. Unrealistic demands on the patient by family members.
8. Unrealistic demands on the patient by institutions or agencies.
9. Financial factors limit therapy and/or change.
10. The patient lacks support.
11. Cognitive dissonance based on conflicting resources or demands.
12. The patient is in a physically, mentally, or psychologically abusive environment.

Patient problem/pathology factors
1. Patient rigidity foils treatment compliance.
2. Significant medical or physiological problems.
3. The patient has difficulty in establishing trust.
4. The patient's need for autonomy and independence precludes forming a therapeutic relationship (autonomy press).
5. Significant affective, verbal, or behavioral impulsivity.
6. The patient may be demented or confused.
7. The patient has limited cognitive ability.
8. Symptom profusion on Axes I, II, III, and IV.
9. The patient is very dependent.
10. No matter the data, the patient's minor thought disorder involves constant self-devaluation.
11. The patient is emotionally drained and has limited energy to devote to therapy.
12. There may be dissociation.

THERAPY TECHNIQUES

Cognitive-behavioral therapy for personality disorders progresses in the same manner as cognitive-behavioral therapy for other disorders. The therapist working with the patient to test the meaning, reality, or validity of the thoughts and perceptions follows the identification of the patient's distorted thinking. The techniques can be somewhat arbitrarily divided into cognitive and behavioral techniques. The particular mix of cognitive and behavioral techniques is, of course, related to the needs of the patient. As discussed earlier, the more severe the pathology, the more behavioral the approach. The less severe the behavioral pathology, the more cognitive the approach (Figure 19.3).

Cognitive and behavioral techniques play complementary roles in the treatment of personality disorders. Behavioral techniques serve to move the patient into a new position, and the cognitive ones serve to develop new schemas and to modify or reinterpret old ones. Ultimately, of course, the cognitive techniques probably account for most of the change that occurs (Deffenbacher, Story, Stark, Hogg, & Brandon, 1987). The cognitive work, like its behavioral counterpart, requires more care and precision than usual when clients have personality disorders. The schemas of these patients are often unusually defective, even when the behavior has been corrected, and a larger variety and longer duration of cognitive reworking is typically required. While the first principle of treatment for personality disorders is to emphasize behavioral methods, *the final principle is to follow up with thorough cognitive ones.*

The goals of using the behavioral techniques are threefold. First, the therapist may need to work very directly to alter self-defeating behaviors. Second, patients may be skills deficient, and the therapy must include a skills building component. Third, the behavioral assignments can be used as homework to help to test out cognitions. Behavioral techniques that can be helpful include (1) activity monitoring and scheduling, which permits

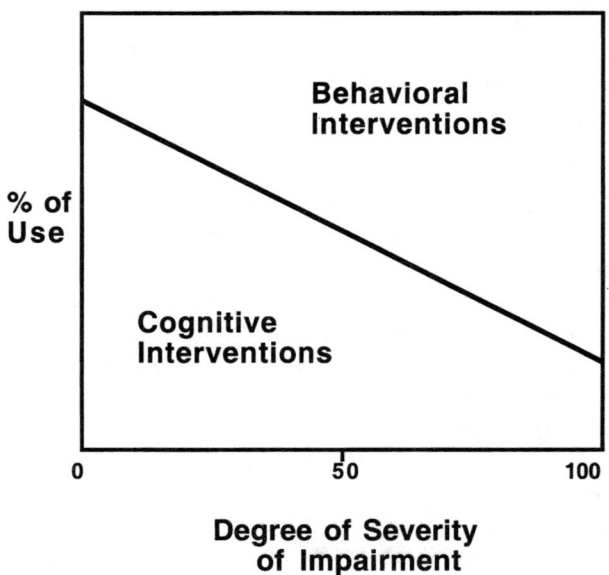

FIGURE 19.3. Relative use of cognitive and behavioral techniques.

retrospective identification of briar patches and prospective planning of changes; (2) behavioral rehearsal, modeling, assertiveness training, and role playing for skills development prior to early efforts to respond more effectively, either in old problematic situations or in new ones; (3) relaxation training and behavioral distraction techniques for use when anxiety becomes an imminent problem during efforts to change; (4) *in vivo* exposure, either by arranging conditions for a problematic situation by appointment in a consultation setting, or by arranging for the therapist to go with the client to a problematic setting to help him or her deal with dysfunctional schemas and actions that have, for whatever reason, not been tractable in the ordinary consultation setting; (5) graded task assignment, so that the patient can picture the process of changes as an incremental, step-by-step process, during which the difficulty of each part can be adjusted and mastery is achieved in stages; (6) mastery or pleasure ratings, so that the patient can validate the successfulness and pleasure from changed experiences, or lack thereof.

CASE EXAMPLE: COGNITIVE-BEHAVIORAL TREATMENT OF ANTISOCIAL PERSONALITY DISORDER

In this final section, case material is presented and then discussed to illustrate how the typical schema manifests itself in the behavioral style of a patient. The patient chosen meets criteria for the diagnosis of antisocial personality disorder. The typical schema underlying the disorder is presented along with the treatment goals to indicate the direction of the therapy. As part of the discussion, a new typology for understanding antisocial personality disorder is presented.

Joe, a 24-year-old male referred by his probation officer, had been in trouble with both school and legal authorities since the age of 15. He was convicted of auto theft, after stealing a car, being stopped by the police, and then driving away. Joe was reported at times to have reached a speed of 100 miles per hour in his attempt to escape. When finally caught and searched, Joe was found to have a large amount of cocaine in the car. He contended that the cocaine belonged to the person whose car he stole. Despite his conviction, he had been given a choice of either going to jail or being on probation and involved in therapy. It was not a great surprise that he chose therapy.

At the initial session, Joe was 15 minutes late. He was friendly and announced that this was the last time that he would come. Joe informed the therapist that attendance in therapy was not required and that he only had to come for this initial session, then never again. When the therapist informed him that he was required to come every week for a year, Joe stated that this was not the case. In any event, he stated, even if it *were* true, no one was held to that requirement. When the therapist persisted, Joe became angry and stated that forcing him to come to therapy against his will was a violation of his constitutional rights. When informed by the therapist that the constitutional question would have to be resolved while he was in jail, Joe tried a different approach.

Joe then made it clear that the state would pay the therapist whether or not he came for therapy. All the therapist had to do was to sign the monthly attendance report and the therapist could get paid for doing nothing. When told that this was equally unacceptable, Joe seemed angry.

Joe then said that he had nothing more to say. He told the therapist that since his was a federal drug conviction, his session records were confidential and that the therapist could not share what went on in the session with anyone. (Note: This is, in fact, correct.) Joe then took out a newspaper and started to read. He did not answer any questions and when the time was up, he left. The next week he came in with a sports magazine. Despite the therapist's questions and comments, Joe said nothing. The same scene was repeated in the third session. At the end of Session 3, on his way out of the office, Joe commented to the therapist, "Next week, Doc, bring work." In an attempt to better understand Joe, the therapist examined the following various schemas that are part of the disorder:

"Rules are meant for others."
"Only fools follow all of the rules."
"Rules are meant to be broken."
"Look out for number 1."
"My pleasure comes first."
"If others are hurt, offended, or inconvenienced by my behavior, that is their problem."
"Do it now!"
"I will not allow myself to be frustrated."
"I will do whatever I must to get whatever I want."
"I'm really smarter than most everybody else."

The therapist decided to use the last schema, "I'm really smarter than most everybody else" as an entry point into Joe's "system." It seemed clear to the therapist that Joe was frequently working to "put one over" on almost everybody. His treatment of the therapist and the therapy requirement was consistent with his rule-breaking style. When Joe came in for the fourth session, he came in with his magazine. The therapist started the session by saying, "I've been thinking about what has been happening here for the past 3 weeks. It impresses me how dumb you are."

Joe's reaction was to look at the therapist over the top of his magazine and inquire, "How would you like a punch in the mouth?"

The therapist's response was that he would not like a punch in the mouth, but Joe was still dumb.

Joe asked, "What makes you so friggin' smart?"

The therapist responded: "I didn't say that I was smart, I said that you were dumb."

This piqued Joe's interest enough that he put the magazine down and asked, "And what makes me dumb?"

"What makes you dumb is that people pay a great deal of money to talk to me. You can do it for nothing, and you're too dumb to use me."

"And just how can I *use* you?" Joe asked.

"See those books over there? Those are all my books. I am an internationally known psychologist and you haven't yet figured out how to use me."

"Like . . . what do you do? How could I use you?" Joe asked.

"I am an expert on behavior change. I would find it hard to believe that there isn't someone whose behavior you would like to change."

Joe thought briefly and said, "Yeah, my girlfriend."

"What about her would you like to change?" the therapist asked.

"I would like her to cook dinner more often and be more sexually available."

"Fine" the therapist said. "I need some information about her."

The therapist spent the next half-hour obtaining data about Joe's girlfriend, Gloria, a 32-year-old waitress. Joe and Gloria had lived together for almost a year. She was divorced and had no children.

When asked how he had tried to get Gloria to comply with his demands for more dinner and sex, Joe stated that he would insult, demean, or curse at her. When asked if this worked, Joe stated that it sometimes had an effect but largely seemed to not work.

The therapist asked Joe if he and Gloria had nice moments that were soft and affectionate. Joe replied that they occasionally did. When asked if he ever brought Gloria gifts, Joe asked, "You mean like Christmas or birthday?"

"Yes" stated the therapist. "Like that."

"No, not really."

"Okay, then let's make out a plan. What does Gloria like, candy flowers . . . ?"

"Yeah, she likes flowers."

"What do you think would happen if you brought her flowers? Really an experiment."

Joe was baffled. "I don't know."

"Would you be willing to try it?"

"Sure, what do I have to lose?"

Leaving the session, Joe seemed pleased. He appeared for the next session without a magazine or newspaper. When asked how the experiment had gone, Joe's response was, "F . . . . . g fantastic!" He reported that on the way home he stole flowers for Gloria by picking them out of someone's garden. When he came into the house and offered the flowers to Gloria, she was suspicious and asked, "What are these for?"

Joe responded that he knew that she loved flowers and thought that she would like them. Gloria kissed him. One thing led to another and they ended up in bed. After making love, she asked, "Are you hungry?"

Joe was impressed. When the therapist asked what he learned from the experiment, Joe stated, "So all I have to do is be nice to her. That's it?"

The therapist helped Joe to extract other "morals" from the experiment. Joe then asked, "Does this work on anyone?"

"Who else's behavior do you want to change?"

"My PO [probation officer]."

The therapy evolved to helping Joe make choices rather than react. Treatment with Joe focused on building prosocial behaviors. The therapist was gentle but firm in not accepting Joe's constant excuses. Joe became extremely anxious when his "clever and cool" persona was threatened. The difficulty had he had in changing was that he did not see his behavior as a mask, but as the only way to behave. For example, although told that he must come weekly, Joe came in for therapy on the average of three times a month. He always had a reason for missing his sessions. His excuses were often so simple as to be naive: "I had to go to another city to get a part for a truck that I am thinking of buying from some guy I just met, and it took 2 days to get the part." When the therapist attempted reality testing, Joe became offended that he was not being believed. "If you don't trust me, how can you help me?" he asked the therapist.

Joe's behavior was identified as being a situation of stimulus → response. He wanted something so he took it. The therapy involved the use of self-instructional techniques to help Joe to intersperse several steps between the stimulus ("I see something that I want") and the response ("Grab it!"). The steps involved his learning a sequence of stimulus → attention to what was going on → awareness of his perception → evaluating his thoughts → making a decision → responding. A typical sequence involved the following:

Stimulus ("I see a car with the keys in the ignition.")
Attention ("There is nobody around.")

Awareness ("I could just jump in and get away.")
Evaluating thoughts ("I could get away, but I might get caught.")
Decision making ("If I'm caught, my probation is revoked and I go to jail. Not worth it for this car.")
Responding (Walking away.)

When Joe could see that he could get even more from the world by becoming part of the system rather than trying always to fool the system, he began to act more adaptively. His goal of getting the most that he could for himself did not waver. One could argue that learning that he could "use" people only made him a better antisocial personality rather than "curing" him. This would be true. The therapist's goal was to use Joe's schema in the service of the therapy. He learned that he could get more by being prosocial or "nice" than he could from his take-it-and-run style that put him in jail.

On follow-up over 2 years, Joe continued to stay out of legal problems, though sometimes he was skirting legality.

DISCUSSION OF THE TREATMENT OF ANTISOCIAL PERSONALITY DISORDER

Lykken (1995) states, "Although antisocial personality disorder (APD) is treated in the *Diagnostic and Statistical Manual of Mental Disorders* (DSM-IV; American Psychiatric Association, 1994) as if it were a single entity, most knowledgeable people, whether they hold the union card of a psychiatrist, psychologist, or criminologist agree that APD is a heterogeneous category. People can meet the criteria for this diagnosis in a variety of ways and for different reasons" (p. vii).

Terms such as "psychopath" or "sociopath" attempt to delineate the area of concern. The term "sociopath" is used to denote those whose behavior is a result of a failure to acquire or accept the social norms of the society. Lykken (1995) claims that the individuals with antisocial personality disorder responsible for most crime are sociopaths and reserves the term "psychopath" for those whose behavior is a result of biological or genetic causes. Others (Gacono, 2000; Walters & DiFazio, 2000) choose to use "psychopath" as an all-inclusive term.

Joe would be, according to Lykken, a sociopath. But even this term is far too broad for clinical use.

SUMMARY

The Axis II problems exemplify Beck's idea of schemas being a central issue in the formation of these disorders. In fact, the personality disorder is basically a result of undeveloped or unevolved schemas. These schemas evolve through the process of adaptation (the interaction of assimilation and accommodation). Schemas are neither good or bad, adaptive or maladaptive, but must be judged by the "goodness of fit." A particular guiding principle may be functional at one point in time but dysfunctional at another point. When schemas are questioned, challenged, or threatened, anxiety (survival-related perception of danger) results. Schemas designated as personal, gender, age-related, social, family, religious, or cultural can be most easily modified or reinterpreted. The more active the schema, the greater the effect on day-to-day behavior. The earlier in life a schema is acquired, the harder it will be to modify. The more credible the source of a schema, the more powerful and difficult it will be to modify. The more the schema was modeled or reinforced by significant others, the harder it will be to modify.

The unique features of the personality disorder represent the exaggeration *or* deficit in the individual's style of responding to stimuli. What makes the "style" a disorder is that the response style differs markedly from that of the general population. The difficulty in changing these styles has to do with individuals' perceptions of their behavior as having long-term, high survival value, despite any short-term pain, difficulty, or problems. The greater the individual's belief in the survival value of the schema(s), the harder it (they) will be to modify. Most often, personality disorders are viewed as unitary phenomena regarded as mild, moderate, or severe. Personality disorders are heterogeneous patterns.

The therapeutic alliance will be a central factor in the treatment of the individual with a personality disorder. Within this context, the patient is first taught the necessary skills for dealing with the personality disorder by dealing with the Axis I problems.

Homework is important, so that the patient can become his or her own therapist; changes to the environment help the individual maintain change.

Because of the difficulty in working with individuals with personality disorders, the therapist must be attuned to their countertransference.

Finally, patients with personality disorders are challenging. They can be helped and, in the process, help the therapist to become a far better therapist.

REFERENCES

American Psychiatric Association. (1994). *Diagnostic and statistical manual of mental disorders* (4th ed.). Washington, DC: Author.

American Psychiatric Association (2000). *Diagnostic and statistical manual of mental disorders* (4th ed., text rev.). Washington, DC: Author.

Beck, A. T., & Emery, G. (1985). *Anxiety disorders and phobias: A cognitive perspective.* New York: Basic. Books.

Beck, A. T., Freeman, A., & Associates. (1990). *Cognitive therapy of personality disorders.* New York: Guilford Press.

Beck, A. T., Rush, A. J., Shaw, B. F., & Emery, G. (1979). *Cognitive therapy of depression.* New York: Guilford Press.

Bullard, D. D. (Ed.). (1959). *Psychoanalysis and psychotherapy: The selected papers of Frieda Fromm-Reichmann.* Chicago: University of Chicago Press.

Costello, C. G. (1996). *Personality characteristics of the personality disordered.* New York: Wiley.

Deffenbacher, J. L., Storey, D. A., Stark, R. S., Hogg, J. A., & Brandon, A. D. (1987). Cognitive-relaxation and social skills interventions in the treatment of general anger. *Journal of Counseling psychology, 34*(2), 171–176.

Foon, A. E. (1985). The effect of social class and cognitive orientation on clinical expectations. *British Journal of Medical Psychology, 58*(4), 357–364.

Freeman, A. (1987). Understanding personal, cultural and religious schema in psychotherapy. In A. Freeman, N. Epstein, & K. M. Simon (Eds.), *Depression in the family.* New York: Haworth Press.

Freeman, A. (1998). *Freeman Diagnostic Profiling System.* Philadelphia College of Osteopathic Medicine, Unpublished test.

Freeman, A., & Leaf, R. (1989). Cognitive therapy applied to personality disorders. In A. Freeman, K. M. Simon, H. Arkowitz, & L. Beutler (Eds.), *Comprehensive handbook of cognitive therapy* (pp. 403–433). New York: Plenum Press.

Freeman, A., & Simon, K. M. (1989). Cognitive therapy of anxiety. In A. Freeman, K. M. Simon, H. Arkowitz, & L. Beutler (Eds.). *Comprehensive handbook of cognitive therapy.* New York: Plenum Press.

Freeman, A., Pretzer, J., Fleming, B., & Simon, K. M. (1990). *Clinical applications of cognitive therapy.* New York: Plenum Press.

Gacono, C. B. (Ed.). (2000). *The clinical and forensic assessment of psychopathy: A practitioner's guide.* Hillsdale, NJ: Erlbaum.

Gunderson, J. G. (2001). *Borderline personality disorder: A clinical guide.* Washington, DC: American Psychiatric Publishing.

Gunderson, J. G., & Gabbard, G. O. (2000). *Psychotherapy for personality disorders.* Washington, DC: American Psychiatric Publishing.

Kernberg, O. (1984). *Severe personality disorders.* New Haven, CT: Yale University Press.

Layden, M. A., Newman, C. F., Freeman, A., & Byers-Morse, S. (1993). *Cognitive therapy of borderline personality disorder.* Boston: Allyn & Bacon.

Lykken, D. T. (1995). *The antisocial personality.* Hillsdale, NJ: Erlbaum.

Merbaum, M., & Butcher, J. N. (1982). Therapists' liking of their psychotherapy patients: Some issues related to severity of disorder and treatability. *Psychotherapy: Theory, Research and Practice, 19*(1), 6–76.

Rosen, H. (1989). Piagetian theory and cognitive therapy. In A. Freeman, K. M. Simon, H. Arkowitz, & L. Beutler (Eds.), *Comprehensive handbook of cognitive therapy* (pp. 189–212). New York: Plenum Press.

Rosenbaum, R. L., Horowitz, M. J., & Wilner, N. (1986). Clinician assessments of patient difficulty. *Psychotherapy, 23*(3), 417–422.

Rosenthal, H. (2000). *Favorite counseling and therapy homework assignments: Leading therapists share their most creative strategies.* Philadelphia: Brunner/Routledge.

Stone, M. H. (1993). *Abnormalities of personality.* New York: Norton.

Walters, G. D., & DiFazio, R. (2000). Psychotherapy and the criminal lifestyle: Similarities and differences. In C. B. Gacono (Ed.), *The clinical and forensic assessment of psychopathy: A practitioner's guide.* Hillsdale, NJ: Erlbaum.

20

Short-Term Dynamic Psychotherapy

Resolving Character Pathology by Treating Affect Phobias

NATHANIEL S. KUHN
LEIGH MCCULLOUGH

This chapter presents a model of short-term dynamic psychotherapy (STDP) developed by Leigh McCullough that conceptualizes psychodynamic conflict as "affect phobia" (McCullough Vaillant, 1997; McCullough et al., in press). Patients' problems and diagnostic symptoms are hypothesized to be caused by fears or shame leading to defensive avoidance of underlying feelings.

This integration of psychodynamic thinking with the principles of learning theory implies that conflict-based psychopathology can be treated by a process of systematic desensitization, and gives a coherent theoretical basis for the combination of dynamic, cognitive, and expressive/gestalt techniques into a unified and therapeutically powerful whole. Just as bridge-phobic patients in behavior therapy can be incrementally "exposed" to crossing a bridge, so can patients in a dynamic therapy be exposed to conflicted and thus warded-off inner experiences of anger, grief, closeness, or positive feelings about the self.

Two clinical trials have demonstrated the effectiveness of this treatment for Axis II personality disorders (Svartberg & Stiles, forthcoming; Winston et al., 1991, 1994).

Prior to these clinical trials, abundant research had shown that patients with less severe and more acute problems responded readily to most types of psychotherapy (Luborsky, 1984; Strupp & Binder, 1984). Both clinical trials of STDP selected subjects with Axis II disorders as the focus of treatment because these patients are burdened with lifelong, treatment-resistant problems with symptoms, relationships, and job functioning. It was thought that a more discriminating test of the effectiveness of specific psychotherapeutic techniques would be to demonstrate an impact on these more unrelenting problems of relationships and adaptation that cause enormous suffering yet have been repeatedly shown to be intractable to treatment (Luborsky, 1984; Strupp & Binder, 1984).

Specific DSM-III-R diagnoses in both these trials included predominantly cluster C diagnoses: avoidant, dependent, obsessive–compulsive, passive–aggressive, and self-defeating. One cluster B disorder—histronic—was also included. Diagnoses of borderline, narcissistic, paranoid, schizoid, or schizotypal personality disorder were excluded, although some patients had traits in these categories. Patients could also have additional Axis I disorders: affective disorder, anxiety disorder, or adjustment disorder.

Patients with cluster C disorders were chosen as the predominant focus, because these anxious and withdrawn individuals have defensive structures that need active attention to restructuring or "getting through" the defensive barrier to be able to expose the underlying affects. In contrast, the more severe cluster B disorders involve more problems with impulse control and self-structure that often can require building defenses rather than tearing them down. Patients with cluster A disorders (paranoid, schizoid, and schizotypal) have issues concerning distrust of relationships that often necessitate more alliance building and supportive therapy.

However, it is important to remember that patients rarely present with a single diagnostic category. It is far more common for patients to have more than one Axis II disorder plus traits of many others, also accompanied by Axis I disorders. This was the case in both clinical trials. Because of this inevitable mix of disorders, it was discovered that STDP could be effective in resolving a number of Axis I and Axis II disorders—especially when the overall patient functioning was above 50 on the Global Assessment of Functioning (GAF) scale (which meant that (1) functioning was only moderately impaired, (2) impulses were fairly well under control, and (3) the patient had sufficient strengths to tolerate a rapid uncovering treatment such as STDP). Patients in both trials had to have a GAF score above 50; the average score for both studies was about 55.

The techniques of actively focusing on defenses and experiencing warded-off affects in STDP was hypothesized to offer more concentrated and efficacious methods of change for these more resistant problems. Such interventions provided ways of "exposing" patients to the feelings that they were avoiding.

The results of both clinical trials demonstrated strong improvement in the selected Axis II disorder. STDP (40 sessions in each study) also proved effective for the accompanying Axis I mood and anxiety disorders. Not only was strong improvement noted at termination but continued improvement was also observed at 2-year follow-up; that is, the improvement did not decay after treatment ended, but patients appeared to have acquired new life skills on which they could continue to build over time. These results, combined with our ongoing clinical experience, increasingly indicate that the STDP model—with appropriate modifications—can be helpfully applied to the conceptualization and treatment of not just Axis II personality disorders but of most "neurotic" psychopathology.

To illustrate the change mechanisms in STDP, the bulk of this chapter is devoted to presenting a case example and demonstrating a few of the basic treatment interventions.

CASE EXAMPLE

The patient is a 39-year-old, married mother of three, whom we refer to as "the Unexcited Wife." On the Psychotherapy Assessment Checklist (PAC forms; in McCullough et al., in press), the patient listed her three main problems as (1) "[my husband] going through a severe depression," (2) "pulling myself away emotionally from [my husband]

and the kids (turning into myself)," and (3) "difficulty feeling excited about things." Based on the PAC forms and further evaluation, the patient met criteria for major depressive disorder, dysthymia, social phobia, and generalized anxiety disorder on Axis I; she also met criteria for obsessive–compulsive personality disorder on Axis II.

The Initial Evaluation

To open the therapy, the therapist asks about the main problems that have brought the patient to therapy, then for concrete examples of these problems, looking for patterns of maladaptive behaviors, feelings, and thoughts. Here is the opening of the initial evaluation with the Unexcited Wife:

THERAPIST: Well, I was able to look that [the PAC forms] over briefly, and I will look it over more, but it would help if you tell me the main problems that brought you here for this.

PATIENT: I just think I'm at a point in my life where there's a lot going on. There's a lot going on with [my husband] but there's also a lot about myself that I would like to change, that's just years of a pattern. I see a lot of what I've done is my survival, and I do what I do, and I act the way I act because it works for me. I'm not sure it's healthy but it's done what it's needed to do. I think [my husband] going through all he's going through has sort of clicked off in me the need—or actually the want—to make some changes that will not only be better for him but also better for me.

Already the patient has identified the existence of a maladaptive pattern of behavior, and some motivation to change it, but she is being vague about specifics, perhaps defensively.

THERAPIST: Can you say a little more about . . .

PATIENT: About what they are?

THERAPIST: Yeah, what those things are . . .

PATIENT: I think about me. I've just spent years being responsible for myself and sort of locking myself up and not really letting myself get close to people. That doesn't mean I don't have tons of friends, but it's not that kind of closeness. I think it's just (*dabbing eyes with tissue*) that I let people get so close and then I just lock myself up and go into my own protection mode.

Even with this small amount of information, the therapist can begin a tentative formulation of the psychodynamic conflict (or affect phobia). To help with this rapid formulation process, McCullough turned to David Malan's "two-triangle" schema, which is summarized in his masterful book *Individual Psychotherapy and the Science of Psychodynamics* (1979, 1995). Before going further with this patient, we take a moment to review this work.

Observing many different psychodynamic schools, Malan concluded that the "universal technique of psychodynamic psychotherapy" is to explore how *defenses and anxieties block the adaptive expression of feelings.*

Malan's "Two Triangles" and Affect Phobia

Malan used two triangles as a simple pictorial representation to formulate psychodynamic conflict (see Figure 20.1). The "triangle of conflict" has three poles, which represent defense (D), anxiety (A), and underlying adaptive feeling (F). The "triangle of person" has poles representing the relationships in which these conflicted patterns originate and are played out: the therapist (T), current persons (C), and past persons (P). (These labels represent a slight shift from Malan's original lettering.)

To broaden the applicability of this concept beyond the Freudian "dual-drive" theory, McCullough Vaillant (1994, 1997) turned to Silvan Tomkins's work on affect (1962, 1963, 1991, 1992), and slightly modified his list of basic affects to better fit with clinical work. There are eight "activating affects" over which patients may have conflict, and which appear on the feeling (F) pole of the triangle of conflict (see Figure 20.2). Of these, the four most common conflicts in clinical work are assertion/anger, grief, closeness/tenderness, and positive feelings toward the self (McCullough et al., in press; McCullough Vaillant, 1997). In the case of our patient, she states quite clearly that she does not let herself get close to people, so "closeness" would go on the feeling (F) pole of the triangle of conflict.

When a patient has a psychodynamic conflict, these adaptive activating affects have become associated with excessive "inhibitory affects." For example, assertion might be inhibited by excessive fear, or, grieving may be inhibited by excessive shame. The inhibitory affects, which go on the anxiety (A) pole of the triangle of conflict, include anxiety, guilt, shame, and (emotional) pain. (There is a long-standing terminological ambiguity in the STDP literature because the anxiety [A] pole can refer not only to anxiety [fear] in the narrow sense but also to the other inhibitory affects.) So far, our patient has not given us any information about what inhibitory affect is involved in her conflict (i.e., what she might experience if she *did* allow herself to get close to someone).

As mentioned earlier, a psychodynamic conflict—in which an activating feeling has become blocked due excessive inhibitory feeling—can be thought of as an "affect phobia." In the same way that an external stimulus (e.g., an elevator) might for some patients automatically evoke anxiety, an internal stimulus such as grief can for other patients automatically evoke shame (or some other inhibitory affect).

Of course, a key feature (and often the most functionally debilitating aspect) of phobias is that patients will go to great lengths to avoid the phobic stimulus. In the affect

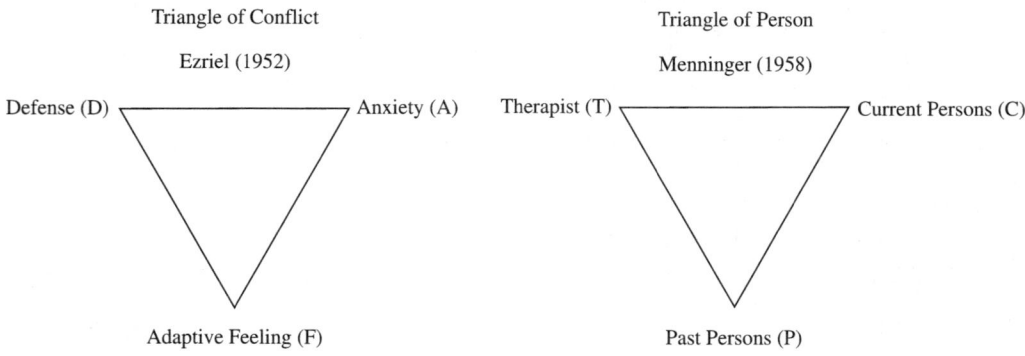

FIGURE 20.1. David Malan's (1979, 1995, Chap. 10) two triangles.

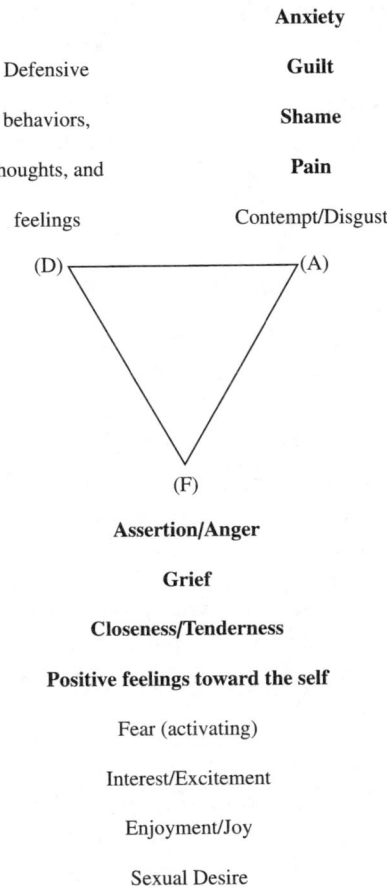

FIGURE 20.2. The affect families, represented on the appropriate poles of the triangle of conflict. Those that are most common in clinical practice are in boldface.

phobia model, *defenses* are seen as behaviors, thoughts, and/or feelings that allow patients to avoid the inner phobic stimulus, that is, the conscious experience of the conflict between activating and inhibitory affects. These behaviors, thoughts, and feelings go on the defense (D) pole of the triangle of conflict. Our patient's last statement contains many examples of defenses that she uses to avoid closeness: "locking myself up," "not letting myself get close to people," a tendency to keep her relationships superficial, and "going into my own protection mode."

In transcript material, the abbreviations of the poles of the two triangles—D, defense; A, anxiety or inhibitory feeling; F, underlying adaptive feeling; T, therapist; C, current persons; and P, past persons—are used to annotate the transcripts. This illustrates how the two-triangles schema can be used not only to organize the complex material that a patient presents but also to suggest ways to intervene rapidly. Returning to that last statement:

PATIENT: I think about me. I've just spent years being responsible for myself and sort of **locking myself up** (D) and **not really letting myself** (D) get **close** (F) to **people** (C). I mean, that doesn't mean I don't have tons of **friends** (C), but it's not that kind of closeness. I think it's just (*dabbing eyes with tissue*) that I let people get so **close** (F) and then I just **lock myself up** (D) and **go into my own protection mode** (D).

So already, with the patient's first statement, the therapist can note defensive behaviors (identified by "D") and underlying feelings ("F"), and thus begin to formulate several elements of a psychodynamic conflict.

The Initial Evaluation (Continued)

The most helpful way for the therapist to continue the formulation process is to ask for specifics:

THERAPIST: Can you give me an example when that happens?

PATIENT: A really good example is actually with my kids (C). I adore my kids. I've always wanted kids. As a child, any TV program [I was interested in] was filled with kids. I've always gotten along well with kids, but . . . I know I back away from (D) [my own kids] (C). You know, they would love to spend time cuddling with me (F, closeness); they'd like me to lie down with them when they go to sleep at night, and I do that, but it's really painful (A). It's hard (A) for me to just sit there or lie there with them . . . I can't sit still (D).

In this segment, the patient finally arrives at a more specific example—closeness with her children (F)—and begins to speak of the excessive inhibitory affect (A) (in this case, emotional pain) that closeness evokes in her, though the basis of this pain is still unexplained. The formulation up to this point is represented on the two triangles in Figure 20.3.

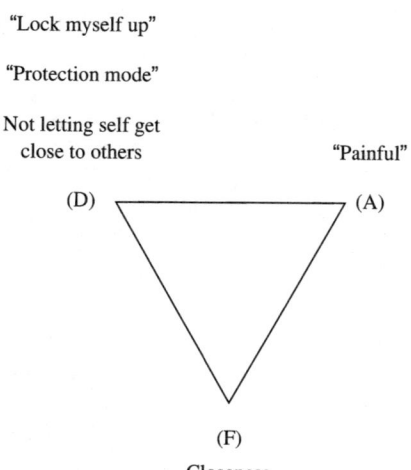

FIGURE 20.3. Preliminary formulation for "the Unexcited Wife."

In the following exchange, the therapist tries to gather more information about the inhibitory affect by staying focused on the underlying phobic adaptive feeling (F, closeness), which generally tends to bring up the inhibitory affect (A). In this case, it mainly brings up descriptions of the patient's defensive avoidance, as well as some of the inhibitory affect causing the phobia.

THERAPIST: What happens to you inside when you try to [sit still with your children]?

PATIENT: It's almost like I get impatient (D), it's like "I can't lie here, I can't lie here and just relax." I have to think about what I have to do. I have to think about doing the laundry, I have to think about doing things (D). It's not that I'm so compulsive and my house is so neat and clean, but I'm always trying to do the next thing, to sort of keep things organized (D) so that I don't totally lose control (A) . . . it's just all trying to be in control (D). And I've done that since I was a kid.

The patient speaks about her defenses, primarily obsessional ones. Although she alludes to the origin of the defenses in childhood, the therapist continues to pursue the fears—or phobia—about feeling, similar to cognitive therapy interventions that ask, "What is the worst thing that might happen?" Questions of this sort are used throughout this therapy to help patients deal with inhibitory affects (fear, shame, etc.) as they arise. (See the later discussion regarding "anxiety regulation.")

THERAPIST: What do you feel would happen (A) if you weren't in control in that way?

PATIENT: I don't know, I don't sort of get to that point. (*Chuckling*, D.) It's so many years of keeping myself in control that . . . you know, as a little kid, that's how I survived, growing up.

The patient says—quite straightforwardly—that her defenses function so well that she cannot even imagine experiencing the inhibitory affect.

Spontaneous associations to childhood often lead to important material, and this time the therapist follows up:

THERAPIST: Tell me more about that, what that was like.

PATIENT: I'm the youngest of three kids. My brother (P) is 8 years older than I am; my sister (P) is 5 years older than I. My father (P) was an alcoholic. I had a horrible relationship with him. We were both like the youngest children actually. I always tried to get close (F) to him (P) and he always pushed me away . . .

Though less than 5 minutes of the initial evaluation has elapsed, an astute therapist might wonder whether the pain inhibiting the patient's closeness with her children has to do with her unmet needs and longings for closeness with her alcoholic father (and perhaps others) in childhood.

Pain of this sort is reduced by a process of grieving, and the fact that the patient may still be experiencing the effects of this pain suggests that there is another affect phobia (psychodynamic conflict) around the adaptive feeling of grief. We have very little information about this conflict, but we can surmise as part of our formulation that one way the patient defends against this grief is by avoiding closeness, which would bring up the sadness over what she did not get as a child (see Figure 20.4). Of course, a formula-

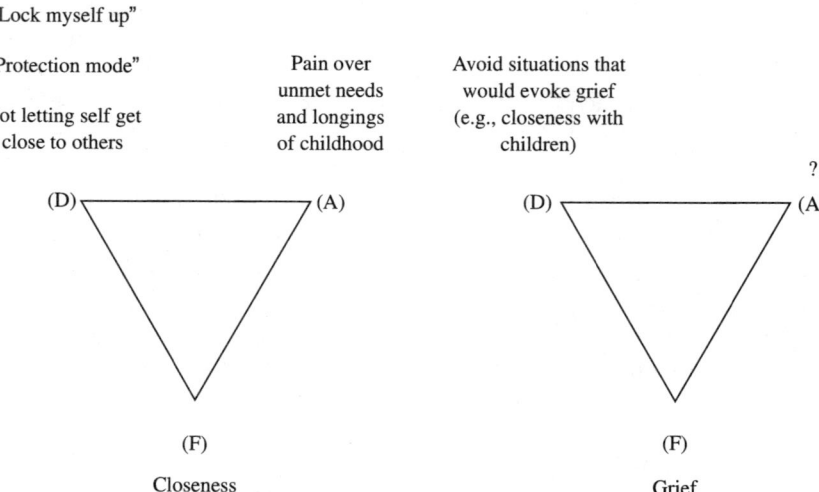

FIGURE 20.4. More detailed formulation for "the Unexcited Wife."

tion arrived at so early and on such slim data would be tentative to say the least; it would need to be either confirmed or modified by later therapy material.

Treatment Implications of the Affect Phobia Concept

As we have just seen in the realm of formulation, the concept of affect phobia gives us a new way to think about and discuss psychodynamic conflict. In the realm of treatment, thinking of psychodynamic conflict as affect phobia has significant implications: that psychodynamic conflict—like other phobias—can be treated by a process of desensitization, that is, exposure and response prevention.

Of the methods of desensitization in common practice, systematic desensitization (Wolpe, 1958) was selected for this therapy because it is effective and well-tolerated.[1] In systematic desensitization, the patient is exposed to the phobic stimulus in a graded fashion, with small increases of intensity between the steps. With each exposure, the patient is helped to bear and reduce the anxiety in an adaptive way, a process known in this psychodynamically based model as *anxiety regulation*.

For a phobia or other anxiety treatment to be effective, simply experiencing less anxiety when confronted with the phobic stimulus is not sufficient. Patients must also reduce their avoidant behaviors and maladaptive responses. For example, in obsessive–compulsive disorder, patients often wash their hands excessively as a (maladaptive) way of coping with fear of contamination. *Response prevention* involves learning to master the (contamination) anxiety *without* the maladaptive coping mechanism (hand washing).

With affect phobias, the defenses are the maladaptive coping mechanisms, and response prevention means helping patients see and give up their defenses (defense restructuring; see McCullough Vaillant, 1994). In the case at hand, the patient needs to prevent shutting down or distancing herself from people close to her.

In terms of the use of systematic desensitization in STDP, we can see that, at almost any point in treatment, the therapist is weighing three choices:

1. Increase the intensity of exposure to the conflicted adaptive affect, which is likely to increase the level of anxiety or defensiveness.

    THERAPIST: I'd like you to imagine lying quietly in bed and enjoying your kids' company. How does it feel?

2. Reduce the anxiety with anxiety-regulating techniques (mostly cognitive exploration).

    THERAPIST: What would be the most difficult thing about lying down with your kids?

3. Prevent the defensive response by confrontation or clarification to help patients see their defenses and give up their use.

    THERAPIST: Can you see how that urge to get up and clean things keeps you from being close to your children? What would it be like just to say, "I'll deal with that stuff later. Right now it's more important for me to just be there with them."

Sometimes it is clear which of these three options is most needed; at other times, therapists need to proceed by trial and error. Generally, though, by staying attuned to the patient and maintaining the therapeutic alliance, the therapist develops a "feel" for the direction in which to move at any given moment.

Returning to our case, in the following extended transcript from a later session in the therapy, the patient discusses how hard it is for her to spend time just playing with her daughter, which gives the therapist an entry into exploring the conflict around closeness.

PATIENT: It's harder to do something that's more imaginative. It's not that I can't. I can do it, I've done it, but it's not relaxing or fun for me.

THERAPIST: Just to watch her imagination at work . . .

PATIENT: No, it's fun to watch her imagination, it's fascinating. I love it. But to actually sit there and get immersed in it, I find I'm really restless (D). Sitting there with the horsey, I know all the parts to do and I do them, but . . . I just get restless.

THERAPIST: So what is that restlessness? [Tries to explore the anxiety/defense.]

PATIENT: I can't relax, I'm racing, and it's like, "When is this going to end?"

THERAPIST: What would happen if you just did that and just got totally into it and absorbed in it? [Tries to explore the anxieties that would come up if the defense were not in place.]

PATIENT: I don't think my inner voice would allow me to do it, I truly don't. I mean, if you're asking, I think that's where I'm . . . [As in the initial material, the patient's defenses are too entrenched to allow her to imagine this.]

THERAPIST: What I'm asking is what is the feeling, or whatever, that inner voice is helping you to avoid? [Making no progress looking at defenses or anxieties, the therapist tries to look at the underlying feeling, with an almost explicit statement about the triangle of conflict.]

PATIENT: I don't know. I don't have a clue. It's just a total, it's a, you know, I mean, it's a physical feeling. (*Affect becomes sad.*) It's not . . .

THERAPIST: You looked very sad as you . . . [Stays with patient's affect, which could easily have been passed over.]

PATIENT: I am, I can't stand the feeling . . . I feel very badly for [my daughter]. I do other things [with her], but I feel badly that . . . I'm not even thinking about her. I'm so *mad* that it's so painful for me to do. I can't stand the fact that it's so painful for me to do. It makes me crazy that I . . . . Sometimes I can sit back and relax, and sometimes I just can't do it. It's like, "Okay, we're doing this. How long have I been doing it, should I do it for a few more minutes, can I get away now, when can I get away from this?" She used to try engage me a good deal. She doesn't really engage me in it much anymore, and I feel bad about that, but it's just . . .

THERAPIST: So, getting back to the idea that maybe there's a feeling (F) that tries to come up when you do this, and . . . that there's something about the feeling that's uncomfortable (A), and the voice (D) stops that . . .

PATIENT: It's like I don't have a clue. When I was little, I remember being afraid of the dark. [It is interesting that now—when a lot of painful feeling has come up—the patient has another spontaneous association to her past.] My bedroom was the first bedroom at the top of the stairs, and they'd leave the hall light on and leave my door open. I was just terrified that someone was going to break into the house and somehow hurt me. My sister used to laugh because I was the first to go to bed. I would sit there telling stories out loud for hours . . . a lot of the stuff that [my daughter] does, and it wasn't a bad thing. I did it as a *little* kid. I didn't do it as I got older, but I remember I would just sit there going on and on, and talking a mile a minute. It was okay for me to do, [so] I don't understand why it's so hard . . . being a participant [with her]. . . . It's as much a physical as an emotional response, and I don't know why. It's a very simple thing . . . it doesn't involve a whole lot. I've gotten a little bit better at lying down with the kids. [This is a response to a more purely behavioral suggestion that the therapist had given early on in the therapy, and the patient reports mild change from it.] It doesn't seem to be as painful as it was for a while. Lately I've been trying to avoid it a little bit more, but when I do it, it's not as painful as it had been, but I do find certain activities just really painful to do. Some of them I don't want to do, but others are painful. I haven't a clue.

THERAPIST: You know, it strikes me that the things that you're talking about—you know, how you would tell imaginative stories to yourself—it sounds like you must have longed so much for a parent who *could* sit with you and play with you . . . [Links the childhood association to the hypothesized underlying conflict over grief.]

PATIENT: By the way, while I'm listening to you, it's amazing what's going through my head. I'm just sitting here saying, "This is just silly, this is so ridiculous." I'm just trying to push away (D) everything you're saying. It's like, "Yeah, it does make me feel bad, but so what?" [Has a sharp increase in defensiveness but is also able to observe it and report it with some detachment, a marker of her ability to form a strong therapeutic relationship.]

THERAPIST: That longing (F) is something that you really do push away and hold at a distance (D). It must have been so strong in you as a child. [Holds focus on the sadness/longing to expose the patient to the underlying feeling that she is avoiding and thus desensitize the conflict.]

PATIENT: It was. So if I have a person now who longs for it and wants it, and it's something I want, then why do I push it away (D)? If it's everything I want? (*Blows nose.*)

THERAPIST: Maybe it would make you feel that longing (F) you felt as a child. [Interprets the patient's behavior as a defense against the sadness.]

PATIENT: I mean, I wanted it, but I didn't get it. I know that. (*Shrugs—defensive nonchalance.*)

THERAPIST: To be a child and not be able to get that is so . . . to have that longing that goes on day after day, month after month, and year after year. [Maintains focus on exposure.] That longing is such a difficult feeling, I think that as a child you would do anything to keep it away. And that grief over all those things that you couldn't get as a child, and how much you missed your father *and* your mother, how much you missed having a father and a mother who could relate to you.

PATIENT: Yeah, but at such an intellectual level. But it just seems like, "I know." There's so much of what you're saying, maybe not the specifics of it, but the general flavor of it. . . . I *know* I raised myself, I was on my own. Yeah, people have rough lives. There are a lot of things I didn't get, there are a lot of things I did get. It just infuriates me that it has such an effect on me now.

THERAPIST: It sounds like it's more comfortable to feel fury (D, defensive affect)—which is very understandable [validates the defense]—than it is to feel the grief (F).

PATIENT: Oh, absolutely.

THERAPIST: What would happen if you let yourself really feel that grief? [Returns to helping to regulate the anxiety around the exposure to grief.]

PATIENT: Actually I go back to what I said to you that first time we met. It would just be very embarrassing (A, shame).

THERAPIST: Embarrassing how?

PATIENT: I'm 39 years old, it's like "just get a life." You hit a point where I know your past affects you. On one level, it's good to go back and get rid of things, or just put them to rest and move on, and the other part says, "You can't live in the past, and you just have to pull up your bootstrings and move on." To be this age and be that vulnerable is terrifying (A); it just feels totally humiliating and embarrassing (A). I can't even put it into words. Sometimes I drive home and I'm just so embarrassed at being the age I am and being where I am, it just feels very demeaning. [Note multiple examples showing the enormous shame that makes her run from the underlying feelings.]

THERAPIST: You know I think the paradox of this is that . . . I don't think it's *having* those feelings of grief that's keeping you where you are. I think it's *pushing away* those feelings of grief that's keeping you where you are. [This is a gentle confrontation of the defenses and a cognitive reframing that can help patients increase motivation to relinquish their defenses. Patient might also benefit from more exploration of just why she finds the therapy process so humiliating.]

PATIENT: But I felt like I was in pain (A) most of my childhood. Or, not in pain, I was in real good numbness-land (D).

THERAPIST: Yeah, of course you were [numb]. Because the alternative was to be in incredible pain (A). [Validates the defense in the past.] But I'm not trying to suggest you go back and have all that pain, I'm trying to suggest that you . . .

PATIENT: But it feels like it's either numbness (D) or pain (A). Or not pain (A), just incredible sadness (F).

THERAPIST: Sadness, yeah. [Tries to stay with adaptive feeling (F).]

PATIENT: It goes back to the intellectual part . . . I *know* all that. [Returns to defensive stance.]

From this exchange, it was clear that the patient had a significant conflict over grief, and that resolving that conflict would likely help her be closer to others, especially her children. At the following session, the therapist focused on that patient's grief over her childhood, attempting to expose her to as much affect as possible.

In the following transcript of a brief segment from that session, the therapist refers back to an episode the patient had mentioned during the initial evaluation. This episode took place when the patient was in elementary school. She and her father had returned to the family house after an enjoyable outing, and she inadvertently kicked open the car's glove compartment, revealing his stash of hidden cigarettes. He was supposed to have given up smoking for health reasons, but he lost his temper and blamed her.

THERAPIST: What were you thinking about that scene where he got angry like that? What would you want to say to him now? What would you want to tell him?

PATIENT: (*Blows nose.*) Um, I don't know where to start. I mean, actually, I would probably tell him that I had a good day with him. [Grieving involves experiencing both positive and negative aspects of the memories, so this positive statement about the father is not seen as denial or purely defensive.] You know, it was nice being with him. That I liked going to the place we went to, and that it held a lot of really good memories. (*Starts to cry.*)

THERAPIST: (*quietly*) Just stay with that. [Simply encourages the patient to remain with the affect.]

PATIENT: And he just had to ruin it (*tearing up*).

THERAPIST: Stay with that . . . [Continued encouragement, almost whispered.]

PATIENT: It's so unfair (*tearing up again*).

THERAPIST: Stay with that. It wasn't fair . . . [Reflects back the patient's statement, then allows a long pause, so as not to step on affective material. When none is forthcoming, the therapist prompts the patient again, in an open-ended way.] What else would you tell him?

PATIENT: That he ruined the day. That he messed things up. That I was just a kid. Probably now I'd tell him that he had no right to yell at me.

THERAPIST: Uh huh . . . he really hurt you. [More reflective listening.]

PATIENT: Probably because there wasn't a "me." There was just a "him."

THERAPIST: Uh huh.

Although this was about the highest level of grief elicited in that session, the intensity is not extremely high: A few tears ran down the patient's face, but she did not sob. In addition, the fact that she was able to cry with the therapist implies that she experienced a moderately high level of trust and closeness. This sustained experience of grief (and closeness) throughout the session was enough to lead to significant change. In the following session (which for unrelated reasons did not take place for a number of weeks), the patient recounted a significant shift in her relationships with her children:

PATIENT: ... Lately, I've felt a lot closer with the kids and a lot more relaxed around them.... You know, I can keep a lot more intact around them and just be a little more aware. They seem a lot more relaxed, which is really good. We were at the Cape. I tried to take them to the beach pretty much every day, and they obviously wanted to spend all their time in the water. Normally, for me to go to the beach would be this big stressed-out thing: packing up, getting there, and trying to keep my eye on everyone. I end up making more work for myself rather than enjoying it for myself, and [this time] I really felt that I enjoyed it with them. I ... liked being around them. I had fun with them and enjoyed going in the water with them.

THERAPIST: It sounds great.

PATIENT: Yeah, it was really, really nice.... The other thing is, they'll joke around and they'll do things, and I'll chuckle at some of the things they say. At times [my son] really ticks me off, but he'll say something that will just really crack me up, and I really have to work at not laughing out loud, because I really *need* to be annoyed at him at that moment, and that sort of, you know, surprises me 'cause I don't do *that* too often. I'm being entertained.

THERAPIST: That's something that you think wouldn't have happened before.

PATIENT: I think part of it is me and part of it is also their age. They're getting more sophisticated in their humor. But certainly, it wouldn't matter how sophisticated their humor was, I could sort of just block them out. So I'm definitely finding more little bits that help me enjoy being with them.

The patient reports a very significant shift in a long-standing, entrenched, disturbing, and destructive pattern of behavior and emotion. She reported improvement in the two main problems that had to with her own behavior: closeness with family members, and her ability to enjoy and get excited about things. Our understanding of the change mechanisms in this treatment points to the desensitization of conflicts around closeness and grief, thus freeing the patient to be closer to her children and to enjoy her life more.

It is worth noting that there is still some defensiveness present: the idea that she is finding her children funnier because their senses of humor have grown more "sophisticated" over 2 months is put forward but then appropriately dismissed as an explanation for the change. The defense here is malleable and the patient has some awareness of it, so there is no need to point it out.

At termination, the patient had received 25 hours of therapy: one 3-hour initial evaluation and 11 2-hour therapy sessions. (Generally, the therapy is done in 1-hour sessions, but this patient had to travel a considerable distance.) Her rating of the target complaints at termination reflected the substantial improvement reported earlier. At 2-year follow-up, there had been some modest further improvement in the target complaints. At termination (and at 2-year follow-up), she no longer met criteria for major depressive disorder, generalized anxiety disorder, social phobia, or obsessive–compulsive personality disorder; she continued to meet criteria for dysthymia.

RESEARCH RESULTS

As noted earlier, the effectiveness of this style of STDP for Axis II cluster C personality disorders has been demonstrated in two clinical trials. The first trial, conducted at the Beth Israel Brief Psychotherapy Research Program in New York, compared two types of brief dynamic treatment: an anxiety-provoking therapy based on high confrontation of defenses, and a more anxiety-regulating style, as we have discussed here. In this difficult population of patients with personality disorders—typically unresponsive to treatment—both therapies proved effective, with an average of 1 standard deviation change in outcome measures after 40 sessions of brief, active, focused psychotherapy. There were no significant differences between groups (Winston et al., 1991, 1994). At 18-month follow-up, these gains had not only been maintained, but also there was in fact slight improvement (Winston et al., 1994).

In the second trial (Svartberg & Stiles, forthcoming), at the University of Trondheim in Norway, this anxiety-regulating model of STDP has been compared to cognitive therapy in a repeated-measures comparative process–outcome design. Fifty patients meeting DSM-III-R criteria for cluster C personality disorders were randomized to 40 sessions of either STDP or cognitive therapy. Results at termination and 2-year follow-up (in preparation for publication) were similar to the Beth Israel clinical trial; there were strong improvements in both groups but no significant difference between them. Ongoing research at the Norwegian Technical and Scientific Institute in Trondheim will examine the processes and change mechanisms in both treatments.

In addition to these outcome studies, a number of process studies have suggested that an empathic approach with an emphasis on clarification of defenses is more effective in reducing defensive behavior than an approach that relies more on strong confrontation (McCullough Vaillant, 1997, pp. 438–439).

CROSS-CULTURAL VALIDITY

The cross-cultural applicability of this model of STDP is an area that is ripe for research. In some ways, the therapy could be viewed as highly culturally bound: The therapist is not "neutral" but constantly assesses which of the patient's behaviors, thoughts, and feelings are adaptive and which are maladaptive; this assessment will vary depending on the cultural context. (Of course it is also important to remember that "neutrality" will have varying impacts depending on the cultural context, among other things). In this active model, the therapist must explore what seems maladaptive, and must do so in a spirit of humility, understanding that he or she may well be wrong. Although the stance toward the patient needs to be nonjudgmental, the therapist cannot escape the need for discernment. Because adaptive expression of affect may be radically different in New York, Trondheim, Tokyo, Rome, and Minneapolis, good therapists would not do the same thing in each of those cultural milieus.

On the other hand, the model rests on a foundation that we believe will give it great cross-cultural robustness: affect theory and learning theory. Tomkins's affect theory has been validated cross-culturally (e.g., Ekman, 1992a, 1992b). The principles of learning theory, such as conditioning, are so basic to us that they are highly conserved throughout the course of evolution. For these reasons, we believe that this model, with appropriate modifications and allowances, will be universally effective.

CONCLUSIONS

We have presented a research-validated model of STDP that integrates principles and practices from many other schools into a coherent whole. We believe that this sort of integration helps therapists select helpful interventions on a moment-to-moment basis at the many choice points within a therapy session. It is our hope that this quick summary has piqued readers' curiosity enough that they will want to explore other resources—our main text *Changing Character* (McCullough Vaillant, 1997), and the accompanying therapist's guide *Treating Affect Phobia* (McCullough et al., in press)—to learn more.

NOTE

1. Systematic desensitization is one of a number of types of desensitization. In *flooding*, patients are exposed to high levels of the phobic stimulus. As with systematic desensitization, the exposure needs to continue until anxiety is reduced—otherwise, the phobia can be increased (i.e., sensitized rather than desensitized). Because of the high levels of anxiety provoked in flooding, many patients either drop out or otherwise refuse to continue. Patients who flee treatment in the middle of exposure may find the treatment itself traumatizing.

    There are highly confrontational, anxiety-provoking models of STDP (e.g., Davanloo, 1980) that use "flooding" paradigms to expose patients to intense feelings. These therapies are effective for patients who are able to tolerate them, but such patients seem to be a minority, and the risks of dropouts and sensitization of conflict appear to be real.

    In addition, eye movement desensitization and reprocessing (EMDR; Shapiro, 2001) is another form of treatment that involves some desensitization and some information reprocessing, with documented effectiveness in the treatment of posttraumatic stress disorder. EMDR techniques have been incorporated into affect phobia treatment and appear to be an effective complement or alternative to systematic desensitization (McCullough, in press).

REFERENCES

Davanloo, H. (Ed.). (1980). *Short-term dynamic psychotherapy*. New York: Jason Aronson.
Ekman, P. (1992a). Facial expressions of emotion: New findings, new questions. *Psychological Science, 3*, 34–38.
Ekman, P. (1992b). An argument for basic emotions. *Cognition and Emotion, 6*, 169–200.
Ezriel, H. (1952). Notes on psychoanalytic group therapy: II. Interpretation. *Research Psychiatry, 15*, 119.
Luborsky, L. (1984). *Principles of psychoanalytic psychotherapy: A manual for supportive-expressive treatment*. New York: Basic Books.
Malan, D. M. (1979). *Individual psychotherapy and the science of psychodynamics*. London: Butterworth.
Malan, D. M. (1995). *Individual psychotherapy and the science of psychodynamics* (2nd ed.). London: Butterworth–Heinemann.
McCullough, L. (in press). Exploring change mechanisms in EMDR applied to "small t trauma" in short term dynamic psychotherapy: Research questions and speculations. *Journal of Clinical Psychology*.
McCullough, L., Kuhn, N., Andrews, S., Kaplan, A., Wolfe, J., & Lanza, C. (in press). *Treating affect phobia: A therapist's manual for short-term dynamic psychotherapy*. New York: Guilford Press.
McCullough Vaillant, L. (1994). The next step in short-term dynamic psychotherapy: A clarifica-

tion of objectives and techniques in an anxiety-regulating model. *Psychotherapy, 31,* 642–654.

McCullough Vaillant, L. (1997). *Changing character: Short-term anxiety-regulating psychotherapy for restructuring defenses, affects and attachment.* New York: Basic Books.

Menninger, K. (1958). *Theory of psychoanalytic technique.* London: Imago.

Shapiro, F. (2001). *Eye movement desensitization and reprocessing: Basic principles, protocols, and procedures* (2nd ed.). New York: Guilford Press.

Strupp, H. H., & Binder, J. L. (1984). *Psychotherapy in a new key: A guide to time-limited dynamic psychotherapy.* New York: Basic Books.

Svartberg, M., Stiles, T. C., & Seltzer, M. H. (forthcoming). Effectiveness of short-term dynamic psychotherapy and cognitive therapy for cluster C personality disorders: A randomized controlled trial. *American Journal of Psychiatry.*

Tomkins, S. S. (1962). *Affect, imagery, and consciousness: Vol. I. Positive affects.* New York: Springer.

Tomkins, S. S. (1963). *Affect, imagery, and consciousness: Vol. II. Negative affects.* New York: Springer.

Tomkins, S. S. (1991). *Affect, imagery, and consciousness: Vol. III. Negative affects.* New York: Springer.

Tomkins, S. S. (1992). *Affect, imagery, and consciousness: Vol. IV. Cognition.* New York: Springer.

Winston, A., Laikin, M., Pollack, J., Samstag, L., McCullough, L., & Muran, C. (1994). Short-term psychotherapy of personality disorders: 2 year follow-up. *American Journal of Psychiatry, 151*(2), 190–194.

Winston, A., McCullough, L., Trujillo, M., Pollack, J., Laikin M., Flegenheimer W., & Kestenbaum, R. (1991). Brief psychotherapy of personality disorders. *Journal of Nervous and Mental Disease, 179*(4), 188–193.

Wolpe, J. (1958). *Psychotherapy by reciprocal inhibition.* Stanford, CA: Stanford University Press.

Concluding Remarks

STEFAN G. HOFMANN
MARTHA C. TOMPSON

The goal of this handbook is to provide the reader with a practical guide to some of the most efficacious psychological treatments for severe mental disorders that psychologists have to offer, irrespective of the particular theoretical orientation. Editing this text has been a tremendously enjoyable, rewarding, and educational experience. At the same time, it has underscored the difficulties in making fair judgments about the efficacy of a particular treatment. However, despite these problems, this volume has demonstrated that a number of effective psychological interventions exist to treat a range of mental disorders.

Unfortunately, only a few therapists are familiar with these interventions, and efficacious psychotherapy is only available to a few individuals suffering from such disorders. Sometimes, clinical scientists are able to secure funding from the National Institute of Mental Health to study ways to disseminate such interventions. Developers of psychological treatments lead workshops and seminars at professional conferences in order to train other clinicians. And sometimes, treatment protocols are converted into therapist guides or chapters published in professional books, such as this one. However, aside from these notable exceptions, there is little incentive and guidance to develop, test, and disseminate psychological treatments.

In addition to finding more and better strategies to disseminate these interventions, future treatment research will also need to address a number of additional issues. First, although the treatment outcome literature reports encouraging results on the efficacy of various psychological treatments for severe mental illnesses, little is known about the underlying treatment mechanism or the patient variables that predict good or poor treatment outcome. Identifying these variables is important, in that it will enable researchers to further increase the efficacy, shorten the treatment duration, and thereby maximize the cost-effectiveness of the intervention. Research to identify the mechanism of action (i.e., the mediators of change) and predictors of outcome (i.e., the moderators) requires a different design than traditional outcome studies. Mediators and moderators are typically studied by employing regression models and structural equation models. These studies are more costly than traditional outcome research, because they often require a relatively greater number of subjects tested at numerous times during the treatment phase.

Second, among individuals with severe mental disorders, comorbidity is more the norm than the exception. For example, substance abuse and dependence are common problems in individuals with schizophrenia and bipolar disorders; depressed persons often have co-occurring anxiety disorders; and those with severe personality disorders frequently experience depression. Treatments for specific psychopathologies frequently need to be combined to address the range of difficulties and complications individuals face. Therefore, more research needs to be conducted on strategies for combining psychological treatments that holistically address our patients' needs. Should treatments be sequentially or serially applied? Do particular treatments have effects on multiple problems? These are among the many questions to be addressed when effectively treating individuals in which comorbidity so often occurs.

Third, as stated earlier, psychological interventions are typically developed for treating particular DSM-IV disorders. New findings on the psychopathology of a mental disorder lead to revisions of the defining diagnostic criteria, which may then also lead to modifications of the particular treatment approach. However, certain patient characteristics, which are not part of the diagnostic definition but are nevertheless important moderators of treatment change, remain unrecognized, including gender, sexual orientation, ethnicity, cultural background, and socioeconomic status. Future psychotherapy research needs to examine whether such variables effect the response to a particular treatment. If they do, the treatment for a particular subgroup of patients will need to be revised to maximize its efficacy.

Fourth, for most individuals with severe mental illnesses, medication treatment is not only an alternative or useful adjunct but also a necessary form of intervention. At the same time, noncompliance to medication treatment is a significant problem in many of these patients for a number of reasons. Psychological techniques can be very useful to enhance compliance to drug therapy. For example, cognitive strategies, motivational interviewing, or a reinforcement plus voucher plan might be potentially useful techniques to increase compliance to drug therapy.

These are only some of the examples of areas for future psychotherapy research for severe mental disorders. We have come a long way but still have a long way to go. We hope this volume reaches not only practicing psychotherapists and psychiatrists but also policymakers and funding agencies with the power to encourage and actively support such research and dissemination.

Index

Page numbers followed by "f" indicate figure, "n" indicate note, "t" indicate table

active listening, 163, 169
activity levels, 82, 117–120, 396–397
addiction. *See* substance abuse
adolescent depression, 141, 152
adolescent suicide, 191–192
  emergency room treatment of, 192–199
  See also suicide
"affect phobia," 403, 406
  case example, 405
  treatment, 410–415
  "two-triangle" schema, 405, 406f, 407f, 408
  See also short-term dynamic psychotherapy
Al-Anon, 261. *See also* twelve-step facilitation therapy
alcohol abuse, 252–253
  case example, 307–308
  cocaine use and, 301
  cognitive impairments, 235–236
  treatment, 242, 302
  See also Alcoholics Anonymous; coping and social skills training; substance abuse; twelve-step facilitation therapy
Alcoholics Anonymous, 260–261, 264–268, 278–279. *See also* twelve-step facilitation therapy
anger, 87, 182
antepartum depression, 141
antidepressants, 134
  compared to interpersonal psychotherapy, 132
  marital therapy and, 186
  See also pharmacotherapy
antipsychotics, 1, 54–56
  bipolar disorder, 160
  maintenance dose, 63
  research, 64
  social skills training, 47
  See also pharmacotherapy
antisocial behavior, 316, 365, 367
  See also multisystemic therapy
antisocial personality disorder, 400
anxiety disorder, 116, 318
anxiety regulation, 410–411
arousal system, 74–76, 87, 196–197, 334
  belief modification strategies, 84–85
  dearousing techniques, 83, 86. *See also* cognitive-behavioral therapy
  dialectical behavior therapy, 327
  regulation dysfunction, 76
  See also psychotic experience; Successful Negotiation/Acting Positively
assertiveness training, 299, 300, 397
assessment
  of alcohol abuse, 238–240, 279
  case example, 88–90, 187, 304, 373–375, 374t, 404–410
  cognitive-behavioral therapy, 78, 385–388
  cognitive conceptualization diagram, 104
  Community Reinforcement Approach, 298–299
  conceptualization, 388–389
  dialectical behavior therapy, 327–333
  family, 5–7, 91, 181–182, 351–353
  following, 393
  Global Assessment of Relational Functioning, 166
  interpersonal approach, 131–132, 135
  interview instruments, 21–23, 78
  multisystemic therapy, 367, 367–368
  obtaining history, 21–22
  role play, 34
  social skills training, 45–47
  suicidality, 200
  techniques, 78

assessment (*continued*)
   twelve-step facilitation therapy, 262, 268–270, 269t
   See also interview instruments
assignments. *See* homework
attachment, 358–359
attribution, 84–86, 103
auditory hallucinations, 44, 70, 78, 85–86. *See also* hallucinations
automatic thoughts, 100, 102–105, 110f. *See also* internal dialogue
avoidance, 80
   belief modification strategies, 84–85
   coping, 83
   cue exposure treatment, 249
   social skills training, 60
   suicide attempts, 195
awareness training, 83–84. *See also* symptoms

Beck, Aaron, 99–100. *See also* cognitive model of depression
Beck Depression Inventory, 101
   case example, 309
   Community Reinforcement Approach, 298
   depression and marital discord, 177
   research, 185–186
   See also assessment; depression; symptoms
behavior
   cues, 60
   defenses, 406–407
   emotions, 79
   modification, 201–202, 383
   schemas, 389–392
   therapy, 105–106, 185–186
   See also social skills training
behavioral rehearsal, 23, 85–86
   cognitive-behavioral therapy, 397
   family-focused therapy, 163
   See also cognitive-behavioral therapy; social skills training
beliefs, 70, 84–86, 87
bereavement, 135
   depression, 179
   interpersonal psychotherapy, 136–137
   loss of healthy self, 149
biological clock, 143. *See also* circadian rhythm
biological vulnerability, 74
   alcohol abuse, 235, 260
   mood disorders, 132, 162
   psychotic experience, 74–76, 79, 87
   schizophrenia, 1
   See also vulnerability-stress model
biosocial theory, 323–325
bipolar disorder
   borderline personality disorder and, 153
   geriatric population, 171
   symptoms, 159, 166–167
   treatment, 97–98, 119, 146, 160–162
   See also specific treatment methods
booster sessions, 56, 105, 301. *See also* personal therapy
borderline personality disorder, 316, 317–318, 323–325
   bipolar disorder and, 153
   family factors, 345
   pattern recognition, 356
   psychoeducational approach, 345–346
   sexual abuse, 324
   statistics, 343
   suicide, 320
   See also dialectical behavior therapy; multiple family group treatment; *specific treatment methods*
brainstorming, 356–357. *See also* problem-solving
brief therapy, 53
   adolescent suicide, 191–192, 193–198
   marital discord, 185

case management, 76, 118
   dialectical behavior therapy, 338–339
   integration of, 10
   personal therapy, 55, 63
   training centers, 91–92
chain analysis, 385, 386f. *See also* assessment
circadian rhythm, 143, 146, 147. *See also* patterns; sleep
cocaine dependence, 296–297, 299–301. *See also* Community Reinforcement Approach; substance abuse
cognitive-behavioral therapy, 3, 99, 316, 396f, 400–401
   assessment, 78–81
   automatic thoughts, 102–105
   background of, 69–71
   bipolar, 117–120, 127
   case example, 87–91, 397–400
   case formulation, 101–102, 121–122, 123f, 124f, 388–389
   clinical issues, 87, 113, 394–395
   comorbidity, 125–126
   compared to twelve-step facilitation therapy, 258
   depression, 99–100
   dialectical behavior therapy, 317–318, 327–333
   explained, 4–5, 77t, 100
   family therapy, 3–4, 10, 14–15, 205–206
   goals, 76, 101, 120–121
   homework, 394
   interventions, 12, 53, 81–86, 86–87, 88f
   personality disorders, 315, 344, 392–394
   population, 106
   relapse, 122, 124
   research, 71–74, 73t, 105–106, 292
   schemas, 389–392
   substance abuse, 216–217, 234, 277
   Successful Negotiation/Acting Positively, 192, 209

techniques, 76–77, 396–397
therapeutic relationship, 382–385
training centers, 91–92
treatment model, 74–76, 75f
See also psychoeducational approach
cognitive conceptualization diagram, 104, 120, 121f
cognitive continuum, 104–105
cognitive differentiation, 43. *See also* integrated psychological therapy
cognitive distortions, 103
cognitive distraction, 249, 250
cognitive enhancement therapy, 63
cognitive impairments
  alcohol abuse, 235–236
  social skills training, 42–43, 46–47
cognitive model of depression, 99–100. *See also* Beck, Aaron
cognitive-perceptual abilities, 19. *See also* social skills
cognitive responses, 76
cognitive restructuring, 117, 118–120, 127
cognitive themes. *See* core assumptions
cognitive triad, 100, 118–119, 320, 407. *See also* Beck, Aaron; cognitive-behavioral therapy
communication
  analysis, 137, 140
  bipolar disorder, 162
  emergency room staff, 194–195
  family, 346, 355–356, 357–358
  interpersonal, 8, 9
  marital therapy, 183
  positive, 164, 184, 203, 300
  reciprocal, 338
  restructuring patterns of, 168
  role disputes, 137
  validation, 336. *See also* validation
communication training
  alcohol abuse, 237
  bipolar disorder, 118
  family-focused therapy, 8, 159, 163, 168–169
  marital therapy, 185
  research, 163–164
Community Reinforcement Approach, 296
  case example, 303–310
  goal of, 298
  intake assessment, 298–299
  refusal training, 303
  research, 302–303
  therapy sessions, 299–301
  voucher program, 301–302
  See also cocaine dependence
community reintegration, 61–62
community supports, 5, 235
  case example, 47
  cocaine-refusal skills, 299–300
  social skills training, 42, 44, 47, 49
comorbidity, 151, 420. *See also* diagnosis, multiple

compensation strategies, 81–83. *See also* cognitive-behavioral therapy
compliance, 77
  assessment, 385
  cognitive-behavioral therapy, 394–395
  drug therapy, 420
  family detoxification, 287–288
  lack of, 56, 326
conflict resolution skills, 59
  interpersonal, 141, 383
  multiple family group treatment, 357–358
  social skills training, 60, 245t, 247t
  substance abuse and, 62
  Successful Negotiation/Acting Positively, 200, 203–205
  as suicide risk factor, 197, 200
consequences
  aversive, 322
  cue exposure treatment, 249–250
  psychotic disorder, 76
  substance use, 269–270
  symptoms, 80
controlled drinking experiment, 289–290
coping, 80–81
  assessment, 238–240
  cue exposure treatment, 237, 249–250
  improving, 81–83, 206–207
  internal, 58–59
  negative predictions, 103
  strategies, 70, 86, 230
  Successful Negotiation/Acting Positively, 192
  See also coping and social skills training
coping and social skills training, 234–235
  assessment, 238–240
  cognitive impairments, 235–236
  considerations, 250–251
  effectiveness of, 252
  overview, 240–243
  session modules, 244–247t
  therapy, 237–238
  See also cue exposure treatment; social skills training
core assumptions, 119
  case example, 108–109
  cognitive-behavioral therapy, 102, 104–105
  cognitive triad, 100
  Core Belief Worksheet, 105
  See also schemas
corrective feedback, 23, 33–34. *See also* feedback; social skills training
couple alcoholism treatment, 277
  background of, 278–279
  consultation, 279–286
  family detoxification, 286–288
  individual sessions, 283–284, 290
  interventions, 289–291
  phases of, 280t

couple alcoholism treatment (*continued*)
  problem-solution loops, 288–289
  relapse prevention, 290–291
  research, 291–293
couple therapy
  alcohol abuse, 277
  Community Reinforcement Approach, 303
  coping and social skills training, 234
  depression, 98
  See also couple alcoholism treatment
crisis management, 10, 13, 163–164
criticism management, 59
  marital therapy, 184
  social skills training, 60, 244t, 246t
cue exposure treatment, 235, 236–237, 248–250
  assessment, 238–240
  effectiveness of, 252
  overview, 243
  rationale, 247–248
  See also coping and social skills training
curriculum planning, 40–41

deficits, interpersonal, 135, 138–139. *See also* interpersonal psychotherapy
delusions, 74, 82
  beliefs, 70, 86–87
  grandiose, 159
  therapy and, 9, 72, 77, 78
denial, 261, 264, 279. *See also* twelve-step facilitation therapy
depression
  adolescent, 186, 191–192, 197
  approaches to, 97–98, 318
  HIV-positive patients, 151
  marriage, 175–180, 182–184, 186
  medical model of, 134
  psychotic experience and, 87
  symptoms, 97
  unipolar vs. bipolar, 142
diagnosis, 404
  determining, 165, 420
  multiple, 87, 318, 321–322, 337–338, 383, 420
  reviewing with client, 77, 386, 388
dialectical behavior therapy, 317–318, 320–321, 360
  borderline personality disorder, 323, 344
  domestic violence, 318–319
  functions of treatment, 321–323
  philosophy, 319–321
  problem-solving, 327–333
  research, 318–319
  stages of treatment, 325–327
  strategies, 337–339
  validation, 333–337
  See also bipolar disorder; dialectical behavior therapy
dialogue, internal
  automatic thoughts, 100, 102–105, 110f
  modification of, 83, 84, 86. *See also* coping

didactic instruction, 23, 28. *See also* social skills training
differentiation, cognitive, 43. *See also* integrated psychological therapy
disability, 58, 80
discrimination modeling, 34
disease model approach, 302
distortions, cognitive, 103
distraction, 86. *See also* symptoms
disulfiram therapy. *See* pharmacotherapy
"Drinker's Check-Up," 216–217, 224
  client resistance, 217–218
  coping and social skills training, 234
  See also feedback; substance abuse
Drinking Triggers Interview, 239–240
  cue exposure treatment, 243, 248
  See also triggers
drug abuse. *See* substance abuse
DSM Checklist, 298. *See also* diagnosis
dysfunctional thoughts, 102–104, 110f
dysthymic disorder, 141
  interpersonal psychotherapy, 138–139, 151
  marital discord, 178
  See also interpersonal psychotherapy

eating disorder, 116, 318
education, 4, 7–8, 11, 14, 55. *See also* psychoeducational approach
emergency room. *See* dialectical behavior therapy
emotions
  arousal, 334
  dysregulation, 315, 316, 333
  learning, 360
  physical reaction to, 79
  regulation, 323–325, 331–332. *See also* borderline personality disorder
  responses, 74–76, 79, 83, 110f, 119
empathy, 8, 55, 101, 217, 335, 359. *See also* motivational interviewing
employment, 54, 60–62, 99, 300
enabling, 261–263. *See also* twelve-step facilitation therapy
engagement
  case example, 88–90
  cognitive-behavioral therapy, 76–77
  home-based crisis intervention, 366
  multiple family group treatment, 350–351
environmental stress
  personal therapy, 54, 55
  personality disorders, 315
  schizophrenia, 1
  See also stress; vulnerability-stress model
ethnicity, 251, 297
evaluation
  group therapy, 25
  interpersonal psychotherapy strategies, 135
  social skills, 20, 21–22, 45–47
expressed emotion, 5, 15, 161–162

family
  blame within, 201–202
  boundaries, 355–356
  detoxification, 286–288, 291
  interventions, 72, 91–92
  problem hierarchy, 204–205, 206, 208
  problem-solving, 14–15
  systems perspective, 3, 6, 161, 205–206, 292
family-focused therapy, 159, 346
  alcohol abuse, 237, 278
  applications, 171
  assessment, 165–166
  bipolar disorder, 118, 127, 162
  case example, 208–209
  communication training, 168–169
  discussing treatment, 167–168
  history, 3–4, 162–163
  problem-solving skills training, 169–170
  relapse prevention, 168
  research, 163–165
  setting, 165, 195–196
  Successful Negotiation/Acting Positively, 192, 209
  termination, 170–171
  See also couple alcoholism treatment; multiple family group treatment; psychoeducational approach
feedback, 33–34, 59, 76, 80
  cognitive-behavioral therapy, 101
  coping and social skills training, 236, 241–243, 244t, 246t
  corrective, 33–34
  couple alcoholism treatments, 279, 281
  delivering, 163
  "Drinker's Check-Up," 216–217
  example of, 36
  homework, 37
  inconsistent, 334
  maintaining symptoms, 74–76
  mechanism, 86
  multiple family group treatment, 354–355
  multisystemic therapy, 367
  negative, 33–34, 60
  positive, 33–34, 141, 149
  role play, 28, 32–33
  substance abuse, 224–227, 225t, 231
  See also social skills training
"Feeling Thermometer," 196–197, 197f, 205. See also Successful Negotiation/Acting Positively
flooding, 417n. See also systemic desensitization
focusing, 84. See also cognitive-behavioral therapy
framing, 359
Freeman Diagnostic Profile System, 386, 387f
functional analysis, 5, 385
  case example, 306
  cocaine use, 299
  Community Reinforcement Approach, 303
  See also assessment
functioning, interpersonal, 99, 141, 148, 151

generalization strategies, 28, 30t, 46–47
genogram, 284, 292
Global Assessment of Functioning, 404
Global Assessment of Relational Functioning, 166
goal-directed behavior, 97, 146, 159
goal-oriented therapy, 99. See also cognitive-behavioral therapy
goal setting
  behavior, 83
  borderline personality disorder, 324–325
  collaborative nature of, 389
  defining, 8, 102
  family therapy, 7, 353
  personal therapy, 56, 61–62, 120–121, 139, 328
  social skills training, 59–60
  therapeutic, 101, 108
goals
  case example, 375
  emotional arousal, 334
  multiple diagnosis, 383
  social/recreational, 299–300
  substance abuse, 225–227
  treatment, 354t, 367, 392–393
grief, 135
  depression, 179
  interpersonal psychotherapy, 136–137
  loss of healthy self, 149
group therapy
  cohesion, 359–360
  disruptive behaviors, 44
  social skills training, 23–27, 237, 240–243
  See also multiple family group treatment
guided imagery, 59. See also internal coping

hallucinations, 74, 77–78, 82
  cognitive-behavioral strategies, 9, 72
  disruptive behaviors, 44
  See also auditory hallucinations
handouts. See homework
Higher Power, 264, 266, 272–273. See also twelve-step facilitation therapy
historical storytelling, 351–352
history. See assessment
HIV/AIDS education, 300
home-based crisis intervention, 6, 9, 366, 378. See also multisystemic therapy
homework, 23, 28, 41, 103, 263–264
  cognitive-behavioral therapy, 101–102, 122, 394, 396–397, 401
  communication training, 8
  couple alcoholism treatments, 183–184, 283
  cue exposure treatment, 238
  dialectical behavior therapy, 322
  functional analysis, 385
  noncompliance with, 43–44
  pacing, 26
  positive reinforcement, 28
  recovery tasks, 267, 268, 273–274

homework (*continued*)
  "self-sessions," 105
  social skills training, 28, 30t, 36–37, 236
  Successful Negotiation/Acting Positively, 203, 205, 206, 207
  symptoms, 79–80
  thought record, 102, 109
  twelve-step facilitation therapy, 262
  See also social skills training
hypomania, 120, 126f

imitative learning principles, 3–4
impulsive behavior, 146, 159, 198, 343
in vivo exercises, 28
  coping strategies, 81
  pacing, 26
  therapy, 39, 47, 62, 243, 397
  See also homework
insight
  borderline personality disorder, 356
  group therapy, 25
  internal coping, 58–59
  lack of, 55
  marital discord, 181–182
  substance abuse, 62, 282–283
insomnia. *See* sleep
integrated psychological therapy, 43
internal coping, 58–59
internal dialogue
  automatic thoughts, 100, 102–105, 110f
  modifying, 83, 84, 86. *See also* coping
internal rules. *See* schemas
interpersonal and social rhythm therapy, 118, 143–149, 144t, 152–155. *See also* interpersonal psychotherapy
interpersonal deficits, 135, 138–139. *See also* interpersonal psychotherapy
interpersonal functioning, 99, 141, 148, 151
interpersonal psychotherapy, 131, 154–155
  bipolar disorder, 127, 162
  described, 131–135, 141–142, 151–153
  grief, 136–137
  vs. interpersonal and social rhythm therapy, 144–149, 144t
  interpersonal deficits, 138–139
  personality disorders, 315
  phases of, 135–136, 139–141
  predictors of response to, 153–154
  research, 149–153
  role structuring, 137–138
  See also interpersonal and social rhythm therapy
interpersonal relationships, 60, 61, 132
interpersonal role transitions, 135. *See also* interpersonal psychotherapy
interventions
  case example, 90–91, 187
  couple alcoholism treatments, 289–291
interview instruments, 78–81

isolation, 76, 80, 347
  belief modification strategies, 84–85
  decreasing, 24
  dialectical behavior therapy, 326
  social skill development, 19–20
  See also symptoms

learning theory, 74, 403, 416
life events
  bipolar disorder, 162
  depression, 132–133
  interpersonal psychotherapy, 133–134
  relapse rates, 124
  rhythms, 143
  stress, 99–100, 161
limbic system, 162
lithium, 9. *See also* pharmacotherapy
loneliness, 76, 80. *See also* symptoms

managed care, 343
marijuana use, 301. *See also* substance abuse
marriage
  alcohol abuse, 237
  bipolar disorder, 161
  case example, 186–188
  depression and, 132, 176–182, 186
  discord, 98
  treatment, 106, 164, 182–185
medication
  addiction, 252–253
  adherence, 124–125, 149, 168, 169
  bipolar disorder, 116–117
  discontinuing, 56
  See also pharmacotherapy
metacommunications, 57
metaphors
  bipolar disorder treatment, 119
  couple alcoholism treatments, 281, 282, 285
  patient, 384
miracle question, 283
mirroring, 358–359. *See also* modeling
modeling, 23, 59
  cognitive-behavioral therapy, 119, 397
  dialectical behavior therapy, 319
  discrimination, 34
  family therapy, 4
  group therapy, 23–24
  reframing, 201–202
  social skills training, 27
  Successful Negotiation/Acting Positively, 192
  supplementary, 34
  See also social skills training
mood
  disorders, 97, 143, 159–161, 318. *See also* bipolar disorder
  therapy techniques, 101, 105, 160
motivation, 25, 47, 58, 265–266. *See also* insight
motivational enhancement therapy, 216–217, 230, 234

motivational interviewing, 231–232
  building motivation, 219–228
  cognitive-behavioral therapy, 72
  commitment to change, 228–230
  compliance, 77, 420
  Decisional Balance Sheet, 222t
  rationale, 216–217
  self-efficacy, 219
  special populations, 230–231
  See also substance abuse
multimodal teaching method, 353–355. See also multiple family group treatment
multiple family group treatment, 316, 344–345, 361
  cohesion, 349–353, 359–360
  family communication patterns, 346–347
  goals, 345–346, 347–348, 355–361
  structure of treatment, 348–349, 353–355, 354t
  See also borderline personality disorder
multisystemic therapy, 364–365, 370–371
  case example, 372–377, 374t
  effectiveness of, 364, 366–367
  principles, 366, 367–372
  research, 377–378
  theoretical basis, 365
mystification, 352

naturalistic observation, 22, 38. See also observation
negative thoughts, 119, 194. See also automatic thoughts
negotiation, 202, 206–207, 300
neurocognitive impairments, 21, 42–43, 71
noncompliance, 56, 326. See also compliance
nonverbal communication, 19, 20, 32–33, 59

observation, 22, 27, 55
opiate dependence, 301. See also substance abuse

patterns
  of family behavior, 3, 356
  of symptoms, 79–80
peer relations, 28, 33, 57
personal therapy, 53–54
  patient responsibility, 56, 58–59, 60–61
  phase transitions, 62–64
  principles, 54–57
  principles of, 57–62, 61–62
  rehabilitation agencies, 55
  research, 64–67, 65f
  social skills training, 59–60
personality disorders, 400–401
  case example, 397–400
  conceptualization, 388–389
  defining, 315
  homework, 394
  problems with treating, 382–383
  schemas, 389–392

  treatment, 250–251, 383–385, 392–394, 396–397, 403–404
  See also specific treatment methods
pharmacotherapy, 9, 49, 53–54
  bipolar disorder, 116–117, 118, 124–125, 159, 160
  case example, 307–308
  Community Reinforcement Approach, 297, 302
  with other therapies, 10, 54–56, 105–106, 165, 186, 322
  patient responsibility, 44, 149, 160–161, 162
  personality disorders and, 1, 153
  social skills training, 47
  See also pharmacotherapy
phobias. See "affect phobia"
post-partum depression, 141, 152. See also interpersonal psychotherapy
present-focused therapy, 99. See also cognitive-behavioral therapy
problem analysis, 5, 8
problem-focus, 122, 288–289
problem-solution loops, 282, 287, 288–289. See also couple alcoholism treatment
problem-solving, 15, 120
  ability to, 12, 14, 20, 23
  behavior therapy, 105, 327–333
  case example, 208–209
  cocaine use, 300
  Community Reinforcement Approach, 303
  emotional dysregulation, 324
  family therapy, 8–9, 159, 163, 169–170
  interpersonal, 43, 97, 132–133. See also integrated psychological therapy
  marital therapy, 183
  multiple family group treatment, 347, 354t, 356–357, 360
  multisystemic therapy, 369
  orientation, 103
  pharmacological treatment and, 9
  psychoeducation, 355
  relapse prevention, 168
  research, 163–164
  social skills training, 39
  specific disorders and, 117, 118, 119, 162, 324–325
  strategies, 9
  Successful Negotiation/Acting Positively, 192, 200–205, 207–208
  as a suicide risk factor, 126–127, 197
psychodynamic conflict, 403, 405, 406. See also short-term dynamic psychotherapy
psychoeducational approach, 100, 361
  assessment, 14–15
  behavior therapy, 101, 322, 325, 327
  bipolar disorder, 117, 118–120, 163
  borderline personality disorder, 323–324, 344, 345–346, 352–353
  family therapy, 4, 159, 166–167, 166t

psychoeducational approach (*continued*)
    interpersonal and social rhythm therapy, 143
    joining, 349
    personal therapy, 57–58
    pharmacotherapy and, 9, 149
    research, 64–67
    responsibilities, 61
    therapist role, 134
    See also cognitive-behavioral therapy; education
psychological treatment, 419–420
psychological vulnerability, 74
psychomotor agitation, 159
psychosocial functioning
    difficulties, 18
    evaluation, 21–22
    theoretical models, 19–20
    See also social skills training
psychosocial treatment
    alcohol abuse, 277
    bipolar disorder, 117, 118, 143, 159
    integration of, 14
    vs. medication, 162
    research, 64–67
    schizophrenia, 53
    social skills training, 49
psychotherapy
    common factors, 135
    dialectical behavior therapy and, 322
    goals, 162
    specific disorders and, 53, 142–143
psychotic experience, 74–76, 79, 87

rapport building, 101, 140, 366
reality testing, 85, 86, 87. *See also* cognitive-behavioral therapy
reciprocity, 4. *See also* systems therapy
recovery tasks. *See* homework
reflection, 59, 77, 101, 218, 351
reframing, 192, 201–202. *See also* Successful Negotiation/Acting Positively
rehearsal, 59. *See also* social skills training
reinforcement, 23, 76
    cocaine produced, 298
    contingent, 322
    desired affects of, 27, 420
    positive, 4, 8, 28, 369
    praise, 28
    procedures, 9
    role play, 241–243
    survey, 7
    within treatment, 38, 47, 55, 297, 369
    unreinforced behavior, 28
    See also social skills training
relapse, 139
    alcohol abuse, 239–240
    behavior change, 216
    bipolar disorder, 117

cognitive-behavioral therapy, 69
couple treatment, 183, 290–291
cue exposure treatment, 239
depression, 144–145
family therapy, 163, 347
internal coping, 58–59
life events, 55
multiple, 164
personal therapy, 54
pharmacological treatment, 56
prevention, 105, 160, 168, 235, 296–297, 303
rates, 74, 122, 124, 346
research, 64–67
resources, 62–63
risk factors, 124
stress, 161–162
treatment plan, 120
warning signs, 7–8, 45
relationships, 60, 61, 132
relaxation techniques, 59, 60
    cognitive-behavioral therapy, 105, 397
    substance abuse, 62, 300
    See also internal coping
resistance, 217–218, 385, 394–395. *See also* motivational interviewing
Response Generation Task, 23
restructuring, 117, 118–120, 127
rhythms, 146, 147. *See also* interpersonal and social rhythm therapy; patterns
risk taking, 97
role disputes, 135
role play, 59
    assessment, 238
    cocaine-refusal skills, 299
    cognitive-behavioral therapy, 397
    communication training, 169*t*
    coping and social skills training, 81, 236, 237, 241–243
    family therapy, 4, 169
    generalization strategies, 38
    homework, 37
    interpersonal psychotherapy, 140
    mirroring, 359
    negotiation skills, 206–207
    noncompliance with, 43
    pacing, 26
    positive feedback, 28
    prompting, 34
    rational-emotional, 104
    role disputes, 137
    social skills, 22–23, 28, 30*t*, 32–36
    Successful Negotiation/Acting Positively, 192, 205
    task, 22–23, 47
    therapist role, 134
    See also social skills training
role structuring, 60, 135, 137–138, 151. *See also* interpersonal psychotherapy; social skills training

scheduling
  adapting to change, 148
  case example, 304–305, 306–307
  cognitive-behavioral therapy, 105, 396–397
  time management, 300
schemas, 100, 389–392, 393
  case example, 108, 397–400
  personality disorders, 400–401
  "two-triangle," 405, 406f, 407f, 408
  See also core assumptions
schizophrenia
  borderline personality disorder, 345–346
  impact of, 1
  psychoeducational approach, 57–58
  See also specific treatment methods
self-blame, 359
self-esteem, 80
  bipolar disorder, 159
  emergency room, 194
  increasing, 183, 184
  low, 87
  mood disorders, 97
self-regulating strategies, 54, 83–84, 159. See also cognitive-behavioral therapy
serotonin reuptake inhibitors, 9. See also pharmacotherapy
sexual dysfunction, 9, 270
shaping, 23, 28, 42, 47. See also social skills training
short-term dynamic psychotherapy, 417
  case example, 404–405
  personality disorders, 403–404
  research, 416
  treatment implications, 410–415
  "two-triangle" schema, 405, 406f, 407f, 408
short-term therapy, 99, 403–404. See also cognitive-behavioral therapy; short-term dynamic psychotherapy
short-term verbal memory, 55
skills training, 40, 163, 303, 322. See also social skills training
sleep
  cocaine use, 300
  cycles, 124, 143
  interpersonal and social rhythm therapy, 146
  mood disorders, 97, 159
social anxiety, 300
social cues, 20
social disengagement, 82–83. See also coping
social ecological theory, 365, 367. See also multisystemic therapy
social engagement, 82–83. See also coping; engagement
social functioning, 20–23. See also social skills training
social learning theory
  assessing family patterns, 3–4
  functional analysis, 228–229

social skills training, 27–28
  substance abuse, 234, 252, 297
social marginalization, 76
social perception, 43, 60, 62, 63. See also integrated psychological therapy
social rhythms, 143, 145, 161. See also interpersonal and social rhythm therapy
  disruption, 146
  therapy, 147–148, 162
social skills, 43, 76. See also integrated psychological therapy
  cocaine use, 300
  evaluating, 20–21, 22–23
  interpersonal psychotherapy, 138
  Successful Negotiation/Acting Positively, 200
  theoretical models, 19–20
social skills training, 8, 18, 53
  attendance, 28–29, 41–42
  case example, 47
  cognitive-behavioral strategies, 9
  common problems, 41–45
  dysthymic disorder, 151
  generalization strategies, 38–39
  homework, 36–37
  interpersonal psychotherapy, 133
  logistics, 23–27
  other techniques, 39
  personal therapy, 59–60
  prosocial response, 60
  rationale for, 29–31, 45–47
  role play, 22–23, 32–36
  skill steps, 30t, 31–32
  structure of treatment, 20–23, 27–29, 40–41, 42
  See also coping and social skills training; group therapy; social functioning
social withdrawal, 76, 80, 83. See also symptoms
Socratic questioning, 102–103, 104
source monitoring, 83–84. See also cognitive-behavioral therapy
speech-processing mechanisms, 70–71. See also auditory hallucinations
stigma, 76
strengths, identifying, 368–369
stress, 76
  comorbidity, 62, 74, 161–162, 197, 235, 369
  management, 58–59, 133, 184
  marital, 176, 180, 183
  relapse, 56, 124
  situational, 60
  treatment of, 4, 132
  See also environmental stress; social skills training
stress-vulnerability model, 19–20
substance abuse
  Addiction Severity Index, 298
  Change Plan Worksheet, 230f
  patient responsibility, 161, 227–228, 420
  social ecological theory, 365

substance abuse (*continued*)
    specific disorders and, 116, 126, 343
    suicide and, 191–192, 197
    treatment, 62, 72, 87, 213–214, 318
    See also addiction; alcohol abuse; motivational interviewing; twelve-step facilitation therapy
Successful Negotiation/Acting Positively, 192, 199–201, 209
    case example, 208–209
    "Feeling Thermometer," 196–197
    structure of treatment, 197–198, 201–208, 202t
    See also adolescent suicide
suicide, 87, 159
    dialectical behavior therapy, 316, 317–319, 322, 326, 337–338
    family therapy, 9, 98, 344
    marital therapy, 182
    prevention, 126–127
    risk factors, 328
    specific disorders and, 97, 116, 315, 320, 343
    See also adolescent suicide; dialectical behavior therapy
supportive therapy, 64–67, 72, 74
survival analysis model, 164
symptoms, 404
    alcoholism, 260
    assessment of, 135
    bipolar disorder, 159, 166–167
    consequences of, 80
    context of, 79–80
    depressive, 140
    life events and, 122, 124
    maintaining, 74–76, 80–81, 86–87
    measurement of, 101, 134
    mood, 97, 138, 143
    psychotic, 78–79
    reduction, 59–60, 105, 183
    relapse prevention, 168
    research, 65f
    status of, 63
    treatment, 24–25, 133–134, 143, 145, 154, 164
systematic skills training, 253. *See also* social skills training
systemic desensitization, 410–411, 417n
systemic theories, 278. *See also* couple alcoholism treatment
systemic training, 70
Systemic Treatment Enhancement Program, 118, 127, 171
systems therapy, 4

termination
    case example, 415–416
    family-focused therapy, 170
    interpersonal psychotherapy, 133
    marital therapy, 183

Successful Negotiation/Acting Positively, 207
    twelve-step facilitation therapy, 261, 274
therapeutic alliance, 6, 101, 411
therapeutic goals, 108
therapist role, 145–146, 183
Thorn Nurse Training Project, 91–92
time management. *See* scheduling
tokens, 201, 206–207. *See also* Successful Negotiation/Acting Positively
tranquilizers, 9. *See also* pharmacotherapy
treatment
    challenges, 1
    dialectical behavior therapy functions, 321–323
    integration, 10
    manuals, 184–185
    mood disorders, 97–98
    phases, 63
    planning, 56, 121–122, 135–136, 305–310
    readiness, 353
    research, 419–420
    See also specific treatment methods
tricyclics, 9. *See also* pharmacotherapy
triggers
    cue exposure treatment, 243
    rhythm disruption, 146
    substance abuse, 229–230, 229t, 239–240
    symptoms, 79–80
twelve-step facilitation therapy, 261–264, 264–268, 278–279
    Lifestyle Contract, 271t
    patient responsibility, 270–271, 273–274
    research, 258–259
    spirituality, 266t
    stages of treatment, 268–270, 269t, 272–273, 274
    substance abuse, 216–217
    theoretical basis, 259–261
"two-triangle" schema, 405, 406f, 407f, 408, 410f. *See also* schemas

urge reduction imagery, 249, 250
urinalysis monitoring, 301, 306, 307f. *See also* alcohol abuse

validation, 333–337
verbal communication, 43. *See also* integrated psychological therapy
violence, 9, 347
vocational environment
    cocaine use, 300
    depression, 99
    personal therapy, 60–62
    schizophrenia, 54
voucher program, 301–302, 306, 420
vulnerability-stress model, 1, 167–168